AF567161

The
Reticuloendothelial System
and Atherosclerosis

ADVANCES IN EXPERIMENTAL MEDICINE AND BIOLOGY

Volume 1
THE RETICULOENDOTHELIAL SYSTEM AND ATHEROSCLEROSIS
Edited by N. R. Di Luzio and R. Paoletti • 1967

In Preparation
Volume 2
THE PHARMACOLOGY OF HORMONAL POLYPEPTIDES AND PROTEINS
An International Symposium
Edited by Nathan Back, Luigi Martini, and Rodolfo Paoletti

The Reticuloendothelial System *and* Atherosclerosis

Proceedings of an International Symposium on Atherosclerosis and the Reticuloendothelial System, Held in Como, Italy, September 8–10, 1966

Edited by

N. R. Di Luzio

Department of Physiology and Biophysics
University of Tennessee Medical Units
Memphis, Tennessee

and

Rodolfo Paoletti

Institute of Pharmacology
University of Milan
Milan, Italy

Springer Science+Business Media, LLC

DOI 10.1007/978-1-4684-7796-2

Originally published by Plenum Press in 1967
Mycopy version of the original edition 1967

Foreword

The circulatory system is usually considered to be composed of tubes of various diameters, characterized by collateral and terminal branches. There is also a tendency to treat blood vessels merely as conducting tubes in which the various structures of the wall act as mechanical pumps which modify their diameter. This is, of course, not so.

In fact, we know that blood vessels, and in particular arteries, are organs with personalities of their own and a particular susceptibility to several diseases. In addition, blood vessels differ in structure, according to their localization, and age at differing rates. The experimental work carried out so far clearly confirms the data that have come from spontaneous human pathology; experimentally induced arterial lesions have a definite tendency to appear in certain arteries and not in others, depending on the experimental procedures used, and in each specific artery the lesions appear to have a specific location. We now know that the arterial wall is a metabolically active structure, in which a number of enzyme activities have been clearly demonstrated. It possesses a sensitive vasa vasorum apparatus and a specific reactivity to various lesion-inducing stimuli.

We must also remember that the arterial wall is in continuous contact with the blood circulating through the endothelial cells lining the vascular bed. It is obvious, therefore, that any variation in the circulating blood mass can modify the morphology as well as the function of the vessel wall. Numerous studies of "spontaneous" human atherosclerosis and experimental atherosclerosis in various animal species have verified this.

I am certain that in the near future vascular pathology will be investigated with even greater interest, and it will become even more necessary to study it in strict relationship to the general pathological situation. This volume represents one of the first attempts in this direction.

One of the principal aims of the Italian Society for the Study of Atherosclerosis, in close collaboration with the Reticuloendothelial Society and the European Society for Biochemical Pathology, has been to stimulate research and the discussion of problems relating to vascular pathology in relation to reticuloendothelial physiology and pathology, hematology, pharmacology, allergy, and other points of contact. Round table discussions have shown that there is a real relationship among these various fields of research.

It is our hope and conviction that studies in this direction will contribute significantly to the clarification of the many unanswered questions in the field of vascular diseases in general and atherosclerosis in particular.

We wish to acknowledge the kind collaboration of Professor N. R. Di Luzio, President of the Reticuloendothelial Society, Professor E. Trabucchi, Vice President of the International Society for Biochemical Pharmacology, and Professor R. Paoletti, Secretary of the Italian Society for the Study of Atherosclerosis. We are also greatly indebted to Drs. Butti and Rossi of Crinos Pharmacological Industry for the organization of this meeting, and to various other organizations for their financial support.

Cesare Cavallero
President, Italian Society for
the Study of Atherosclerosis

Pavia
April 12, 1967

Preface

The International Symposium on the Reticuloendothelial System and Atherosclerosis was held in the Villa Olmo in Como, Italy, from September 8th to 10th, 1966. This volume contains papers presented at the Symposium, which was the Fifth International Symposium on the Reticuloendothelial System.

The Symposium was designed to bring together outstanding investigators in various disciplines to present recent developments in the area of reticuloendothelial research and to provide for a unique opportunity to exchange ideas and opinions regarding methodology, morphology, and factors influencing and regulating reticuloendothelial activity. The involvement of the reticuloendothelial system (RES) in host defense and the role of the reticuloendothelial system in lipid metabolism and atherosclerosis were also stressed. The Symposium admirably served to integrate recent knowledge and to stimulate future progress in these areas.

A perusal of the table of contents of this book will indicate the versatility, uniqueness, diversity, and multipotential nature and activity of the reticuloendothelial system. Because of its multiple functions, many scientific disciplines converge on the reticuloendothelial system. This volume proves that the area of participation of the reticuloendothelial cells is so broad as to capture the interest of a wide variety of scientists. Still, the subject to which it is devoted is very young. Less than a century has elapsed since the classic studies of Metchnikoff delineated the role of the fixed phagocytic cell as a major component of the host-defense system, and less than half a century has elapsed since Aschoff united the morphologically distinct groups of cells under the name "reticuloendothelial system" because of their common functional property of phagocytosis. Indeed, the remarkable capacity of these cells to distinguish "self" from "nonself" forms the basic attribute of the reticuloendothelial system and one of the major bases for its investigation.

A common method of elucidating the functional activity of an organ or system is to study the effects of its removal on the physiology of the organism. In the case of the macrophage system, this is impossible because of the widespread anatomical distribution of cells comprising the system.

Attempts to remove these cells by physically loading them with various inert materials have generally met with failure. Since the agents employed to induce blockade are relatively crude and generally toxic, and since the macrophage cells proliferate, enlarge, and become hyperfunctional very rapidly, the techniques of blockade are fraught with numerous pitfalls. Thus this approach should be abandoned since it has led to fallacious concepts regarding the participation of the reticuloendothelial system in a variety of situations.

Because it had not been possible to extirpate the reticuloendothelial system or to induce an effective, nonspecific, and prolonged blockage, knowledge of the multiple contributions of the reticuloendothelial cells has developed only gradually over the past 75 years. However, it is obvious that with the recent development of techniques for measuring reticuloendothelial function and activity, as well as the introduction of purified, nontoxic chemical agents capable of inducing either reticuloendothelial stimulation or depression, proliferation or atrophy of the system, future progress in research will be rapid.

The papers in this volume constitute a broad but well-balanced portrayal of the spectrum of reticuloendothelial involvement. The potential importance of this system in atherogenesis as well as the accent on the possible and provocative immune nature of the atherogenic process are stressed. The newer techniques which are presented will permit the investigation of important clinical and experimental aspects which have hitherto escaped investigation and will contribute to the elucidation of the role of the reticuloendothelial system in health and disease. Indeed, the key to the elimination of many diseases of man may well be found within the cells which comprise this system, as more and more of their diverse and versatile activities become known. Clearly, the reticuloendothelial system is one of the major frontiers in clinical and experimental investigation and fully merits exploration.

On behalf of the Advisory Committee, I should like to express our sincerest appreciation to all the participants in the Symposium and the contributing authors for their cooperation.

A particular word of thanks goes to Plenum Publishing Company for their splendid work and assistance in publishing the proceedings, which made the editing of this first volume of "Advances in Experimental Medicine and Biology" a highly gratifying experience.

Nicholas R. Di Luzio
President, Reticuloendothelial Society

Memphis, Tennessee
June 15, 1967

Contents

METHODOLOGY

Application of a Mathematical Model to the Study of RES Phagocytosis in Mice 1
Richard K. Fred and Moris L. Shore

The Use of Radioiodinated Latex Particles for In Vivo Studies of Phagocytosis 18
J. M. Singer, S. Lavie, L. Adlersberg, E. Ende, E. M. Hoenig, and Y. Tchorsh

Interaction of Charged Colloids with the RES. 25
David J. Wilkins

The Potential Use of Glutaraldehyde-Fixed Liver Cells in the Study of Hepatic Reticuloendothelial and Parenchymal Cell Metabolism 34
N. Baker and M. Cohen

The Function of the Reticuloendothelial System Studied with Isolated Perfused Rat Livers 46
H. Schimassek and J. Helms

Reticuloendothelial Excretion Via the Bronchial Tree 58
T. Nicol and J. L. Cordingley

Kinetics of the Phagocytosis of Repeated Injections of Colloidal Carbon: Blockade, A Latent Period or Stimulation? A Question of Timing and Dose 63
Ernest L. Dobson, Lola S. Kelly, and Caroline R. Finney

MORPHOLOGY

Comparative Morphology of Macrophages in Tissue Culture. 74
Boyce Bennett

Fine Structural Aspects of Reticuloendothelial Blockade 85
Joseph Wiener

The Cellular Basis of RE Stimulation: The Effects on Peritoneal Cells of Stimulation with Glyceryl Trioleate, Studied by EM and Autoradiography 98
Ian Carr and M. A. Williams

Cytodynamics of Rat Lung in Response to Freud's Adjuvant 108
Louis J. Casarett, George V. Metzger, and Margaret G. Casarett

Esterase Histochemistry of Reticuloendothelial Cells 121
Bryan Ballantyne

Comparative Cytology of Alveolar and Peritoneal Macrophages from Germfree Rats 133
Eva S. Leake and Eugene R. Heise

FACTORS INFLUENCING AND REGULATING ACTIVITY

The Role of the Environment in Determining the Discriminatory Activity of the Human Phagocytic Cell 147
A. E. Stuart

Some Effects of Divalent Cations on In Vitro Phagocytosis 163
G. V. Metzger and L. J. Casarett

The Engulfing Potential of Peritoneal Phagocytes of Conventional and Germfree Mice 175
E. H. Perkins, P. Nettesheim, T. Morita, and H.E. Walburg, Jr.

Pharmacological Stimulation and Depression of the Phagocytic Function of the RES 188
Kurt B. P. Flemming.

The Action of Some Natural Substances on RES 197
L. Bolis, and R. W. I. Kessel, and G. Petti

Effect of Bacillus Calmette Guerin on the Metabolism of Alveolar Macrophages 203
Quentin N. Myrvik and Dolores G. Evans

Reticuloendothelial System Stimulation by Estrogens and Thorium Dioxide Retention in Rat Liver 214
Giuseppe Grampa

The Effects of Steroid Hormones on Local and General Reticuloendothelial Activity: Relation of Steroid Structure to Function 221
T. Nicol, D. C. Quantock, and B. Vernon-Roberts

INVOLVEMENT IN HOST DEFENSE; ENDOTOXIN AND CARDIOVASCULAR SHOCK, INFECTION, AND IMMUNE REACTIONS

The Quantitative Response of the Host Defense System after Stimulation 243
John H. Heller and Emile G. Bliznakov

The Dissimilar Effects of Two RES Stimulants on Shock 256
Gottfried Lemperle

Comparative Effect of Endotoxin and Reticuloendothelial "Blocking" Colloids on Selected Inducible Liver Enzymes 266
L. Joe Berry, Manjul K. Agarwal, and Irvin S. Snyder

On the Nature of Some Nonspecific Host Responses in Endotoxin-Induced Resistance to Infection 275
Monique Parant, Francine Parant, Fernand Boyer, and Louis Chedid

The Effect of Opsonized Colloids on the Enhancement of Endotoxin Lethality. 285
I. MacKay Murray

The Effect of a Reticuloendothelial-Depressing Substance on Survival from Shock 293
Benjamin Blattberg and Matthew N. Levy.

Effect of Dextrans on Bacterial Infections in Mice 300
G. M. Fukui and M. Cardinale

Prevention and Treatment of Friend Leukemia Virus (FLV) Infection by Interferon-Inducing Synthetic Polyanions 315
W. Regelson

Immunoglobulin Synthesis in the Rat 333
Mariano F. La Via, William S. Hammond, Barbara H. Iglewski, Albert E. Vatter, Michael Bean, and Patricia V. Northup

Modifications of Antibody Synthesis by Chloramphenicol 345
Melvin D. Schoenberg, Richard D. Moore, and Austin S. Weisberger

Arthritis - An Example of Inflammation Based on Particles 357
Jeanne M. Riddle, Gilbert B. Bluhm, and Marion I. Barnhart

A Major Fault in Diabetic Inflammation: Failure of Leucocytic Glycogen Transfer to Histiocytes 369
J. W. Rebuck, F. W. Whitehouse, and S. M. Noonan

ROLE IN LIPID METABOLISM AND ATHEROSCLEROSIS

Participation of Hepatic Parenchymal and Kupffer Cells in Chylomicron and Cholesterol Metabolism 382
N. R. Di Luzio and S. J. Riggi

Importance of the Aging in the Relationships between the Reticuloendothelial System and Cholesterol Transport 404
F. M. Antonini

Arteriopathy Induced by Reticuloendothelial Blockade 413
P. R. Patek, S. Bernick, and V. A. de Mignard

A Form of Immunological Atherosclerosis 426
Louis Levy

Synthetic Cholesterol-Ester Antigens in Experimental Atherosclerosis 433
J. Martyn Bailey and Jean Butler

Atherosclerosis Induced Experimentally by Repeated Intravenous Administration of Hypercholesterolemic Serum and of Lipoproteins 442
A. N. Klimov, L. G. Petrova-Maslakova, L. P. Rodionova, and T. A. Sinitzina

Experimental Arteriopathy Induced in the Rabbit Through Rat Aorta Homogenate Injections: A Study of the Aortic Tissue Specificity. 451
L. Scebat, J. Renais, N. Groult, and J. Lenegre

Enzymatic Activity of the Serum and the Aortic Wall in Animals Immunized by Homologous and Heterologous Aortic Extracts 468
M. Dallocchio, R. Crockett, G. Razaka, F. A. Gandji, H. Bricaud, R. Pautrizel, and P. Broustet

Phagocytosis of Platelets by Monocytes in Organizing Arterial Thrombi 484
J. C. F. Poole

Platelets, Atherosclerosis, and Lipid Metabolism 488
Giorgio Ballerini

Plasma Clearance of Products of Fibrinolysis. 492
Marion I. Barnhart and D. C. Cress

* * *

Subject Index 503

Author Index 508

Application of a Mathematical Model to the Study of RES Phagocytosis in Mice

Richard K. Fred and Moris L. Shore

*U. S. Public Health Service**
U. S. Department of Health, Education, and Welfare
Rockville, Maryland

ABSTRACT. A mathematical model of RES phagocytic function has been developed. Data obtained using this model are compatible with results obtained from animal experimentation. Following administration of a large dose of colloidal carbon, the clearance observed in the "blood" is initially zero order, gradually changing to first order as the concentration in "blood" decreases. It may therefore be invalid to accept the previous conclusions that colloid clearance follows first-order kinetics, with rate constants that are dependent upon initial concentration. Short segments of model clearance curves may appear to be first order when in fact they may be zero order.

Analysis of model behavior suggests that at low and intermediate concentrations of carbon the RES does not exhibit its maximal functional capacity. By using high doses of carbon, however, the maximum functional capacity of the RES is measured. The effect of radiation on the maximum functional capacity of the RES in CD-1 mice was tested. ^{137}Cs gamma radiation ($LD_{05/30}$) decreased the phagocytic capacity of the RES by approximately 13%. Experiments with puromycin suggest that protein synthesis does not limit the functional capacity of the RES. Doses of puromycin that profoundly decreased protein synthesis were without effect on phagocytosis.

INTRODUCTION

It has been reported [1, 2] that the clearance of colloidal carbon from the circulation follows first-order kinetics, i.e., $C_t = C_0e^{-kt}$. These workers also found that the rate constant "k" was dependent on the initial dose of colloid injected into the animal. This finding is inconsistent with

* Biophysics Unit, Research Branch Laboratory, Division of Radiological Health.

the fundamental principle of first-order kinetics, which requires that "k" be independent of initial concentration.

During the course of studies on the effect of radiation on RES phagocytic function we have developed a mathematical model of reticuloendothelial phagocytic function [3]. This model is based on the view that phagocytosis involves a rate-limiting interaction between the colloidal particle and the phagocytic cell surface, followed by either engulfment of the particle into the cell, or release of the particle into the circulation [4]. In this model the number of binding sites for colloid on the cell surfaces constitutes the rate-limiting factor for RES phagocytosis. This contrasts with the view of other workers who have suggested that the limiting factor in phagocytosis is the availability of some plasma protein which is believed to interact with the colloidal particle prior to phagocytosis [5-11].

The observed kinetics of colloid clearance in our model are dependent upon the number of colloidal particles in the circulation relative to the number of binding sites for colloid on the surface of phagocytic cells. When the number of particles in the circulation greatly exceeds the number of binding sites on RE cells, i.e., at high concentrations of colloid, zero-order kinetics will be observed, and colloid clearance will be linear. When the number of particles in the circulation is approximately equal to the number of binding sites on RE cells, i.e., at intermediate concentrations of colloid, quasi-first-order kinetics will be observed. At low concentrations of colloid in the blood, clearance becomes blood-flow dependent, and first-order kinetics are observed [3]. The behavior of this model is generally consistent with experimental data published by other investigators [1, 2, 12-15].

The model has been used to design and to interpret experiments on RES phagocytic function in normal and irradiated mice. Experiments with mice have been performed to resolve altered colloid clearance in terms of either alteration in phagocytic efficiency or altered number of binding sites on phagocytic cell surfaces. Considerations of the experimentally observed effect of puromycin on colloidal carbon clearance have formed a basis for discussion of alternative models of RES phagocytosis. In accordance with practical considerations derived from the analysis of model behavior, the concept of maximum functional capacity of the RES has been utilized to demonstrate a radiation-induced impairment of RES phagocytic function.

MATERIALS AND METHODS

CD-1 specific-pathogen-free male mice were used in this study. The average weight of the mice was 35 gm.

Animals received colloidal carbon by injection into a caudal vein with the appropriate dose of Gunther-Wagner suspension C11/1421A [16]. This was prepared for injection according to the method described by Halpern et al. [17]. Serially timed samples were obtained from the tip of the tail. Immediately prior to sampling, the tail was "milked" to remove stagnant blood and 15 seconds were allowed for fresh blood to enter, at which time the blood sample was obtained for analysis. Five lambda of blood was diluted with 1 ml of 0.2 N NaOH. The optical density of these samples was then determined with a spectrophotometer at a wavelength of 750 mμ. When necessary, each mouse was used as its own control to provide a background blank.

Since large doses of carbon were employed in this study, the linearity of the carbon concentration versus optical density was tested. Over the range of concentrations encountered experimentally, a linear relationship existed. Since the mature rat has a constant blood volume independent of the total body weight [18], the same may be true for the mature mouse. For this reason, the dose of carbon administered to mice in any experiment was not adjusted to body weight. When the same carbon dosages were administered to mice in the range of 25-45 gm, no correlation between body weight and the rate of carbon clearance was found.

Animals received puromycin [19] by intraperitoneal injection. The dose was 7.5 mg of the antibiotic dissolved in 0.15 ml distilled water. Protein synthesis was determined by measuring the 15-min incorporation of ^{14}C-leucine into the acid-insoluble fraction of mouse liver homogenate. At various times up to 155 minutes after puromycin administration, a dose of 10 μc of ^{14}C-leucine [20] was injected i.v. Fifteen minutes after leucine administration, the animals were sacrificed by cervical translocation, and the livers were excised and placed in isotonic saline at 0°C. Approximately 1 gm of liver was weighed and homogenized in 10 ml of cold saline using a Potter–Elvehjem homogenizer. Protein was precipitated by adding cold concentrated $HClO_4$ (61%) in an amount equal to 10% by volume of the homogenate. After 15 min in the cold, precipitated homogenate was centrifuged and the supernatant was decanted and saved. The precipitates were washed three times with 5 ml of 0.6 N $HClO_4$.

For each sample the supernatants were combined and subsequently analyzed for precursor amino acid specific activity. The precipitates constituted the acid-insoluble fraction of liver. Lipid was removed from each of the precipitates by three extractions with boiling ether in acetone (3:7). The precipitates were dried and then dissolved in 7 ml of Hyamine hydroxide in methanol [21] at 65°C. After the precipitates were completely dissolved, they were diluted to 25 ml with methanol. An aliquot of the dissolved precipitate was pipetted into the counting fluid described by Meade and Steiglitz [22], and assayed for radioactivity using liquid scintillation counting techniques. The counting efficiency was determined for each sample using external standardization methods [23] and the appropriate corrections were made.

In order to determine the specific activity of precursor amino acid, analyses of amino acid were performed on aliquots of the supernatant fractions. Perchlorate was largely removed from these samples by precipitation at pH 2.0, and 0°C, with methanolic KOH. Precipitated $KClO_4$ was removed by filtration and the filtrate was evaporated in vacuo to a volume of 2-3 ml. A 2-ml aliquot of the concentrate was pipetted into 6 ml of sodium citrate buffer (pH 2.2). Aliquots were analyzed for leucine using a 150-cm column according to the method of Moore, Spackman, and Stein [24]. A one-micromole norleucine standard was added, on the column, to each sample to determine total recovery during the amino acid analysis. Aliquots of each concentrated supernatant sample were also analyzed for ^{14}C-leucine in Bray's liquid scintillation counting fluid [25]. Corrections for counting efficiency were made as previously described.

Glucan-treated mice [26] were injected intravenously with 1 mg of the polysaccharide in 0.1 ml isotonic saline. Four days later RES phagocytic function was tested with colloidal carbon. Endotoxin-treated animals were given 25 μg of S. typhosa endotoxin [27] in 0.1 ml isotonic saline i.p. and RES phagocytic function was determined four days later.

In the radiation studies mice were irradiated with 700 R ($LD_{05/30}$) of ^{137}Cs gamma.

The model of reticuloendothelial phagocytic function was simulated using digital analog simulation techniques as previously described [3].

RESULTS AND DISCUSSION

The diagrammatic representation of our model is given in Fig. 1. When a large initial dose of colloid is introduced into the body blood compartment of this system, the disappearance of colloid from this compartment will initially be zero order. The constant amount of colloid disappearing per unit time has been shown to be dependent upon the product of the probability of phagocytosis (P4) and the number of sites for binding of colloid on the surface of phagocytic cells (B3). This is expressed by the following equation [3]:

$$\frac{dCl}{dt} \cong -P4 \cdot B3$$

Doses of colloid which are cleared in this manner are considered to be "saturating doses." Such saturating doses force the clearance of colloid to the maximum functional phagocytic capacity of the RES. The term "saturating dose" should not be confused with "satiation" or "blockade" of the RES.

It has been shown that at blood colloid concentrations lower than those produced by saturating doses, the disappearance of colloid will be either

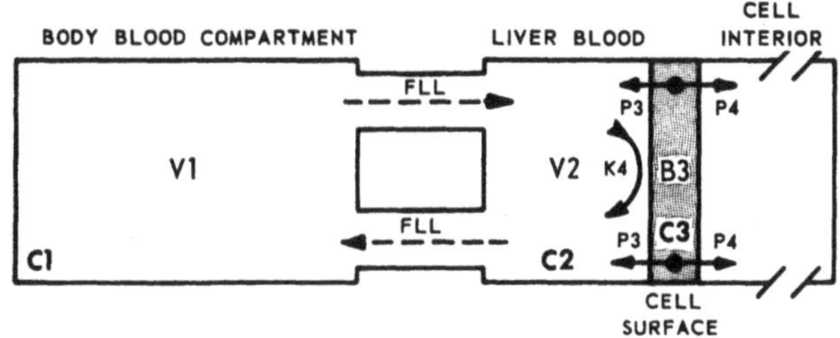

Fig. 1. A diagram of our model of the RES. Colloid (C1) is introduced into the extrahepatic body blood compartment (V1). Blood with a colloid concentration of C1/V1 flows into the hepatic compartment (V2) where part of the flow (K4), now with colloid concentration C2/V2, contacts the RE cell surface (dotted compartment, which has a total of B3 binding sites). Depending on the number of binding sites that are occupied (C3), colloid will attach at an available site. P3 is the probability of release of a bound colloidal particle from a binding site into the circulation, and P4 is the probability of engulfment of the particle into the cell interior.

quasi-first order or first order, depending on the concentration [3]. Figures 2a and 2b present the results of a simulated model experiment in which the disappearance of an initially saturating dose of colloidal carbon was followed through the zero-order, quasi-first-order, and first-order phases of colloid clearance. To permit demonstration of both the zero- and first-order characteristics of the clearance curve, linear and semilogarithmic plots of the same data are given. Although it might appear from the semilogarithmic plot that the initial portion of the curve is linear, suggesting first-order kinetics, this is not the case. Theoretical analysis of the model that produced these data shows that the initial portion of the clearance curve follows zero-order kinetics. Also, the apparent exponential rate constant "k" in model experiments would have to be dependent upon the initial concentration. Such a finding is inconsistent with first-order kinetics.

The apparent linearity of the semilogarithmic plot is an artifact, and results from examination of a short segment of a gradually falling curve over a portion of the logarithmic cycle which is approximately linear. This can be seen in Fig. 3 which is a plot of the same data presented in Fig. 2. However, in Fig. 3, 30-min segments of the 18 mg curve corresponding to initial doses of 12, 6, and 3 mg of colloidal carbon are plotted with each segment transposed to zero time. Both semilogarithmic and linear plots are presented.

If we assume that the semilogarithmic plots describe a first-order process and should therefore be plotted as best-fit straight lines, the data obtained is similar to that of Biozzi et al. [1,2] when different initial doses of carbon were administered to rats and colloid clearance was measured.

Similar data were obtained with mice by Parker et al. [14]. Figure 4 shows typical data obtained in our laboratory from the disappearance of a large dose of colloidal carbon (18 mg/animal). These experimental data show characteristics similar to data obtained from the model of the RES (Fig. 3). The semilogarithmic plots of the transposed segments of the clearance curve (Fig. 4b), as in the case of the model experiments, bear a strong resemblance to the data obtained by Biozzi et al. [1, 2] and Parker et al. [14].

Examination of linear plots of RES model data (Fig. 3a) and mouse data (Fig. 4a) shows that as the carbon concentration increases, the absolute amount of colloid cleared per unit time also increases. A point is reached, however, beyond which further increases in colloid concentration produce no increase in the absolute amount of colloidal carbon cleared per unit time. The segments of the disappearance curves are linear and approximately parallel within this range of concentrations. This indicates that the RES is operating at its maximum functional phagocytic capacity.

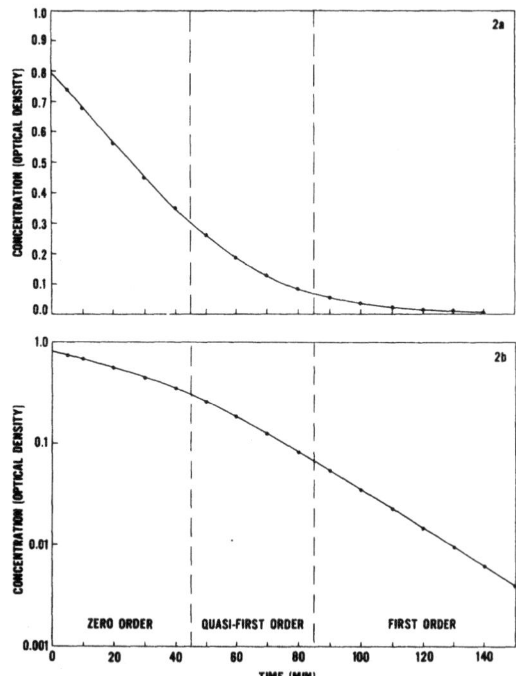

Fig. 2. A plot of carbon clearance data obtained using analog-digital simulation of the RES model. The linear portion of the curve in Fig. 2a is indicative of zero-order disappearance kinetics as was suggested by mathematical analysis of the differential equations describing the RES model. The middle portion of the curve appears more nearly exponential than linear, thus the term "quasi-first order" is used to describe its kinetics. The final portion is definitely exponential, as seen in Fig. 2b, which is in agreement with theoretical considerations of the RES model.

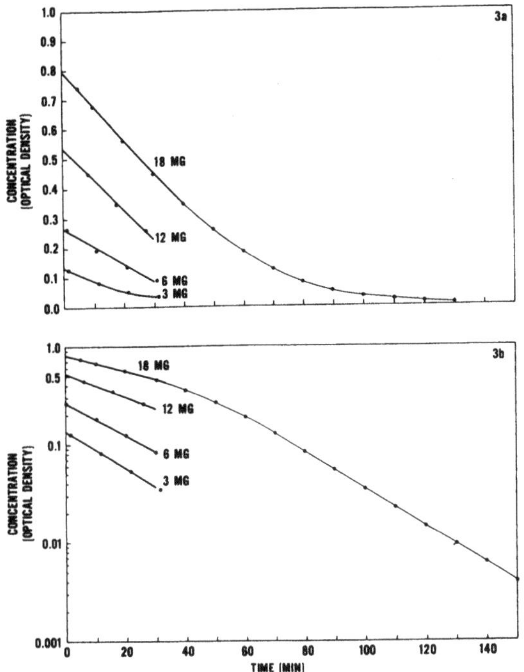

Fig. 3. A plot of analog-digital simulation data, which indicates the effect of injecting various doses of colloidal carbon. The dosage values are given in mg of colloidal carbon per mouse. Fig. 3a shows that saturation, i.e., linear removal, is predicted to occur with a 12-mg initial dose of colloidal carbon.

Figure 5 shows the data obtained in an experiment in which 12- and 18-mg doses of colloidal carbon were administered to two groups of six mice each. Clearance of colloid was measured for 30-60 min after carbon administration. Best-fit lines through the linearly plotted data for each of the two doses are parallel within the limits of error. This suggests, as previously discussed, that these are saturating doses of carbon, and that the RES in these normal mice is operating at its maximum functional capacity.

The suggestion has been made by other workers that an interaction between the colloidal particle and a plasma protein is essential to phagocytosis and that the availability of this plasma protein constitutes the rate-limiting factor in the phagocytic process [5]. Considerable evidence exists that plasma proteins are involved in the phagocytic process [5-11]. However, no definitive evidence has been provided to show that the availability of a plasma protein does, in fact, constitute a rate-limiting factor in the phagocytic process in vivo. In order to investigate this possibility, experiments were performed testing the effect of puromycin inhibition of protein synthesis on the maximum functional phagocytic capacity of the RES.

Figure 6 shows the effect of puromycin on the 15-min incorporation of ^{14}C-leucine into the acid-insoluble fraction of liver. The amount of activity appearing in the acid-insoluble fraction, and the specific activity of the precursor amino acid were determined. The following calculation was employed to provide a measure of the 15-min incorporation of amino acid into protein:

$$\text{15-min incorporation} = \frac{\text{Activity incorporated into acid-insoluble fraction}}{\text{Specific activity of the acid-soluble fraction}}$$

15-min incorporation is expressed as μmoles leucine incorporated into the acid-insoluble fraction per gram of liver during the 15-min interval. This calculation assumes that: (1) instantaneous mixing of ^{14}C-leucine occurs in the amino acid pool (acid-soluble fraction), (2) there is random utilization of labeled and unlabeled precursor, (3) the specific activity of the precursor 15 min after the administration of the labeled amino acid approximates the average specific activity of the precursor during the 15-min incorporation interval, and (4) no loss of label from the acid-insoluble fraction occurs during the course of the 15-min incorporation. Although these assumptions may not all be entirely correct, the calculation that was performed provided the

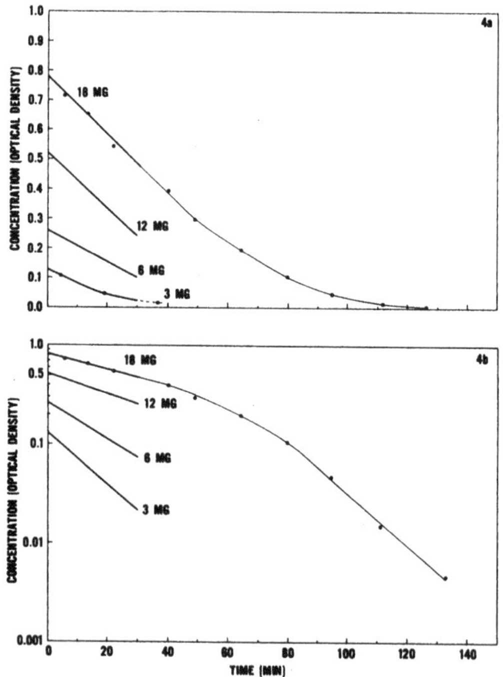

Fig. 4. A plot of typical experimental data showing the disappearance of a large dose of colloidal carbon (18 mg/mouse). As can be seen, this experimental result is very similar to the RES simulation data of Fig. 3.

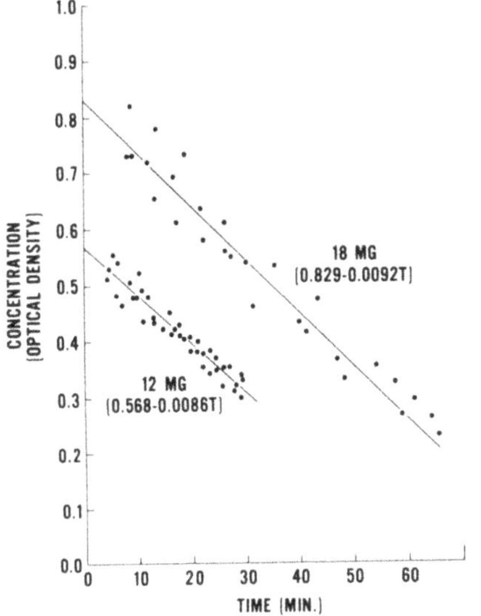

Fig. 5. The experimentally observed clearance of saturating doses of colloidal carbon is demonstrated. The clearance rates for each of these doses are approximately the same, as was predicted by the shape of the principal clearance curve of Figs. 3 and 4.

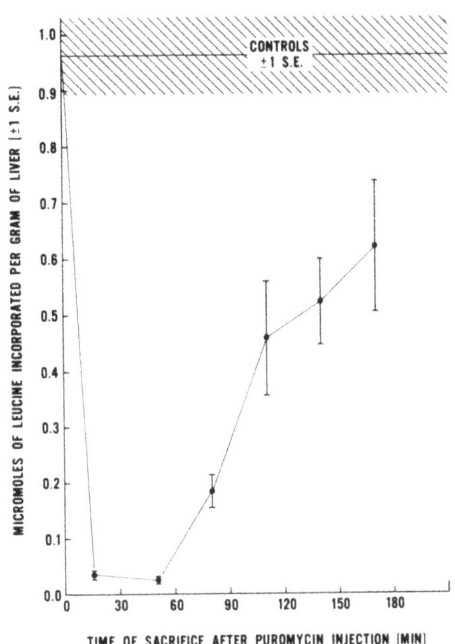

Fig. 6. The effect of 7.5 mg of puromycin on the 15-minute incorporation of ^{14}C-leucine into the acid-insoluble fraction of liver.

best available index of the amount of amino acid incorporated into protein of liver during the 15-min interval measured. It can be seen that puromycin caused a profound depression of protein synthesis for the first 50 min after its administration. Substantial depression in protein synthesis was still apparent 150 min after administering puromycin.

If protein synthesis were a rate-limiting factor in phagocytosis, it might be expected that, under conditions in which a saturating dose of colloid is administered to an animal, some effect on colloid clearance would be observed after puromycin administration. Figure 7b shows the results of an experiment in which 7.5 mg of puromycin was administered, followed immediately by a saturating dose of colloidal carbon (18 mg/mouse). No difference in colloid clearance was observed between experimental animals receiving puromycin and the controls (Fig. 7a) receiving sterile water. Figure 8 shows the results of a similar experiment using a puromycin dose of 5 mg per animal. The same findings were obtained with this dose of puromycin as with the dose of 7.5 mg of the antibiotic (Fig. 7).

It is interesting to consider the consequences of the hypothesis that protein is the rate-limiting factor in phagocytosis, and that the limit is defined by the rate at which this protein is replaced through synthesis or exchange. The hypothesis can be described in terms of the following reaction:

$$C_{total} + P \longrightarrow C_bP + C_u$$

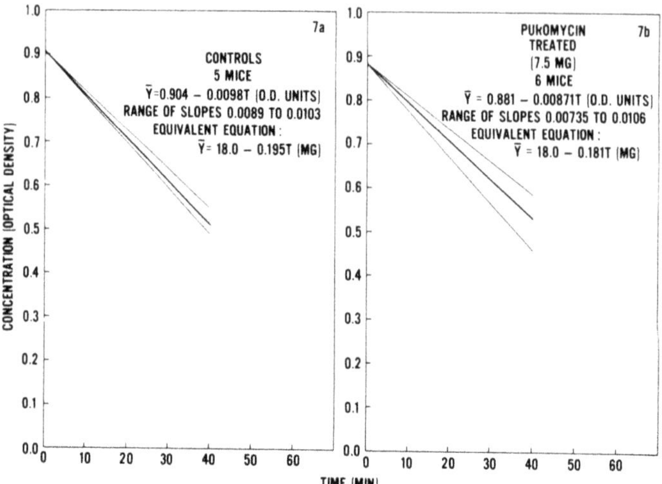

Fig. 7. The effect of 7.5 mg of puromycin on the clearance of a dose of 18 mg of colloidal carbon is seen by comparing Figs. 7a and 7b. The mean slope is shown by the heavy line, the extreme values by the lighter lines. The range of values of the slopes is given in each case. The equivalent equation describes the carbon clearance in terms of mg of colloidal carbon, instead of optical density units.

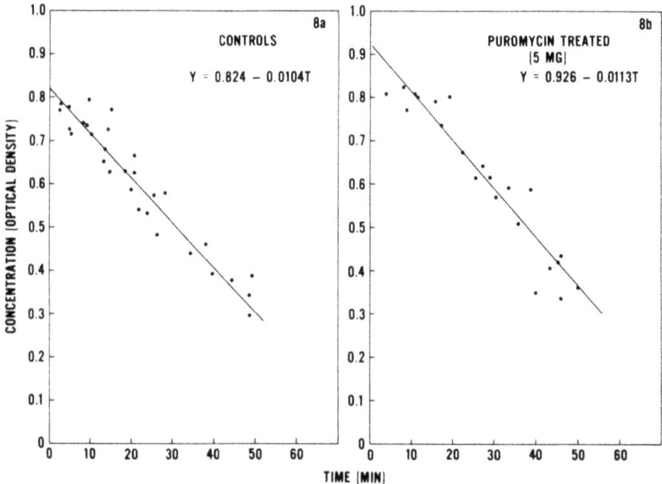

Fig. 8. The effect of 5.0 mg of puromycin on the clearance of a dose of 18 mg of colloidal carbon can be seen by comparing Figs. 8a and 8b. The equations for the best-fit lines are given in terms of optical density units.

where C_{total} is the total amount of carbon injected (in this case $C_{total} > P$), P is the total pool of protein which interacts with colloid, C_b is the colloid which is bound by protein, C_bP is the colloid-protein complex, and C_u is the unbound colloid remaining in the plasma.

It is assumed that when a large dose of colloid is introduced into the plasma, the rate of interaction of colloid particles with the plasma protein is rapid, and therefore not limiting. The hypothesis implies that all of this plasma protein pool interacts with the colloid, and that there is an excess of colloid (C_u) for which there is no protein available for interaction. As the colloid–protein complex (C_bP) is phagocytized, the protein that is lost will be replaced either through synthesis or exchange. If protein replacement requires synthesis and synthesis is stopped, then no new protein will be available and therefore no new complex will be formed. If we assume that there are no other rate-limiting factors in the phagocytic process, the amount of complex present will disappear exponentially. The predicted exponential disappearance curve should be asymptotic to C_u, since carbon, which is not complexed with protein, will not be cleared. The last statement is a necessary consequence of the hypothesis that a plasma protein is rate-limiting.

The rate of colloidal carbon clearance for the first 30 min in normal mice (Figs. 5, 7a, 8a) is about 0.20 mg colloid per min. A predicted exponential rate constant and the value of C_u (asymptotic concentration) can be calculated for the case where protein synthesis is stopped immediately before carbon administration. C_u depends on the fraction of the 18-mg dose of carbon which is required to bind all of the necessary plasma protein pool. The linear decrease in the concentration in Figs. 5, 7a, and 8a suggests that less than 50% of the 18 mg is required. The turnover time for the protein pool can also be estimated.

Figure 9 is a plot showing some of the calculated colloid clearance curves and a table of values which might be expected after puromycin treatment. It can be seen that the smaller the size of the plasma protein pool which interacts with carbon, i.e., the smaller the fraction of the 18-mg dose required for total binding, the more rapidly it must turn over in order to maintain the constant rate of clearance observed in normal mice. Turnover times of approximately 80 min or less are predicted, depending on the size of the protein pool. The effect of stopping protein synthesis is predicted to be most pronounced for the smallest pool sizes. If protein replacement depends more upon exchange than on synthesis, then these values suggest a relatively short turnover time for this plasma protein pool.

The puromycin experiments suggest that <u>de novo</u> protein synthesis is not the rate-limiting factor in phagocytosis. However, there still exists the possibility that the rate of re-utilization of the protein in question is the limiting factor. In order to satisfy the observed dynamics of colloid clearance, however, it would appear necessary for this protein to be stripped from the colloid at the cell surface prior to engulfment of the particle. To establish definitively that a re-utilizable protein is the rate-limiting factor in phagocytosis, it would be necessary: (1) to identify this protein, (2) manipulate the levels of the protein in the plasma, and (3) note the effect of such manipulation on colloid clearance in an experiment in which the maximum functional capacity of the RES is expressed, i.e., with the use of a saturating dose of colloid.

Examine the alternate model in which a re-utilizable plasma protein would constitute the rate-limiting factor in RES phagocytosis. The following conditions would appear essential for such a model: (1) the plasma protein in question exists in limiting quantity, (2) the protein is not phagocytized with the colloid, but is stripped from the colloid at the cell surface, becoming immediately available for re-utilization. If it is phagocytized, the protein must have a rapid rate of exchange from the cell back into the plasma, (3) the number of binding sites on the phagocytic cell surface is not limiting, (4) the colloid–protein complex which is formed in the plasma is brought into contact with phagocytic cells by liver blood flow. The clearance of a saturating dose of colloid in such a model would follow zero-order kinetics and would be dependent on three factors: (1) the amount of colloid complexed with the protein, which is constant for a saturating colloid dose, (2) the constant rate at which the carbon–protein complex is brought into contact with the surfaces of phagocytic cells, which is dependent upon liver blood flow, and (3) the probability of engulfment of the carbon (from the carbon–protein complex) coming into contact with the phagocytic cell surfaces. Such a model would require that clearance of saturating doses of colloid be liver-blood-flow dependent. This requirement is not consistent with current concepts of colloid clearance kinetics [2, 30]. This model may therefore also be an invalid description of the RES.

It is possible that some factor other than the availability of a plasma protein constitutes the rate-limiting factor in the phagocytic process. In our model of RES function we suggest that the magnitude of the dose of colloid that will constitute a saturating dose is dependent only upon the total number of binding sites for colloid on phagocytic cells. The maximum rate at which a saturating dose of colloid will be cleared, however, is dependent upon the product of the total number of binding sites and the probability (per unit time) of engulfment. In order to investigate the possibility that the number of binding sites on RE cells and the probability of engulfment limit the maximum rate of RES phagocytosis in the mouse, experiments were performed in which these two factors were manipulated nearly independently, and the effect of such manipulation on colloid clearance was noted under the condition in which the maximum functional capacity of the RES was expressed, i.e., with the use of a saturating dose of colloid.

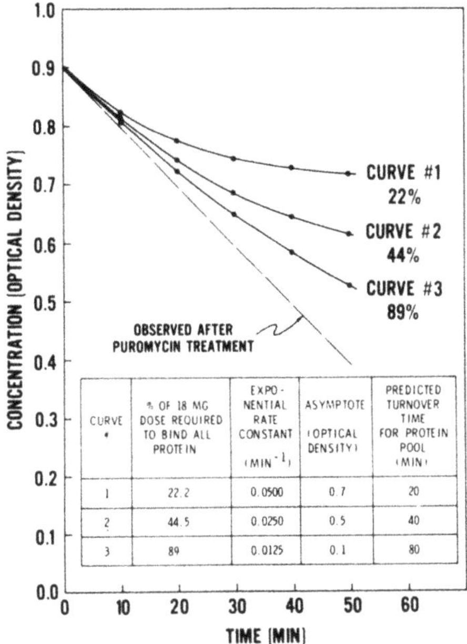

CURVE #	% OF 18 MG DOSE REQUIRED TO BIND ALL PROTEIN	EXPONENTIAL RATE CONSTANT (MIN^{-1})	ASYMPTOTE (OPTICAL DENSITY)	PREDICTED TURNOVER TIME FOR PROTEIN POOL (MIN)
1	22.2	0.0500	0.7	20
2	44.5	0.0250	0.5	40
3	89	0.0125	0.1	80

Fig. 9. The predicted result of stopping protein synthesis. These are the calculated clearance curves for a saturating dose of colloidal carbon, if colloidal carbon clearance is assumed to be limited by the rate of <u>de novo</u> replacement of some plasma constituent. The values for curves 1, 2, and 3 are given in the insert and are explained in the text. The dashed straight line of colloid clearance is observed experimentally and is only for comparison.

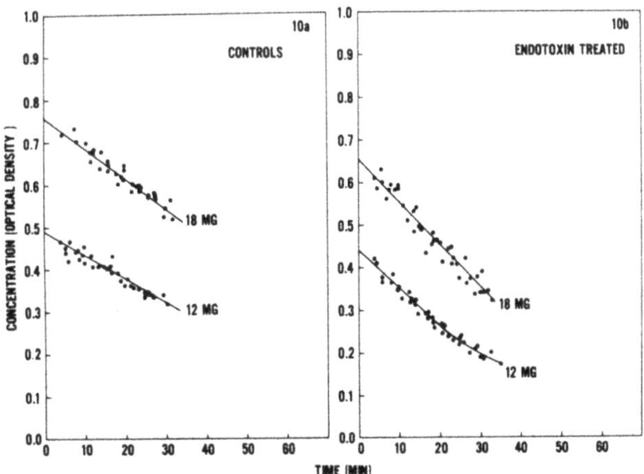

Fig. 10. The change in the characteristics of the clearance of a 12-mg and an 18-mg dose of colloidal carbon four days after S. typhosa endotoxin treatment (10b). The best-fit lines in each set are initially straight and approximately parallel, i.e., both 12 mg and 18 mg are saturating doses of colloid. However, the slopes of the lines for the endotoxin-treated mice are steeper than for the controls.

Figure 10b contains carbon clearance data from an experiment in which the mice were previously treated with S. typhosa endotoxin. Control animals did not receive endotoxin (Fig. 10a). In the control animals it can be seen that both the 12- and 18-mg doses of carbon meet the criteria for saturating doses (Figs. 3a, 4a, 5, and accompanying discussion). The 12-mg and 18-mg doses of carbon were similarly found to be saturating doses for the endotoxin-treated animals. However, the rate of clearance of colloid in the animals receiving endotoxin was greater than that observed in the controls. This suggests that the probability of engulfment (phagocytic efficiency of RE cells) has increased, without a noticeable change in the number of binding sites on RE cells. This conclusion is in agreement with the work of Kelly et al. and Dobson et al., in which it was demonstrated that endotoxin exerted its stimulatory effect on the RE system principally by activation of existing RE cells [28, 29].

Figure 11 presents the results of a similar experiment in which glucan was given to stimulate the reticuloendothelial system. This experiment was performed in conjunction with the previous experiment (Fig. 10), and the same controls were utilized for both experiments. Doses of 12 or 18 mg of colloidal carbon were administered to mice which had previously received glucan. In this case, it can be seen that the 18-mg dose of carbon was initially cleared with zero-order kinetics and at a rate greater than that ob-

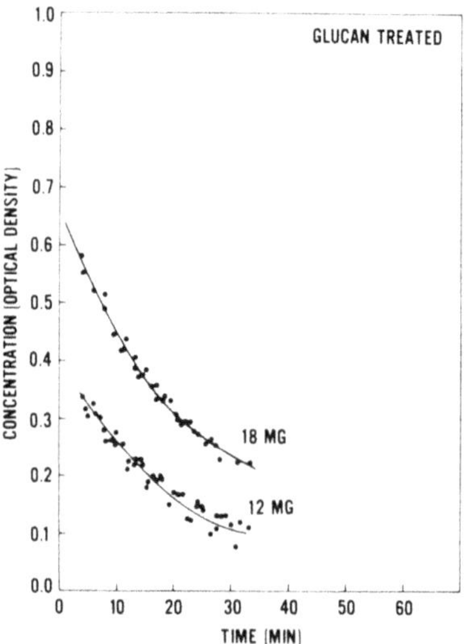

Fig. 11. The effect of glucan on the characteristics of the clearance of a 12-mg and an 18-mg dose of colloidal carbon four days after glucan treatment. The 18-mg curve is approximately linear for the first 15 min and then bends. The 12-mg curve is not linear and is not initially parallel to the 18-mg curve, which indicates that 12 mg is not a saturating dose. See text for further discussion of this. Both curves have slopes that are steeper than the comparable controls (Fig. 10a), which reflects the hyperactivity of the RES produced by glucan.

Table I. The Effect of Sublethal Radiation ($LD_{05/30}$, ^{137}Cs-gamma) on the Maximum Functional Phagocytic Capacity of the RES. The Results of Two Separate, but Identically Performed, Experiments Are Shown. The Colloidal Carbon Test Dose Was 18 mg per Mouse

Experiment	No. of mice	Controls (mg/min) ± S.E.	Irradiated (mg/min) ± S.E.	No. of mice	P (t-test)
1	14	0.195 ± 0.0148	0.172 ± 0.0090	34	.09
2	29	0.178 ± 0.0086	0.157 ± 0.0041	67	<.01
1 and 2 combined	43	0.184 ± 0.0075	0.162 ± 0.0041	101	<.005

served for the controls. However, in Fig. 11, it can be seen that the 12-mg dose of carbon was no longer an initially saturating dose. Since it has been suggested by our RES model data that the magnitude of the dose of colloidal carbon constituting a saturating dose is dependent only upon the total number of binding sites on RE cells, these experimental results suggest that in the glucan-treated animals the total number of binding sites has increased. This conclusion is in agreement with the work of Kelly et al. [28], which demonstrated that zymosan (a crude glucan) stimulated RE function primarily by inducing cellular proliferation of the RES, i.e., increasing the total number of binding sites in the RES. The investigators also suggested that zymosan might produce a portion of its effect through activation of RE cells.

In terms of our model of RES phagocytic function, a change in the probability of engulfment could be differentiated from a simultaneous change in the number of binding sites by first determining the change in the magnitude of the saturating dose. This can be done either by determining the clearance of multiple increasing doses of colloid (Fig. 5 and accompanying discussion), or by examining the clearance of a single large dose of colloid and determining the lower limits of concentration at which zero-order kinetics are no longer followed (Figs. 3a, 4a). Having determined the relative change in the number of binding sites, a calculation can be made predicting the relative change in the rate of clearance of a saturating dose of carbon. A comparison of the expected rate with the observed rate of clearance will then provide an estimate of any relative change in the probability of colloid engulfment by RE cells.

As a practical application of the concept of maximum functional capacity of the RES, an investigation of the effect of radiation on RES phagocytic function was performed. Table I shows the results obtained in two separate experiments in which normal and irradiated mice were tested with a saturating dose of colloidal carbon (18 mg/animal), at various times up to four days after irradiation. The normal control animals were compared with the irradiated animals without regard to the time after irradiation.

A decrease in the rate of colloid clearance in irradiated mice as compared to controls was observed in both experiments as shown. The differences were statistically significant, as indicated in the last column of Table I. In both experiments, at each time tested, the irradiated mice had lower mean clearance rates than the controls. These data show that sublethal doses of gamma radiation cause a statistically significant injury to the RES which can be detected as a decrease in the maximum functional phagocytic capacity.

SUMMARY

The weight of evidence which has been presented strongly supports the principle, incorporated in our model, that an interaction at the phagocytic cell surface constitutes the rate-limiting factor in RES phagocytosis.

A method has been suggested, based on the RES model, for resolving changes in colloid clearance in terms of either alteration in phagocytic efficiency or altered number of binding sites on phagocytic cell surfaces.

The results of the radiation experiments indicate that the concept of maximum functional phagocytic capacity of the RES can be utilized to investigate altered RES function which may not be detectable when smaller than saturating test doses of colloid are employed.

ACKNOWLEDGMENTS

Thanks are due to J.F. Williams, and Dr.H.A. Sober, ICR, NIH, for assisting with the amino acid analysis; Mr. J.G. Harris who helped prepare the manuscript; and to Miss T.M. Greene who assisted with the animal experiments.

REFERENCES

1. G. Biozzi, B. Benacerraf, and B.N.Halpern, Brit. J. Exptl. Pathol., 34:441, 1953.
2. G. Biozzi and C. Stiffel, in: H. Popper and F. Schnaffiner, Eds., Progress in Liver Diseases, New York, Grune and Stratton Inc., 1965, p. 166.
3. R.K. Fred, J.G. Harris, and M.L. Shore, J. Reticuloendothelial Soc., 2:344, 1965. (Abstract) Full text to be published.
4. W.O. Fenn, J.Gen.Physiol., 4:373, 1922.
5. E.R. Gabrieli and F.M. Snell, J.Reticuloendothelial Soc., 2:141, 1965.
6. T.M. Saba and N.R. Di Luzio, J.Reticuloendothelial Soc., 2:437, 1965.
7. S.J. Normann and E.P. Benditt, J.Exptl.Med., 122: 709, 1965.
8. B. Benacerraf, E. Kivy-Rosenberg, M.M. Sebestyen, and B.Zweifach, J.Exptl.Med., 110:49, 1959.

9. B. Benacerraf, M.M. Sebestyen, and S. Schlossman, J. Exptl. Med., 110:27, 1959.
10. J.P. Filkins, R.E. Chase, and J.J. Smith, J. Reticuloendothelial Soc., 2:287, 1965.
11. C.R. Jenkin and D. Rowley, J. Exptl. Med., 114:363, 1961.
12. E.L. Dobson, in: B.N. Halpern, B. Benacerraf, and J.F. Delafresnaye, Eds., Physiopathology of the Reticuloendothelial System: A Symposium, Oxford, Blackwell Scientific Publications, 1955, p. 80.
13. B. Benacerraf, G. Biozzi, A. Cuendet, and B.N. Halpern, J. Physiol., 128:10, 1955.
14. H.G. Parker and C.R. Finney, Am. J. Physiol., 198:916, 1960.
15. S.J. Riggi and N.R. Di Luzio, Am. J. Physiol., 200:297, 1961.
16. Gunther–Wagner Pelikan Ink Works, Hanover, Germany.
17. B. N. Halpern, B. Benacerraf, and G. Biozzi, Brit. J. Exptl. Pathol., 34:426, 1953.
18. W.R. Keene and J.H. Jandl, Blood, 26: 157, 1965.
19. Puromycin Dihydrochloride, M.W. 544.5, M.P. 175-177°, Nutritional Biochemicals Corp., Cleveland, Ohio, Refs.: (i) Waller et al., J. Am. Chem. Soc., 75:2025, 1953, (ii) Porter et al., Antibiot. Chemotherapy, 2:409, 1952.
20. L-Leucine–C^{14} (uniformly labeled), 1.7 mc/mg, Lot No. 190-117c-46, New England Nuclear Corporation, Boston, Mass.
21. Hydroxide of Hyamine*^{R} 10-x, p-(diisobutyl-cresoxyethoxyethyl) dimethylbenzylammonium hydroxide, 1 molar in methanol, Lot No. 1193, Packard Instrument Co., Inc., LaGrange, Ill.
22. R.C. Meade and R.A. Steiglitz, Intern. J. Appl. Radiation Isotopes, 13:11, 1962.
23. F.N. Hayes, in: S. Rothchild, Ed., Advances in Tracer Methodology Vol. 3, New York, Plenum Press, 1966, p. 81.
24. S. Moore, D.H. Spackman, and W.H. Stein, Anal. Chem., 30(7):1185, 1958.
25. G.A. Bray, Anal. Biochem., 1:279, 1960.
26. Glucan, Lot No. IF 5500, Fleischmann Laboratories, Division of Standard Brands, Inc., Stamford, Conn.
27. S. typhosa endotoxin (DiFco). Kindly furnished by Dr. W.W. Smith, National Cancer Institute, Bethesda, Md.
28. L.S. Kelly, E.L. Dobson, C.R. Finney, and J.D. Hirsch, Am. J. Physiol., 198:1134, 1960.
29. E.L. Dobson, L.S. Kelly, and C.R. Finney, The Physiologist, 3:50, 1960.
30. R.W. Brauer, in: R.W. Brauer, Ed., Liver Function, Washington, D.C., American Institute of Biological Sciences, 1958, p. 113.

The Use of Radioiodinated Latex Particles for In Vivo Studies of Phagocytosis*

J. M. Singer, S. Lavie, L. Adlersberg, E. Ende, E. M. Hoenig, and Y. Tchorsh

Montefiore Hospital and Medical Center
Department of Microbiology and Neuropathology
Laboratory Division
Bronx, New York

ABSTRACT. Polystyrene latex particles were radioiodinated, and combined radioisotope, histologic and electron microscopic studies traced the fate of these particles in vivo. Particular emphasis has been given to the role of charge and stability in determining distribution of the colloid. Nonphagocytic aspects of blood clearance and evidences for recirculation of phagocytized particles are discussed.

The functions of the reticuloendothelial system have been studied using a variety of test materials [1-4]. Although much information has been obtained, there have always been discrepancies among the results of workers using different test substances. The obvious conclusion is that the nature of the particles presented to the RES is one of the most important features governing response of the phagocytic system. Some of the variables which influence the choice of a test colloid include the physicochemical characteristics of the substance and the stability of the material in vitro and in vivo. The latter variable would appear, from our work, to be of considerable significance in governing the behavior of the colloid in the blood and in various organs containing phagocytic cells.

Polystyrene latex particles have been used by a number of workers to study phagocytosis, reticuloendothelial proliferation, and interaction of charged particles with the RES [3, 5]. Latex particles are unique among colloidal materials used to test the RES in that their surface properties may be modified without changing the chemical structure of the particles, they may be manufactured in a wide range of sizes while retaining the same chemical properties, and they may be quantitatively coated with serum pro-

*Aided, in part, by Grant Nos.: AM 06052-06, AI 05604-03 and 2F 11 NB 1104-03 NS RB of National Institutes of Health.

teins. In addition, these particles are readily identified in electron microscope sections because of their size and electron density. They may be directly visualized by phase contrast and darkfield microscopy. In paraffin sections they may be stained with Oil Red 0 in propanol. By this method latex particles stain reddish, whereas fat droplets remain unstained.

Because of their particular physicochemical properties, monodisperse latex particles were used to investigate the effect of charge and stability on phagocytosis by cells of the RES.

Latex particles were obtained from Dr. J. Vanderhoff, Dow Chemical Company. These particles were prepared by the polymerization of styrene with relatively small amounts of butadiene. The polymerization of standard latex particles in the presence of butadiene was necessary because radioiodination must be accomplished through the butadiene double bond. Iodination was performed according to the procedure developed in this laboratory [6].

The amount of radioisotope incorporated into the structure of the particles is so small that the physicochemical properties, charge, stability, and homogeneity of size are not detectably altered. The level of radioactivity (^{125}I or ^{131}I) may be varied within certain limits according to experimental requirements, and particles are obtained which have no deleterious effect on the test animal and yet are readily detected in a gamma scintillation counter [6].

Latex particles are prepared by emulsion polymerization. The nature and amount of detergent used in this process are primarily responsible for the net surface charge of the particles. Charge may be simply and conveniently determined by using a moving boundary four-compartment micro-Tiselius cell developed in our laboratory [7]. Since it is the detergent that confers surface charge on the latex, it has been possible to reverse this charge by the use of different detergents [7, 8]. All commercially available latex particles are negatively charged. Following iodination, the particles have an electrophoretic mobility toward the anode of $2.3 \cdot 10^{-4}$ cm/sec/V per cm at 4°C corresponding to a zeta potential of −46 mV. Positive particles, prepared by exchange dialysis in benzalkonium chloride have a mobility toward the cathode of $1.47 \cdot 10^{-4}$ cm/sec/V/cm (zeta potential +29.4 mV). The nonionic particles prepared in Tween 80 are slightly electronegative having an electrophoretic mobility toward the anode of $0.63 \cdot 10^{-4}$ cm/sec/V/cm (zeta potential −12.6 mV). Stability is controlled by the amount of emulsifier used, and may be checked by observing the particles by dark field or phase contrast microscopy. Stable preparations are monodisperse. Particles of 2200-Å size were tested in vivo, using CF_1 male mice for blood clearance, organ localization, histology, and electron microscopy studies.

Studies of reticuloendothelial function and of phagocytosis have given much attention to the rate at which injected test colloids are removed from the blood. In general, the shape of the clearance curve has been interpreted in terms of phagocytic activity and its relation to particle size and dosage [1-4]. Clearance curves have been obtained for various concentrations of latex particles. In all cases, there was an initial rapid clearance, followed by a gradual slope ending in an asymptotic line continuing for at least 12 months The shape of the curve and rate of clearance is unlike that described for carbon and chromium phosphate, but similar to that described by Schoenberg for nonradioactive anionic latex [1, 2, 4, 9]. The "tailing effect" found with chromium phosphate has been attributed to slower clearance of smaller size particles present in suspensions with a nonuniform size distribution. Latex suspensions are uniform with respect to size, yet still show this "tailing effect." Schoenberg [9] attributed the residual amount of latex in the blood to the presence of circulating leukocytes and macrophages containing latex particles, suggesting that the low circulating level of latex reached and maintained in the experiments may be explained by a constant renewal of reticuloendothelial cells that have participated in phagocytosis. It was suggested that clearance of particles may be used as a rough estimation of the half-life of RE cells. The concept of reverse phagocytosis, i.e., reappearance of previously phagocytosed material in the circulation, is supported by Gabrieli et al. [10].

Histological evidence gathered in our laboratory would tend to support Schoenberg's explanation of the "tailing effect" as being due to recirculation. In the first minute, although the majority of Kupffer cells are free of latex particles, a few cells, mainly in the periportal region, are loaded with latex. After 30 min, most of the particles have been phagocytized but a number of free particles, either singly or in clumps adjacent to the Kupffer cells, remain in some of the sinusoids. Not all of the sinuses contain latex particles. The majority of the particles are in the midportion of the lobules from 10 to 30 min after injection, but many are still at the periphery. After 4 h, latex particles may be seen in enlarged sinusoids in all parts of the liver. A few are now seen in polymorphonuclear leukocytes as well as free in the sinusoids. The histological pattern obtained after 6 months is completely different. At this stage, the hepatic phagocytes are loaded with latex particles. Plaques of these loaded cells (epitheloid-like) obscure the lumens of the sinuses, adjacent to the central lobular veins. Plaques are also present in the vicinity of the portal vein. Some of the plaques appear to be completely detached from the sinusoidal wall. They may be contained in Kupffer cells which have been transformed into free macrophages. This transformation suggests a mechanism whereby latex particles are made available for recirculation, either within the macrophages, or as free particles if these cells are destroyed. The mesenchymal cells of the liver are known to localize the majority of foreign colloidal particles. Yet, a definite role in immunology has never been assigned to this organ. It may be speculated that recirculation of phagocytized particles provides a constant source of antigen for the immune

Table I. Latex Activity per Whole Blood Following Administration of Nonionic, Anionic, and Cationic ^{125}I-Latex Particles

Sampling time, min	Nonionic latex		Anionic latex		Cationic latex	
	micrograms	per cent	micrograms	per cent	micrograms	per cent
1	2526	31.5	1326	16.6	1496	18.7
3	663	8.3	986	12.3	–	–
5	496	6.2	748	9.3	952	12.0
10	403	5.0	629	7.8	816	10.2
15	342	4.3	535	6.7	760	9.5
20	299	3.7	459	5.7	775	9.7
30	243	3.0	433	5.4	612	7.7
40	212	2.6	340	4.2	–	–
50	196	2.4	289	3.6	585	7.3

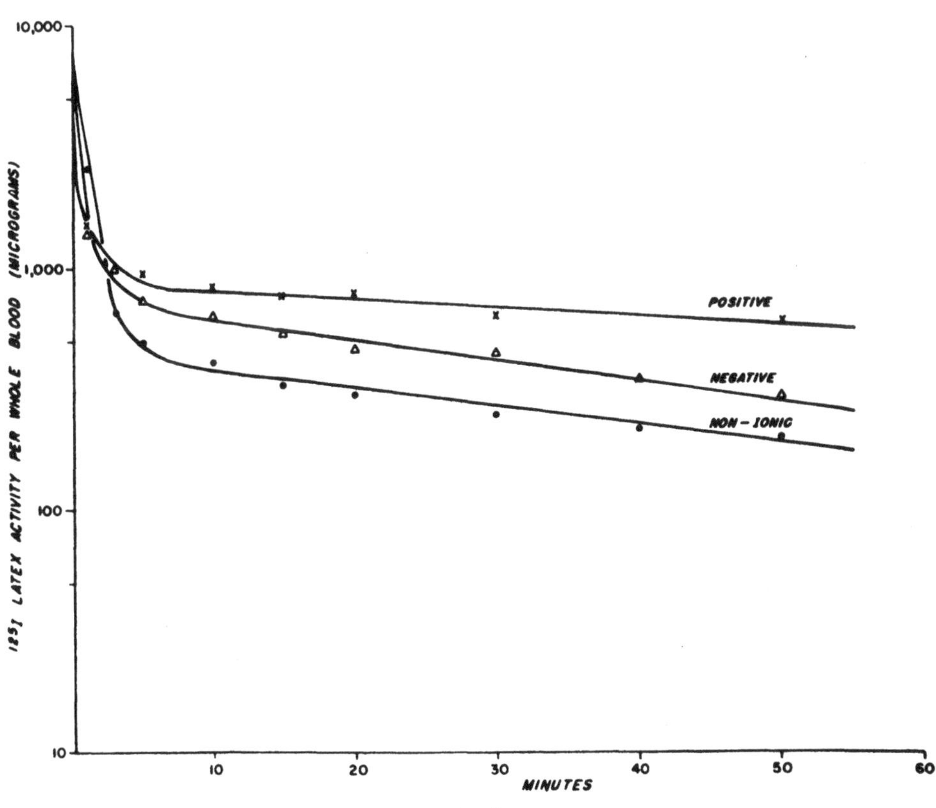

Fig. 1

mechanism. This might be correlated with theories requiring the persistence of antigen for immunity.

The response of the reticuloendothelial system to particles of varying charges has been investigated by a number of workers [1, 2, 3, 5]. A major problem in such experiments is the fact that test substances used to study the effect of charge differ also in their chemistry, size, and stability so that it becomes difficult to attribute variations among such materials to charge alone. Because the amount of detergent coverage responsible for the charge of latex particles is as low as 5%, the particles remain quite similar in all respects except net surface charge. Blood clearance data obtained following intravenous administration of an 8-mg dose of anionic, cationic, and nonionic latex particles are presented in Table I and plotted in Fig. 1. More detailed information concerning organ localization, histology, and electron microscopy is presented in another publication. The initial clearance rates are similar for anionic and cationic particles; approximately 85% of the initial dose is removed from the blood in the first minute after injection. For nonionic latex the initial rapid fall in blood concentration is not so abrupt, the clearance being 68.5% in 1 min. However, in the case of the nonionic particles, the first component of the clearance curve lasts longer, so that after 3 min, particles with a nonionic surface are at a lower blood concentration than either anionic or cationic particles. Radioactivity counts of the lung 1 min after injection reveal that from 15-20% of the injected positive and negative particles are localized in that organ. Only 6% of the initial nonionic dose is to be found in the lung. Nonionic particles are most rapidly localized in the liver despite the fact that they show the slowest decline in blood concentration. This discrepancy seems to be due to a temporary retention of the charged particles by the lung. Radioactivity counts and histological observations show that latex has been removed from the lung 20-50 min after injection.

In our series of experiments, in vivo stability has been a function of the net surface charge of the injected particles. Latexes closer to electrical neutrality are more stable than those which have either a stronger negative or positive charge.

Charge cannot be treated as an isolated characteristic because it seems to affect stability in vivo. The physicochemical characteristics of test substances require more detailed explanation in terms of stability. Carbon particles, chromium phosphate, and other materials including latex particles are hydrophobic colloids. By definition, such materials are metastable in vitro. Addition of small amounts of a hydrophilic material to these colloids will destabilize them by neutralization of the surface charge of the particles. Upon addition of larger amounts of the hydrophilic material the particles will acquire a net charge and surface chemistry due to the adsorbed hydrophilic material and thereby be stabilized. The properties given to the test particles by the hydrophilic coat will then determine their behavior both in vitro and in vivo, particularly in terms of stability. Gold particles will be stabilized by relatively small amounts of hydrophilic colloids, whereas most other hydrophobic colloids require a larger amount of stabilizing agent. Particles in vivo will interact with plasma constituents according to the properties acquired from the coating or stabilizing agent, and relative stability will be quite similar to that observed in vitro. Surface adsorption of any polymer molecule to solid surfaces is based on Van der Waals forces and the polymer molecule will be broken up, by contact with the surface, into short sequences of segments [11]. This discontinuity in the adsorbed layer indicates that the chemical nature of the colloidal particle is still important in determining physicochemical behavior of the particles. For the most productive interpretation of the results obtained with the different colloidal materials used to study the RES, the particles would best be described in terms of: electrical charge of the test material before and after the addition of stabilizer, chemical formula and amount of stabilizing agent used, the gold number of the protective colloid, and the degree of dispersion of the particles before injection. This knowledge should permit some degree of predictability of the in vivo behavior of test particles. One cannot say whether particles of a given charge or stability in vivo are most suited to reticuloendothelial studies. The choice of material must, of course, be suited to the aims of the investigator. Studies concerning the lung might call for more unstable particles, whereas the more stable, nonionic particles might be better suited for investigation of various parameters of phagocytosis.

For most studies of phagocytosis, the kinetics of blood clearance have been treated as a direct function of phagocytic activity [1, 2, 4]. Our studies indicate that, for latex particles, removal from the circulation does not necessarily reflect only phagocytosis. Most obviously, the unstable positive and negative particles cleared from the blood are temporarily retained in the lung in association with thrombocytes. Both ionic and nonionic particles have been visualized by histology and electron microscopy in the spleen, lymphatics, and hepatic sinuses in the unphagocytized state. This observation holds true for all phases of the clearance curve although the number of these free particles is greatly diminished with time.

All the information concerning phagocytic and extraphagocytic distribution of latex particles in plasma and various organs has been further investigated and a set of mathematical assumptions has been formulated. The clearance curve of latex particles has been dissociated into three exponential functions corresponding to a three-compartment distribution. Variation in stability in the blood of the latex particles due to changing emulsifiers has been found markedly to influence the distribution between these compartments, as well as the uptake by RE cells.

REFERENCES

1. B. W. Halpern et al., Physiopathology of the RE system, Springfield, Illinois, Charles C. Thomas, 1957.
2. J. H. Heller, Reticuloendothelial Structure and Function, New York, Ronald Press, 1958.
3. See References in C.H. Rouiller, Liver: Morphology, Biochemistry, Physiology, New York. Academic Press. Vol. I, 1963. Vol.II, 1964.
4. E.L. Dobson, Acta Med.Scand., 273, 275, 1952.
5. D.J. Wilkins, Nature, 202:798, 1964; J. Reticuloendothelial Soc., 1: 343, 1964; this volume, p. 25.
6. J.M. Singer, C.J. van Oss, and J.W. Vanderhoff: To be published.
7. C.J. van Oss and J.M. Singer, J. Colloid Interface Sci., 21:117, 1966.
8. C.J. van Oss and J.M. Singer, J. Reticuloendothelial Soc., 3:29, 1966.
9. M.D. Schoenberg, P.A. Gilman, V. Mumaw, and R.D. Moore, Brit. J. Exptl. Pathol., 42:486, 1961.
10. E.R. Gabrieli, F.M. Snell, and E.J. Meyer, J. Reticuloendothelial Soc., 1:343, 1964.
11. A. Silverberg, J. Phys. Chem., 66: 1884, 1962.

Interaction of Charged Colloids with the RES

David J. Wilkins

New England Institute for Medical Research
Ridgefield, Connecticut

INTRODUCTION

The involvement of plasma factors in the clearance of colloids from the circulation by the RES has been suggested by many authors, both in a general way [1, 2] and from the point of view of finding specific phagocytosis-promoting factors [3]. In the course of our own work, data obtained by the microelectrophoresis of model colloids in serum [4] (see also Table I) would also indicate an interaction between the colloid surface and serum. It has been further suggested that fibrin or fibrin-like macromolecules may be adsorbed on the surface of injected colloids [5], but the involvement of the blood coagulation system in the RES clearance mechanism of colloids has never been firmly established. Circumstantial evidence for this idea comes from several authors. For example, Smith and his co-workers [6] showed that rapid injections of colloidal silica into dogs lowered the fibrinogen content of the blood to less than measurable levels. Biozzi et al. [7], in experiments on blockade, suggested that blood coagulation factors interfered with their measurements but these effects could be reversed by adminstration of heparin. Lee [8] was able to show that fibrin itself produced by slow intravenous infusion thrombin into dogs is cleared by the RES. Finally, it has been shown [9] that calcium ions, known to be essential for blood coagulation, affect phagocytosis in a manner that cannot be explained in terms of its effect on the surface charge of the colloid.

Table I. Uptake of Positive and Negative Polystyrene Latex 2 min after Intravenous Injection (Dose 0.73 mg/100 g of rat)

Surface	Electrophoretic mobility		Percent injected dose				
	Isotonic Michaelis buffer. pH 7.5	Serum	No. of animals	Blood	Liver	Lungs	Spleen
P. Lys. G.	+0.82	−0.65	5	19.62	39.66	27.99	5.41
P. Glu. G.	−1.65	−0.72	5	7.67	70.77	5.75	5.02

In the course of experiments to establish the mechanism whereby the RES is able to distinguish a "foreign," e.g., bacterial, from a "native," e.g., red blood cell, a model system was prepared in which it was possible to alter the surface properties of an injected colloid. This colloid consisted of isotopically labeled polystyrene latex [4, 10] which by adsorption of certain macromolecules could be given a positive or negative surface charge or ζ-potential. One of the findings of this work was that particles with a positive ζ-potential showed an initial rapid accumulation in the lungs. Preliminary experiments showed that this effect was not shown by previously heparinized animals. This paper considers a more detailed examination of this experimental system in an attempt to elucidate the interaction of the colloid surface with blood. Preliminary data are also presented on the effect of Dicumarol on the system.

METHODS AND MATERIALS

The model system consists of polystyrene latex of 1.305 μ diameter which has been labeled with iodine 125. The surface properties are modified by the adsorption of poly-L-lysyl gelatin (P. Lys. G.) to give an electrophoretically positive surface or by the adsorption of poly-L-glutamyl (P. Glu. G.) gelatin to give an electrophoretically negative surface. Preliminary details of the preparation of the labeled PSL and the synthesis of and coating with the gelatin derivatives have already been presented elsewhere [10] and will shortly appear in more detail [4]. The positive (P. Lys. G. / PSL) colloid and negative (P. Glu. G. / PSL) colloid were suspended in isotonic saline and the dose administered was 0.73 mg/ 100 g of rat (approximately $6 \cdot 10^8$ particles/ 100 g).

Electrophoresis Measurements

The electrophoretic mobility of the particles was measured using a cylindrical cell similar to that described by Bangham et al. [11]. For ease of operation, a closed-circuit television camera and monitor were linked to the microscope. The colloids were suspended in 0.145 M NaCl or Michaelis buffers of constant ionic strength for mobility measurements unless otherwise noted. Each experimental point represents the mean of ten readings and all measurements were made at 25° ± 1°. Electrophoretic mobilities are expressed as mobility per unit field strength, i.e., microns/sec/v/cm. This may be converted to ζ-potential by use of the Smoluchowski equation [12], but in the present paper the results will be recorded as mobilities. The adsorption of heparin by P. Lys. G. / PSL was obtained by following the change in electrophoretic mobility when suspended in different concentrations of heparin. This was carried out by adding a few drops of colloid to a suitable solution of heparin in 0.0145 M NaCl at its natural pH of approximately 5.2 and taking the mobility measurement after 5 min to allow for equilibration.

Measurement of Organ Uptake

Colloids were injected into the saphenous vein of Nembutal-anesthetized (0.1 ml/100 g) adult male rats* (200-250 g), and the incision closed with a wound clip. Two minutes after injection, the chest cavity was opened and 1.0 ml of blood withdrawn from the heart into a heparinized syringe. The liver, lungs, and spleen were removed, rinsed in isotonic saline, blotted dry, and weighed. The radioactivity of the blood and organ samples was determined, using a γ-ray spectrometer counting in the region 20-90 kev. The results were expressed as a percentage of the injected dose. In all animal experiments the results are the mean value for at least five animals.

Administration of Anticoagulants

Heparin,† suitably diluted with 0.145 M NaCl to the desired concentration, was injected into the saphenous vein of Nembutal-anesthetized animals four minutes before injection with colloid or before taking a blood sample for determination of prothrombin time. The volume injected was always 0.15 ml/100 g of rat. The incision was closed with a wound clip and the contralateral branch of the vein used for injection of the colloid. Dicumarol was administered orally as a suspension in water of the desired concentration by means of a syringe and a flexible silver cannula, 24 h before injection of colloid or removal of a blood sample.

Prothrombin Time

After experimenting with other methods, the prothrombin time was found to be the most convenient measure of the coagulation status of rat blood. 2.25 ml was withdrawn from the anesthetized rat by cardiac puncture into a siliconized syringe. This was immediately added to 0.25 ml of 0.1 M sodium oxalate solution and inverted several times for mixing. After centrifuging at 1500 rpm for 5 min, the prothrombin time of the plasma was determined with Simplastin‡ by Quick's method [13].

RESULTS

Table I shows the uptake by the various organs 2 min after injection of P. Lys. G./PSL and P. Glu.G./PSL together with their electrophoretic mobilities in buffer and rat serum. It will be noted that there is considerable difference of distribution between the positive and negative colloids. From the blood concentration it is clear that the negatively charged material is removed from the circulation more rapidly. It has been noted elsewhere that the distribution val-

---

* CFN – Nelson-Wistar Strain. Carworth Farms, New City, New York.

† Eli Lilly, Indianapolis, Indiana.

‡ Warner-Chilcott Labs, Morris Plains, New Jersey.

ues for the negative colloid do not alter substantially over a period of several days, whereas, with the positive colloid, the material accumulating in the lungs is rapidly lost (less than 1% after 72 h) and accumulates in the spleen [4].

Figures 1 and 2 show the distribution 2 min after injection of the colloid as a function of the concentration of previously administered heparin. The heparin was administered 4 min before the colloid, since this was felt to give adequate time for mixing, and insufficient time for significant elimination from the vascular system. Heparin in sufficient concentration has a marked effect upon the distribution of P. Lys. G. / PSL but has little effect on the distribution of P. Glu. G. / PSL. Heparin could be acting here as an anticoagulant or as a strongly acidic macromolecule which is in effect changing the P. Lys. G. / PSL from a positive to a negative colloid. The effect of different heparin concentrations on both blood coagulation and electrophoretic mobility was therefore examined. Figure 3 shows the effect of different doses of heparin on the prothrombin time of the plasma. This curve parallels Fig. 1 in its effect, but the concentrations to produce optimum effect are different (see Table II). Since Dicumarol is unlikely to be strongly adsorbed at the particle surface, since it acts on the liver to decrease prothrombin production, the effect of this material on the distribution of the two colloids was also examined. Figure 4 shows the effect of Dicumarol on the prothrom-

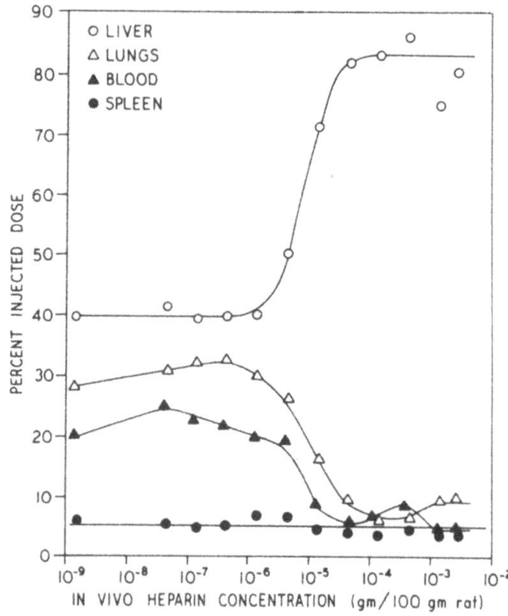

Fig. 1. Organ distribution of PLG-coated PSL 2 min after injection vs injected dose of heparin (heparin injected 2 min before PSL-PSG).

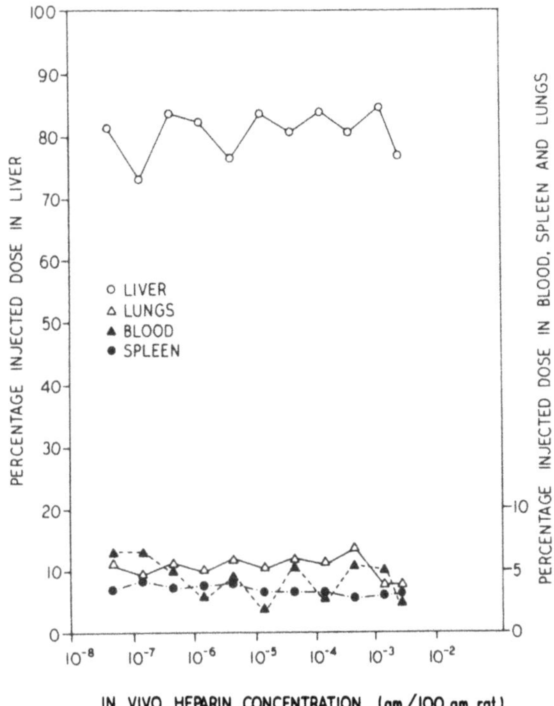

Fig. 2. Organ distribution of P. Glu. G.-coated PSL 2 min after injection vs injected dose of heparin (heparin injected 4 min before P. Glu. G.-PSL).

Table II. Minimum Concentrations of Heparin Required to Produce the Maximum Physiological Effect

Effect	Concentration in gm/ml	
Prothrombin time	$8.2 \cdot 10^{-6}$	in vivo
Maximum change in liver uptake of P. Lys. G./PSL. .	$5.5 \cdot 10^{-4}$	in vivo
Charge reversal of P. Lys. G./PSL.	$1 \cdot 10^{-7}$	in vitro

bin time of rat blood 24 h after oral administration. Figure 5 shows the effect of various concentrations of heparin on the electrophoretic mobility of P. Lys. G. / PSL. It can be seen that at a low concentration in vitro the charge on the colloid is reversed.

DISCUSSION

It is clear from Table I that the surface properties of these colloids markedly affect their distribution after intravenous injection. In previous

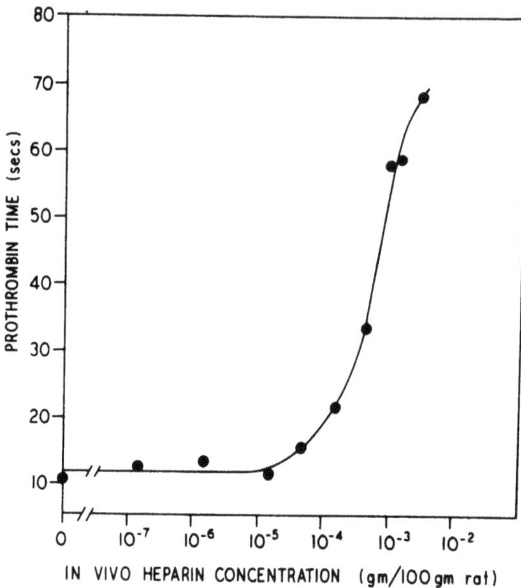

Fig. 3. Prothrombin time vs heparin concentration.

reports the negatively charged particles were produced by adsorption of gum arabic rather than polyglutamyl gelatin [10] and it is interesting to note that although these two macromolecules are chemically very dissimilar, they affect the organ distribution in a similar manner. It should be pointed out, however, that the surface parameter measured, i.e., electrophoretic mobility, is only a net measure of surface properties. As pointed out by Wright and Dodd [14], it would be preferable to know the exact distribution of the various charge groups. Thus it is not meant to imply that surface charge alone is responsible for the mechanism of the discrimination between these two colloids. Further, it will be noted that when these two colloids were suspended in fresh rat serum, they showed very similar mobilities. From preliminary electrophoretic studies the adsorbed protein behaves similarly to albumin, but this finding is probably of minimal interest. The important question would seem to be: What is the mechanism of interaction of a foreign surface with whole blood in vivo? This question is of obvious importance to other fields such as the design of nonthrombogenic materials for artificial organ fabrication [15].

As mentioned briefly in the introduction, there seems to be a body of indirect evidence which gives strong support to the idea that the blood coagulation system may be important here and that whether or not a particle becomes coated with fibrin may determine whether it is recognized as different. The experimental evidence presented here does not allow us to settle this question however.

By assuming a blood volume for the rat of 5.5 ml/ 100 g, it is possible to express the heparin concentrations in Figs. 1, 3, and 5 in the same units.

Table II shows the minimum concentrations of heparin required to produce the maximum change in the observed effect, converted to the same concentration units. It will be noted that at the concentration of heparin required to produce the maximum change in organ distribution, the prothrombin time would be normal (see Fig. 3). This would indicate that heparin is not acting as an anticoagulant in this case. Preliminary experiments on the distribution of both colloids in animals given 10 mg of Dicumarol 24 hr previously, showed no difference in distribution of positive or negative colloid as compared to untreated control animals. This would make it appear that the coagulation mechanism is unimportant here, since this concentration can be seen from Fig. 4 to exert a powerful effect on the prothrombin time. However, Fig. 4 shows that a dose of Dicumarol of 10 mg/ rat still gives a finite, though elevated, prothrombin time. Thus, the blood level of prothrombin is lowered, not eliminated, and hence it is possible that this concentration would be adequate for coagulation on a local scale, such as at a particle surface.

An alternative explanation would be that heparin being a strongly acidic macromolecule, adsorbs to the surface of the positively charged P. Lys. G./ PSL and reverses the charge. That this happens in vitro is strongly suggested from the fact that the positive colloid injected into a heparinized animal behaves in a similar manner to the negative colloid injected into a non-heparinized animal (see Figs. 1 and 2). This is further supported by the finding that heparinization of the animal has no effect on the distribution of the negatively charged colloid, since even if heparin were adsorbed it would not substantially alter the surface charge. However, note that a concentration of heparin in vitro as low as $1 \cdot 10^{-7}$ gm/ ml is sufficient to reverse the

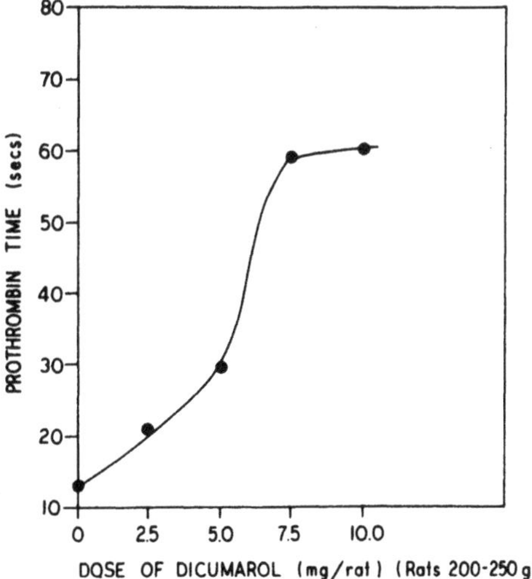

Fig. 4. Prothrombin time vs dose of Dicumarol administered.

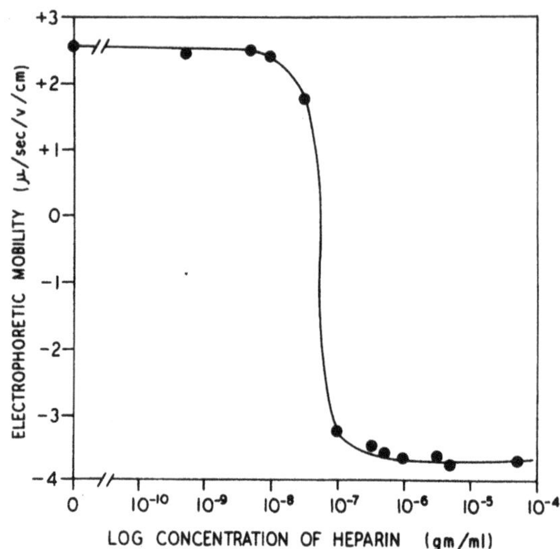

Fig. 5. Uptake of heparin on positive PSL in 0.0145 M NaCl.

surface charge on P. Lys. G. / PSL, whereas it requires a much higher concentration ($5.5 \cdot 10^{-4}$ gm/ml) of heparin in the blood before any change in distribution of colloid occurs. Even allowing for such possibilities as competition between heparin and other macromolecules for adsorption, and complexing of heparin with blood elements, it is difficult to interpret this discrepancy. Certainly it is important to consider the charge determining properties of heparin when interpreting data obtained from heparinized animals.

Neither the heparin results nor the albeit preliminary Dicumarol results rule out the possibility that fibrinogen can adsorb specifically to a foreign surface introduced into whole blood, with or without subsequent polymerization to fibrin. If this is the case, the interesting question, of course, is: What is the surface difference that causes some particles to be coated and others uncoated? In this connection it is interesting to note that the erythrocyte surface seems incapable of adsorbing proteins [16]. Further, although glassware used in hematological procedures is usually rendered hydrophobic with silicone or paraffin wax, in order to slow coagulation and also adsorption of proteins and platelets, it was shown by Lovelock et al. [17] that a sulphonated and hence highly negative surface was far more useful in retarding coagulation.

Further work in this area is being done using rats slowly perfused with dilute thrombin solutions [18]. This has been shown [8] to cause microthrombi which are then removed by the RES, effectively lowering the blood fibrinogen levels. In experiments in which such animals are injected with model colloids, consideration will have to be given to the possibility that any changes seen could be due not only to the lowered fibrinogen concentrations, but also to the elevated thrombin levels and possible "blockade" of the RES by fibrin.

ACKNOWLEDGMENTS

It is a pleasure to acknowledge the skilled technical assistance of Phyllis Myers, Linda Roig, and Margaret Stewart. Thanks are due also to Dr.J.H. Heller for his continuous support and encouragement.

This work was supported in part by Office of Naval Research Grant Nonr-4170(00), NR 301-740 and by the John A. Hartford Foundation, Inc.

REFERENCES

1. T.M. Saba and N.R. DiLuzio, J. Reticuloendothelial Soc., 2:437, 1965.
2. S.J. Normann and E.P. Benditt, J.Exptl. Med., 122:693, 1965.
3. J.L. Tullis and D.M. Surgenor, Ann.N.Y.Acad.Sci., 66:386, 1956.
4. D.J. Wilkins and P. Myers: In press.
5. M.H. Knisely, E.H. Bloch, and L. Warner, D.Kgl.Danske Vidensk. Selskab, Biologiske Skrifter, 4:1, 1948.
6. J.J. Smith: Personal communication.
7. G. Biozzi, G. Mene, B.N. Halpern, and B. Benacerraf, Compt.Rend. Soc.Biol., 145: 499, 1951.
8. L. Lee, J.Exptl.Med., 115:1065, 1962.
9. D.J. Wilkins and A.D. Bangham, J.Reticuloendothelial Soc., 1:233, 1964.
10. D.J. Wilkins and P. Myers, J.Reticuloendothelial Soc., 1:344, 1964.
11. A.D. Bangham, R. Flemens, D.H. Heard, and G.V.F. Seaman, Nature, 182:642, 1958.
12. A.E. Alexander and P. Johnson: Colloid Science, New York, Oxford University Press, 1949, p. 302.
13. A.J. Quick, J.Biol.Chem., 109:73, 1935.
14. C.S. Wright and M.C. Dodd, Ann.N.Y.Acad.Sci., 49:945, 1955.
15. R.I. Leininger, C.W. Cooper, R.D. Falb, and G.A. Grode, Science, 152:1625, 1966.
16. H.A. Abramson, L.S. Moyer, and M.H. Gorin, The Electrophoresis of Proteins, New York, Reinhold, 1942.
17. F.E. Lovelock and J.S. Porterfield, Nature, 167:39, 1951.
18. F.C. Monkhouse and S. Milojevic, Am.J. Physiol., 199:1165, 1960.

The Potential Use of Glutaraldehyde-Fixed Liver Cells in the Study of Hepatic Reticuloendothelial and Parenchymal Cell Metabolism

N. Baker

Radioisotope Research
Veterans Administration Center, Los Angeles, California

and

Department of Biological Chemistry
UCLA School of Medicine, Los Angeles, California

and

M. Cohen

Electron Microscopy Research Laboratory
Veterans Administration Center, Los Angeles, California

Glutaraldehyde has been widely used to fix tissue for electron microscopic, histochemical, and biochemical studies [1-3]. This dialdehyde not only has the capacity to stabilize subcellular structures, but it does so without completely inhibiting certain enzymes. These are properties which make glutaraldehyde a desirable tool in tissue structure-function studies.

We have been particularly interested in the metabolism of liver cells and have recently developed a technique for homogenizing mouse liver in the presence of glutaraldehyde for combined electron microscopic and biochemical studies of the subcellular particulates [4]. In the course of this work, we observed that fixation of the liver with glutaraldehyde in vivo resulted in the liver's displaying some rather unusual properties, which permit the preparation of fixed liver cell suspensions that may be especially useful for some unique types of biochemical investigation. We shall describe them in this communication.

When liver tissue is suspended in 5-20 times its weight of aqueous solutions and subjected to the hydrostatic pressure and shearing forces produced by various homogenizers, the cells are fragmented into their constituent, subcellular particulate components. Some of these, e.g., microsomes, are, in part, artifacts of the homogenization procedure.

If glutaraldehyde is included in the homogenizing medium, then a similar homogenate is obtained. However, the particulates are stabilized as they are released from the cells, so that they appear to be in a state resembling that of the corresponding structure in the unhomogenized tissue [2, 4].

On the other hand, if liver is soaked for many hours in a glutaraldehyde-containing buffer and then subjected to comparable homogenization, a heterogeneous suspension is obtained which, according to Janigan [3], can be pipetted only with difficulty. Its microscopic appearance has not been described in the literature to our knowledge, but we may assume from its sedimentation and size that the suspension is composed of pieces of tissue. It is not surprising that tissue soaked in glutaraldehyde should be difficult to homogenize; such tissue becomes hard and leathery. Indeed, glutaraldehyde has been used to tan leather.

However, electron microscopists know that the liver may also be made hard and leathery by a 30-sec perfusion, in vivo, with glutaraldehyde, We have found that liver, fixed in this fashion, can be subjected to extremely high shearing forces with only a slight suggestion of cell breakage. Instead, 90-95% of the liver may be subdivided rapidly into its component cells, most of which are either single, double, or in very small groups. The technique which we have used is given in Table I. The resulting suspension is easily and uniformly suspended even after centrifugation at 900 g for 20 min, and reproducible aliquots may be obtained readily, in contrast to the preparation of Janigan.

Cell suspensions were examined by phase microscopy and by ordinary light microscopy after staining them either with methyl green-pyronin (MGP) or with Lugol's stain for glycogen [5]. An extremely well-dispersed preparation, stained with MGP, is shown in Fig. 1. Although reticuloendothelial cells are not recognizable in this figure, they could be seen floating freely at times but, frequently, closely associated with parenchymal cells (Fig. 2). Occasionally, preparations were highly clumped. However, clumping was most notable when glutaraldehyde-perfused livers had been soaked in cold buffered glutaraldehyde for 40 min or longer instead of the usual 20 min (Table I). Deposition of glycogen in fixed liver cell suspensions of mice was easily demonstrated (Fig. 3). The mice had been fasted overnight and then injected intraperitoneally with 3 ml of 0.26 M glycerol. Two to six hours after glycerol injection, using Lugol's stain [5], deposition could be seen.

Fixed cell suspensions were also examined by electron microscopy. The following steps, until otherwise indicated, were in the cold. The cell dispersions of glutaraldehyde-fixed liver were treated with 1% w/v OsO_4 in veronal-acetate buffer (pH 7.3) containing 25% v/v Carbowax 200, then centrifugally passed through increasing aqueous concentrations of hydroxyethylmethacrylate [6] or ethanol. On reaching full strength of each solvent,

Table I. Technique for Preparing Glutaraldehyde-Fixed Liver Cells

1. Anesthetize mice with ether.
2. Perfuse liver through portal vein with 5 ml buffer (pH 7.4) containing:

10% $NaH_2PO_4 \cdot H_2O$	4.0 ml
2.3% NaOH	4.4 ml
40% Glucose	1.3 ml
50% Glutaraldehyde	0.6 ml
Water	25.7 ml

3. Excise liver (without gall bladder) and place for 20 min in perfusion medium at 0°C.
4. Cut liver into 8 pieces, blot, and weigh (approximately 500 mg).
5. Place in very loose-fitting homogenizer (Dounce type) in ice bath and disperse liver in 13.5 ml glutaraldehyde-free perfusion medium for about 1 min (approximately 30 strokes; no appreciable resistance).
6. Homogenize partially dispersed liver in Ten Broeck, very tightly fitting homogenizer, 10 strokes, 0°. Approximately 5-10% of tissue remains at bottom after last down-stroke.
7. Pour suspension from upper reservoir (contains approximately 0.50 ml packed cells per 10 ml).

the cells were treated with 1% w/v uranyl acetate in the respective solvents, then centrifugally passed through the respective solvents once more. The cells were passed through a 1:1 mixture of the respective solvents and a catalyzed [7] mixture of four volumes of ethyl to six of n-butyl methacrylate. After two changes of the catalyzed ethyl-butyl methacrylate mixture, the preparations were warmed to room temperature, and then the cells were embedded in very viscous prepolymerized ethyl-butyl methacrylate mixture for 60° polymerization. Ultrathin sections were stained with alkaline lead citrate [8].

Most of the single cells obtained by our technique have been found by electron microscopy to show little, if any, signs of damage (Fig. 4). The cytoplasm is compact and the organelles are not swollen (Fig. 5). Frequently RE cells are found freed from one parenchymal cell but still attached to another (Fig. 6), which confirms our impressions of methyl-green pyronin-stained cells examined by light microscopy. One portion of the RE cell shown in Fig. 6 has probably been separated from a parenchymal cell which does not appear in the section. Occasionally, partially separated groups of cells are found (Figs. 7 and 8). Less frequently, broken cells can be found after considerable searching (Fig. 9). Cell breakage may best be observed by phase microscopy. In every instance, some cell breakage has occurred, but this has been greatest when the procedure given in Table I was not followed closely. The majority of cells, as stated above, seem to be very well preserved. Attachments, where they exist, are sufficiently loose (Fig. 10) to suggest that further "homogenization," perhaps with other agents added,

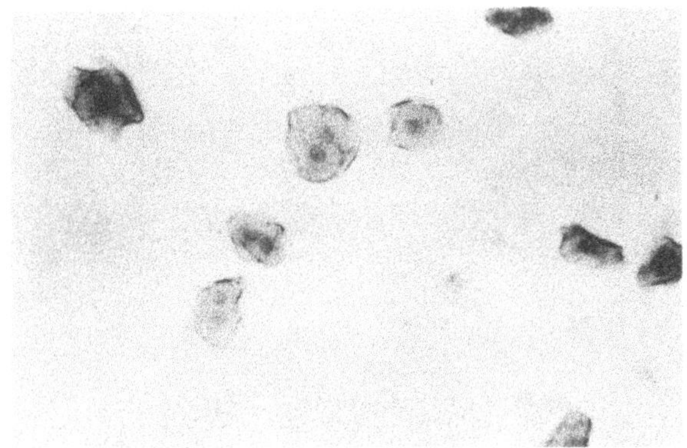

Fig. 1. Suspension of glutaraldehyde-fixed liver cells prepared according to the technique described in Table I.

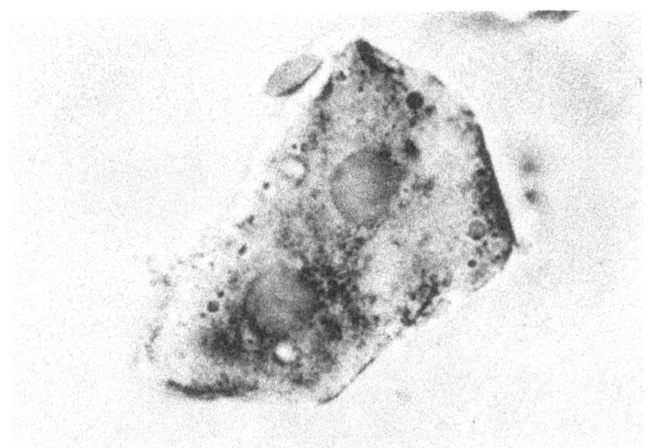

Fig. 2. Reticuloendothelial cell closely associated with binucleated parenchymal cell in glutaraldehyde-fixed suspension of mouse liver.

may increase significantly the yield of single cells, and, in particular, the separation of RE cells from parenchymal cells.

We are particularly interested in the separation of structurally well-preserved parenchymal and RE cells so that we may study biochemical function in each type of cell and determine whether the RE cell plays a quantitatively important role in the production of lactate from glucose. However, if the present cells are to prove useful for this purpose, we must be able to demonstrate that glutaraldehyde itself does not damage enzymatic function or, if it does, find out whether and how the inhibition may be reversed.

We have carried out a variety of studies, all of which we consider preliminary at this time. We show in Figs. 11-14 that tracer quantities of acetate-2-C^{14}, and perhaps glycerol-1, 3-C^{14}, may be oxidized to $C^{14}O_2$ by fixed liver slices to about the same extent as in unfixed slices. We also show that

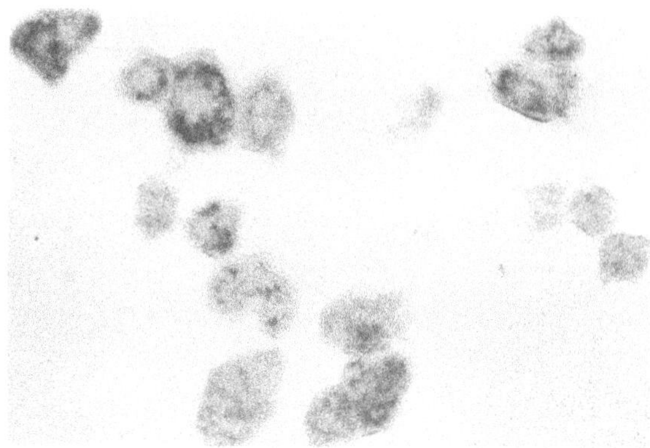

Fig. 3. Liver cell suspension stained with Lugol's stain to show net glycogen deposition following injection of glycerol. Fat droplets which accumulated following the overnight fast (which preceded glycerol injection) are also visible. Note the large number of poorly separated groups of cells.

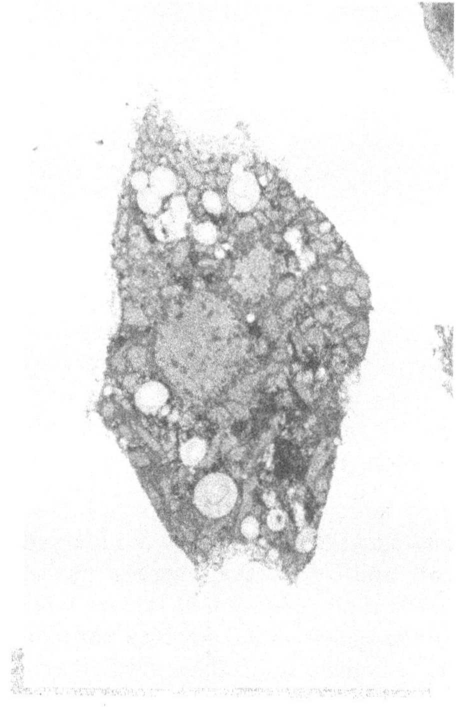

Fig. 4. Electron micrograph of a parenchymal cell from a suspension of glutaraldehyde-fixed, mouse liver cells (1500 ×).

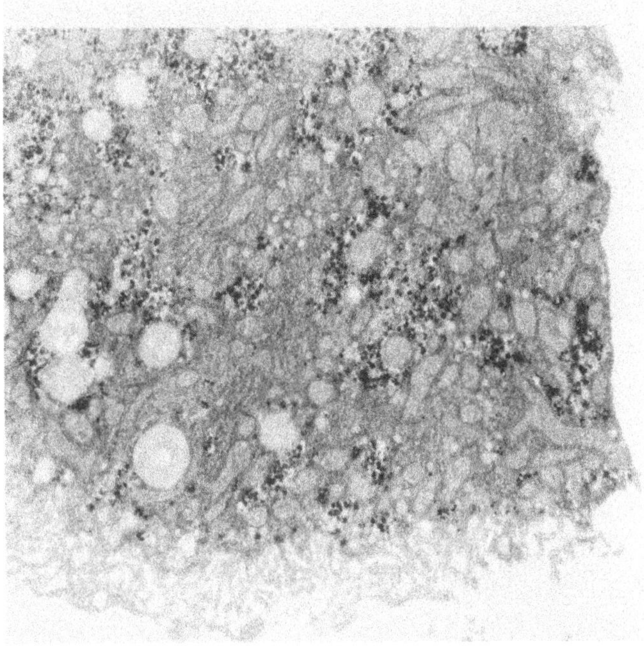

Fig. 5. Electron micrograph of a portion of a parenchymal cell from a suspension of glutaraldehyde-fixed mouse liver cells (4500 ×).

acetate may be converted to fatty acids at about as rapid a rate in fixed as in unfixed liver slices, but that a marked inhibition of glyceride synthesis from glycerol results from perfusion of mouse liver with glutaraldehyde. Under fixation conditions other than those given in Table I, we have found considerable inhibition of glycerol oxidation to CO_2, the cause of which is as yet undetermined.

Several properties of our liver cell preparation make it potentially useful for a variety of studies. First of all, the yield of well-preserved cells is almost quantitative, and the method of preparation is rapid. Separation is still incomplete, but if it can be improved, we may be able to isolate the different cell types and study metabolism separately in liver parenchymal and reticuloendothelial cells.

Second, we have observed that slices of fixed liver release much less acid-precipitable material (protein?) after incubation at 37° than unfixed liver. This property, coupled with that of possibly increased permeability to small molecules resulting from fixation, could make suspensions of fixed cells particularly useful for a variety of histochemical studies. Dispersion of fixed tissue into cell suspensions is a rapid means for obtaining material suitable for cytochemical studies without the complications of structural bar-

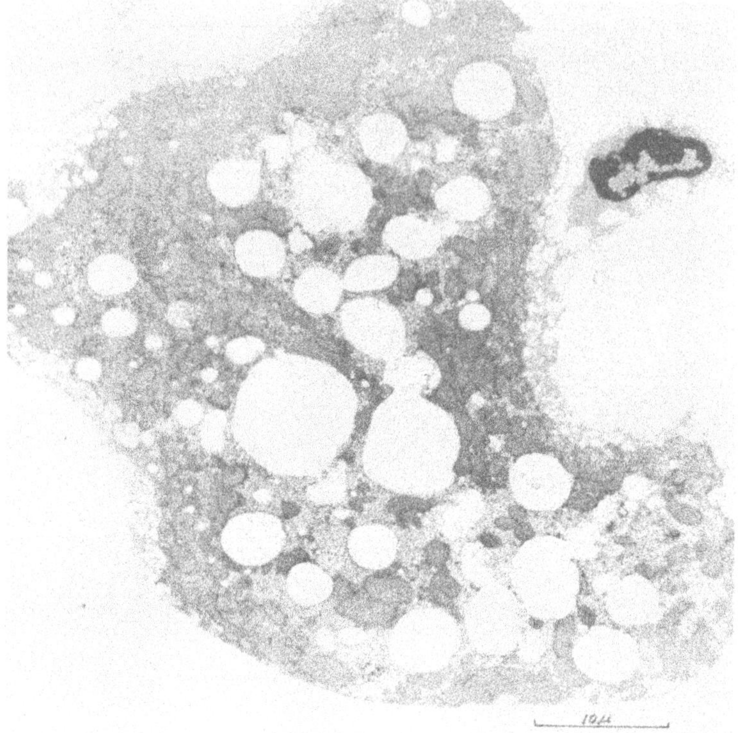

Fig. 6. Electron micrograph of a parenchymal cell and partially dissociated RE cell from a suspension of glutaraldehyde-fixed mouse liver cells. The mouse had been fasted overnight to deplete liver of glycogen and then injected with glycerol (see text). Note large fat droplets (induced by fasting) and the densely packed areas of newly synthesized glycogen in the parenchymal cell.

riers to uniform movement of substrates or enzymes, ordinarily encountered with tissue slices.

Moreover, the preparation described here may serve as a unique means for investigating the nature of materials which are adsorbed to the exterior of both hepatocytes and Kupfer cell plasma membranes. The treatment with glutaraldehyde results in the cells' being able to withstand forces which ordinarily result in the release of intracellular material from the interior of unfixed cells. It seems feasible now, perhaps for the first time, to attempt to scrape off the material which adheres to the outside of the cells by using forces which could never be employed with cells that have not been stabilized.

In conclusion, we have described a rapid method of preparing liver cell suspensions from mouse livers that have been perfused briefly with glutaraldehyde dissolved in a phosphate buffer. Although the liver from which the

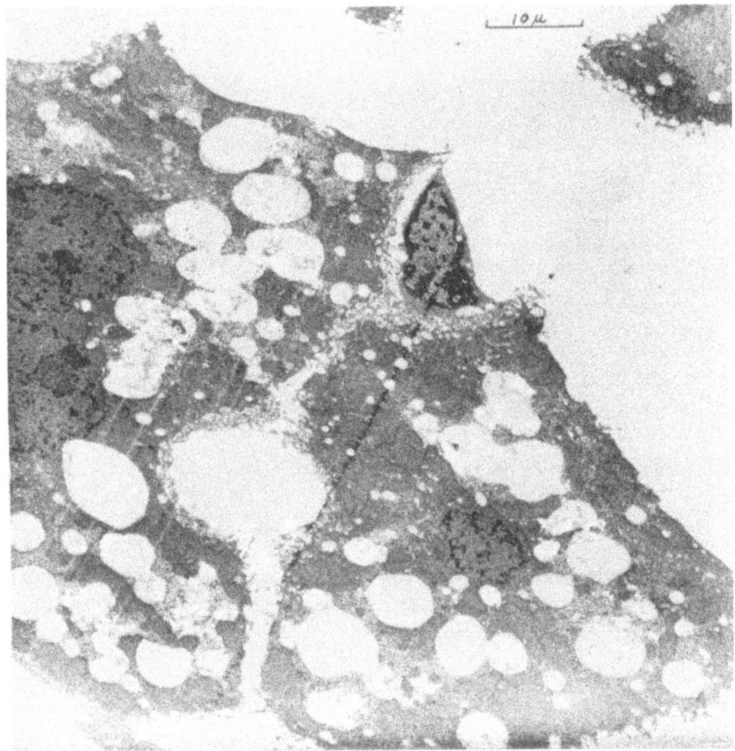

Fig. 7. Electron micrograph showing incompletely separated group of parenchymal cells and an RE cell. Mouse treated as in Fig. 6. Diagonal lines are artifacts.

cell suspension can be derived is hard and leathery, it still retains the capacity to oxidize tracer acetate-2-C^{14} and glycerol-1, 3-C^{14} to $C^{14}O_2$ and to convert acetate-2-C^{14} to fatty acids, based upon studies using liver slices. Fixed liver is highly resistant to cell breakage. When subjected to forces which ordinarily cause unfixed liver to be reduced to homogenates of subcellular particles, the glutaraldehyde-perfused liver separates into a suspension of single, double, and small groups of cells, most of which appear to be remarkably well preserved. Several potential uses of the fixed-cell suspensions in the study of liver biochemistry, cytochemistry, and physiology have been indicated. Among them, the most important, we feel, may be in the study of materials adsorbed to plasma membranes. Further studies are required to determine whether complete separation of reticuloendothelial cells from parenchymal cells can be accomplished. If so, can the high level of enzymatic activity found in our preliminary studies of fixed liver slices be maintained in the suspension of cells?

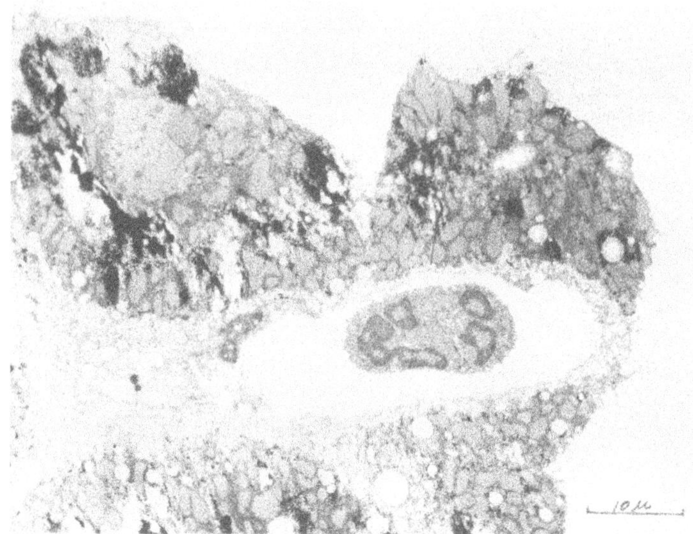

Fig. 8. Electron micrograph of fixed-liver cell suspension showing a clump of liver cells surrounding a blood cell. The heavily stained areas in the parenchymal cells are rich in glycogen.

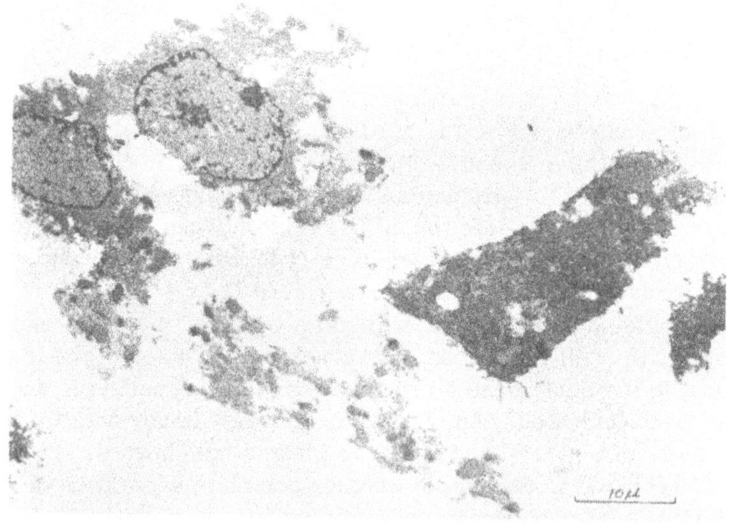

Fig. 9. Electron micrograph showing both a broken cell and an intact parenchymal cell from a suspension of glutaraldehyde-fixed mouse liver cells.

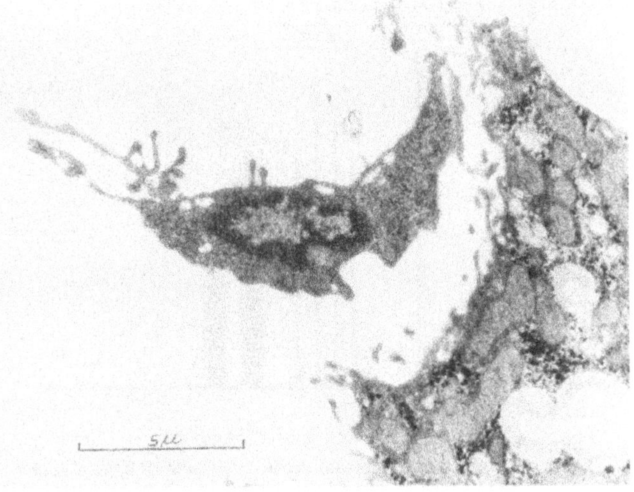

Fig. 10. Electron micrograph of an RE cell loosely associated with a parenchymal cell from a suspension of glutaraldehyde-fixed mouse liver.

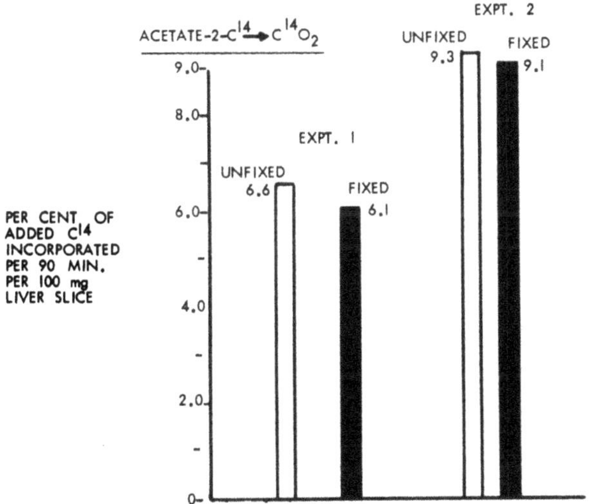

Fig. 11. Incorporation of acetate-C^{14} into CO_2 by liver slices prepared from glutaraldehyde-fixed and unfixed mouse livers. Unfixed livers were perfused with glutaraldehyde-free buffer. Each bar represents a single mouse (duplicate incubations averaged). Incubations were in Krebs phosphate buffer, pH 7.4, containing 10^5 cpm tracer acetate-2-C^{14}; gas phase, air.

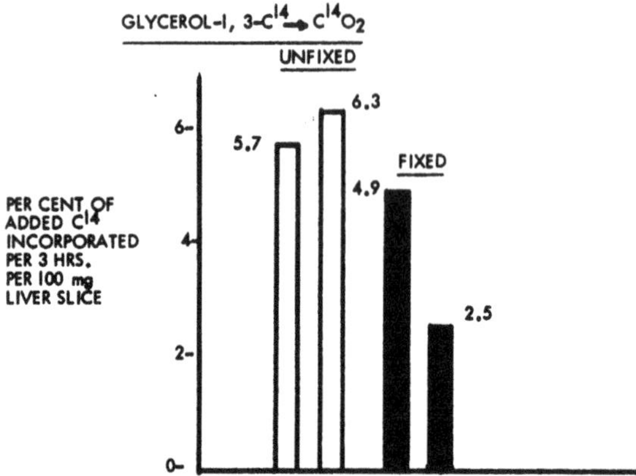

Fig. 12. Incorporation of glycerol-C^{14} into CO_2 by liver slices prepared from glutaraldehyde-fixed and unfixed mouse livers. Unfixed livers were perfused with glutaraldehyde-free buffer. Each bar represents a separate mouse (other than those used for experiment shown in Fig. 11). Incubation conditions as in Fig. 11, except 10^6 cmp glycerol-1, 3-C^{14} used in place of acetate-2-C^{14}.

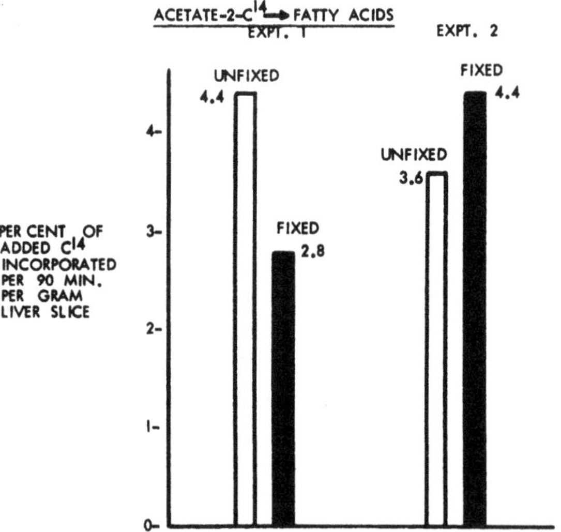

Fig. 13. Incorporation of acetate-C^{14} into total lipid fatty acids by liver slices prepared from glutaraldehyde-fixed and unfixed mouse livers. Same mice as in Fig. 11. See legend to that figure.

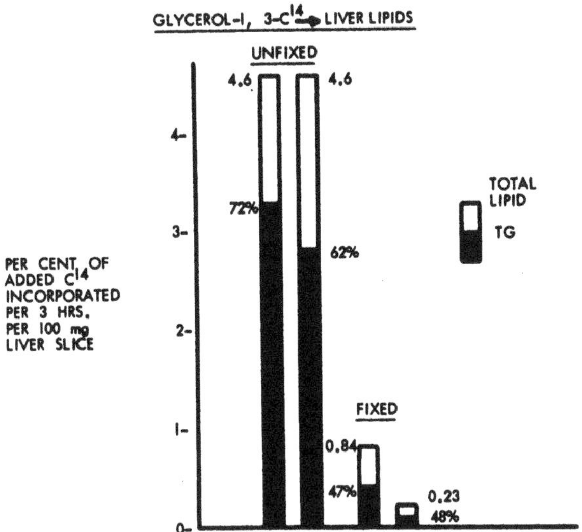

Fig. 14. Incorporation of glycerol-C^{14} into total lipid and triglyceride (TG) by liver slices prepared from glutaraldehyde-fixed and unfixed mouse livers. Same mice as in Fig. 12. See legend to that figure.

ACKNOWLEDGMENTS

Supported in part by NIH grants AM 4705 and AM 4706. We wish to thank Mrs. Monica Jacobson for her excellent technical assistance in the preparation of thin sections for electron microscopy.

REFERENCES

1. D.D. Sabatini, K. Bensch, and R.J. Barrnett, J.Cell Biol., 17:19, 1963; D.D. Sabatini, F. Miller, and R.J. Barrnett, J. Histochem. Cytochem., 12:57, 1964.
2. D.J. Morré, H.H. Mollenhauer, and J.E. Chambers, Exp.Cell Res., 38: 672, 1965.
3. D.T. Janigan, Lab.Invest., 13:1038, 1964; J.Histochem.Cytochem., 13:476, 1965.
4. M. Cohen, N. Baker, and M.C. Schotz, J. Ultrastruct.Res., 13:561, 1965.
5. V.M. Emmel and E.V. Cowdry, Laboratory Technique in Biology and Medicine. 4th Ed., Baltimore, Williams and Wilkins, 1964, p. 245.
6. A.E. Vatter and J. Zambernard, Proc. San Francisco Mtg. Electron Microscopy Soc.Am., 1966.
7. F.H. Shipkey and A.J. Dalton, J.Appl.Phys., 30:2039, 1959.
8. E.S. Reynolds, J.Cell Biol., 17:208, 1963.

The Function of the Reticuloendothelial System Studied with Isolated Perfused Rat Livers

H. Schimassek and J. Helms

Physiological Chemistry Institute
University of Marburg
Marburg, Germany

Among the biological cell systems of higher organisms, the reticuloendothelial system (RES) offers an unequalled scope for research, and to study its function is as interesting from the point of view of electron microscopy, biochemistry, or physical chemistry as it is from that of bacteriology, immunology, and genetics. It is a study which, more than any other, is predestined for good team work and for a team comprising numerous specialists. The complex functions of this cell formation and its importance for the complete organism also require the most versatile and accurate methods of investigation to be employed. In essence, the question of the function of the RES is one of metabolism.

In the following, we shall discuss the RES with respect to one organ only, i.e., the liver, although to study the cell system itself separately is impossible in any one organ. The RE cells form a very close functional unit with the parenchymal cells of the liver. This functional correlation is already pointed out clearly by Jaffe and Berman in 1928 [1] in a study on the uptake of fat by the liver. They write that "from the histologic picture it is also evident that the function of the Küpffer cells cannot be separated from that of the liver. Both cells are a functional unit." Today, with a good basic knowledge in biochemistry, it is impossible to ignore this fact. As mentioned before, the RES function is also a question of metabolism, and the best method to be employed in the study of the liver metabolism is doubtless that of liver perfusion. The time allotted to my presentation is not very long but it will suffice to substantiate this claim, to demonstrate to you the good functional state of an isolated perfused liver, and also to show you the great many possibilities that this technique offers for RES studies.

The method of liver perfusion is easy to handle, but as it is absolutely essential to apply it with great care and accuracy, it is a time-consuming process.

One might ask if the advantages of this technique compensate for the time spent on the experiment. But bear in mind that the main object of any in vitro experiment is to simplify experimental conditions as much as possible. In the biological field, we frequently have to work under unfavorable experimental conditions, measuring systems the type, extent, and network of which are but vaguely known. To cite an example, it is impossible to measure in vivo the metabolism of an individual organ, or the effects of a particular drug or substance. What we measure in this case is the reflection of a given effect by the entire organism, the sum of interference and cross regulation by hormones or substrates of the body. In our particular study, which investigates the liver RES, the otherwise common in vitro methods employing homogenates or liver slices are not satisfactory. We have stressed earlier that the RE cells and the parenchymal cells of the liver form a functional unit, and it is important for experiments to maintain this unit. The RE cells are an essential part of the blood sinusoids in the liver [2, 3]. In order to study their function it is necessary to preserve the structure of the sinusoids and the physiological pathways for the transport of metabolites and other substances. It will not be difficult to demonstrate that these prerequisites are given in the technique of liver perfusion, and that this technique in many respects combines the advantages of in vivo and in vitro experiments.

Basically, the technique is well known from the papers of Miller [4] and Schimassek [5]. To help you understand the following more readily, a few data on our method will suffice: the technique in question is that of recirculation in a closed circulatory system. Influx of blood into the liver goes via the portal vein, output by the hepatic vein via the vena cava superior. Bile is also collected from the bile duct. The blood pressure is adjusted hydrostatically according to the portal pressure of about 18 cm of water. As perfusion medium many investigators use pooled blood of donor animals which they dilute to a greater or lesser degree with saline solutions. This blood contains a great number of metabolically active but mostly unknown constituents. As was pointed out before, however, the purpose of isolating a system is to achieve accurate and consistent experimental conditions. Thus, we prefer to use a semisynthetic perfusion medium consisting of a saline solution which contains highly purified albumin and in which red cells are suspended [5]. To test the function of the liver we have used highly sensitive functional criteria, as the criteria commonly used, viz., examination of the histologic picture and of bile production, give incomplete results. Experimental and clinical studies have shown that the slightest damage incurred by the cell, even before it becomes visible under an electron microscope, leads to a loss of enzymes. We have therefore tested enzyme activities before and after perfusion and also in the perfusion medium, and have established that the enzyme pattern and enzyme activities do not change in the isolated organ during perfusion [5]. This means that the isolated organ retains its full metabolic capacity in vitro. Beyond that we have, at various stages of the

Table I. Comparison of the Metabolic State of Isolated Perfused Rat Liver with the In Vivo State

Ratios of substrate couples	In vivo (Hohorst)	In vitro after perfusion for		
		0 min	30 min	180 min
Lactate / Pyruvate	10	239	13	10.5
Glycerol-1-P / Dihydroxyacetone-P	6.7	72	6.7	7.0
ATP / ADP	3.3	0.4	3.3	3.8
Σ adeninenucleotides (mμ moles/gm wet weight)	4200	–	3160	3690

Table II. Comparison of the Lactate/ Pyruvate Ratio in the Perfused Rat Liver and in the Outer Medium under Different Experimental Conditions

Experiment	Lactate/pyruvate ratio	
	Liver	Perfusion medium
Control	10	10
Hypoxia	24	26
Glucagon	7	6
Prednisolone	17	18
Hypothyreosis	16	17

experiment, measured the contents of major substrates of the energy metabolism in the liver, and have compared them with in vivo findings [5]. Some details of this are shown in Table I. The period of anoxia during the operation causes an extremely reduced metabolic state in the liver, but in spite of this the substrate and energy ratios revert back to in vivo values after less than 30 min perfusion and remain constant for 3-4 hr perfusion [5].

A particular point of interest in the study of the RES is, for various reasons, the uptake or exchange of substances and drugs by the organ. In the isolated liver, we shall study exchange capacities with regard to important blood substrates, especially those which appear inside and outside the cell membrane. At present, the special points of passage and the process of exchange of these blood substrates are unknown.

For this purpose we have measured the levels of lactate, pyruvate, and glucose in the liver and in the perfusion medium. Immediately as perfusion begins, the isolated organ releases all three substrates into the perfusion medium. For lactate and pyruvate, it establishes physiological levels corresponding to those in rat blood. We know from experiments with ^{14}C-labeled lactate [6] that the liver takes up lactate continuously from the outer medium and, as it is adjusting levels, releases it again in respective quantities. The extent and direction of this continuous substrate exchange depends on the metabolic state of the isolated organ [7]. Our investigations brought another important fact to light: in the isolated system, the levels of lactate and pyruvate, and thus also the ratio of lactate to pyruvate, were the same in the liver as in the perfusion medium under any experimental conditions [7]. Lactate and pyruvate are partners of an important NAD/NADH-dependent system in liver metabolism [8]. So the agreement in the ratios lactate/pyruvate inside and outside the cell is of interest in many aspects, and also with regard to the study of the RES. Drugs and substances used to investigate the function of the RE cells can affect the metabolism of the entire organ. Stuart and Cooper [9] pointed out that many agents used to modify phagocytic function may be relatively nonspecific, but the concentrations used are very high and toxic. Under these circumstances there is some uncertainty whether death of the animals results from phagocytic depressions and resulting inability to remove endotoxin or to some other unrelated factors. And we can add that many of the investigators did not measure metabolic or functional parameters in these experiments. In liver perfusions repeated measurements of the contents of lactate and pyruvate in the outer medium are simple, reliable, and almost constant indicators of the changes that take place in the system in the isolated organ. In most cases this system will also change when the energy state of the isolated organ is affected.

It is interesting in some cases to compare the performance of the RE cells in a hypoxic or almost anoxic state. The perfusion technique makes it possible to induce a defined hypoxic state in the isolated organ by changing the blood flow through the liver. As hypoxia is linked by changes in the lactate/pyruvate ratio, we can ascertain the extent of this hypoxia and observe the degree of variation in the metabolic state by measuring lactate and pyruvate in the perfusion medium [5]. The autonomous regulation of these two substrates, lactate and pyruvate, which, by a single enzyme step, can be converted into one another, seems quite simple and easy to understand, although the phenomenon of the regulation of levels alone gives rise to a great many interesting problems. However, the fact that during 30-60 min perfusion the rat liver releases into the outer medium the entire range of free amino acids, and in the same order of magnitude as in the rat plasma, is probably even more remarkable. Under standard conditions, our perfusion medium contains no free amino acids. The only substrates added to the medium are lactate, pyruvate, and glucose. Then, after only 30 min of perfusion, all detectable free amino acids in rat plasma, including the so-called essential acids, are present in the outer medium. The isolated organ itself loses no free amino acids in the process [10]. Yet the regulation

Table III. Effect of Changes of the Hormonal State In Vivo on the Metabolic State of the Isolated Rat Liver Perfused In Vitro

	Control (untreated)	Pretreatment	
		hyperthyreosis (by inj. of TJT)	hypothyreosis (by thyroidectomy)
Oxygen consumption (μmoles/g/min)	2.2	4 (+80%)	1.9 (–15%)
Glycogen (μmoles/g)	185	2.6	160
ATP/ADP	3.3	2.3	3.3

Table IV. Influence of Hormones on the Uptake of L-Lactate by the Isolated Perfused Rat Liver

Experiment	L-lactate uptake (μmoles/gm liver/h)	Remarks
Control	20	Untreated rats, hormones
Glucagon	60	added into perfusion
Epinephrine	50	medium
Prednisolone	5	
Hypothyreosis	3	Pretreated rats
Hyperthyreosis	60	

of substrate levels by isolated livers is not a generally applicable fact. The isolated organ produces consistent substrate levels only as far as it is responsible for the steady state of blood substrates. It releases, for example, too much glucose into the medium and, on the other hand, takes up free fatty acids from it very rapidly.

The RES is controlled, or at least influenced, by hormones. Thus, RE cells can be activated by estradiol [11, 12] and, conversely, they participate in the control of the blood levels of corticosteroids [13, 14].

Therefore, let us consider how the isolated organ reacts to hormones. Our first question is: Which is the hormonal state that we measure in vitro? By means of thyroidectomy or a single injection of triiodothyronin we have produced a hypo- or hyperthyroid state in vivo. Table III contains the essential data to demonstrate that the metabolic state measured in vitro corresponds exactly to the one achieved by the pretreatment in vivo. The oxygen consumption in the isolated liver of a hyperthyroid animal is, for instance, increased by 80%, whereas it is reduced by 15% in the isolated livers of hypothyroid animals, and the list of differences in the content of metabolites could easily be extended [15]. This means that in vitro we actually measure the same hormonal state as in vivo. The liver also remains susceptible to the direct effects of hormones, as can be seen in Table IV, which summarizes data of the uptake of lactate by perfused livers under differing hormonal conditions. Glucagon, for example, causes an increase in the lactate uptake as well as epinephrine, whereas hormones of the adrenal cortex cause it to decrease. The effect of a hyperthyroid influence on the lactate metabolism is in inverse relation to that of a hypothyroid influence.

So far we have concentrated on investigating the function of the cell system as a whole. For a number of experiments, however, it is important to study in more detail the subcellular particles of different isolated cells. The possibility for further and more detailed investigations following perfusion must therefore be examined, and, together with Dr. Klingenberg, we have, to this end, isolated mitochondria from the liver after 3 hr perfusion. The mitochondria thus obtained show the normal P/O ratio of 3 (for hydroxybutyrate as substrate) and, as a more sensitive criterion, they also retain respiratory control [5].

The perfusion technique is undoubtedly the best in vitro method of investigating metabolic problems. At present, our data are the only data available to characterize the metabolic state of an isolated organ on a comparably large scale. Anyone interested in liver metabolism can use our findings as a basis for his particular studies. It is, however, essential to apply this perfusion technique with care and precision in experiments which are to characterize complex metabolic and functional phenomena. It is further of importance to check the function of the isolated organ and to characterize its metabolic state under the given experimental conditions (and these conditions may differ for individual scientific problems). Without some of the above-mentioned basic data it is impossible to compare and to discuss effects on the perfused system with other authors. Liver perfusions which are conducted without regard for the essential basic requirements may be likened to measurements of a well-defined substance in a spectrophotometer adjusted to the wrong wavelength.

Filkins and Smith [16] investigated the carbon phagocytosis in isolated perfused rat livers. For a period of 3 hr they perfused first one, and later, in the same medium, another rat liver. As perfusion medium they employed rat blood. They established that the half-time of carbon clearance was considerably prolonged in the liver perfused last. An equally prolonged half-time value was produced in experiments in which they used our semisynthetic perfusion medium. They suggested, on the basis of these experiments, the existence of an exhaustible plasma factor operative in Kupffer cell phagocytosis of colloidal carbon gel. In a second paper [17], published in the same year, they enlarged on their earlier findings in two respects. They had found that the gelatin used to stabilize the carbon suspension brought about a considerable prolongation of carbon phagocytosis. Many investigators have demonstrated the difficulties in experiments with unspecific particles by the manifold interactions of plasma constituents or the pre-

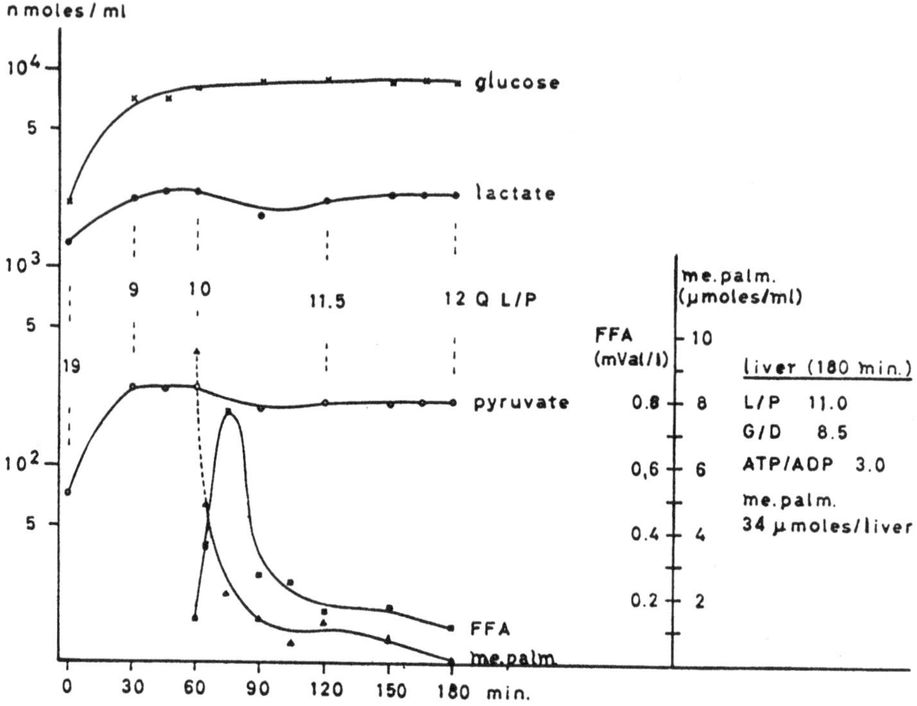

Fig. 1. Influence of methyl palmitate (me. palm) on the substrate levels in the perfusion medium and (after 3 h perfusion) in the liver.

treatment of particles [18-20]. The second addition referred to the perfusion medium employed. Pooled rat blood contains a great quantity of heparin to prevent blood clotting. Heparin has long been known to activate RE cells in vivo [21,22]. If one replaces a part of the semisynthetic medium with heparin-plasma, the half-time of carbon clearance is as short as that found in experiments with pooled rat blood when used for the first time. It is more advisable to use a perfusion medium of known constituents and calculate to suit particular requirements.

I feel that we have passed the stage of counting carbon particles, and that more satisfactory results can be obtained by the use of biological radioactive labeled material or particles [23-29]. This should facilitate the observations of special metabolic pathways of the RE cell. Bonventre and Oxman [30] have used isolated perfused livers to investigate the kinetics of the phagocytosis and also the rate of survival of *Staphylococcus aureus* and *Salmonella enteritides* in the RE cells under differing immunologic conditions. They perfused livers from immunized or nonimmunized rats with plasma from immunized or nonimmunized rabbits. They found that the immunologic status of the animals was without effect on the phagocytosis and intracellular disposition of S. aureus but S. enteritides was found to be quite sensitive to either humoral or cellular immune factors. Immune serum enhanced markedly both the rate and extent of phagocytosis. But the recovery of viable organisms was the smallest in a complete immune system, which means immune serum and immune rat livers. We missed some further special indications of these experiments and cannot enlarge on these findings. But, the data may indicate the possibility also of studying immunologic problems and phenomena with the perfusion technique.

^{14}C-labeled chylomicrons are an interesting example for the study of the absorption of radioactive labeled biological particles by the liver. The investigation of the uptake and the way of entrance of these particles and their further degradation is an excellent program for liver perfusions, studied at first by Morris or Chaikoff et al. [31, 32]. Edgren and Zilversmit reported further data using $^{14}C/^{32}P$ phospholipid labeled chylomicrons [33]. They compared the uptake of the doubled labeled particles by the liver with two in vitro techniques: liver slices and perfused livers. They reported, moreover, that in liver slices as well as in perfusion experiments the uptake of chylomicrons is not inhibited by cyanide. Measuring the ratio of the radioactivity of $^{32}P/^{14}C$, they brought the best evidence that the chylomicrons are taken up by the liver as a unit. But the uptake of the chylomicrons without changes in the ratio $^{32}P/^{14}C$ was found only in perfusion experiments. The authors pointed out there is some doubt of the validity of experiments with tissue slices for the study of chylomicron transport into the liver.

In our laboratory we have concentrated, in the study of the RES, mainly on the field of the biological transformation of drugs and substances. Particular attention has been paid to simple fatty esters such as methyl palmitate [34, 35]. As is known and described in detail [36], methyl palmitate reduces the phagocytic and immunologic activity of the RE cells. Di Luzio and coworkers investigated [37] further the metabolism of different ^{14}C-labeled methyl palmitate, labeled in the methyl group or in the fatty acid portion. They found that the methyl palmitate rapidly disappears from the blood stream, and that the C14 of the methyl group and of the fatty acids could be measured as labeled carbon dioxide shortly afterwards, which means that the ester linkage was split very rapidly.

We have studied the effects and the metabolism of methyl palmitate in various experiments. We are starting with these investigations and I can exhibit only preliminary notes.

By sonification, a microsuspension of methyl palmitate was prepared in a physiological salt solution containing purified albumin. We took albumin instead of Tween as we know from other experiments that surface-active substances disturb the in vitro metabolism of the liver. The concentration of methyl palmitate in the perfusion fluid or in the perfused organ was measured by gas chromatography. First we measured the distribution of methyl

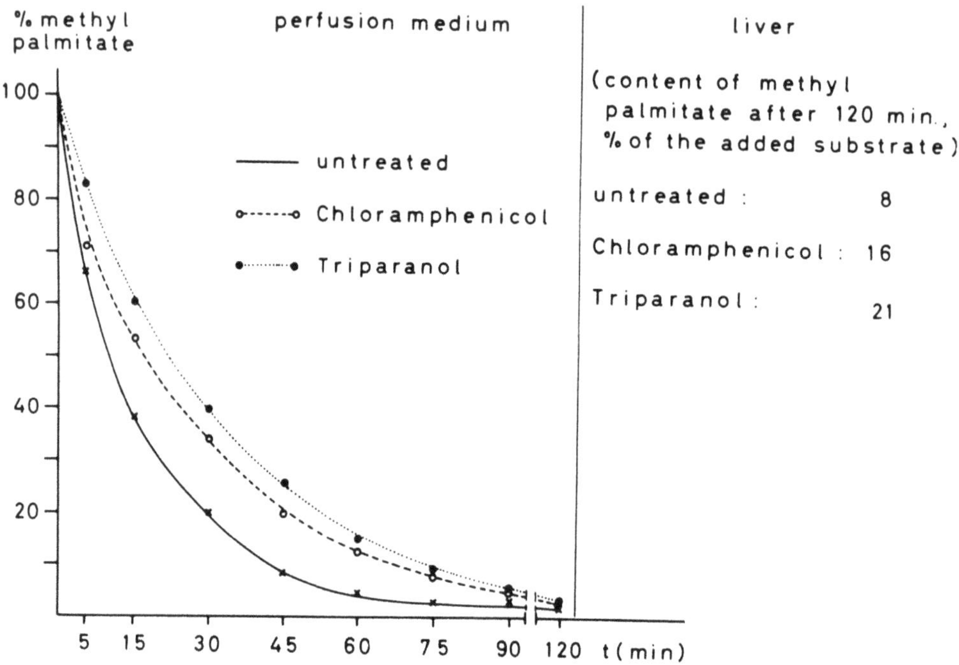

Fig. 2. Effect of chloramphenicol and triparanol on the uptake and metabolism of methyl palmitate by isolated perfused rat livers (standard conditions).

palmitate suspension in the complete perfusion system excluding the liver. In previous investigations, no splitting of the ester linkage had occurred in the perfusion plasma or in the red cells of the medium. After short circulation of the medium in the perfusion system, we found a decrease in the concentration of methyl palmitate. This decrease amounted to about 10%. It is likely that part of the microsuspension is absorbed by the large surface area of the tubes and glass containers of the circulation system. In perfusion experiments with livers of untreated rats, the disappearance of methyl palmitate from the perfusion medium is very rapid (Fig. 1). With the decrease of methyl palmitate in the perfusion medium we measured a simultaneous increase in the levels of free fatty acids in the medium which were taken up by the liver at a normal metabolic rate. It seems very significant to us that the disappearance of methyl palmitate is accompanied by a rise in the levels of free fatty acids outside the cell. It is possible that the splitting process of the ester linkage is localized in the membrane of the cell itself or in its immediate vicinity. This question of reciprocal levels of methyl palmitate and fatty acids liberated from methyl palmitate also enters the observations made by DiLuzio and coworkers. They measured the disappearance of radioactive material from the blood, and it is likely that they measured both the disappearance of methyl palmitate and of the splitting products. Our next experiments were directed at influencing the metabolism of methyl palmitate. We chose two substances for this purpose, one of which, chloramphenicol, is reported to disturb protein synthesis [34-40], to inhibit the synthesis of antibodies [41, 42], and to diminish the biological transformation of drugs [43]. The other substance, Triparanol {1-[4(Diethylaminoethoxy)phenyl]-1-(p-toloyl)-2-(p-chlorophenylethanol)}, is known to disturb lipid metabolism. As can be seen in Fig. 2, both substances reduce the rate of disappearance of methyl palmitate from the perfusion medium. This could be of interest for further investigations on the effects and the metabolism of methyl palmitate with regard to the action of both drugs in different metabolic pathways.

Another use of the perfusion technique is to investigate the kinetics of blood clearance. As an example, consider the work of Gabrielli and Snell [44] as it is connected with our present subject. Gabrielli and Snell discuss many processes to be considered in the study of clearance kinetics. There is the injection of test substances with respect to their disappearance rate. There are many possibilities of interactions of test substances with blood constituents. Finally, there is their entrance into different compartments in the organs of the body. It is the purpose of these studies to describe the kinetics of the different processes by means of mathematical models. Perfusion experiments with isolated organs have special advantages for these mathematical analyses. In perfusion experiments, we also have some interactions with medium constituents and components, but, as pointed out earlier, as long as one knows the medium and the system one has constant and reproducible conditions and the sum of the components is much smaller than in vivo.

In summarizing, one might say that the technique of isolated perfused livers offers many advantages for studies concerning the function of the RE cells in the liver. The isolated perfused liver retains a metabolic state which is directly comparable with in vivo conditions. The isolated organ is maintained in a good functional state and one can expect to measure its metabolism adjusted in vivo by the hormonal state of the animal.

Differences between in vivo and in vitro measurements are not due to damage. They may indicate metabolic steps or interactions in which regulation takes place by hormone substrates or plasma constituents. We feel that this technique opens a wide field for further studies of the reticuloendothelial system.

ACKNOWLEDGMENTS

The authors thank Miss Jutta Feuerstein for her excellent assistance. This work was supported by the Deutsche Forschungsgemeinschaft.

REFERENCES

1. R.H. Jaffe and S. L. Berman, Arch. Pathol., 5:1020, 1928.
2. J.H. Heller, Reticuloendothelial Structure and Function, New York, Ronald Press, 1960.
3. Ch. Rouiller, The Liver, New York, Academic Press, 1963, p. 61.
4. L.L. Miller, C.G. Bly, M.L. Watson, and W.F. Bale, J. Exptl. Med., 94:431, 1951.
5. H. Schimassek, Life Sci., 1962; 629, 635; Biochem. Z., 336:460, 468, 1963.
6. H. Schimassek, Unpublished.
7. H. Schimassek, Ann. N. Y. Acad. Sci., 119:1013, 1965.
8. H.J. Hohorst, F.H. Kreutz, and Th. Bücher, Biochem. Z., 332:18, 1959.
9. A.E. Stuart and G.N. Cooper, J. Pathol. Bact., 83:227, 245, 1962.
10. H. Schimassek and W. Gerok, Biochem. Z., 343:407, 1965.
11. F.J. DiCarlo, B. Dubnick, L.J. Haynes, and G.E. Phillips, J. Reticuloendothelial Soc., 2:40, 1965.
12. T. Nicol and B. Vernon-Roberts, J. Reticuloendothelial Soc., 2:15, 351, 1956.
13. D.L. Berliner, Ch.J. Nabors, and Th.F. Dougherty, J. Reticuloendothelial Soc., 1:1, 1964.
14. J. Nabors, N.J. Mutungi, and D.L. Berliner, J. Reticuloendothelial Soc., 2:349, 1965.
15. H. Schimassek, H.J. Mitzkat, and J. Feuerstein, Biochem. Pharmacol., 15:129, 1966.
16. J.P. Filkins and J.J. Smith, Proc. Soc. Exptl. Biol. Med., 119:1181, 1965.
17. J.P. Filkins and J.J. Smith, J. Reticuloendothelial Soc., 2:287, 1965.
18. R.F. Kampschmidt et al., Proc. Soc. Exptl. Biol. Med., 108:216, 1961; J. Reticuloendothelial Soc., 2:256, 347, 1965.
19. E.R. Gabrielli, T. Pyzikiewicz, and P. Mlodozeniec, J. Reticuloendothelial Soc., 2:344, 1965.
20. S.J. Normann and E.P. Benditt, J. Reticuloendothelial Soc., 1:346, 1964.
21. R.G. Higginbotham and G.J. Murillo, J. Reticuloendothelial Soc., 2:352, 1965.
22. N. Panagiotis, G. Schneebeli, and Th.F. Dougherty, J. Reticuloendothelial Soc., 2:362, 1965.
23. A.R. Roberts and F. Haurowitz, J. Exptl. Med., 116:420, 1962.
24. Z.A. Cohn, J. Exptl. Med., 117:27, 43, 1963.
25. L. Chedid, C. Robert, and M. Parant, J. Exptl. Med., 117:561, 1963.
26. E. Rubin, J. Reticuloendothelial Soc., 1:345, 1964.
27. N.R. Di Luzio and S.J. Riggi, J. Reticuloendothelial Soc., 1:248, 1964.
28. St. Marcus and B.D. Thorpe, J. Reticuloendothelial Soc., 1:343, 1964.
29. R.S. Jones and I.R. Ward, J. Reticuloendothelial Soc., 1:352, 1964.

30. P. F. Bonventre and E. Oxman, J. Reticuloendothelial Soc., 2 : 313, 1965.
31. B. Morris and J. E. French, Quart. J. Exptl. Physiol., 43 : 180, 1958.
32. L.A. Hillyard, C.E. Cornelius, and I. L. Chaikoff, J. Biol. Chem., 234 : 2240, 1959.
33. B. Edgren and D.B. Zilversmit, Proc. Soc. Exptl. Biol. Med., 119 : 64, 1965.
34. A.E. Stuart et al., Brit. J. Exptl. Pathol., 41 : 599, 1960; 64 : 24, 1963.
35. W.R. Wooles and N.R. Di Luzio, Science, 142 : 1078, 1963.
36. D.A. Blickens and N.R. Di Luzio, J. Reticuloendothelial Soc., 2: 187, 1965.
37. D.A. Blickens and N.R. Di Luzio, J. Reticuloendothelial Soc., 2 : 60, 1965.
38. E.F. Gale and J.P. Folkes, Biochem. J., 53 : 493, 1953.
39. R. Schweet, J. Bishop, and A. Morris, Lab. Invest., 10 : 992, 1961.
40. A.I. Shihama, N. Mizuno, M. Takay, E. Otaka, and S. Osawa, J. Mol. Biol., 5 : 251, 1962.
41. Ch.T. Ambrose and A.H. Coons, J. Exptl. Med., 117 : 1075, 1963.
42. M.D. Schoenberg, this volume, p. 345.
43. W. Schmid, Sitzber. Ges. Befoerder. Ges. Naturw. Marburg, 1966. In press.
44. E.R. Gabrielli and F.M. Snell, J. Reticuloendothelial Soc., 2 : 141, 1965.
45. R.K. Fred and M.L. Shore, this volume, p. 1.

Reticuloendothelial Excretion Via the Bronchial Tree

T. Nicol and J. L. Cordingley

The Hambledon Department of Anatomy
King's College, University of London
London, England

The importance of the alveolar phagocytes in the defense of the lung against infection and in the removal of inhaled harmful substances from the bronchial tree is generally accepted. The origin of the alveolar phagocytes is, however, still a matter of controversy. It is stated that they may be derived from the cells of the alveolar septa, the epithelial lining of the alveoli, the liver and spleen, and the monocytes of the blood (Cappell [1], Bertalanffy [2]).

In the present research, after the administration of carbon intravenously and trypan blue subcutaneously, we examined the alveolar phagocytes of the same animal in the collapsed lung, the expanded lung, and in washings from the bronchial tree. For this purpose we devised an atraumatic method using the apparatus shown in Fig. 1.

MATERIALS AND METHODS

The lungs and trachea were first removed en bloc and placed in the apparatus. The pressure around the lungs in chamber A was then reduced to −20 cm H_2O by using the negative pressure pump and the lungs were thus made to expand and suck the saline from chamber B. The pressure in chamber A was then increased to +20 cm H_2O and the lungs were compressed and returned the saline to chamber B. This procedure of expansion and contraction was carried out six times for each specimen and the bronchial tree was thus washed out by the saline in chamber B. The saline washings were centrifuged and smears made for histological examination. Chamber B was then replaced by a vessel containing fixative and the lung made to expand again to suck in the fixative and thus become fixed in expansion. In order to examine the collapsed lung, a lobe was removed for fixation and

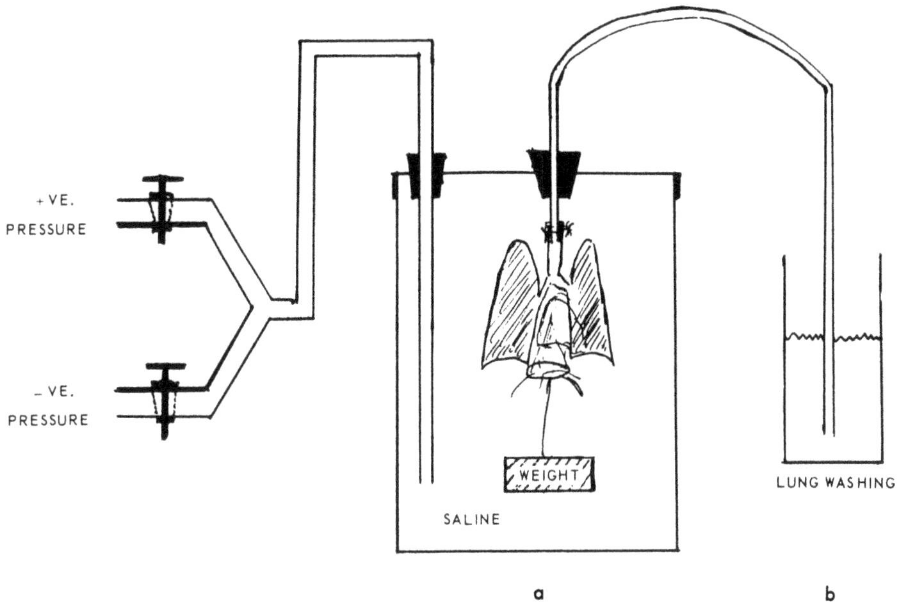

Fig. 1. Schematic representation of the atraumatic method for harvesting alveolar macrophages and subsequently fixing the lung in the fully expanded state.

the stump ligated before the commencement of the above procedure. Thus, in the same animal the collapsed and expanded lung and the washings of the bronchial tree could be examined.

One hundred and twelve male albino rats (Chester Beatty strain), aged about 6 weeks, were used for this research. Half the animals were given carbon intravenously; the other half received trypan blue subcutaneously. The carbon was obtained from Gunther–Wagner and had an average particle size of 250 Å. The dose of carbon was 8 mg/100 g body weight given into the dorsal vein of the penis in one injection. The method of preparation of the carbon is a modification of that of Biozzi et al. [3]. The dose of trypan blue was 0.8 ml 1% aqueous solution/100 g body weight given subcutaneously in one injection.

Two rats were killed daily for the first week, then weekly up to 12 weeks, and monthly up to one year. Paraffin sections of the lung were stained with H and E and eosin alone. The smears made from the centrifuged lung washings were air dried, fixed in alcohol–ether, and stained with hematoxylin and eosin and eosin alone. The slides were examined and a subjective estimate made of the amount of carbon or trypan blue present in the cells. The results are shown in Fig. 2.

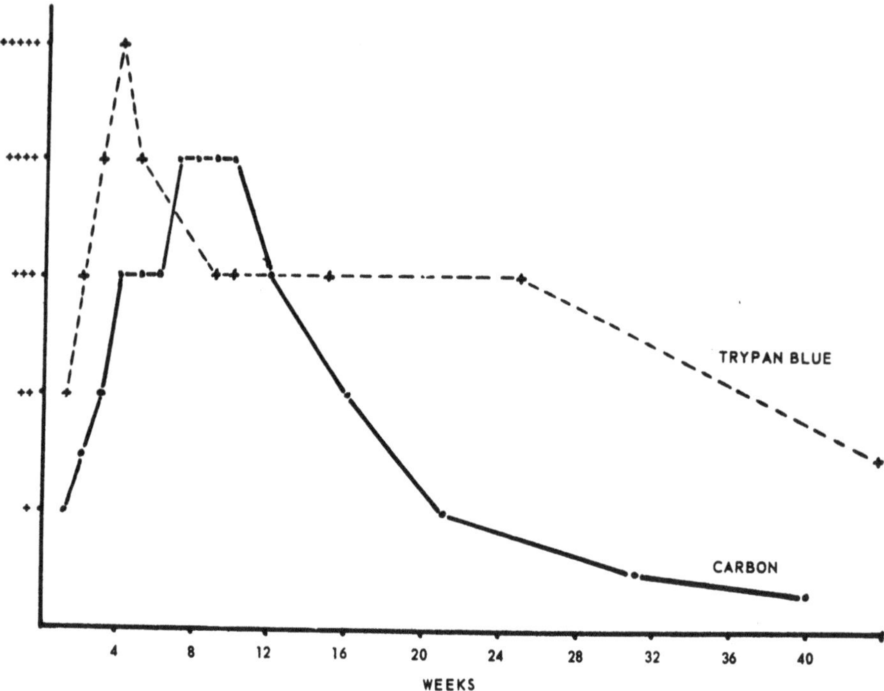

Fig. 2. Subjective estimation of the relative concentration of carbon and trypan blue present in the cells obtained from the lung washings.

RESULTS

Carbon-Treated Rats

In the present research, a few carbon-containing phagocytes were present in the lung washings during the first 10 days after the carbon injection. Thereafter, they increased in number and reached a peak about the third month, after which they became gradually reduced. The amount of carbon in the cells varied and some of the cells were degenerating, and thus free carbon was also present in the washings. A considerable number of free cells which did not contain carbon were also seen in the lung washings, and these appeared to be identical with the carbon-containing phagocytes.

Meanwhile, the carbon in the liver had become reduced in amount and that which remained in the sinusoids had become aggregated into larger masses. At nine months many of the Kupffer cells were completely free of carbon, whereas at the commencement of the experiment almost all these cells contained carbon. Similar changes were also seen in the spleen.

Trypan Blue-Treated Rats

It is well known that trypan blue given subcutaneously is taken up by the phagocytes of the body generally. During the first 10 days after injection of the dye the number of vitally stained cells in the lung washings gradually increased. Thereafter, there was a rise in the proportion of dye-containing cells until it reached a peak at the 4th week. This continued at a somewhat reduced level until the 24th week, and then the number became gradually reduced. One year after the injection of trypan blue, many dye-containing phagocytes were still present in the lung washings, although the dye had been completely cleared from the liver and spleen at the 10th week.

Histological examination showed that 2 days after the injection of dye the tissue histiocytes of the body generally were vitally stained, including those in the peribronchial tissue. The alveolar macrophages, however, were devoid of dye. At 10 days, vitally stained alveolar macrophages were much in evidence. In sections of the collapsed lung they appeared to be in the alveolar septa, but in the expanded lung of the same animal they had disappeared from the septa and were now seen free in the lumen of the alveoli. This suggests that these phagocytes were in fact lying between the folds of the alveolar wall and that they became free when the alveoli were expanded. It is interesting to note that at the time of maximum elimination of the phagocytes only a few cells of the trypan blue animals were free of dye. In the carbon-treated animals a considerable number of the cells were without carbon, but the others were heavily laden.

DISCUSSION

It is well known that carbon injected intravenously is taken up exclusively by the intravascular phagocytes chiefly of the liver and spleen, that about 90% of the carbon can be recovered from the liver and about 5% from the spleen, and that many of the carbon-containing phagocytes become mobilized into the circulation. The present results demonstrate that at least some of the alveolar phagocytes are derived from the liver and spleen. This was previously indicated by Irwin [4], who showed in rabbits that after the administration of Thorotrast there was a migration of Kupffer cells to the lungs; and by Nicol and Bilbey [5], who found carbon-containing phagocytes in the trachea of mice four days after intravenous administration of carbon.

When trypan blue is injected subcutaneously it becomes diffused throughout the tissues generally, and is taken up by the tissue phagocytes as an insoluble dye-protein complex. The trypan blue results indicate that the tissue macrophages also migrate to the lungs. This is supported by the fact that long after the liver and spleen have become clear of trypan blue, dye-containing cells are present in considerable numbers in the lung washings. Also, at the peak time of elimination of the dye, nearly all the cells in the washings contain dye, whereas in the carbon-treated animals at the corresponding time, a considerable proportion contain no carbon and are probably tissue phagocytes in the course of migration into the respiratory tract.

The results as a whole suggest that the bronchial tree is a normal excretory pathway for tissue phagocytes, and that in the collapsed lung they commonly lie between folds of the alveolar wall instead of within the alveolar septa. They become free when the alveolus expands, and thus both functionally and physically they are on the air side of the alveolar epithelium. The appearances suggest that these phagocytes are not formed locally in the alveolar septa and this aspect is now being examined further by electron microscopy.

The above results are of clinical interest since many of these phagocytes can carry substances such as carcinogens which could become applied to the wall of the bronchial tree after cellular disintegration. These findings point to a possible factor in the initiation of lung carcinoma.

REFERENCES

1. D.F. Cappell, "Intravital and supravital staining," J. Pathol. Bacteriol., 32:675, 1929.
2. F.D. Bertalanffy, "Respiratory tissue: structure, histophysiology, cytodynamics," in: G.H. Bourne and J.F. Danielli, Eds., International Review of Cytology, 1964.
3. G. Biozzi, B. Benacerraf, and B.N. Halpern, "Quantitative study of granulopectic activity of the reticuloendothelial system: study of kinetics of granulopectic activity of the reticuloendothelial system in relation to the dose of carbon injected," Brit. J. Exptl. Pathol., 34:441, 1953.
4. D. Irwin, "Kupffer cell migration," J. Can. Med. Assoc., 27:130, 1932.
5. T. Nicol and D.L.J. Bilbey, "Elimination of macrophage cells of the reticuloendothelial system by way of the bronchial tree," Nature, 182:192, 1958.

Kinetics of the Phagocytosis of Repeated Injections of Colloidal Carbon: Blockade, a Latent Period or Stimulation? A Question of Timing and Dose

Ernest L. Dobson, Lola S. Kelly,
and Caroline R. Finney

Donner Laboratory
University of California
Berkeley, California

ABSTRACT. The phenomenon of "blockade" has been attributed to the satiation of phagocytic cells, to the saturation of the phagocytic mechanism, or to the depletion of opsonins or other serum factors by excessive amounts of colloidal material. The experiments reported indicate that processes are involved which are not readily accounted for by any of these mechanisms. Development of "blockade" was shown by Parker and Finney to occur after a 3- to 4-hr latent period. Four repeated intravenous injections of 6 mg of colloidal carbon given at 2-hr intervals to 25-gm mice prolong this latent period and frequently result in an increased rate of clearance. If the time interval is shortened to 1 hr, and, in addition, the dose of carbon is increased to 12 mg per injection, an even greater increase in colloid removal is observed. This very marked effect, the antithesis of blockade, is evidenced by a rate of removal many times as great as the rate of removal of the first injection. This phenomenon obviously occurs too rapidly to be the result of cellular proliferation, Indeed, it seems too rapid to be the result of synthesis of new opsonins and serum factors. The possibility was envisaged that phagocytic stimulation by particulate injection might provoke the elaboration of new protein for cell membrane or adaptive enzyme synthesis. However, neither actinomycin D nor puromycin treatment had any effect on the stimulation resulting from repeated injections of colloid.

* * *

If a suspension of colloidal carbon is injected intravenously it is found to disappear from the blood in an approximately exponential manner (Fig. 1).

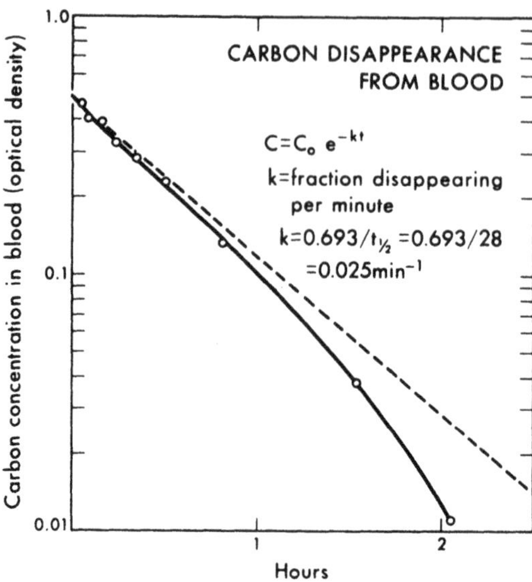

Fig. 1. Typical curve showing the apparent exponential disappearance of colloidal carbon from blood following the intravenous injection of 6 mg in a 25-gm mouse.

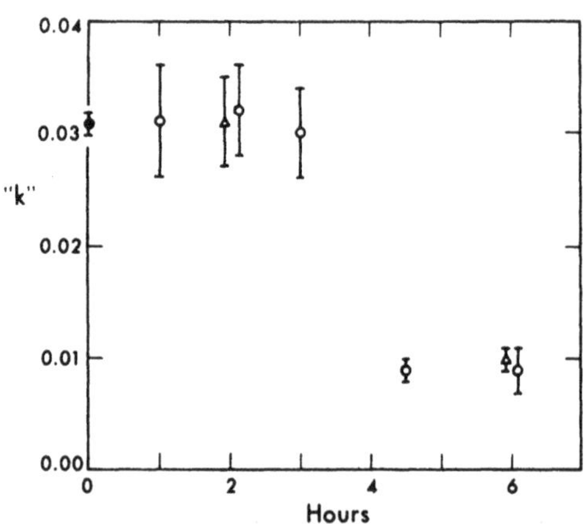

Fig. 2. Disappearance rate constant k of the 6-mg test, second injection, plotted against the time between first and second doses. ● Control, given no prior dose of carbon. ○ First dose, 12 mg carbon. △ First dose, 6 mg carbon. Limits indicated are 1 standard error. From Parker and Finney [11].

The concentration of carbon in the blood as a function of time closely follows the equation

$$C = C_0 e^{-kt}$$

for about 90% of the injected material. In this equation, k is the fraction of carbon present in the blood which is removed per unit time. Why the disappearance should be an exponential function is not clear. In the mouse, with a 6-mg dose of colloidal carbon, * we get a carbon clearance half-time of about 25 min and a chromic phosphate clearance half-time of $\frac{1}{2}$ min. From this, one can calculate that the phagocytes are removing only about 2% of the colloidal carbon as it passes through the liver. Under these circumstances one might expect the phagocytic mechanism to be saturated and operating at full capacity and hence at a constant rate.

Benacerraf and co-workers [1] have employed a related constant which they have called the phagocytic index K, † defined by the equation

$$C = C_0 10^{-Kt}$$

They have shown that the value of K is a function of the dose D of carbon injected. Their observation that KD is a constant indicates that regardless of dose the initial rate of carbon removal is constant. Such a relationship is not consistent with exponential clearance. The exponential function is a description of a process in which the rate of removal is proportional to the amount present. It therefore has a rate constant k which should be, theoretically at least, independent of concentration instead of inversely proportional to it. This contradiction between exponential clearance and a rate constant which is dependent on the injected dose has been explained by Benacerraf [2] as due to "...the opposite effects of two phenomena. The saturation effect of phagocytosed carbon, decreasing the efficiency of clearance throughout the experiment, is counterbalanced by the increased efficiency with which the Kupffer cells can extract particles from the circulation as the blood concentration decreases." Basically, this invokes the concept of a constant phagocytic rate which yields linear instead of exponential kinetics, and the concept of a gradually developing progressive blockade.

This concept of gradual satiation of phagocytic cells was made questionable by the observation of Parker and Finney [11], who reported that a second injection of carbon given 1-3 hr after the first did not show a slowing in the rate of clearance, and that "blockade" occurred only after a latent period of several hours. Parker and Finney show (Fig. 2) a number of measurements of the rate constant of a second injection made at different times after

---

*Gunther—Wagner, Hanover, Germany. Suspension No. C11/1431A, prepared as described by Parker and Finney [11].

† $K = k \frac{\log e}{\log 10} = 0.4343\,k.$

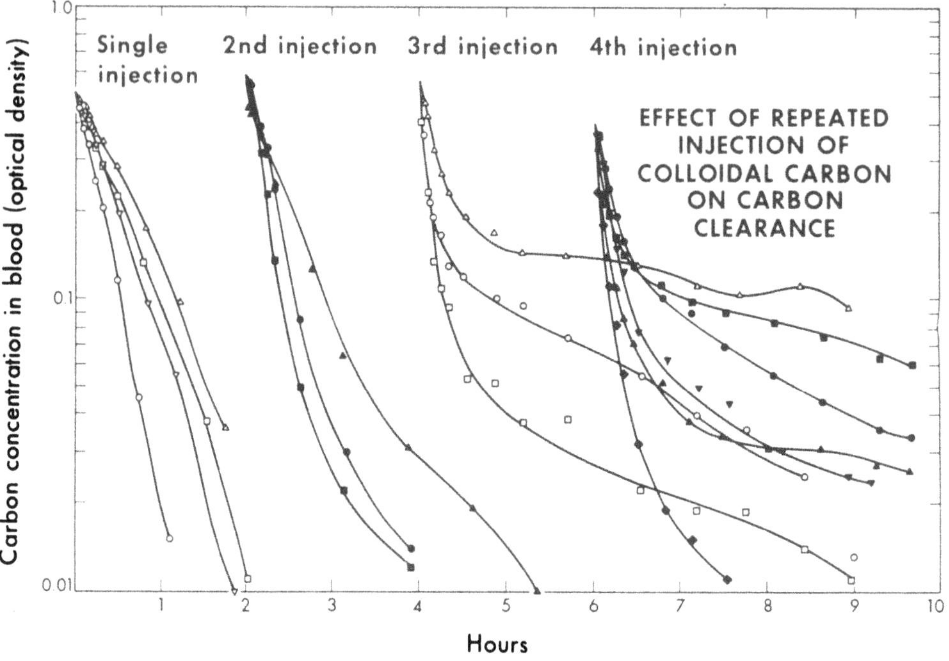

Fig. 3. Six-milligram injections of colloidal carbon were given at 2-hr intervals to mice.

a first injection of colloidal carbon. It can be seen that the so-called "blockading" dose of carbon produced no change in the rate of carbon disappearance until 4 ½ hr after it was given. This behavior did not fit the concept of simple satiation of the phagocytic cells.

Murray [6-8] and Jenkin and Rowley [4], and more recently Normann and Benditt [10], have suggested that blockade is produced by a mechanism in which the first dose depletes opsonins or serum factors in the blood. The second or test dose is then removed at a slower rate because the carbon cannot be opsonized. The evidence which has been presented for the existence of serum factors is very convincing. But, this mechanism for the induction of blockade, like the satiation of phagocytic cells, does not adequately explain the latent period observed by Parker and Finney, nor does it explain the observations we wish to present.

We have studied the kinetics of clearance of multiple injections of colloidal carbon in order to determine whether repeated injections given during the latent period would further prolong the induction of blockade. In our first experiments in this venture [3], we injected mice with 6 mg of carbon every 2 hr for 6 hr and measured disappearance curves at 2-hr intervals. In Fig. 3 the curves at 0 hr are from animals without previous injection, the curves at 2 hr are from animals with one previous injection, the curves at

4 hr are from animals with previous injections at zero time and at 2 hr, and the curves at 6 hr are from animals with three previous injections at 2-hr intervals. This last group, shown at the right, received a total of 24 mg of carbon.

There is an increase in the initial disappearance rate with each successive injection. This is the antithesis of the generally accepted concept of satiation. Though the mechanism of increased rate of disappearance from the blood is unknown, it seems more to be an increase in cell appetite. It is also in marked opposition to the theory of opsonin or plasma factor depletion.

There are other interesting features to these curves. Note that the single injection curves to the left have a tendency to bend down. With the repeated injections, the curves bend the other way and show an increasingly large tail. Yet, another injection is removed rapidly at the time this tail is still in evidence from previous injections. This strongly suggests that carbon exists in two distinct forms in these multiply-injected animals.

We thought for a time that the tail of the curve might be due to carbon in the leukocytes. This idea was strengthened by the observation that an increasing granulocytosis occurred after the injection of carbon. However, estimation of the amount of carbon in the leukocytes indicates that this is too low by two orders of magnitude to account for the tail portion of these curves. We are left, therefore, with evidence for the existence of two forms of circulating carbon but no clue to the nature of the difference between them. The fact that the fourth injection (Fig. 3) was cleared rapidly indicates that a depletion of opsonins was not responsible for the tail of the third injection.

Figure 4 illustrates the marked difference in the shape of the curves seen at 6 hr after multiple injections (the dark curves) and the shape of the curves at 6 hr after a single previous injection (the light curves). These light curves have a slope much less steep than either the single-injection curves or the multiple-injection curves. This slow initial disappearance is the phenomenon usually referred to as "blockade." Note the marked downward bend of these curves. This precipitous drop in carbon concentration 2-3 hr after injection in a "blockaded" mouse is shown in Fig. 5, which shows the behavior of carbon injection 18 $\frac{1}{2}$ hr after a "blockading" dose.

In the course of repeating these early experiments we have found that the behavior of multiple injections is variable. Figure 6 shows the repeated experiments superimposed on those of Fig. 3. Note that the increase in clearance rate with repeated injections is not always evident. In trying to discover the cause of the variability we found that by increasing the dose of carbon from 6 to 12 mg per mouse, and by shortening the time interval between injections, we were able not only to improve the reproducibility of the phenomenon, but were able to greatly magnify the effect.

Figure 7 shows the carbon concentration in the blood of a mouse that received three injections of 12 mg each at the times indicated. These repre-

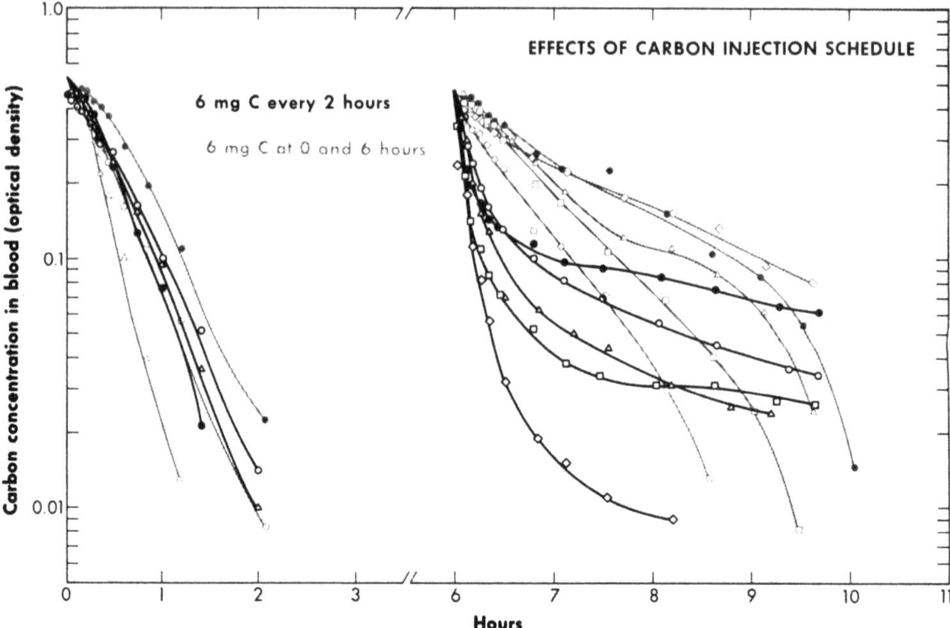

Fig. 4. The dark curves, reproduced from Fig. 3, represent the disappearance of carbon from mice injected every 2 hr. The lightly shaded curves represent the disappearance of carbon from mice injected at 0 and 6 hr only, and show typical "blockade." Note that the omission of two intervening injections has allowed "blockade" to develop.

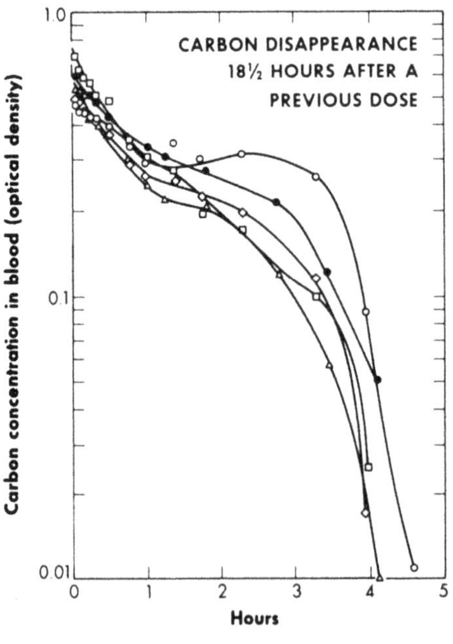

Fig. 5. The disapparance of carbon from the blood of a mouse which had a single previous 6-mg injection of colloidal carbon. When these curves are followed for several hours, a distinct downward bend is observed.

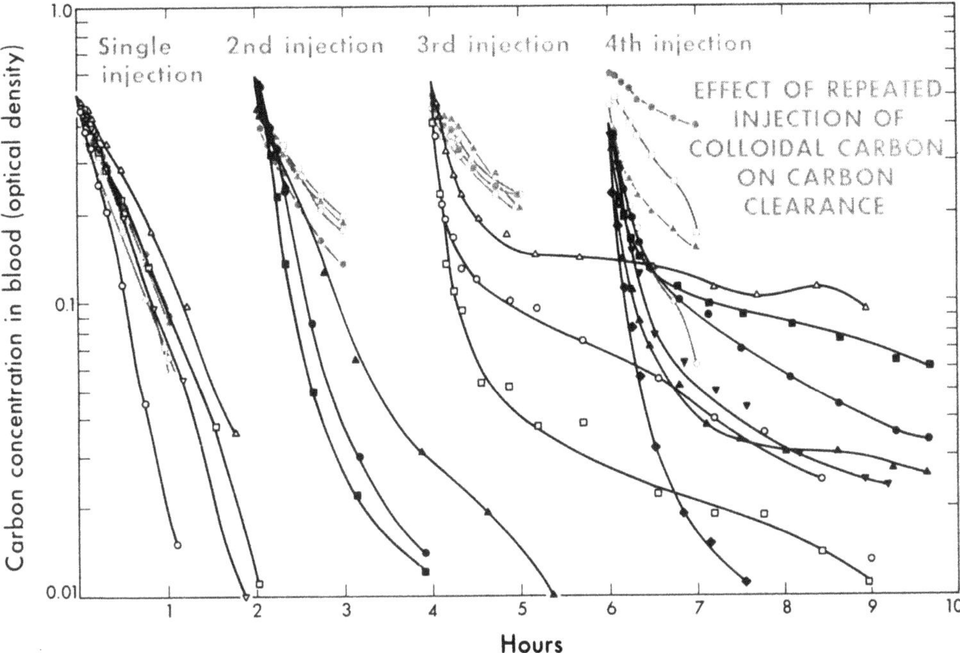

Fig.6. Some inconsistency is shown above in the comparison of two multiple injection experiments.

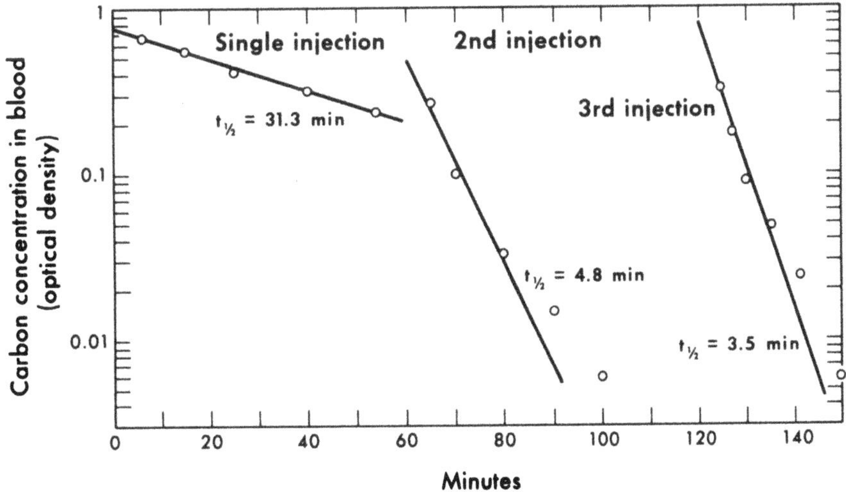

Fig. 7. This experiment was similar to that shown in Fig. 3, except that 12-mg doses of carbon were employed and were repeated every hour.

sent repeat measurements on the same mouse and it appears that the second injection, in addition to being removed faster, has caused the carbon remaining in the blood from the first injection to be cleared at a greater rate. This is typical of the response observed which showed average half-times of 34, 6.2, 3.6, and 5.2 min for the first, second, third, and fourth injections of 12 mg of carbon in a 25-gm mouse.

It must be noted that this represents a very large amount of carbon — 48 mg per mouse, or nearly 160 mg per 100 grams of body weight. We have found this to be toxic. The mice often show persistent tremors following the repeated injections, and many die before the later disappearance curves can be completed. What relation such treatment can have to normal phagocytic challenges is indeed questionable, but it is interesting that such a marked stimulation can be demonstrated at a time when one might expect blockade.

How general a phenomenon this is is not known. Normann and Benditt reported [9] a similar stimulation of carbon clearance by the prior injection of denatured albumin.

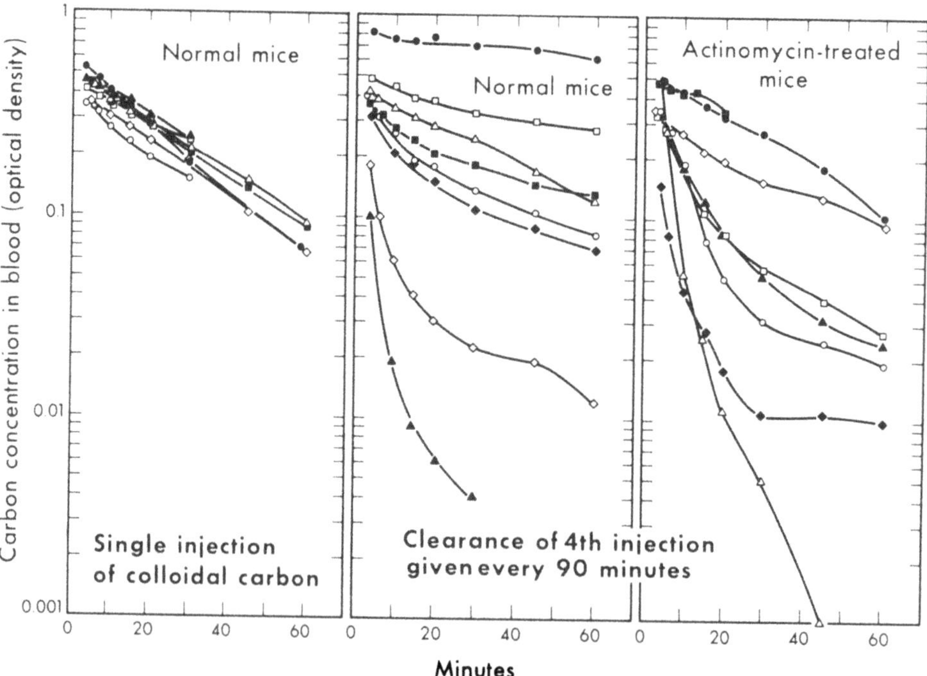

Fig. 8. Six milligrams of carbon was injected every 90 min. Accelerated clearance of the fourth injection was observed regardless of pretreatment with actinomycin D. 100 μg actinomycin D was injected subcutaneously ½ hr before the first carbon injection.

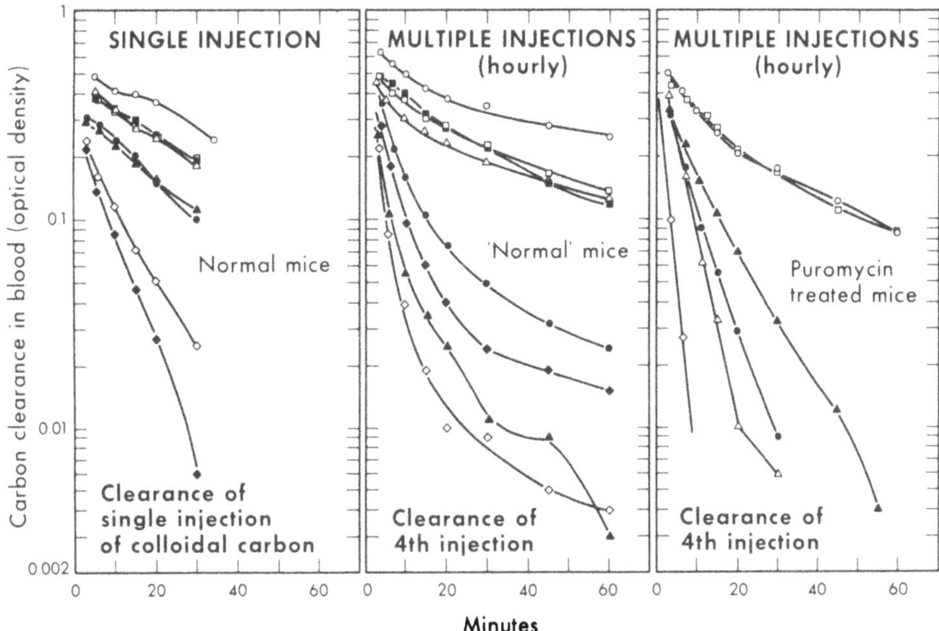

Fig. 9. Six milligrams of carbon were injected every hour. Accelerated clearance of the fourth injection was observed regardless of treatment with puromycin. One milligram puromycin was given i.p. hourly, beginning ½ hr before the first carbon injection.

We have repeatedly tried to reproduce the effect by the injection of the vehicle in which the carbon is suspended. These multiple injections of the vehicle have never produced any modification of the clearance rate. The vehicle was obtained by subjecting the carbon suspension to a centrifugal acceleration of 79,000 g. This produced a clear fluid, free of carbon. Such centrifugation would undoubtedly sediment any endotoxin present. Early stimulation with endotoxin has been reported by Arredondo and Kampschmidt [12].

This phenomenon obviously occurs too rapidly to be the result of cellular proliferation [5]. Indeed, it seems too rapid to be the result of synthesis of new opsonins and serum factors. The possibility was envisaged that phagocytic stimulation by particulate injection might provoke the elaboration of new protein for cell membrane or adaptive enzyme synthesis. Mice were treated with actinomycin D* or with puromycin. Actinomycin D, which interferes with messenger RNA synthesis, was given in doses sufficient to cause all mice to die in 24 hr. No interference with the activation was observed, as can be seen in Fig. 8.

*Actinomycin kindly supplied by Dr. Thomas F. Butler of Merck Sharp and Dohme, Rahway, New Jersey, U.S.A.

Similarly, puromycin, which interferes with protein synthesis at the ribosomal level, did not interfere with the acceleration of clearance produced by multiple injections of colloidal carbon. This lack of effect is shown in Fig. 9. The data of Figs. 8 and 9 were obtained with multiple injections of 6 mg of colloidal carbon rather than with 12-mg injections.

We do not know the nature of the mechanism for this unexpected stimulation by repeated doses of colloidal carbon, but it seems likely that previous concepts of satiation of phagocytic cells and the depletion of serum factors in the induction of blockade is too simple. It is possible to get "blockade," a latent period in its induction, or a marked stimulation in colloid removal by simply adjusting the time sequence and dose injected.

REFERENCES

1. B. Benacerraf, G. Biozzi, B.N. Halpern, and C. Stiffel, "Physiology of phagocytosis of particles by the RES." In: B.N. Halpern, B. Benacerraf, and J.F. Delafresnaye, Eds., Physiopathology of the Reticuloendothelial System, A Symposium, Oxford, Blackwell, 1957, pp. 52-79.
2. B. Benacerraf, "Functions of the Kupffer cells." In: Ch. Rouiller, Ed., The Liver II, New York, Academic Press, 1964, pp. 37-62.
3. E.L. Dobson, L.S. Kelly, C.R. Finney, and H.G. Parker, "Further complications in interpretation of RE system blockade." Federation Proc., 22:399, 1963 (Abstract).
4. C.R. Jenkin and D. Rowley, "The role of opsonins in the clearance of living and inert particles by cells of the reticuloendothelial system." J. Exptl. Med., 114:363-374, 1961.
5. L.S. Kelly, E.L. Dobson, C.R. Finney, and J.D. Hirsch, "Proliferation of the reticuloendothelial system in the liver." Am. J. Physiol., 198:1134-1138, 1960.
6. I.M. Murray, "The effect of a plasma globulin fraction on the rate of phagocytosis." Anat. Record, 139:258-259, 1961 (Abstract).
7. I.M. Murray, "The mechanism of blockade of the reticuloendothelial system." J. Exptl. Med., 117: 139-147, 1963.
8. I.M. Murray, "Clearance rate in relation to agglutinins for gelatin-stabilized colloid in the rat." Am. J. Physiol., 204: 655-659, 1963.
9. S.J. Normann and E.P. Benditt, "Reticuloendothelial blockade: The importance of the sequence and dose of administered particles." J. Reticuloendothelial Soc., 2: 345-346, 1965 (Abstract).
10. S.J. Normann and E.P. Benditt, "Function of the reticuloendothelial system, II. Participation of a serum factor in carbon clearance." J. Exptl. Med., 122:709-719, 1965.

11. H.G. Parker and C.R. Finney, "Latent period in the induction of reticuloendothelial blockade." Am.J.Physiol., 198:916-920, 1960.
12. M.I. Arredondo and R.F. Kampschmidt, "Effect of endotoxins on phagocytic activity of the reticuloendothelial system of the rat." Proc. Soc.Exptl.Biol.Med., 112:78-81, 1963.

Comparative Morphology of Macrophages in Tissue Culture*

Boyce Bennett

Department of Pathology
Albert Einstein College of Medicine
New York, New York

ABSTRACT. Macrophages were obtained in tissue cultures with cells obtained from mouse lung, spleen, bone marrow, peripheral blood, and peritoneal cavity. In addition, macrophages from lung, spleen, bone marrow, and peritoneal cavity of guinea pigs and rats were also cultivated in vitro. Cells from the rat closely resembled those from the mouse, whereas guinea pig cells differed in several respects. In most instances, cells other than macrophages were phagocytized or died with the result that within seven days the cultures consisted entirely of macrophages. Macrophages from all these sources were actively phagocytic, were present as solitary ameboid cells, and, with the exception of certain guinea pig cells, underwent mitosis.

Tissue culture methods have been used in many studies dealing with the behavior and cytology of macrophages [1]. Investigations into the properties of macrophages cultivated in vitro have several apparent advantages over experiments with the intact animal: (1) macrophage activity may be observed directly with live cells; (2) metabolic measurements and histochemical studies may be made under controlled environmental conditions; and, (3) the role of macrophages in certain processes such as the immune response may be ascertained under circumstances where other cell types are not present. In general, macrophages used for these studies were obtained from the peritoneal cavity. In a report [2] from this laboratory, however, it was shown that macrophages may be cultured in vitro from a number of other sources. Furthermore, cells from these various sites differed in certain characteristics. Since this previous work dealt entirely with cells from the mouse, further studies were performed to culture macrophages from

* Supported by U.S. Public Health Service Research Grant CA-08145 from the National Cancer Institute.

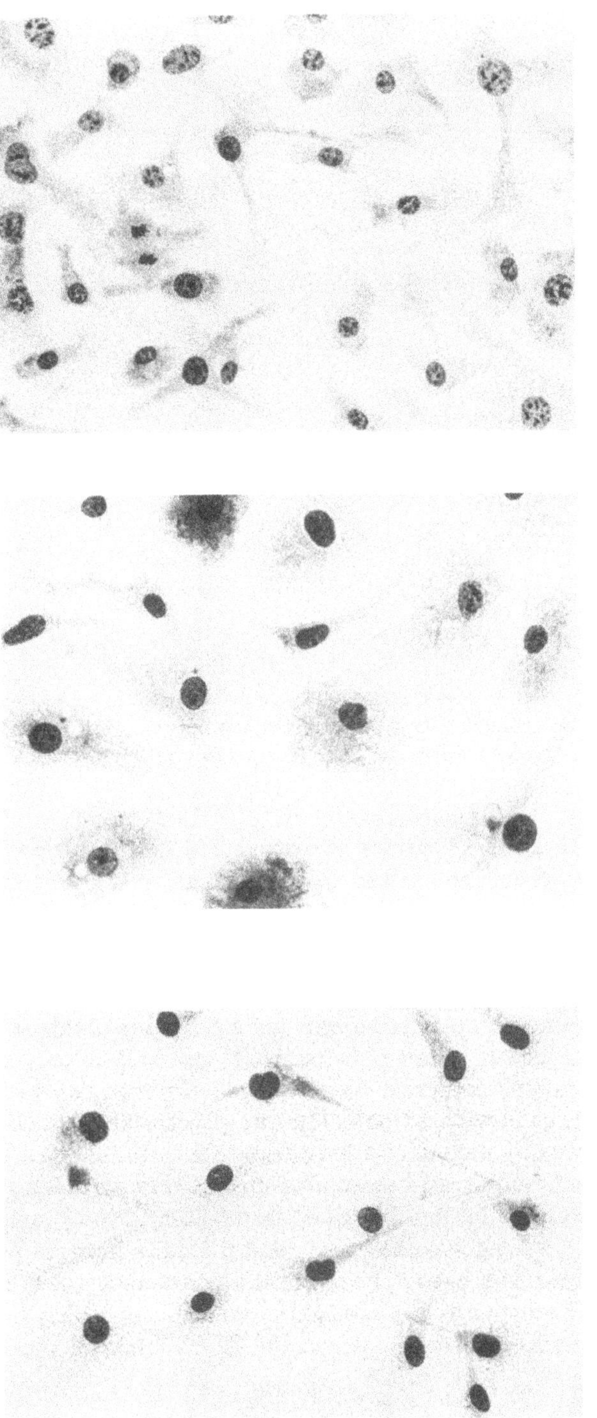

Fig. 1. Mouse peritoneal macrophages cultured for 7 days. The cells have extremely long cytoplasmic processes. × 425.

Fig. 2. Mouse spleen macrophages from 7-day cultures. Some of the cells show long, irregular cytoplasmic processes. × 425.

Fig. 3. Macrophages from 7-day cultures of mouse bone marrow. The nuclei vary in size and shape, but the cells are well spread. One mitosis is present. × 425.

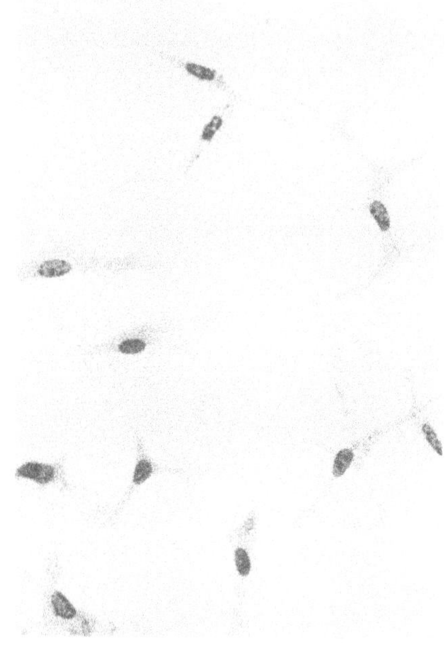

Fig. 4. Mouse peripheral blood macrophages in culture 7 days. The cells possess fully extended cytoplasmic processes. × 425.

other species. At this time, results are presented in which macrophages from several organs from the rat and guinea pig, as well as the mouse,were cultivated in vitro.

TISSUE CULTURES

The methods by which cells from various sites were obtained for culture have been described in detail previously [2] and will be only summarized here. Cell suspensions from lung and spleen were prepared by mincing the respective organs with a fine scissors. Bone marrow cells were forced from the femur by means of a hypodermic needle inserted into the marrow cavity. Peritoneal cells were obtained merely by rinsing the peritoneal cavity with Eagle's Minimum Essential Medium (MEM) containing 100 units penicillin, 0.1 mg streptomycin, and 0.5 units heparin per ml. No exudate-inducing agent was used. Peripheral blood leukocytes were separated from the erythrocytes by differential centrifugation of heparinized blood. Liver cells were prepared for culture by trypsinization of liver fragments.

Leighton tubes, each containing a glass coverslip, were used for the tissue cultures. Cells were suspended in MEM (containing antibiotics and heparin) to which 4 mM of glutamine per 100 ml and 40% serum were added.

In cultures of cells from the mouse, horse serum was utilized. Rat cells were cultured best with fetal bovine or homologous rat serum. Guinea pig cells were cultured in medium containing fetal bovine or horse serum. In all cases special care was taken to remove clumps and fragments of tissue before culture. The cell suspension (1 ml for each tube, with $3 \cdot 10^6$ cells for spleen, bone marrow, or peripheral blood, $5\text{-}10 \cdot 10^5$ cells for peritoneal cells, and $5 \cdot 10^5$ cells for lung) was placed in Leighton tubes. The tubes were gassed with 10% CO_2 in air, and the preparations were incubated at 37°C. The medium was renewed the next day and twice weekly thereafter. At intervals, the coverslips were removed and the cells were stained generally by the May–Grunwald–Giemsa method.

MOUSE CELLS

Macrophages were cultured with cell suspensions from mouse peritoneum, spleen, bone marrow, peripheral blood, and lung (Figs. 1-5). All these sources yielded macrophages with similar properties: they were phagocytic, possessed cytoplasmic acid phosphatase, were present as solitary ameboid cells, and underwent mitosis after 4-6 days in culture. They differed, however, in certain other characteristics. First, peritoneal and peripheral blood macrophages attached in culture within 2 hr and spread fully within 24

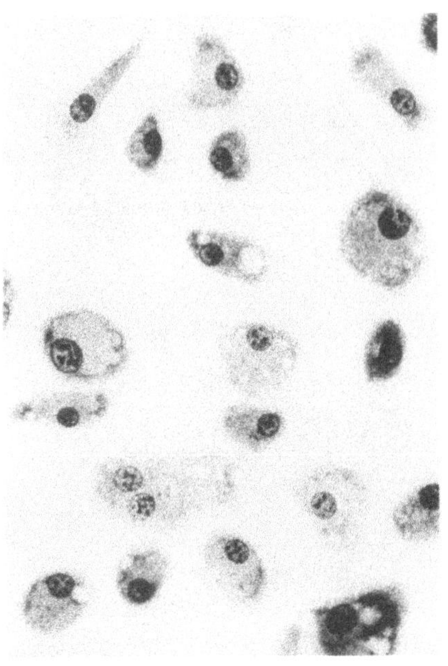

Fig. 5. Mouse lung macrophages from 7-day-old cultures. These cells contain round nuclei and few cytoplasmic processes. x 425.

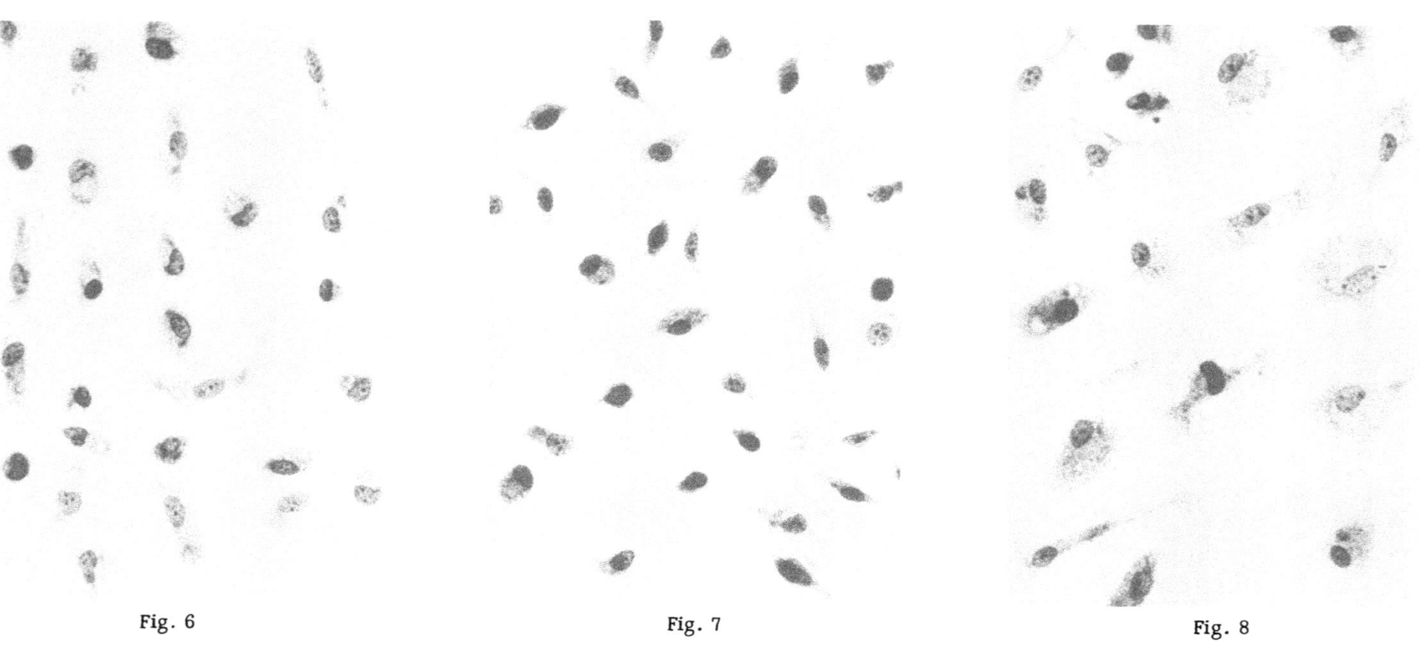

Fig. 6 Fig. 7 Fig. 8

Figs. 6-8. Rat macrophages in 7-day cultures of peritoneal cells (Fig. 6), spleen cells (Fig. 7), and bone marrow cells (Fig. 8). The macrophages from all three sources are morphologically similar with generally oval nuclei and irregular cytoplasmic processes. ×425.

hr, whereas bone marrow and spleen macrophages attached and spread much more slowly. Second, macrophages from peritoneum, spleen, bone marrow, and blood had extended cytoplasmic processes and irregular or oval nuclei. Lung cells, on the other hand, had round nuclei and blunt cytoplasmic processes. Third, the mitotic rate for cells from spleen, bone marrow, and lung was found to be considerably higher (approximately 1%) than for peritoneal or blood macrophages (approximately 0.03%).

In all cases, after 3-7 days in culture, cells other than macrophages died and were removed from the cultures with changes in medium or were phagocytized by the macrophages. As a consequence, essentially "pure" populations of macrophages were present in week-old preparations. Fibroblast proliferation was not generally a problem, probably because these cells did not persist in the medium selected. Macrophages from all sources were maintained in culture for periods up to three months. They remained morphologically virtually unchanged during this time, although the mitotic rate, after reaching a peak in 7-10 days, slowly declined until in one-month-old cultures, cell division had ceased. Neither changes of medium nor subculture resulted in the reappearance of mitoses. Eventually the number of cells slowly diminished as occasional macrophages fell from the culture surfaces and died.

Macrophages were also obtained in cultures of trypsinized liver. In this instance, a variety of nonphagocytic cells were present and proliferated

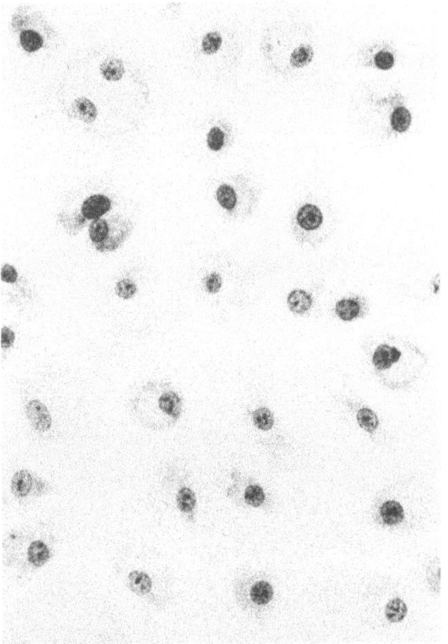

Fig. 9. Rat lung macrophages in 7-day cultures. Like lung macrophages from the mouse, these cells have round nuclei and blunted cytoplasmic processes. × 425.

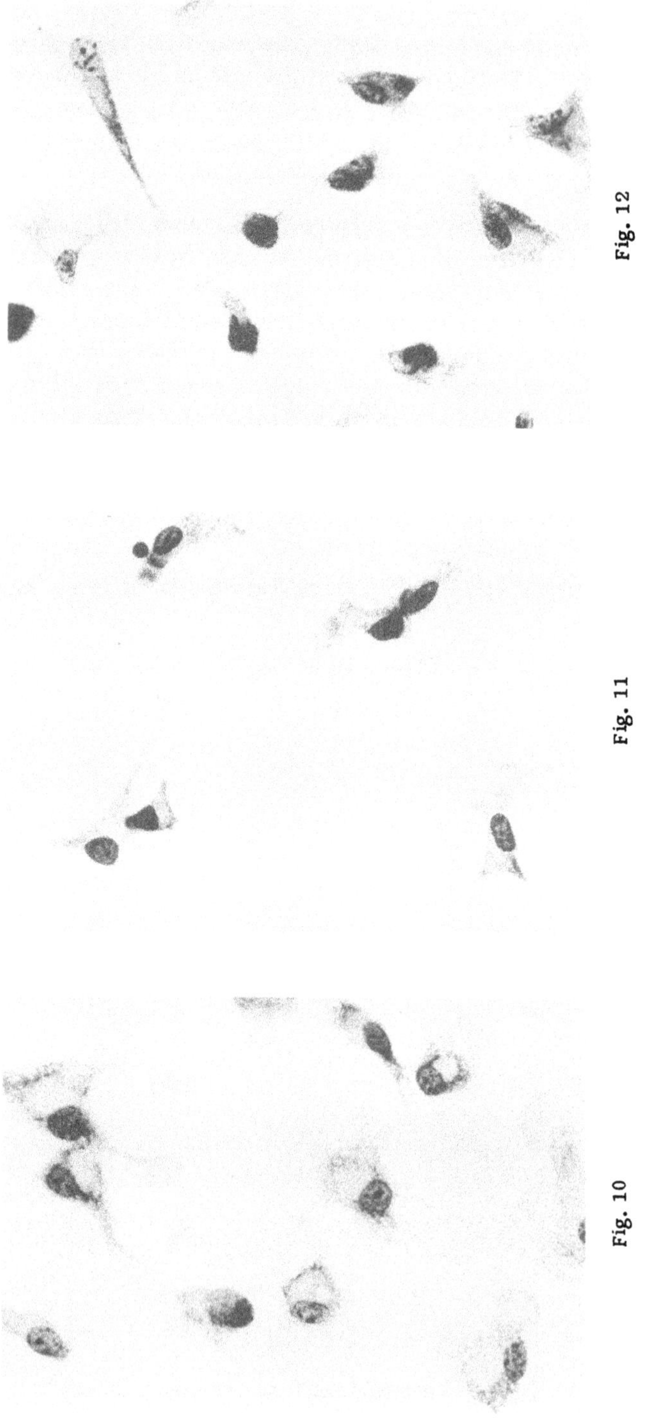

Figs. 10-12. Guinea pig macrophages from 7-day cultures of cells from the peritoneal cavity (Fig. 10), bone marrow (Fig. 11), and lung (Fig.12). Cells from these sources are morphologically alike. × 425.

more rapidly than the macrophages, eventually overgrowing the cultures. Nevertheless, while present, liver macrophages underwent mitosis and were morphologically similar to spleen or bone marrow macrophages.

RAT CELLS

Macrophages were produced in "pure" culture with cells from the peritoneum, spleen, bone marrow, and lung from the rat (Figs. 6-9). These cells resembled their counterpart in the mouse morphologically, attached and spread in a like manner, and underwent mitosis.

GUINEA PIG CELLS

The cultivation of macrophages from the guinea pig was found to be less satisfactory than with the mouse or rat. This was due partly to fibroblast proliferation, especially in lung or bone marrow cultures, and also to the nearly total absence of cell division among the macrophages. Despite this, macrophages were obtained in cultures of peritoneal cells, bone marrow, spleen, and lung (Figs. 10-13).

Peritoneal macrophages attached and spread rapidly, and by 4 hr, a monolayer of macrophages was present. Afterward, the majority of the cells slowly became rounded so that by 24 hr, only about 25% remained well spread. The rounded cells subsequently fell from the culture surfaces, but the remaining cells were maintained in culture for several weeks.

Spleen macrophages from the guinea pig attached and spread, as did cells from the mouse. One unusual aspect in these cultures, however, was that after three days, multinucleated giant cells appeared. These increased in number, and by seven days large cells containing as many as 50 nuclei were present. Mitoses were rare and were present only among the mononuclear cells. The origin of the multinucleated cells was not determined, but the work of Goldstein [3] and of Sutton and Weiss [4] indicate that such cells arise from the fusion of mononuclear cells rather than amitotic division.

Macrophages from bone marrow and lung attached in one day and were fully spread soon afterward. Because of fibroblast overgrowth, however, these macrophages could be maintained in culture for only about 10 days.

Guinea pig macrophages were found to differ in several aspects from mouse or rat cells. First, mitoses were absent in cultures of guinea pig lung and peritoneal macrophages, and were only rarely seen in bone marrow and spleen cell cultures, whereas mitoses were seen with mouse and rat macrophages from all sources. Second, lung macrophages from the guinea pig were morphologically similar to macrophages from other sources; rat or mouse lung macrophages had distinct morphology. Third, multinucleate giant cells, a cell type not encountered elsewhere in these studies, were present in guinea pig spleen cultures. Whether these differences represent

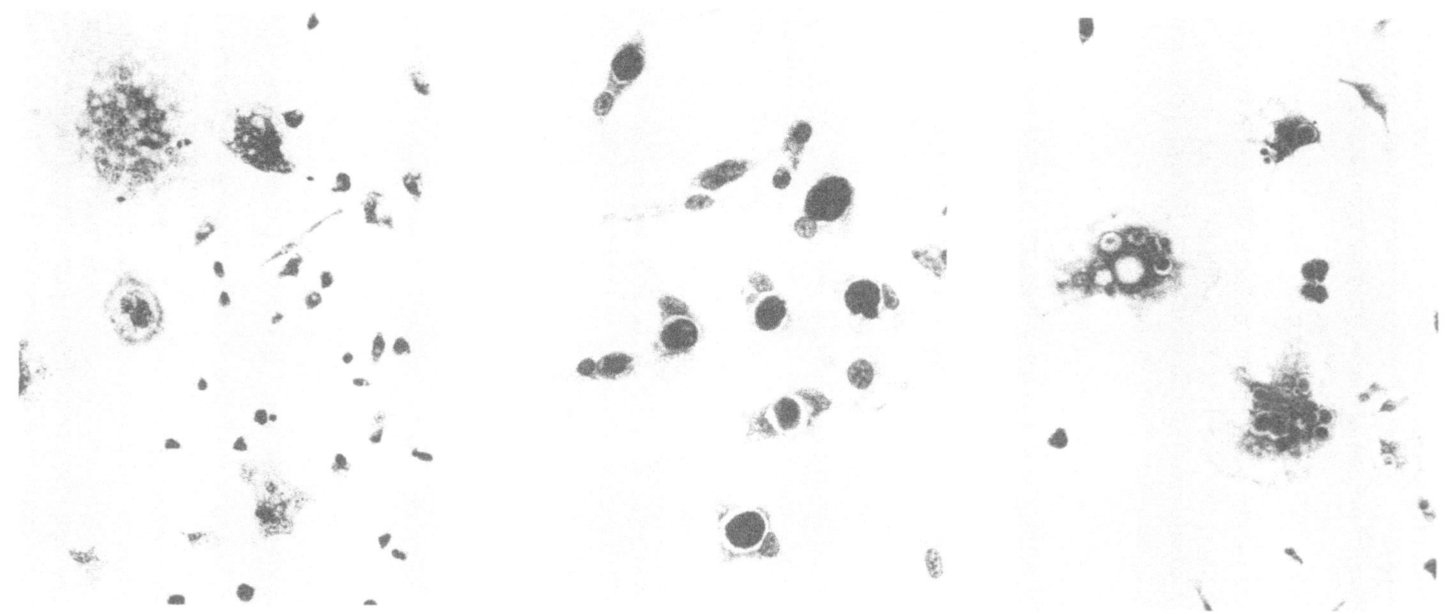

Fig. 13. Guinea pig spleen macrophages from 7-day-old cultures. This population consists of two cell types: (1) mononuclear cells similar to macrophages from other sources in the guinea pig, and (2) multinucleate giant cells. × 175.

Fig. 14. Phagocytosis of Meth A (BALB/c) tumor cells by rat bone marrow macrophages in presence of C57BL/6 anti-Meth A serum. All the tumor cells in this field have been phagocytized by the macrophages. × 425.

Fig. 15. Phagocytosis of Meth A by guinea pig spleen macrophages in the presence of rat anti-Meth A serum. Both the multinucleate and the mononuclear cells are phagocytic. × 175.

intrinsic divergences or are merely the result of tissue culture conditions remains to be established.

PHAGOCYTOSIS IN VITRO

The distinguishing quality that separates the macrophage from other cell types is its great phagocytic potential. To demonstrate the phagocytic nature of the cells described here, they were tested for their ability to phagocytose specifically opsonized mouse tumor cells in vitro [5]. This capacity to phagocytize mouse tumor cells has been shown to be a quality of macrophages alone (and certain reticulum cell sarcomas) and not of any other cell type tested [6]. In brief, the phagocytic test is performed by adding to the macrophage culture a suspension of mouse tumor cells in a medium containing isoimmune serum directed against the tumor cells. Generally, the BALB/c tumor, Meth A [7] was used along with C57BL/6 anti-Meth A serum. Numerous phagocytoses were present in such macrophage–tumor cell–antiserum preparations after incubation for 1-1½ hr (Fig. 14).

Macrophages from all the sources mentioned above were capable of phagocytosis under these conditions. It is interesting to note that phagocytosis of mouse tumor cells opsonized with mouse antiserum was readily accomplished not only by mouse cells but also by rat and guinea pig cells as well. Furthermore, tumor cell phagocytosis could be induced with heteroantiserum as well. Thus, either rat or guinea pig macrophages phagocytized Meth A in vitro in the presence of rat anti-Meth A serum (Fig. 15). (This antiserum was heated to 56°C for 30 min to destroy complement activity, thus avoiding lysis of Meth A cells. Nonspecific opsonins were then provided by adding 10% normal mouse serum; mouse sera do not contain complement in sufficient amounts for cytolysis in vitro [8].) In all cases, phagocytosis was virtually absent in preparations lacking antiserum.

COMMENT

In these experiments, macrophages from several sources and species were cultivated in vitro. The conditions presented favored the persistence of macrophages in most instances rather than other cell types. As a result, after seven days in culture, macrophages generally remained in "pure" culture. Macrophages from all these sources can be cultured not only in Leighton tubes, as described above, but also in glass or plastic Petri dishes or culture vessels, thus allowing the cultivation of large numbers of macrophages. Furthermore, viable macrophages may be released into suspension by treatment with versene (Grand Island Biological Co., Grand Island, N.Y.) followed by vigorous pipetting.

Mitoses were readily observed in cultures of mouse and rat macrophages from all sources tested, but only rarely among guinea pig spleen and bone marrow macrophages. Formerly, much difficulty was encountered in attempts to promote mitosis in mammalian macrophages, with few instances of success being reported [1]. The probable reason for this difficulty was the use of the peritoneal macrophage, a cell type shown here to have a very low mitotic rate. The number of mitoses was found to be substantially greater in cultures of mouse or rat spleen, bone marrow, or lung cells. Unfortunately, no macrophage population continued to undergo mitosis, in that the mitotic rate declined after 10 days, and mitoses were absent in month-old cultures. We have not, therefore, found it possible to maintain these cells in continuous tissue culture passage. Despite this, however, these cultures provide means not only for studying the morphological characteristics and functional capacities in vitro of macrophages from several sites in at least three species, but also for preparing macrophage cultures essentially free of extraneous cell types.

REFERENCES

1. F. Jacoby, In: E.N. Willmer, Ed., Cells and Tissues in Culture. New York, Academic Press, 1965, Vol. 2, p. 1.
2. B. Bennett, Am.J.Pathol., 48:165, 1966.
3. M.N. Goldstein, Anat. Record, 118:577, 1954.
4. J.S. Sutton and L. Weiss, J.Cell Biol., 28:303, 1966.
5. B. Bennett, L.J. Old, and E.A. Boyse, Transplantation, 2:183, 1964.
6. B. Bennett, J. Immunol., 95:80, 1965.
7. L.J. Old, E.A. Boyse, D.A. Clarke, and E.A. Carswell, Ann.N.Y. Acad.Sci., 101:80, 1962.
8. P.A. Gorer and P. O'Gorman, Transplantation, 3:142, 1956.

Fine Structural Aspects of Reticuloendothelial Blockade*

Joseph Wiener

Department of Pathology
College of Physicians and Surgeons
Columbia University, New York, N.Y.

INTRODUCTION

Aschoff first introduced the term "reticuloendothelial system (RES)" to designate cells with marked ability to take up dyes [1]. Much literature has accumulated since the early studies pertaining to the incorporation of both particulate and soluble materials by the cells of the RES. The subject of RES blockade has also attracted considerable attention. The following mechanisms have been proposed for blockade: (1) Saturation of phagocytic cells [2], (2) Clones of phagocytic cells [3] with one substance preventing further phagocytic activities, (3) the blockading agent damages the phagocytic cells' [4-6], (4) RES blockade results from the depletion of serum opsonins [7-8] or other serum factors [9] that are essential for the phagocytic process.

Blockade produced by the injection of various substances is usually demonstrated by observing the degree of incorporation of these injected materials by the RES utilizing histologic and clearance techniques. In the present study, electron microscopic observations have been correlated with the phagocytic activity of the RES as measured by carbon clearance. Two types of blockade have been examined: that induced by Thorotrast [10] (a colloidal blockading agent) [11], and that induced by cortisone [12], a nonparticulate blockading substance [13-15].

MATERIALS AND METHODS

Female rats of the Columbia—Sherman strain, weighing approximately 200 gm, were divided into seven groups of three animals each.

* Supported in part by the General Research Support Grant and Grant HE-5906 of the National Institutes of Health of the U.S. Public Health Service.

Group I rats were not injected, and served as controls.

Group II rats received carbon without a preceding injection of Thorotrast* or cortisone to demonstrate normal carbon clearance. The carbon clearance procedure is described below.

Group III rats were sacrificed 4 hr after receiving intravenously a blockading dose of Thorotrast (3.0 ml/kg body weight), and did not receive carbon or cortisone.

Group IV rats received intravenously a blockading dose of Thorotrast 4 hr prior to carbon clearance.

Group V rats received Thorotrast intravenously 3.0 ml/kg body weight 48 hr prior to carbon clearance.

Group VI rats received 25 mg cortisone acetate (cortone acetate, Merck, Sharp and Dohme, saline suspension) intramuscularly for three days, but did not receive carbon.

Group VII rats received carbon after being treated with 25 mg cortisone acetate intramuscularly for three days.

Carbon clearance studies were performed by injecting 15 mg of a carbon suspension (Pelikan C11/1431a, Gunther–Wagner Co., Hanover, Germany) into three animals of each group via a tail vein catheter. Samples of blood were then obtained with heparinized capillary pipettes from the retro-orbital venous plexus at timed intervals [16-17]. The concentration of carbon in each sample was measured spectrophotometrically. The plasma carbon concentration plotted per unit time resulted in a straight line, the slope of which is a mathematical constant K, the granulopectic or phagocytic index:

$$K = \frac{\log C_1 - \log C_2}{T}$$

in which C_1 is the initial blood concentration of carbon and C_2 is the concentration of carbon at time T. Delayed uptake or clearance is revealed by a smaller slope than is found in normal animals, expressed numerically as a lower value for the granulopectic index K.

The rats in groups II, IV, V, and VII were sacrificed following the carbon clearance studies, i.e., 15 min after the injection of carbon. Small blocks of liver from all the animals were quickly excised and processed for both light and electron microscopy.

---

*24-26% thorium dioxide suspended in dextrin, Testagar & Co., Detroit, Mich.

RESULTS

Measurements of Phagocytic Activity

The numerical value for the granulopectic index K of each animal receiving a carbon clearance test is listed in Table I. The carbon clearance data for each animal are shown in Fig. 1. Carbon clearances are delayed both in the animals receiving cortisone (Group VII), and in the animals receiving Thorotrast four hours previously (Group IV), indicating blockade. The clearance rates in Group V animals escaping from blockade (48 hr after injection of Thorotrast) tend to be greater than those of the controls. (Group II). This augmented rate of clearance is typical of escape from blockade [17].

Electron Microscopic Observations

The Kupffer cells in the control animals which did not receive carbon (Group I), form a discontinuous cellular layer lining the sinusoids which are widely patent. These cells contain relatively few cytoplasmic organelles and exhibit features previously described by numerous investigators [18-20] (Fig. 2). The parenchymal cells contain their usual complements of glycogen, mitochondria, smooth and rough surfaced endoplasmic reticulum, microbodies and dense bodies.

Carbon particles are present in the majority of Kupffer cells in the control animals receiving only carbon (Group II). These particles are approximately 250 Å in diameter and are found within cytoplasmic vacuoles measuring up to 4.5 μ in diameter (Fig. 3). Although most of the carbon is intracellular, smaller numbers of carbon particles are also in intimate contact with the Kupffer cell surface membranes or within superficial invaginations of these membranes. The Kupffer cells containing the colloidal particles are considerably larger than those devoid of carbon. They contain numerous vesicles and vacuoles devoid of carbon, as well as prominent Golgi complexes and dilated cisternae of smooth surfaced endoplasmic reticulum. The largest amounts of carbon are found within the Kupffer cells in the peripheral portions of the lobules.

Table I. Granulopectic Index (K) of Each Animal Receiving Carbon Clearance Test

	Group II (carbon without Thorotrast)	Group IV (Thorotrast 4 h prior to carbon clearance)	Group V (Thorotrast 48 h prior to carbon clearance)	Group VII (carbon and cortisone)
	0.043	0.012	0.079	0.008
	0.052	0.012	0.090	0.005
	0.062	0.020	0.092	0.012
Mean	0.052	0.015	0.087	0.008

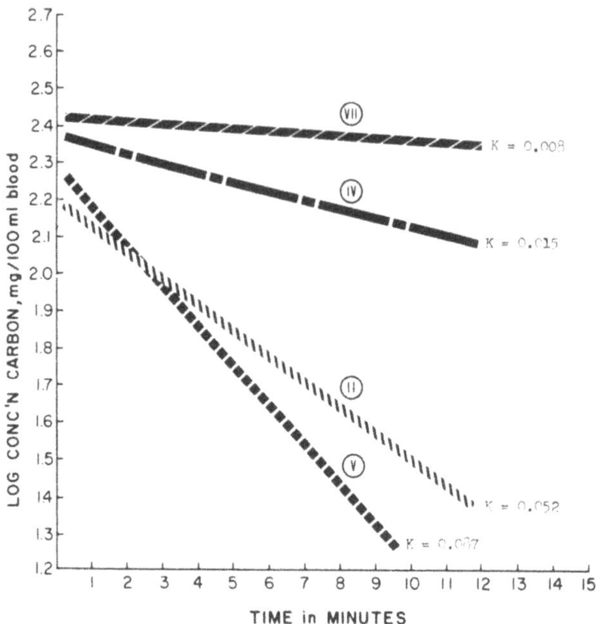

Fig. 1. Carbon clearance in control, Thorotrast, and cortisone-treated rats.

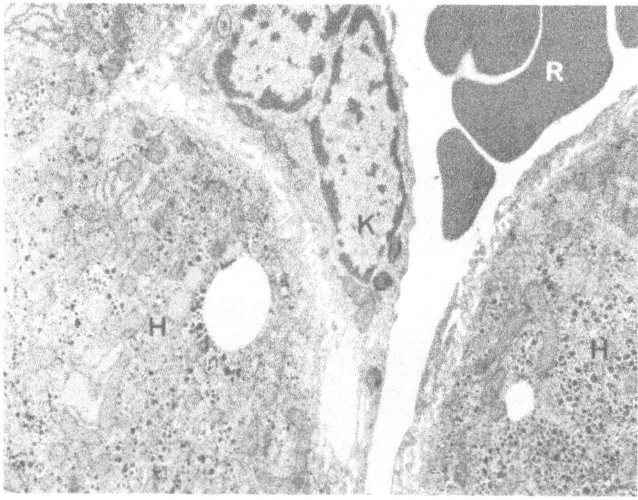

Fig. 2. Uninjected control animal (Group I). A Kupffer cell (K) and several erythrocytes (R) are seen in the widely patent sinusoid which lies between two cords of hepatic parenchymal cells (H). × 10,500, reduced 35% for reproduction.

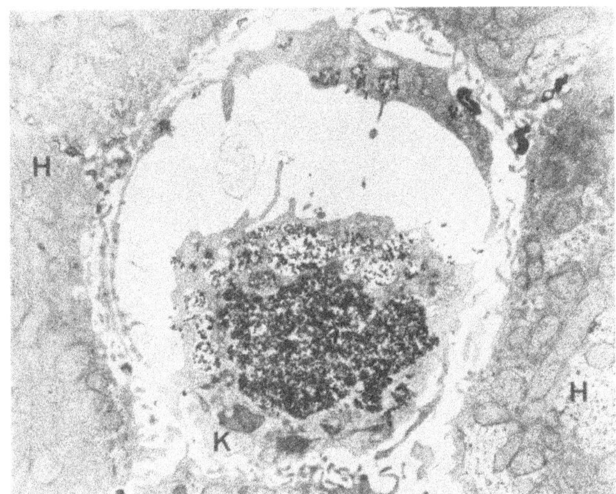

Fig. 3. An animal that received only carbon (Group II). The Kupffer cell (K) contains large numbers of carbon particles within cytoplasmic vacuoles. Small numbers of carbon particles are on the surface membrane. H indicates hepatic parenchymal cell. x 9500, reduced 35% for reproduction.

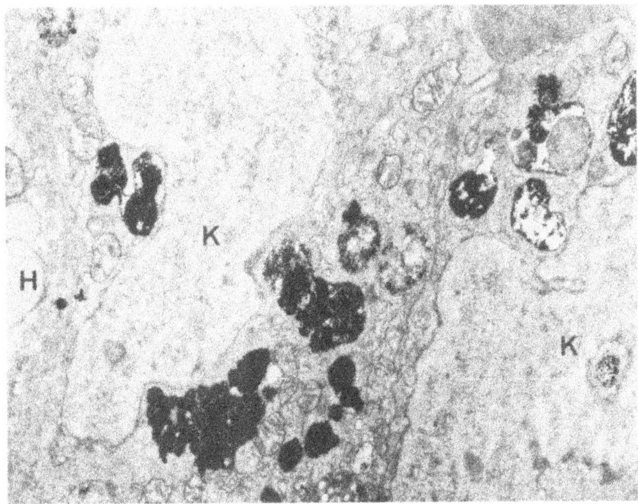

Fig. 4. Animal given Thorotrast (Group III) 4 hr prior to sacrifice. Large aggregates of Thorotrast are seen within cytoplasmic vacuoles of the Kupffer cells (K). H indicates hepatic parenchymal cell. x 12,000, reduced 35% for reproduction.

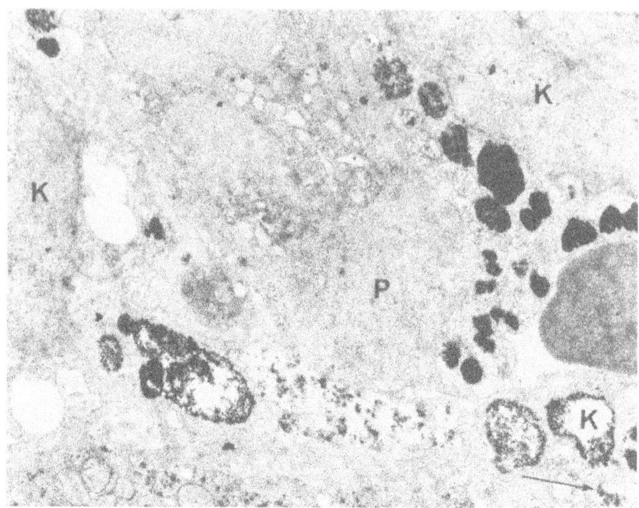

Fig. 5. Animal blockaded with Thorotrast 4 hr before carbon clearance (Group IV). Three Thorotrast-labeled Kupffer cells (K) and a polymorphonuclear leucocyte (P) are seen within the narrowed sinusoid. Although large numbers of carbon particles are seen within the sinusoid, few of these are in actual contact with the Kupffer cell surface membranes. One cytoplasmic vacuole containing carbon is seen (arrow). H indicates hepatic parenchymal cell. × 13,000, reduced 35% for reproduction.

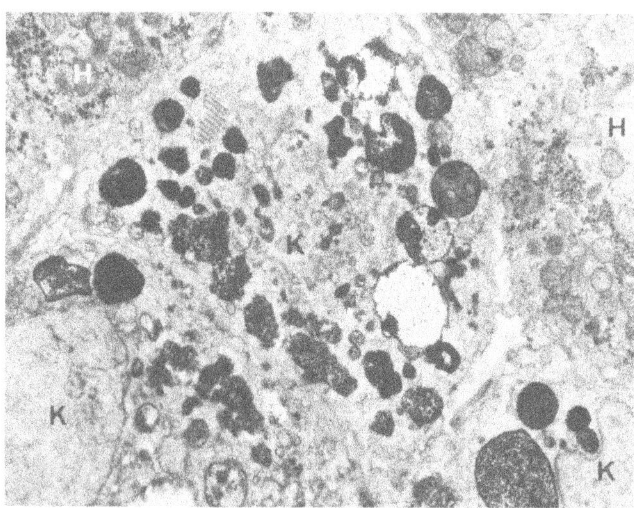

Fig. 6. Rat that has escaped from Thorotrast-induced blockade (Group V). Kupffer cells contain membrane-limited aggregates of Thorotrast and carbon. The sinusoids are free of carbon particles. H indicates hepatic parenchymal cell. × 8000, reduced 35% for reproduction.

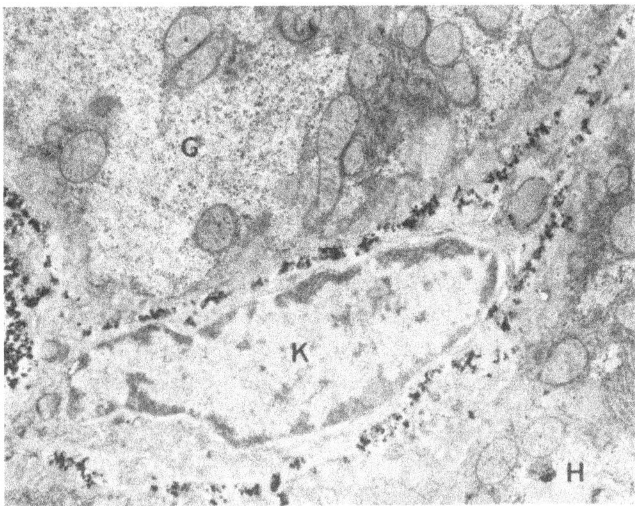

Fig. 7. An animal that received cortisone acetate and carbon (Group VII). The sinusoid is compressed by the parenchymal cells (H) which contain large amounts of glycogen (G). Although large numbers of carbon particles are seen near the surface membrane of the Kupffer cell (K), no carbon is seen within this cell. ×15,000, reduced 35% for reproduction.

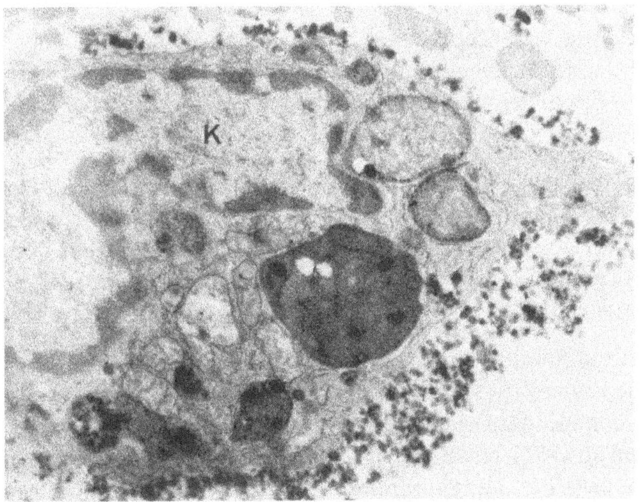

Fig. 8. Similar to Fig. 7. Many carbon particles are seen adjacent to the surface membrane of this Kupffer cell (K). × 20,000, reduced 35% for reproduction.

No carbon is seen within the parenchymal cells of these animals. The cytologic characteristics of the parenchymal cells do not differ from those seen in the uninjected control animals (Group I).

A blockading dose of Thorotrast alone (Group III) labels the majority of Kupffer cells at 4 hr (Fig. 4). Particles of Thorotrast measure approximately 70 Å in diameter, are more electron dense than carbon, and are found as large and small aggregates within cytoplasmic vacuoles of Kupffer cells. Unlike carbon, Thorotrast is never seen extracellularly. The cells containing Thorotrast are enlarged and, in general, similar to those containing carbon. However, the vacuoles containing Thorotrast also have amorphous electron dense material and whorls of membranes. Occasional multivesicular bodies containing Thorotrast are also seen.

The majority of Kupffer cells in animals given carbon at the height of Thorotrast-induced blockade (Group IV), are labeled with Thorotrast in a manner similar to that described in Group III (Fig. 5). In addition, large numbers of carbon particles are present in narrowed sinusoids in the vicinity of the Kupffer cells. However, relatively few carbon particles lie in actual contact with the Kupffer cell surface membranes. Occasional small membrane-enclosed aggregates of carbon are present within the cytoplasm of Kupffer cells in this group of animals.

The Kupffer cells of animals that have escaped blockade (Group V) contain intracytoplasmic collections of Thorotrast comparable to the amounts seen in Groups III and IV. However, in contrast with the Kupffer cells of blockaded animals (Group IV), abundant intravacuolar aggregates of carbon are noted within the cytoplasm of these cells (Fig. 6). On occasion, single vacuoles containing both Thorotrast and carbon are noted. Very little extracellular carbon is present at this time. These cells are again enlarged. It is noteworthy that the cells which phagocytize carbon invariably contain the previously injected Thorotrast.

Occasional hepatic parenchymal cells in all animals receiving Thorotrast (Groups II-V) have vacuoles containing Thorotrast in the regions of the bile canaliculi. Increased numbers of peribiliary bodies, some containing Thorotrast, are also noted. Carbon particles, however, are not found within parenchymal cells.

The hepatic sinusoids of animals treated with cortisone (Group VI) are somewhat compressed by enlarged parenchymal cells that contain large amounts of glycogen, enlarged mitochondria, and numerous lipid droplets [21]. The Kupffer cells in this group of animals do not differ from those of the controls (Group I). Large numbers of carbon particles are present in the narrowed sinusoids in the vicinity of the Kupffer cells in the cortisone-treated animals (Group VII) injected with India ink (Fig. 7). Relatively few carbon particles, however, are in actual contact with the surface membranes of the Kupffer cells (Figs. 7-8). Many of these Kupffer cells contain no carbon particles (Fig. 7), whereas others contain relatively small amounts of intracytoplasmic carbon (Fig. 8) as compared with the carbon clearance controls (Group II).

Necrobiotic changes are not observed in the Kupffer cells of any of the animals examined.

DISCUSSION

The presence of functional blockade of the RES is reflected morphologically by Thorotrast-laden Kupffer cells unable to incorporate significant amounts of colloidal carbon, despite the presence of numerous carbon particles near their cell surfaces. A similar relationship between the carbon particles and the plasma membranes of the Kupffer cells is present in the animals blockaded with cortisone.

The uptake by cells of colloidal particles with presumably varying amounts of dispersion medium is usually regarded as a form of pinocytosis [22-25]. Many investigators have discussed this process in terms of phagocytosis. The precise terminology is of little consequence, inasmuch as phagocytosis and pinocytosis are basically similar processes which differ primarily with respect to the quantities of liquid of the suspending dispersion medium that are absorbed [24, 26]. It has been shown that pinocytosis is a two-stage process [27, 28]. The initial step involves a reversible physicochemical adsorption of the dispersed substance to sites on the cell surface membrane. This phase is independent of temperature and of metabolic inhibitors. The second stage of uptake may be related to membrane synthesis and flow [29] with the resultant incorporation of the adsorbed material into vesicles and vacuoles derived from the surface membrane. This stage is slower, irreversible, and sensitive to metabolic inhibitors and temperature. In this regard, it has been shown that there is increased incorporation of C14-acetate into neutral lipids and phospholipids and of P32 into phospholipids of leukocytes during phagocytosis [30-32]. Karnovsky considers the increased uptake of P32 to be due to the synthesis and disruption of bonds in the membranes actively involved in particle ingestion [33].

Very few carbon particles are in contact with the surface membranes of Kupffer cells in blockaded animals. This is to be compared with the control animals where the carbon particles are found either on the cell surface membranes or within cytoplasmic vacuoles of the Kupffer cells. This suggests that the failure to incorporate carbon during RES blockade is a result, at least in part, of a defect in the first or surface attachment phase of pinocytosis. Opsonins and other substances that alter surface charges and play a role in RES blockade may influence the surface binding of colloidal materials in the first stage of pinocytosis [7, 8, 34-36].

Whether the failure of carbon ingestion is also due, in part, to interference with the second or cytoplasmic uptake phase cannot be ascertained from this study. It should be pointed out that the incorporation of carbon is never completely inhibited inasmuch as small quantities of intracytoplasmic carbon are found at the height of blockade. It has been postulated that destruction of Kupffer cells by the phagocytic material results in RES blockade [4-6]. The absence of degenerative changes in these Kupffer cells is at variance with this concept. Moreover, numerous electron microscopic studies of the pinocytosis of Thorotrast by a variety of cells failed to disclose degenerative changes [19, 37-39]. This study also demonstrates that blockade is not necessarily due to physical saturation of the Kupffer cells by colloidal particles. There is no evidence in this study that the inhibition of phagocytosis is the result of saturation of clones of phagocytic cells which are specific for the particles under study. Such clones have not been observed in the carbon clearance control animals in which the majority of Kupffer cells, rather than a select population, contain carbon.

The mechanism by which large doses of steroids affect the Kupffer cells has not been resolved. Several workers have suggested that steroids regulate cell permeability by either specific interaction with or nonspecific absorption to surface membranes [40-43]. It is well established that steroid hormones also stabilize lysosomal membranes [44]. Since the surface attachment phase of phagocytosis involves a reversible physicochemical adsorption of the dispersed substance to sites on the cell surface membranes [28], it seems possible that alterations in the plasma membranes induced by steroids could result in impaired attachment of the colloidal particles to the plasma membranes. Alternatively, steroid-induced modifications in the surface properties of the colloidal particles themselves might impair surface attachment. The effects of cortisone on opsonins and surface charges [7-9, 34-36] remain to be elucidated. Cortisone-induced alterations in the surface membranes of the Kupffer cells could also interfere with the cytoplasmic uptake phase of colloidal material since, as previously stated, this step involves membrane synthesis and flow [29] and incorporation of adsorbed material into vesicles and vacuoles derived from the surface membranes.

The blockade produced by large doses of steroids could be related to decreased perfusion of the liver. Hepatic blood flow is an important factor regulating the clearance of colloidal particles and other materials from the blood stream [45-46]. The parenchymal cells of blockaded animals are clearly enlarged and there is considerable narrowing of the sinusoidal spaces. This explanation, however, seems unlikely, since large numbers of colloidal particles are present within the sinusoids of these animals.

In animals which have escaped from blockade (carbon clearance performed 48 hr after the injection of Thorotrast), the Kupffer cells contain abundant amounts of Thorotrast and carbon within cytoplasmic vacuoles. Carbon particles are seen on the surfaces of the Kupffer cells in these animals more frequently than in blockaded animals, but far less often than in animals given carbon alone. It therefore appears that in animals which have escaped from blockade the Kupffer cells are once more capable of adsorbing carbon particles. Far fewer adsorbed extracellular carbon particles are seen in the livers of animals which have escaped from blockade than in the animals given carbon alone. This may be related to a more rapid cytoplasmic uptake phase, which is in turn reflected by the extremely rapid carbon clearances seen in the former group.

The mechanism involved in escape from blockade remains obscure. Benacerraf et al. have postulated that the resumption of phagocytic activity in animals which have previously undergone blockade is due to proliferation of a new Kupffer cell population [4]. It has been previously shown that recovery from RES blockade is accompanied by Kupffer cell proliferation, and that such cells are able to divide despite the fact that they contain ingested colloidal material [47, 48]. The latter characteristic is in agreement with the present observations showing that most Kupffer cells in animals which have recovered from Thorotrast-induced blockade contain the previously injected Thorotrast.

SUMMARY

Fine structural observations have been correlated with the phagocytic activity of the RES as measured by carbon clearance. The Kupffer cells of rat liver have been examined following carbon clearance determinations in Thorotrast and cortisone-induced blockade and following escape from blockade, as well as after the injection of carbon, Thorotrast, or cortisone alone. The injection of either Thorotrast or carbon alone labels most Kupffer cells. Large numbers of carbon particles are present in the vicinity of Kupffer cells at the height of blockade, but few particles are in actual contact with the Kupffer cell surface membranes. After Thorotrast-induced blockade has disappeared, the carbon is almost entirely within Kupffer cells and the cells which phagocytose the carbon invariably contain Thorotrast. These observations suggest that blockade of the RES is due, at least in part, to a defect in the first or surface attachment phase of pinocytosis.

ACKNOWLEDGMENTS

The author wishes to acknowledge the collaboration of Drs. David Spiro, William Margaretten, and Thomas S. Cottrell in the work reported here.

REFERENCES

1. L. Aschoff, Lectures on Pathology, New York, Paul B. Moeber, Inc., 1924, p. 1.
2. P.B. Beeson, Proc.Soc.Exptl.Biol.Med., 64:146, 1947.
3. H.N. Wagner, Jr. and M. Iio, J.Clin.Invest., 43:1525, 1964.
4. B. Benacerraf, B.N. Halpern, G. Biozzi, and S.A. Benos, Brit.J. Exptl.Pathol., 35:97, 1954.
5. R.T. McCluskey, B.W. Zweifach, W. Antopol, B. Benacerraf, and A.L. Nagler, Am.J. Pathol., 37:245, 1960.
6. A.E. Stuart, G. Biozzi, C. Stiffel, B.N. Halpern, and D. Mouton, Brit.J.Exptl.Pathol., 41:599, 1960.
7. C.R. Jenkin and D. Rowley, J.Exptl.Med., 114:363, 1961.
8. I.M. Murray, J.Exptl.Med., 117:139, 1963.
9. S.J. Normann and E.P. Benditt, J.Exptl.Med., 122:709, 1965.
10. J. Wiener, D. Spiro, and W. Margaretten, Am.J. Pathol., 45:783, 1964.
11. R.A. Good and L. Thomas, J.Exptl.Med., 96:625, 1952.
12. J. Wiener, T.S. Cottrell, W. Margaretten, and D. Spiro, Am. J. Pathol., 50:187, 1967.
13. J.F. Snell, In: J.H. Heller, Ed., Reticuloendothelial Structure and Function, New York, Ronald Press, 1960, p. 321.
14. J.H. Heller, Endocrinology, 56:80, 1955.
15. T. Nicol, R.S. Snell, and D.L.J. Bilbey, Brit.Med.J., 2:800, 1956.
16. B.N. Halpern, B. Benacerraf, and G. Biozzi, Brit.J.Exptl.Pathol., 34:426, 1953.
17. G. Biozzi, B. Benacerraf, and B.N. Halpern, Brit.J.Exptl.Pathol., 34:441, 1953.
18. H.F. Parks, In: F.S. Sjostrand and J. Rhodin, Eds., Proceedings of the Stockholm Conference on Electron Microscopy, Stockholm, Almqvist and Wiksell, 1956, p. 151.
19. J.C. Hampton, Acta Anat., 32:262, 1958.
20. F.C. Schmidt, Anat. Anz., 108:376, 1960.
21. A.V. Loud, D.V. Kimberg, J. Wiener, and D. Spiro, In preparation.
22. H. Holter, Ann.N.Y.Acad.Sci., 78:524, 1959.
23. H.E. Karrer, J.Biophys.Biochem.Cytol., 7:357, 1960.
24. P.W. Brandt and G.D. Pappas, J.Biophys.Biochem.Cytol., 8:675, 1960.
25. G.E. Palade, Circulation, 24:368, 1961.
26. D.W. Fawcett, Circulation, 26:1105, 1961.
27. P.W. Brandt, Exptl.Cell Res., 15:300, 1958.
28. V.N. Schumaker, Exptl.Cell Res., 15:314, 1958.
29. H.S. Bennett, J.Biophys.Biochem.Cytol., 2 Suppl., 4:99, 1956.
30. P. Elsbach, J.Exptl.Med., 110:969, 1959.
31. A.J. Sbarra and M.L. Karnovsky, J. Biol.Chem., 235:2224, 1960.
32. M.L. Karnovsky and D.F. Wallach, J.Biol.Chem., 236:1895, 1961.

33. M.L. Karnovsky, Physiol.Rev., 42:143, 1962.
34. S. Mudd, M. McCutcheon, and B. Lucke, Physiol.Rev., 14:210, 1934.
35. J.L. Tullis and D.M. Surgenor, Ann.N.Y.Acad.Sci., 66:386, 1956.
36. D.S. Mabry, J.A. Bass, M.C. Dodd, J.M. Wallace, and C.-S.Wright, J.Immunol., 76:54, 1956.
37. G.I. Kaye, G.D. Pappas, A. Donn, and N. Mallett, J.Cell Biol., 12:481, 1962.
38. P.W. Brandt and G.D. Pappas, J.Cell Biol., 15:55, 1962.
39. G.D. Pappas and V.M. Tennyson, J.Cell Biol., 15:227, 1962.
40. A. Munck, Biochem.Biophys.Acta, 24:507, 1957.
41. O. Hechter and G. Lester, Recent Prog. Hormone Res., 16:138, 1960.
42. E.N. Willmer, Biol.Rev., 36:368, 1961.
43. N.L. Gershfeld and E. Heftmann, Experientia, 19:2, 1963.
44. G. Weissmann and L. Thomas, J. Clin. Invest., 42:661, 1963.
45. B. Benacerraf, G. Biozzi, B.N. Halpern, and C. Stiffel, Reticuloendothelial Soc.Bull., 1:44, 1955.
46. B.N. Halpern, B. Benacerraf, G. Biozzi, and A. Cuendet, J.Physiol., 128:1, 1955.
47. L.S. Kelly, E.L. Dobson, C.R. Finney, and J.D. Hirsch, Am.J. Physiol., 198:1134, 1960.
48. L.S. Kelly, B.A. Brown, and E.L. Dobson, Proc.Soc.Exptl.Biol. Med., 110:555, 1962.

The Cellular Basis of RE Stimulation: The Effects on Peritoneal Cells of Stimulation with Glyceryl Trioleate, Studied by EM and Autoradiography

I. Carr and M. A. Williams

Department of Human Biology and Anatomy
University of Sheffield
Sheffield, England

Among the many substances that stimulate reticuloendothelial function, one of the most convenient experimentally is glyceryl trioleate [1]. This substance has been shown to have an effect on individual RE cells. After exposure to it in vitro a population of peritoneal cells had increased phagocytic activity toward bacteria [2], probably due to an increase in the number of active cells [3]. The cellular mechanism of this effect is obscure.

An early demonstration of the fact that individual RE cells could vary significantly in function was the finding that tuberculous macrophages were more actively phagocytic than normal [4]. More recently it has been shown that macrophages stimulated in vitro by various components of the culture medium contain more acid phosphatase and other lysosomal enzymes than normal [5, 6, 7]. These findings have not been related to general RE stimulation.

Glyceryl trioleate appeared to be a suitable substance to use in the study of RE stimulation, since it was readily available in tritiated form. This report describes the effects of treating mouse peritoneal macrophages in vitro and in vivo with glyceryl trioleate (see also [8]).

MATERIALS AND METHODS

The animals used were male white mice of 20- to 25-gm body weight from a closed colony.

Cells were obtained by washing out the peritoneal cavity after abdominal massage. They were examined (a) by phase contrast microscopy, first in a moist chamber, and again after fixing a thick preparation in osmium vapor and mounting in Farrant's medium, (b) after smearing on a glass slide,

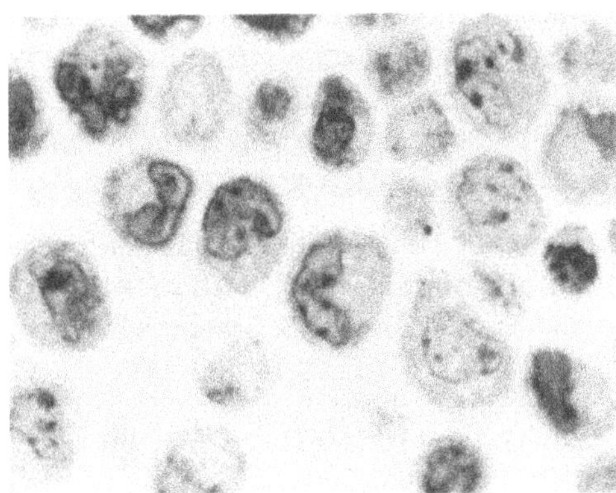

Fig. 1. Control peritoneal cells. The cells have smooth outlines, and contain few granules. Araldite section, toluidine blue, × 1600.

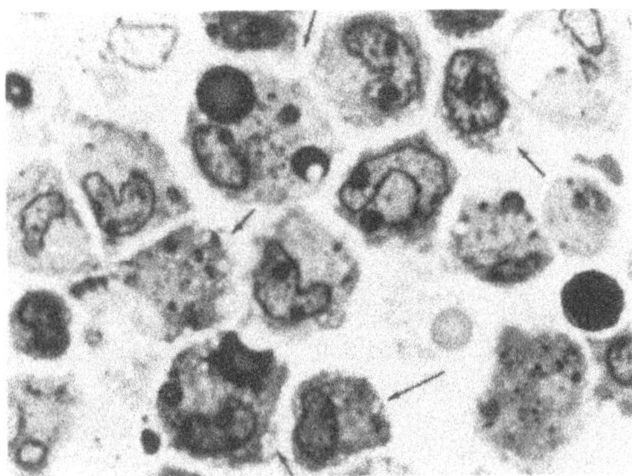

Fig. 2. Peritoneal cells 5 days after intraperitoneal injection of glyceryl trioleate. The cells have irregular microvillous outlines (arrowed), and contain black lipid globules, and small blue-staining granules, presumably lysosomes. Araldite section, toluidine blue, × 1600.

fixing in formalin, and staining with haematoxylin and eosin, or Sudan IV, (c) after smearing on mylar film, without fixation [9] and staining for acid phosphatase by the Gomori technique, and for α-naphthyl esterase [10], (d) after fixation in glutaraldehyde and osmium tetroxide and embedding in araldite [11]. Thick sections stained with hot alkaline toluidine blue were examined with the light microscope, and thin sections stained with lead citrate were examined with the electron microscope.

The experiments were carried out as follows:

(1) In Vivo Stimulation. Animals received intraperitoneally 10 mg glyceryl trioleate (BDH). This was emulsified in Hanks solution containing 0.01% Tween 20, by repeated passage through a syringe and needle. The animals were killed 8 hr to 14 days after injection. Controls were uninjected, or injected with Hanks solution and emulsifying agent only.

(2) In Vitro Stimulation. Cells were stimulated by incubation for 15 min to 4 hr in tissue culture medium 199, with or without 25% horse serum, and/or glyceryl trioleate 0.4 mg/ml with Tween 20.

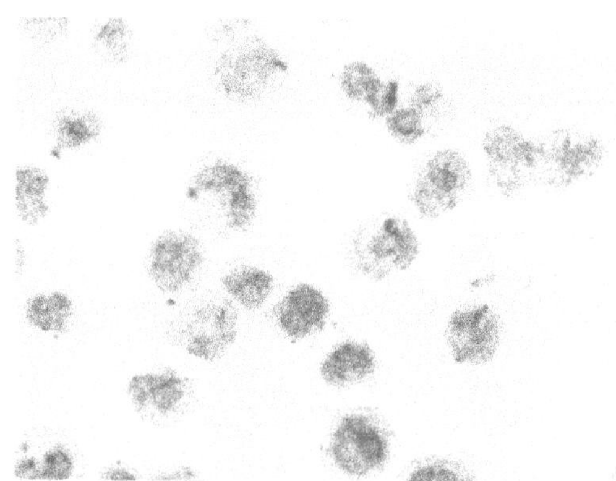

Fig. 3. Control peritoneal cells. Some acid phosphatase reaction is present. Gomori acid phosphatase/haematoxylin. x 1000.

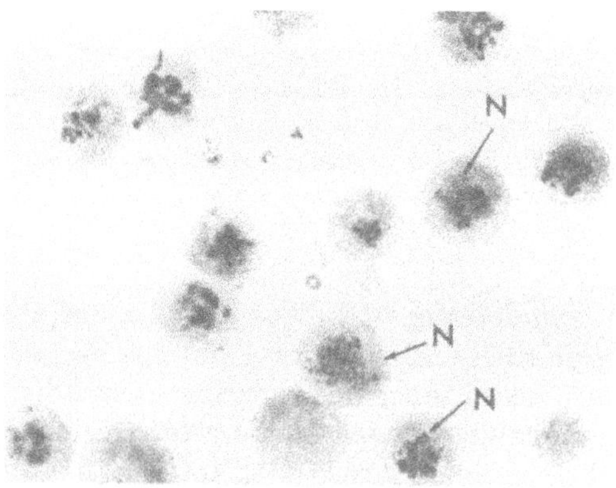

Fig. 4. Peritoneal cells 5 days after intraperitoneal injection of glyceryl trioleate. There is a dense acid phosphatase reaction in the center of the cells. The nucleus (N) shows no deposit. Gomori acid phosphatase/haematoxylin. x 1000.

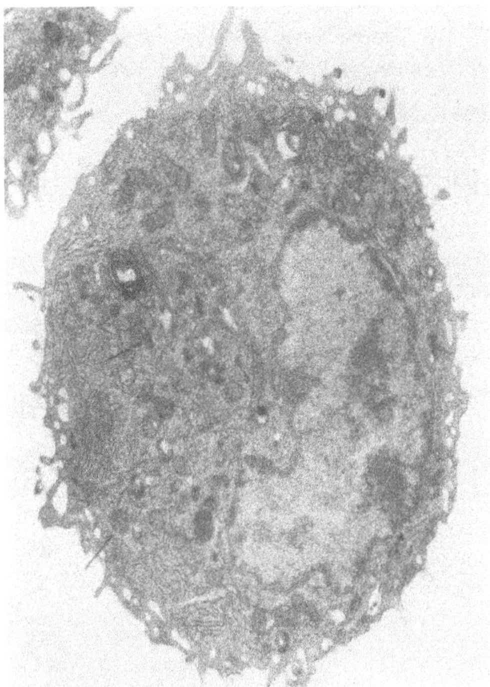

Fig. 5. Control macrophage. The surface is relatively smooth, but processes are visible. Several dense bodies or lysosomes are present (arrowed). × 15,000, reduced 40% for reproduction.

(3) Experiments with Radioactive Triglyceride. Experiments similar to those under 1 and 2 were repeated using tritiated glyceryl trioleate (Radiochemicals Center) in a dose in vivo of 2 mg (0.84 mc) and in vitro of 0.4 mg (0.17 mc) ml. Stripping film autoradiographs were made for light microscopy of cell smears fixed in formalin, and of glutaraldehyde–osmium-fixed araldite embedded blocks. The former were stained with methylene blue; the latter were examined unstained by phase-contrast microscopy. It was found that the most convenient stage affording large numbers of macrophages heavily labeled, and uncontaminated by polymorphonuclears, was after 1 hr incubation in vitro. EM autoradiographs were therefore made of cells incubated in vitro with tritiated glyceryl trioleate for 15 min to 4 hr.

RESULTS

These can be summarized briefly. On incubation in vitro there was an increase in length of cell processes, but no increase in acid phosphatase. This effect was maximal after 1 hr incubation. After stimulation in vivo there was an increase both in length of cell processes and in acid phosphatase. This effect was maximal after five days. The detailed results described below refer, for the sake of brevity, to those seen after 1 hr in vitro stimulation, or five days in vivo stimulation.

(1) Phase Contrast Microscopy. Control cells had smooth, or only slightly scalloped edges. Only a few cells had distinct processes. After stimulation in vivo and in vitro, long processes were seen in many but not in all cells.

(2) Toluidine Blue-Stained Araldite Sections. Control cells had smooth or slightly scalloped edges, and contained few blue granules. After in vivo stimulation, cells showed processes and contained a black lipid globules and blue granules, probably lysosomes (Figs. 1 and 2). After in vitro stimulation, processes were longer, but no increase in lysosomes was demonstrated.

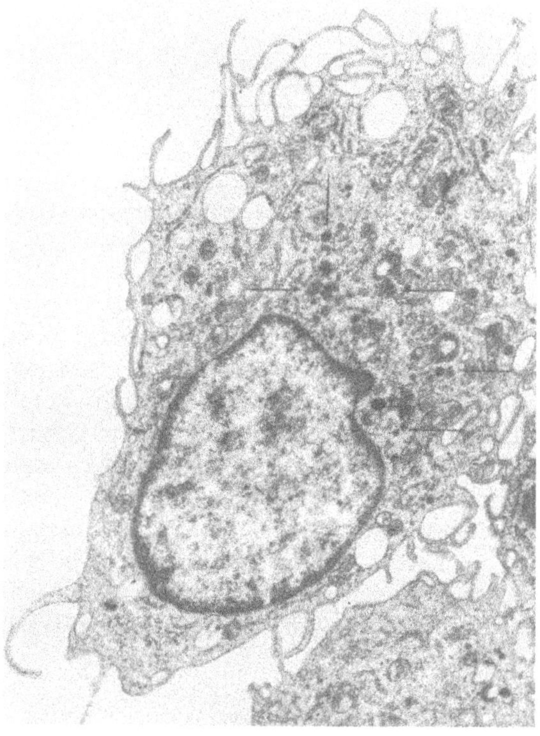

Fig. 6. Macrophage 5 days after intraperitoneal injection of glyceryl trioleate. Many long processes are present, and there are numerous small dense bodies, or lysosomes (arrowed). × 15,000, reduced 40% for reproduction.

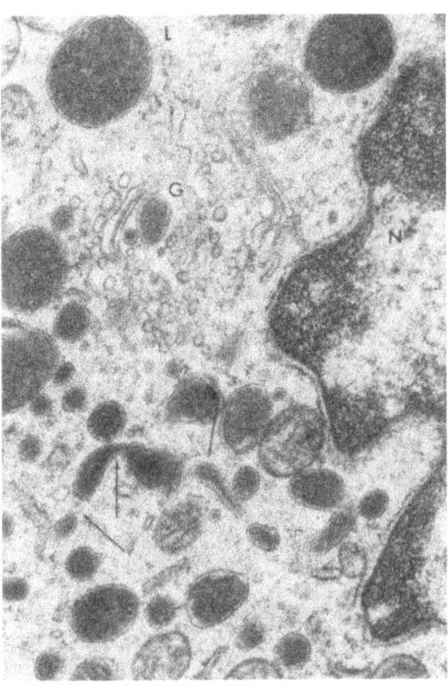

Fig. 7. Cytoplasm of macrophage 5 days after intraperitoneal injection of glyceryl trioleate. There are numerous lysosomes (L). In the Golgi region (G), small bodies of similar structure are present. Elsewhere, lysosomal material is contained within elongated channels (arrowed). Nucleus (N) × 34,000; reduced 40% for reproduction.

(3) Cytochemical Preparations. Control cells showed some reaction for acid phosphatase, and α-naphthyl esterase. Cells stimulated in vivo showed a gross increase in these enzymes (Figs. 3 and 4).

(4) Electron Microscopy. Control preparations (Fig. 5) contained many macrophages, some lymphocytes, and a few mast cells and degenerate mesothelial cells.

After incubation in vitro, macrophages had markedly longer processes; globules of lipid were often closely related to areas where processes were longest.

After stimulation in vivo again macrophages had longer processes (Fig. 6). They now contain more dense bodies. Most of these were clearly primary lysosomes, similar to those seen in control cells, but smaller, and often prominently arranged around the Golgi region of the cell. Granular material was present in the endoplasmic reticulum, and small lysosomes were seen budding from the region of the Golgi apparatus (Fig. 7). A positive acid phosphatase reaction was present in the endoplasmic reticulum, and some, but not all, of the lysosomes.

After intraperitoneal injection of tritiated triglyceride, most cells were labeled after 24 hr, but thereafter the proportion labeled fell off steeply, so that by five days few were labeled, although these were often strongly labeled. After incubation in vitro with tritiated triglyceride, most of the cells in the preparation were strongly labeled at 1 hr. This applied both to macrophages and lymphocytes.

EM autoradiographs of the latter cells showed label associated with the areas of the cell, where the processes were most prominent. Label was also present in nuclei, and less obviously associated with lysosomes, intracellular globules, and mitochondria. Relatively little of the intracellular label was obviously related to particulate lipid. The precise sites of intracytoplasmic lipid await further analysis (Figs. 8 and 9).

DISCUSSION

These experiments show the effect of direct stimulation of a group of RE cells with a potent RE stimulant. It is worth while considering the

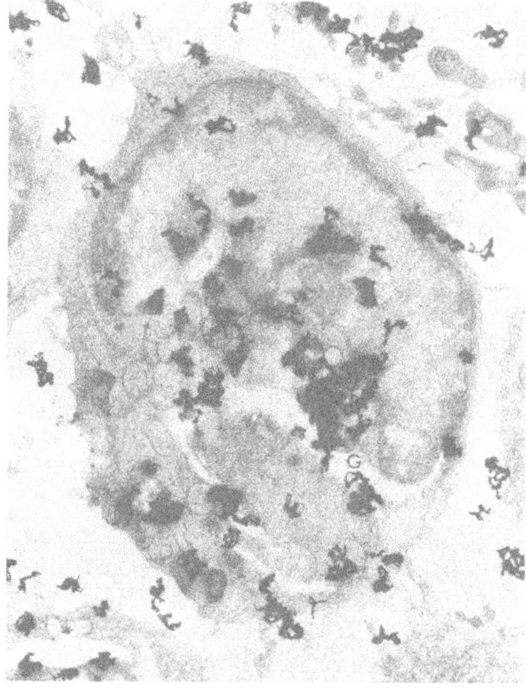

Fig. 8. Macrophage after incubation in vitro for 1 hr with tritiated glyceryl trioleate. Label is present over the nucleus, the Golgi region (G), and apparently over mitochondria. × 20,000; reduced 40% for reproduction.

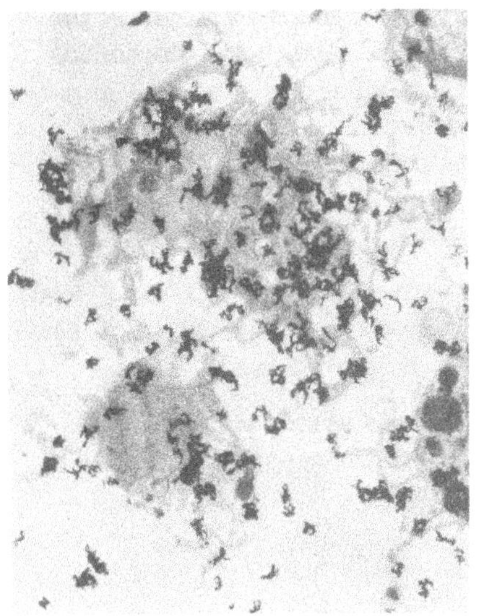

Fig. 9. Tangential section through a macrophage incubated for 1 hr in vitro with tritiated glyceryl trioleate, showing numerous processes, many of them with associated label. × 12,000; reduced 40% for reproduction.

cellular mechanism involved, and the relation between this phenomenon and stimulation of the entire RES.

The stimulated macrophages have much longer processes than normal. The change occurs rapidly, and persists for several days. It may be induced by repeated contact with particles of lipid.

The presence of a high concentration of label where the cellular processes are most prominent suggests that the action of the lipid on the cells is direct. When glucan [12] was used in vitro and in vivo as a stimulant, similar results were obtained [13]. Similar results have been obtained by incubating polymorphs with cocci [14].

The induction of lysosome synthesis by stimulation in vivo with glyceryl trioleate is in general similar to that demonstrated to occur when chicken monocytes are cultured in vitro [15], and when mouse peritoneal macrophages are cultured in vitro or stimulated with lipopolysaccharide [16]. It seems likely that the mode of intracellular production of hydrolytic enzymes is similar to that of other protein products [17-19].

The present experiments also show, despite previous doubts [20], that when glyceryl trioleate acts as a stimulant on RE cells it (or, at any rate, a labeled derivative) enters the cell in considerable amounts. It seems likely that as shown in the case of lymph node cells [21] it would be actively metabolized over a period of 24 hr.

The results produced by stimulation of cells in this experiment conform broadly to those expected on a previous hypothesis on the stimulation of RE cells [6]. Since RE cells all over the body have a basically similar structure, and since, when glyceryl trioleate is administered it is rapidly distributed throughout the body, it seems a reasonable hypothesis for further experiment that similar changes are likely to occur through the RES when it is stimulated.

SUMMARY

When the peritoneal cells of the mouse are stimulated in vitro by incubation with glyceryl trioleate, the cell processes become longer and more prominent. When glyceryl trioleate is injected into the peritoneum of the mouse in vivo, a population of cells appears which have longer processes and more lysosomes. When tritiated glyceryl trioleate is used as a stimulus, label is present in large amounts near the surface of the cells and within them, suggesting that the action on the cells is direct.

ACKNOWLEDGMENTS

This work was made possible by grants to the Department from S. R. C. and M. R. C., and a grant for technical assistance from Unilever, Ltd. One of the authors (M.A. Williams) is supported by a grant from S. R. C.

We are grateful to Professor R. Barer for his advice and criticism, to Dr. G.A. Meek for his guidance on electron microscopy, and to the technical staff of the Department for much help.

REFERENCES

1. A.E. Stuart, G. Biozzi, C. Stiffel, B.N. Halpern, and D. Mouton, Brit.J. Exptl. Pathol., 41: 599, 1960.
2. G.N. Cooper and Dawn West, Austral.J. Exptl. Biol. Med. Sci., 40: 485, 1962.
3. G.N. Cooper and Barbara Houston, Austral.J. Exptl. Biol. Med. Sci., 42: 429, 1964.
4. M.B. Lurie, J. Exptl. Med., 69: 579, 1939.
5. L.P. Weiss and D.W. Fawcett, J. Histochem. Cytochem., 1: 47, 1955.
6. A.M. Dannenberg, Jr., P.C. Walter, and A. Kapral, J. Immunol., 90: 448, 1963.
7. Z.A. Cohn and B. Benson, J. Exptl. Med., 121: 153, 1965.
8. I. Carr, J. Pathol. Bacteriol., in press.
9. A.M. Dannenberg, Jr., M.S. Burstone, P.C. Walter, and J.W. Kinsley, J. Cell Biol., 17: 465, 1963.
10. A.G.E. Pearse, Histochemistry – Theoretical and Applied. London, Churchill, 1961, p. 881.
11. B.G. Achong and M.A. Epstein, J. Roy. Microscop. Soc., 84: 107, 1965.
12. W.R. Wooles and N.R. Di Luzio, J. Reticuloendothelial Soc., 1: 60, 1964.
13. I. Carr, Unpublished.
14. W.R. Lockwood and F. Allison, Brit.J. Exptl. Pathol., 47: 158, 1966.
15. J.S. Sutton and L. Weiss, J. Cell Biol., 28: 303, 1966.
16. Z.A. Cohn, J.G. Hirsch, and M.E. Fedorko, J. Exptl. Med., 123: 747, 1966.
17. C. DeDuve, In: A.V.S. De Reuck and M. Cameron, Eds., Ciba Symposium on Lysosomes. London, Churchill, 1963, pp. 1-31.
18. D. Brandes, J. Ultrastr. Res., 12: 63, 1965.

19. H. Moe, J. Rostgaard, and O. Behnke, J. Ultrastruct. Res., 12:396, 1965.
20. A. Lee and G.N. Cooper, Austral. J. Exptl. Biol. Med. Sci., 42:725, 1964.
21. A.J. Day, N.H. Fidge, P.R.S. Gould-Hurst, M.L. Wahlquist, and G.K. Wilkinson, Quart. J. Exp. Physiol., 51:11, 1966.

Cytodynamics of Rat Lung in Response to Freund's Adjuvant*

Louis J. Casarett, George V. Metzger, and Margaret G. Casarett

Department of Radiation Biology and Biophysics
University of Rochester Medical Center
Rochester, New York

ABSTRACT. This study is part of a larger series related to the origin of the alveolar macrophage and the responsivity of alveolar cells to injected and inhaled stimuli. Alveolar epithelial proliferation has been measured by use of tritiated thymidine in rats which had received one or two injections of Freund's adjuvant. An increase in the rate of DNA synthesis accompanied the proliferative response. Histological and ultrastructural observations are summarized briefly. A similar increase in numbers of alveolar epithelial cells entering mitosis is reported following inhalation of about 25 or 50 μg Fe_2O_3 dust.

INTRODUCTION

The process of clearance of inhaled insoluble particulate material from the lung has an obvious practical significance to public health and environmental toxicology from which has derived a fundamental interest in several facets of pulmonary deposition and retention. Rates of clearance are partially dependent upon the deposition pattern, which is in turn influenced by the physical characteristics of the inhaled material and the physiological parameters of the respiratory system. Clearance pathways are further related to the cellular response of lung parenchyma. Some of the factors influencing pulmonary deposition and retention have been reviewed (Morrow [1], Casarett [2]), and a generalized multifaceted predictive model of lung dynamics has recently appeared (ICRP [3]).

---

* This work was performed under AEC contract W-7401-ENG-49. The technical assistance of Terry McMahon and Karl Emilson is gratefully acknowledged.

Of particular concern in our laboratory has been the role of phagocytosis in lung clearance and the relation of alveolar cells to the etiology of pulmonary disease processes, especially pneumoconioses. It has been shown (LaBelle and Brieger [4]) that increased numbers of alveolar macrophages appear after dust instillation, an event which is consonant with similar observations made by many other investigators and with the frequent observation of accumulated alveolar macrophages around dust deposits prior to development of dust-induced pulmonary lesions (e.g., Schepers et al. [5]).

Based on a variety of experiences with inhalation studies, a working hypothesis was invoked to help explain microscopically observed alveolus-particle relationships (Casarett and Milley [6]). Drawing upon studies in which such small amounts of material were inhaled as to preclude typical pathological responses (e.g. Casarett [7]; Morrow and Casarett [8]), it was postulated that the alveolar epithelium was the source of some of the mobile alveolar cells and that the epithelial cell has a potential phagocytic capability. It was suggested that activation of this potential was accompanied by a cellular differentiation which could be initiated by a variety of stimuli including dust inhalation. This concept was shown not to be inconsistent with electronmicroscopic and autoradiographic observations. Further, preliminary data illustrated a mitotic response of the epithelium to dust loading with microgram quantities of Fe_2O_3. A corollary scheme was presented to relate those physical characteristics of the particle thought to be important in clearance (Morrow et al., [36]) to phagocytosis as a biologically oriented rate-limiting or -determining process for alveolar clearance.

A number of suggestions have been made that stimulation of phagocytic elements of the lung (irrespective of origin) might serve to increase the rate of removal of inhaled noxious agents. Because of the generally described "proliferative" response to adjuvants, these agents were considered despite the pathologic responses reported from them. Among other adjuvants, Hilleman [9] has summarized conclusions about the adjuvant of Freund [10]. Effects of Freund's adjuvant were described by Steiner et al. [11] in rabbits following several routes of administration. Focal granulomas of the lung were described; gross lesions were found only after intravenous injection.

Similar studies have illustrated disseminated lesions in mice, guinea pigs, and hamsters (Laufer et al. [12]) and in rabbits (Ruggs et al. [13]; Moore and Schoenberg [14]). In a particularly pertinent study, Moore and Schoenberg [15] concluded that the increased population of cells in rabbit alveolar spaces in response to adjuvant derived from monocytes of the circulation, mesenchymal cells of the alveolar walls, and epithelial lining cells of the alveoli. Among other findings, these authors pointed out the presence of two types of alveolar living cells similar to those described by Bertalanffy and Leblond [16], and reported a degree of difficulty in distinguishing

Table I. Treatment Schedule

Group	Day of 1st injection	Day of 2nd injection	Days of sacrifice
A	0	none	1, 2, 3, 5, 8, 10, 15
B	0	7	8, 10, 15
C_1*	0	none	1, 3, 5, 8, 11, 13, 15
C_2*	0	7	8, 11, 13, 15
D_1*	0 Saline	none	1, 3, 5, 7
D_2*	0 Saline	7 Saline	8, 11, 13, 15

*Preceded by injection of ^{3}H-thymidine.

them from "macrophages" during some stages after intravenous injection of the adjuvant.

The present study concerns itself with the alveolar response to dust and to Freund's adjuvant in rats at low levels of administration and for short periods after administration. Particular emphasis is on the implications of the response on lung clearance processes.

METHODS AND MATERIALS

A total of 44 male rats of the Rochester strain (Wistar-derived) weighing approximately 200 g were used for the Freund's adjuvant injections. These were divided into three treatment groups, as shown in Table I. Subcutaneous injections of Freund's complete adjuvant* were made on the schedule indicated; the intravenous route was avoided to prevent a high concentration of the adjuvant reaching the lung immediately. Following a series of preliminary injections at levels reported by other workers, 0.01 ml/100 g body weight was selected. It produced no grossly detectable respiratory distress. All injections were made at this level.

Rats were sacrificed by cervical dislocation and sections of lung were taken for light microscopy, fixed in either Susa's fluid, Orth's fixative, or in 10% neutral buffered formalin (for autoradiography). (Other tissues were also taken but are not discussed in this report.) Paraffin sections were made at about 6 μ and were stained routinely in hematoxylin and eosin or Masson's trichrome stain. Rats in series C and D were injected intraperitoneally with 1.0 μc/g body weight of tritiated thymidine 1 hr before sacrifice. Sections were covered with bulk NTB Nuclear Track emulsion,†

*Difco Products Company, Chicago, Ill.
† Eastman Kodak Company, Rochester, N. Y.

exposed from 4 to 14 days at 4°C, and processed in D-19 developer* under proper time and temperature control. Twenty-five randomly selected microscopic fields of lung constituted a single count. A minimum of four counts was made on each animal in the series.

Sections of lung for electron microscopy were fixed either in glutaraldehyde or osmium, or both, embedded in epoxy resin, and sectioned at approximately 500 Å. Some sections were stained with uranyl acetate. Electron microscopic examination was carried out on an RCA-EMU-3 instrument. In an attempt to relate the proliferative response with the postulated multidirectional potential of the alveolar epithelial cell (Casarett and Milley [6]), several histochemical reactions have been applied in this laboratory. Of pertinence here is an ascorbic acid stain, carried out according to the method of Bacchus [17].

Two exposures to Fe_2O_3 dust were carried out. Trace quantities of Fe^{59} permitted estimation of lung burdens as approximately 25 μg for the first and about 50 μg for the second exposure. Both groups were exposed in a chamber described by Leach [18] to an aerosol suspension of the particles with a count median diameter of approximately 0.07 μ and a geometric standard deviation of 1.65. From the first exposure (2 hr, 9 rats),three animals each were sacrificed immediately and at 22 and 122 hr after termination of exposure. From the second exposure (4 hr, 12 rats), three rats were sacrificed at each of the following time intervals: 12, 36, 108, and 278 hr. A control group of 12 rats was similarly "exposed" in the chamber without the addition of the dusty atmosphere. All rats were injected with tritiated thymidine 2 hr before sacrifice and subsequent procedure was equivalent to that described above for the Freund's adjuvant series.

RESULTS

Microscopic findings can be summarized briefly. Generally, early changes were similar to those described for other species. After injection, lungs became hyperemic, alveolar walls became slightly thickened, and small numbers of lymphocytes and polymorphonuclear leukocytes were found in alveolar spaces and septa. Except for a decrease in leukocytes, the response was more pronounced on the second day, subsiding by the fifth to seventh day after the first injection. At this time there were numerous lipoid vacuoles in cells lining alveoli and in cells within alveolar walls. Increased cellularity of the alveolar surfaces became apparent and took the form of more numerous rounded epithelial cells, and was accompanied by increased numbers of cells in alveolar spaces in some areas of the sections examined.

---

* Eastman Kodak Company, Rochester, N.Y.

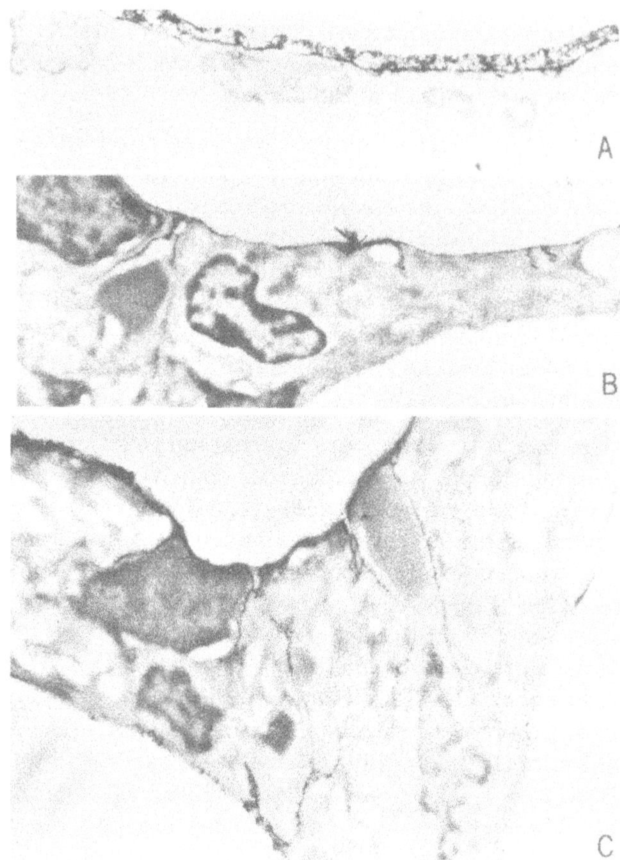

Fig. 1. A. Alveolar epithelial reaction to ascorbic acid stain. B,C. Minimal response to Freund's adjuvant. Ascorbic acid stain.

After the second injection, the changes described above were more pronounced, occurred earlier, and persisted to the end of the time period studied. During this second week, as during the week following the first injection, the alveolar epithelial cells became more rounded and, as the numbers increased, the cells of the lining tended to assume a cuboidal shape.

With the appearance of patches of cells which had become cuboidal in shape, one could find an increase in vacuoles and, more often, bits of osmophilic material contained in the vacuoles. The impression was gained that there was an increasing gradation of vacuolization and appearance of electron-dense material in the vacuoles from the flattened epithelial cell through a transition state of partially rounding cells, those becoming cuboidal to the fully rounded "free" cell. Cells in alveolar walls, other than blood leukocytes, showed an ultrastructure not dissimilar to the partially rounded alveolar epithelial cell. Small collections of cells in interstitial regions were viewed as suggestive of the granulomas reported (Moore and Schoenberg [15]) for longer periods of time after administration of adjuvant to rabbits.

Ascorbic acid-stained material showed a positive reaction in control tissues predominantly along alveolar surfaces. Although there were some cytoplasmic invaginations extending beneath the basement membrane and intra-alveolar membranes which showed positive reactions, these were relatively weak and infrequent. The thin or slightly thickened cytoplasmic extensions of flattened alveolar epithelial cells showed a markedly greater reaction. A typical example is shown in Fig. 1A.

Following Freund's adjuvant, particularly after the second injection, there was an increased frequency of staining within the alveolar walls. Although the intensity of reaction was variable, it appeared that significant parts of cell membranes (often of whole cells) were stained. These cells were generally indistinguishable from alveolar epithelial cells. A representative view of a minimal reaction is shown in Fig. 1B, C. Alveolar epithelial cells continued to show a positive reaction. During periods when there was an increase in the rounded type of epithelial cell with partially retracted cytoplasm, the cell surfaces facing the air interface continued to stain positively. Where an apparent detachment from the basement membrane seemed to be in progress, there was little or no reaction at the underlying surface. Where sufficient numbers of cells were present to give a cuboidal appearance to the cells, there was a reaction at the air surface approximately equivalent to that observed in controls with a less intense reaction in the membranes separating adjacent cells.

The results of measurement of DNA synthetic rate by alveolar epithelial cells is shown in Fig. 2. Control values did not vary significantly and

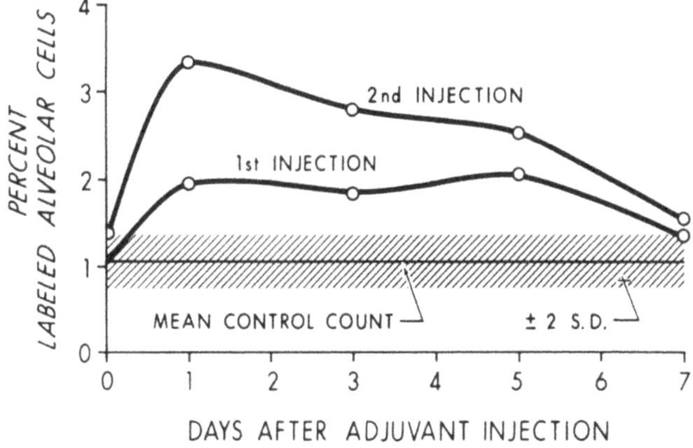

Fig. 2. Labeling of alveolar epithelium with ^{3}H-thymidine after injection of Freund's adjuvant.

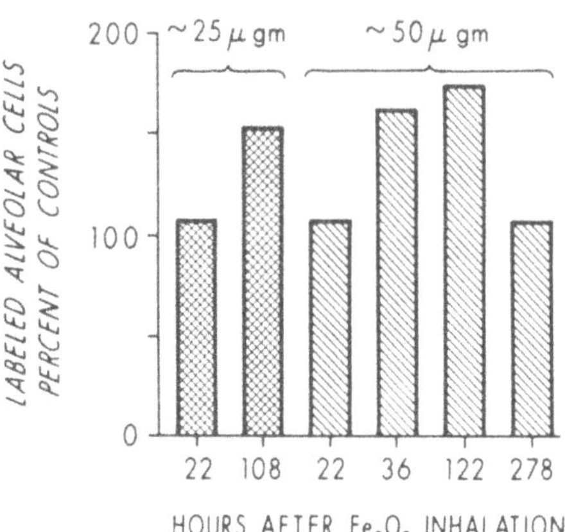

Fig. 3. Alveolar response to Fe_2O_3 inhalation. ^{3}H-tymidine labeling.

are plotted as a mean value ± two standard deviations. It will be noted that there is a significant increase in the percentage of alveolar cells which are synthesizing DNA, presumably preparatory to division. A peak is reached in 3-5 days and the index of mitotic activity falls to control levels by seven days after the first injection.

The 7-day point has been plotted as the zero time value for the second injection series. It appears that the response to the second injection is more prompt, apparently reaching a higher peak at a somewhat earlier time. Although subsiding, mitotic activity has not returned to control levels at seven days after the second injection.

The effects of inhaled dust on the mitotic activity of alveolar epithelium can be seen in Figs. 3 and 4. In the bar graph (Fig. 3) the number of labeled cells found at the specified time intervals after deposition of approximately 25 or 50 μg of the dust in the lung is expressed as a percent of the control values. In both exposures there is a significant increase in thymidine incorporation about five days later with a borderline significance at about 36 hr after the higher quantity of dust. At 10 days after the second exposure, mitotic activity has essentially returned to control values.

In Fig. 4, data are expressed in another way. The mean number of photographic grains in labeled cells is taken as an index of the rapidity of DNA synthesis and therefore a reflection of mitotic activity. Control values for the entire series are plotted on the ordinate (±2 S.D.). Note a significant increase in activity as early as 36 hr after inhalation in the higher-level exposure (II). No equivalent point was obtained for the first exposure (I). Irrespective of the size of the quantity deposited in the lung, this method of expression suggests an equivalent peak of both curves about 5 days after exposure. At 10 days postinhalation, the rate of thymidine incorporation has reached nearly control levels.

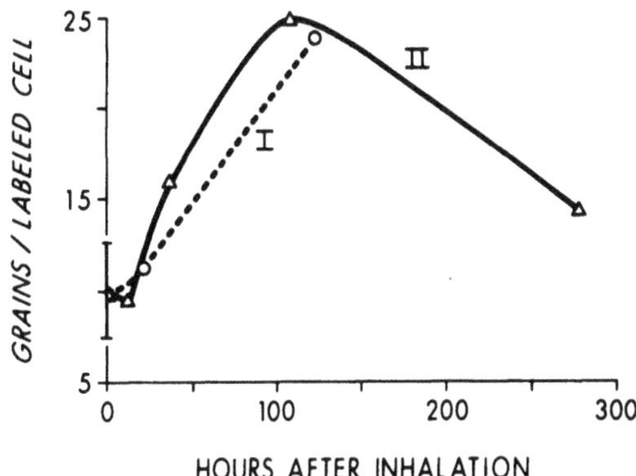

Fig. 4. Rate of ^{3}H-thymidine uptake by alveolar epithelium after Fe_2O_3 inhalation.

DISCUSSION

Although not specifically designed to answer questions about the origin of the alveolar macrophage, these studies have some bearing on the subject. That the alveolar epithelium might be a source of alveolar macrophages has been suggested for some years (Briscoe [19]; Sewell [20]; Carleton [21]). Much evidence has been derived from morphological similarities of cell structure or response to injection of relatively large amounts of particulate material. Inhalation of particles in small quantities has been postulated as an initiation for alveolar epithelial participation in pulmonary clearance processes (Casarett [7] and Casarett et al. [22]). In most studies, the concept of differentiation (or de-differentiation) has been explicitly stated, postulated, or, at least, is implicit in the conclusions drawn from the observations.

There appears to be no question about the phenomenon of "rounding up" and detachment of alveolar epithelial cells. This, in itself, suggests functional change. Along with demonstration of this process in unfixed tissue (Krahl [23, 24]), it has been suggested that the alveolar epithelium has an adaptability to multiple roles. Similar observations have been made in this laboratory with fresh newborn mouse lung subjected to UO_2 particles (unpublished). Questions about these cells as a source of alveolar macrophages usually concern ultrastructural differences in cells found in alveoli, variable degrees of evidence for their phagocytic role, and their relation to embryonic origin. A full discussion of these questions is beyond the scope of this paper, but some aspects of the results complement the view of the alveolar epithelium as a source of alveolar phagocytic cells.

The increase in macrophages after Freund's adjuvant reported for other species (Moore and Schoenberg [15]; Laufer et al. [12]) also occurs in the rat and at short intervals of time after injection. Description of cellular changes have led to conclusions of proliferation of two or more different types of cells. Observations in the present study can as readily be interpreted as a cellular differentiation process. The gradation of ultrastructural change reported here and elsewhere is consonant with a cellular differentiation and multidirectional movement of epithelial cells either into alveolar walls or spaces (Casarett and Milley [6]). This is further supported by descriptions of responses to Freund's adjuvant. Such descriptions point out the inability to distinguish ultrastructural identity of the two cell types at periods of greatest response (i.e., proliferation). It is reasonable to expect that the greater the response, the more rapid would differentiation occur and thus, difficulty would be encountered in identifying two cell types. Before maximal response and upon subsidence, one might postulate a slower or less extensive change and the apparent reemergence of the two cell types. Although the ascorbic acid stain might have no particular specificity or significance in itself, the pattern of staining adds further support to the concept of epithelial proliferation followed by entrance into the alveolar wall.

The observations reported here and elsewhere by the present authors are substantiated by other reports in recent years. For example, the detailed studies of Nagaishi et al. [25] and Kitamura [26], although not entirely confirmatory of the potential phagocytic capability of all alveolar cells, present considerable evidence for a functional differentiation of alveolar epithelial cells, part of which points to response of the epithelium to dust. The excellent ultrastructural studies by Karrer [27-29], although pointing out the differences in relative amounts of phagocytosed material between epithelial cells and macrophages, did, in fact, show presumably phagocytosed material in epithelial cells. Karrer further leaves open the question of transformation of epithelial cell to macrophage while emphasizing that the physiological properties of the two cells types must be quite different.

The observations of Schoenberg and others after Freund's adjuvant, other ultrastructural reports cited above as well as some aspects of studies by other investigators (Low and Sampaio [30]; Woodside and Dalton [37]), support the possibility of a transformation of alveolar epithelial cell to alveolar macrophage. Further indirect support is given by the fact that the mitotic activity of the epithelium was demonstrably responsive to injection of Freund's adjuvant, and that the response paralleled the qualitative observations of cellular change in structure and number.

The distinction between two types of alveolar cells and the two turnover rates described by Bertalanffy and Leblond [16], and presumably confirmed with a ^{3}H-thymidine technique (Shorter et al. [31]) could not be established in the present study. The two turnover rates might have a number of interpretations. One of these must distinguish between flux of labeled cells in connective tissue (and some entry into alveoli) and proliferative activity of dividing or differentiating fixed interstitial forms. Similarly, whether the two morphological types of cells are distinct or differentiated forms of one cell line (e.g., alveolar epithelium), one could also obtain two turnover rates based on a difference between sessile or "germinal" cells and mobile (presumably more highly differentiated) forms of the same cell type.

Perhaps of more pertinence is the response of alveolar epithelium to inhaled dust. The results using tritiated thymidine are comparable to those previously reported using colchicine (Casarett and Milley [6]). Ross [32] had concluded that appreciable response of the epithelium was achieved only with toxic substances, and that the cells were not phagocytic. The amount of dust deposited in this study can hardly be considered large or toxic, and an equivalent mass of radioactive Fe_2O_3 has been shown to produce no response which could be considered "pathologic" (Casarett and Epstein [33]). Thus, the alveolar epithelium must be considered to be responsive to innocuous dusts. It is highly unlikely that such a response could occur without some interaction between particles and cells, and the most reasonable interaction is that of engulfing whether by phagocytic or pinocytotic activity. Although the squamous epithelial cell might not be actively phagocytic, the rounded alveolar epithelial cell might well represent a functionally differentiating cell form with an increased phagocytic potential.

Whatever the cellular interpretation, however, it is clear that priming of the alveolar cell population has an effect on pulmonary clearance of particulate material. LaBelle and Brieger [34] described an increased rate of clearance of radioactive particles following pretreatment with other particle populations. The change of clearance was accompanied by increased alveolar cellularity. Similar increase of clearance was observed by Ferin et al. [35] after pretreatment with trypan blue or TiO_2 up to four days prior to exposure to a test dose of SiO_2. In the latter study, there was also an increase in free cells after the pretreatment.

Contribution to the cell population of alveoli by subepithelial tissue cannot be dismissed. It would appear, however, that some contribution by the alveolar epithelium is also likely and that the differentiation of alveolar epithelial cells into so-called alveolar macrophages remains a distinct possibility. It can be suggested that the relative contributions of cells are dependent upon the type and severity of the stimulus used to bring about a response sufficiently exaggerated to allow study. It can further be offered that, with conditions more closely approaching normalcy, i.e., with less destructive stimuli, the relative contribution of the alveolar epithelium is increased. The extension of this idea suggests, finally, that in the "normal" physiological state, the free cellular constitution of alveoli is comprised of a highly significant fraction of cells derived from the epithelium.

REFERENCES

1. P.E. Morrow, "Some physical and physiological factors controlling the fate of inhaled substances. I. Deposition." Health Phys., 2:379-386, 1960.
2. L.J. Casarett, "Some physical and physiological factors controlling the fate of inhaled substances. II. Retention." Health Phys., 2:379-386, 1960.
3. International Commission on Radiation Protection, Committee II. Report by Task Group on Lung Dynamics, P.E. Morrow, Chairman. Health Phys., 12:173-208, 1966.
4. C.W. LaBelle and H. Brieger, "Basic physiologic mechanisms in the pulmonary response to inhaled particulates." Intern. Congr. on Occup. Health, 13th, 730-735, 1960.
5. G.W.H. Schepers, T.M. Durkan, A.B. Delahant, F.T. Creedon, and A.J. Redlin, "The biological action of Degussa submicron amorphous silica dust." Arch. Ind. Health, 16:125-146, 1957.
6. L.J. Casarett and P.S. Milley, "Alveolar reactivity following inhalation of particles." Health Phys., 10:1003-1011, 1964.
7. L.J. Casarett, "Distribution and excretion of polonium-210. XII. Autoradiographic observations after inhalation of Po-210." Radiation Res. Suppl., 5:187-204, 1964.
8. P.E. Morrow and L.J. Casarett, "An experimental study of the deposition and retention of a plutonium-239 dioxide aerosol," in: Inhaled Particles and Vapors, New York, Pergamon Press, 1961, pp. 167-175.
9. M.R. Hilleman, "A forward look at viral vaccines." Am. Rev. Respirat. Diseases, 90:683-706, 1964.
10. J. Freund, "The mode of action of immunologic adjuvants." Advan. Tuberc. Res., 7:130-142, 1956.
11. J.W. Steiner, B. Langer, and D.L. Schotz, "The local and systemic effects of Freund's adjuvant and its fractions." Arch. Pathol., 70:424-434, 1960.
12. A. Laufer, C. Tal, and A.J. Behar, "Effect of adjuvant (Freund's type) and its components on the organs of various animal species." Brit. J. Exptl. Pathol., 40:1-7, 1959.
13. J.C. Ruggs, R.D. Moore, and M.D. Schoenberg, "Stimulation of the reticuloendothelial system in the rabbit by Freund's adjuvant." Arch. Pathol., 70:43-49, 1960.
14. R.D. Moore and M.D. Schoenberg, "Modification of cellular proliferation of the reticuloendothelial system in the rabbit." Exptl. Cell Res., 30:301-310, 1963.
15. R.D. Moore and M.D. Schoenberg, "Alveolar lining cells and pulmonary reticuloendothelial system of the rabbit." Am. J. Pathol., 45:991-1006, 1964.

16. F.D. Bertalanffy and C.P. Leblond, "The continuous renewal of the two types of alveolar cells in the lung of the rat." Anat. Rec., 115: 515-542, 1953.
17. H. Bacchus, "Cytochemical study of the adrenal cortex of the rat under salt stresses." Am.J.Physiol., 163: 326-331, 1950.
18. L.J. Leach, "A laboratory test chamber for studying airborne materials." University of Rochester Atomic Energy Project Report, UR-629, 1963.
19. J.C. Briscoe, "An experimental investigation of the phagocytic action of the alveolar cells of the lung." J.Pathol.Bacteriol., 12: 66-100, 1908.
20. W.T. Sewell, "The phagocytic properties of the alveolar cells of the lung." J.Pathol.Bacteriol., 22: 40-55, 1918.
21. H.M. Carleton, "The pulmonary lesions produced by the inhalation of dusts in guinea pigs." J.Hyg., 22: 438-472, 1924.
22. L.J. Casarett, P.E. Morrow, and F.R. Gibb, "Autoradiographic study of the distribution of plutonium-239 following inhalation." Industrial Health Conference, Chicago (Abstract), 1959.
23. V.E. Krahl, "The expansion of pulmonary alveoli in the newborn mouse. Motion pictures." Anat. Rec., 115:448 (Abstract), 1953.
24. V.E. Krahl, "Current concept of the finer structure of the lung." Arch. Internal Med., 96: 342-356, 1955.
25. C. Nagaishi, Y. Okada, S. Ishiko, and S. Daido, "Electron microscopic observations of the pulmonary alveoli." Exptl. Med. Surg., 22: 81-117, 1964.
26. H. Kitamura, "The fine structure of lung alveoli and its reactions." Acta Pathol.Japan., 14: 147-167, 1964.
27. H.E. Karrer, "The ultrastructure of mouse lung; general architecture of capillary and alveolar walls." J. Biophys. Biochem.Cytol., 2: 241-252 (1956).
28. H.E. Karrer, "The ultrastructure of the mouse lung; the alveolar macrophage." J.Biophys.Biochem.Cytol., 4: 693-700, 1958.
29. H.E. Karrer, "Electron microscopic study of the phagocytic process in lung." J.Biophys.Biochem.Cytol., 7: 357-366, 1960.
30. F.N. Low and M.M. Sampaio, "The pulmonary alveolar epithelium as an entodermal derivative." Anat.Rec., 127:51-64, 1957.
31. R.G. Shorter, J.L. Titus, and M.B. Divertie, "Cell turnover in the respiratory tract." Diseases Chest, 46: 138-142, 1964.
32. I.S. Ross, "Pulmonary epithelium and proliferative reactions in the lungs." Arch. Pathol., 27: 478-496, 1939.
33. L.J. Casarett and B. Epstein, "Deposition and fate of inhaled iron-59 oxide in rats." Am.Ind.Hyg.Assoc.J. (in press, 1966).
34. C.W. LaBelle and H. Brieger, "Synergistic effects of aerosols. II. Effects on rate of clearance from the lung." Arch.Ind.Health, 20: 100-105, 1959.

35. J. Ferin, G. Urbonkova, and A. Vlckova, "Pulmonary clearance and the function of macrophages." Arch. Environ. Health, 10 : 790–795, 1965.
36. P. E. Morrow, F. R. Gibb, and L. Johnson, "Clearance of insoluble dust from the lower respiratory tract." Health Phys., 10 : 543–555, 1964.
37. G. L. Woodside and A. J. Dalton, "The ultrastructure of lung tissue from newborn and embryo mice." J. Ultrastruct. Res., 2:28, 1958.
38. P. E. Morrow, M. Fisher, and F. R. Gibb, "The use of lung analogs in the study of pulmonary clearance mechanisms." John A. Hartford Foundation Conference on Air Pollution and the Lung, NYU and Bellevue Hospital, 1966.

Esterase Histochemistry of Reticuloendothelial Cells

Bryan Ballantyne

Department of Anatomy, School of Medicine
University of Leeds
Leeds, Yorkshire, England

Although other reports on the histochemical distribution of esterases in lymphoid tissue have been published [1, 2, 3], these have led to some confusion because of differences in (1) the descriptions of the distribution of such esterases and their fine localization, and (2) the interpretation of the possible functional significance of such enzyme systems. Some of these differences are accounted for by species variations [4], and others are possibly results of technical artifacts. This report deals with a controlled histochemical investigation of the distribution of cholinesterases and nonspecific esterases in lymph nodes, spleen, and liver from rabbits. The results are interpreted in terms of a function for macrophage and endothelial esterases in lipid metabolism and detoxification mechanisms.

MATERIALS AND METHODS

Lymph nodes, spleen, and liver were obtained from adult male and female Flemish Giant and albino rabbits killed by an overdose of intravenously administered sodium pentobarbitone. The nodes were taken from the parotid area, mesentery, and axilla. In some animals, specimens were removed immediately after death and transferred to the fixative fluid. In

Table I. Optimum pH_S and Incubation Times for the Histochemical Demonstration of RE Cholinesterases Using a 0.1 M Tris + 0.1 N HCl Buffer System

Tissue	AChE		BChE	
	pH_S	Incubation time, hr	pH_S	Incubation time, hr
Lymph node	5.7	1	5.4	4
Spleen	5.7	1	5.4	5
Liver	5.5	4	5.4	6

others, the vascular pattern of the tissues was first outlined by perfusion with 2% Berlin Blue [5] and the tissues then removed for fixation. After fixation for 16-18 hr in cold 4% formaldehyde-saline, sections were cut at thicknesses of from 16 to 200 μ in a cryostat at −25°C. Sites of cholinesterase activity were demonstrated by a modified [5] Koelle technique [6] using acetylthiocholine iodide as the substrate for acetylcholinesterase (AChE; syn. specific cholinesterase, true cholinesterase, acetylcholine hydrolase 3.1.1.7), and n-butyrylthiocholine iodide for butyrylcholinesterase (BChE; syn. nonspecific cholinesterase, pseudocholinesterase, acylcholine acyl hydrolase 3.1.1.8). Sites of enzyme localization were revealed by the use of fresh, dilute ammonium sulphide, and the sections were mounted in Canada Balsam in tetrachlorethylene [7]. The best localization of enzymes was obtained by the use of an 0.1 M 2-amino-2-(hydroxymethyl)-propane-1:3-diol/ 0.1 N HCl buffer system in the incubating medium [8]. The optimum substrate pH values* and incubation times are shown in Table I. As a check on the types of cholinesterases present, some sections were incubated in the presence of $1 \cdot 10^{-5}$ M physostigmine to inhibit all cholinesterase activity [9], $1 \cdot 10^{-5}$ M 1,5-bis(4-trimethylammonium phenyl)-pentan-3-one di-iodide (BW62C47) to inhibit AChE [10], or $2 \cdot 10^{-5}$ M N,N-diisopropylphosphorodiamidic fluoride (Mipafox) to inhibit BChE [11]. The effect of preincubation in $1 \cdot 10^{-6}$ M tetraethyl pyrophosphate (TEPP) was also determined in some sections.

Sites of nonspecific esterase (NSE) were localized by the α-naphthyl acetate [12], the bromoindoxyl acetate [13], and the hexazonium pararosaniline [14] techniques. Some of the sections were preincubated in $1 \cdot 10^{-5}$ and $1 \cdot 10^{-2}$ M diethyl p-nitrophenyl phosphate (E-600) or $1 \cdot 10^{-6}$ M TEPP.

OBSERVATIONS

In lymph nodes AChE is restricted to the cortex, and is present in the marginal sinus, submarginal vessels, nodules, and the outer diffuse lymphoid tissue (Fig. 1). In the marginal sinus the enzyme is present in high concentration in cells with elongated processes, some of which completely line the inner aspect of the marginal sinus, others extend across the sinus toward the capsule (Fig. 2); the capsule itself is devoid of AChE. In the submarginal cortex AChE is present in the walls of capillaries and post-capillary venules, and appears to be present in the cytoplasm of the endothelial cells (Figs. 1-3). The reaction in nodules is present at the periphery of

---

* The term substrate pH value (pH_S) is used to refer to the pH of the final incubating medium used in a histochemical reaction, and thus gives a true index of the optimum histochemical pH of the enzyme system. The pH of a buffer (pH_B) added to an incubating medium may be only a rough guide to the optimum pH of the enzyme system, since there are often differences between pH_S and pH_B.

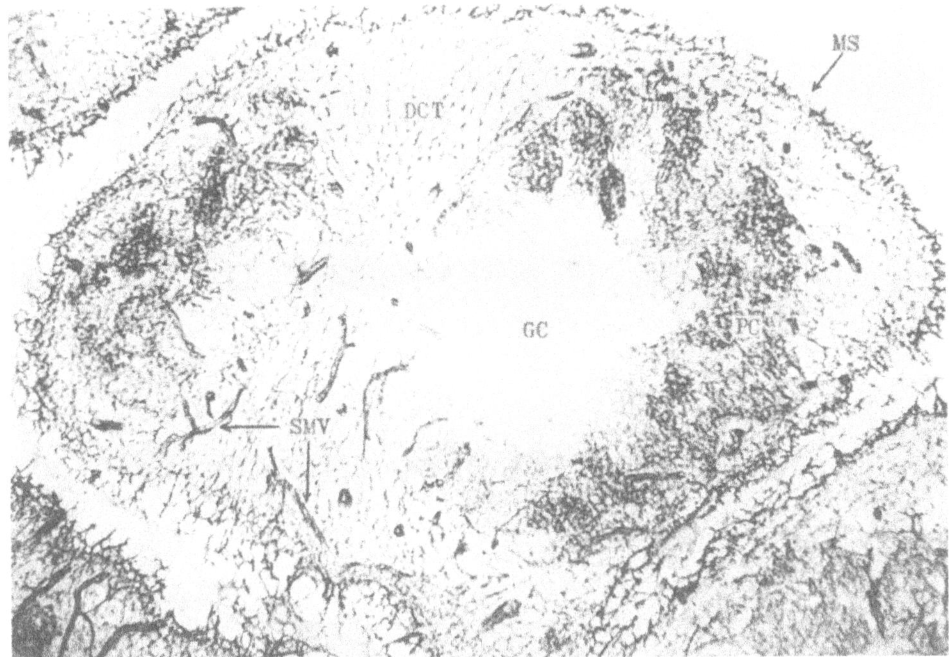

Fig. 1. Section through a portion of the cortex of a lymph node showing the distribution of AChE. Note: (1) activity in the marginal sinus (MS); (2) activity in submarginal vessels (SMV); (3) the reaction in the outer diffuse lymphoid tissue (DCT); and (4) intense activity in the submarginal polar cap (PC) of the nodule, the germinal center being devoid of activity (GC). Section thickness 16 μ; × 101.

these structures, with a marked concentration of AChE positive material toward the capsule, forming a submarginal cap to the nodule; the germinal centers are devoid of activity (Fig. 3). In the outer diffuse cortical lymphoid tissue the enzyme is present in structures arranged in the form of a fine, loose network (Figs. 1, 3). Sections treated with physostigmine, 62C47, and TEPP show no activity; Mipafox does not affect the reaction.

BChE has a distribution identical to that of AChE in the cortex of lymph nodes, but is present in histochemically lower concentrations. The only other site of BChE activity is in nerve fibers which form periarterial plexuses in the medulla (Fig. 4).

NSE, which can be demonstrated with all of the techniques used, and which is sensitive to E-600 and TEPP, is present in the cortex and medulla of lymph nodes. In the cortex, activity is present in cells in the marginal sinus with a distribution like that of AChE. A reaction is also shown by submarginal capillaries and postcapillary venules, and by macrophages scattered through the nodules and diffuse cortical lymphoid tissue (Fig. 5). In the medulla NSE is present in cells which are arranged mainly along the outer borders of the medullary cords (Fig. 6). While all the NSE activity

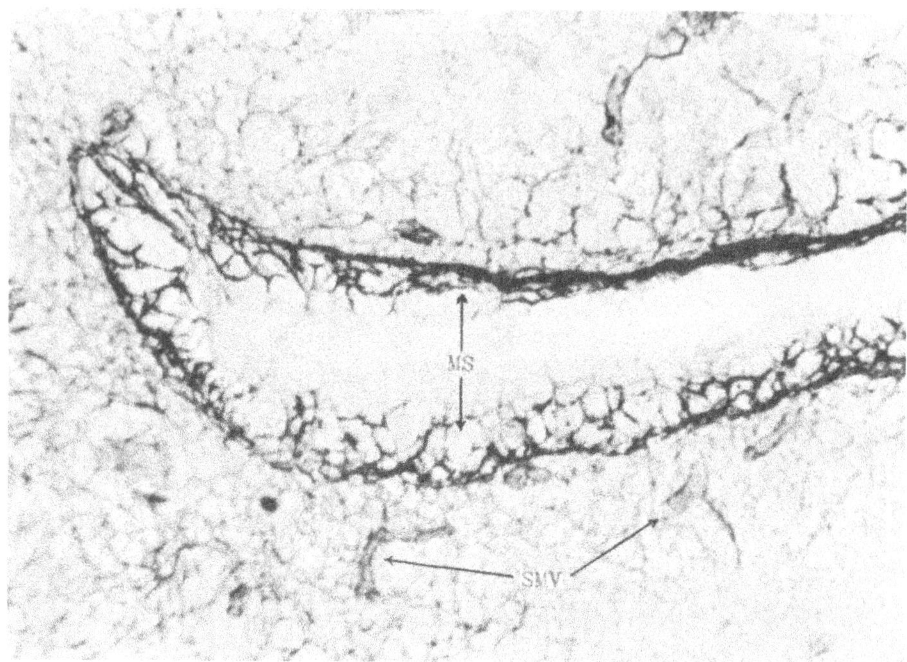

Fig. 2. AChE in the marginal sinus (MS) and submarginal vessels (SMV) of two opposed portions of lymph node cortex. In the marginal sinus, note the activity in the processes crossing the sinus, and the continuous band of activity along the inner side of the sinus. The capsule is devoid of activity. Section thickness 16 μ; × 186.

in the nodes is inhibited by $1 \cdot 10^{-6}$ M TEPP, the cortical enzyme is sensitive to $1 \cdot 10^{-5}$ M E-600 but the medullary enzyme only to $1 \cdot 10^{-2}$ M E-600.

In the spleen, AChE is limited to follicles. It occurs here both in capillaries, where it is apparently localized to the endothelium, and in the cytoplasm of cells with elongated processes (Fig. 7). These processes pervade the whole of the follicle and at its periphery encompass it. The enzyme is sensitive to physostigmine, 62C47, and TEPP; Mipafox has no effect on the development of the reaction. An apparent slight reaction with butyrylthiocholine iodide substrate is shown by the capillaries and reticular processes of the follicle. This reaction, however, is completely inhibited by the incorporation of 62C47 in the incubating medium, indicating that the reaction is due to a breakdown of the substrate by AChE. The only sites of true BChE are in nerve fibers which form periarterial plexuses throughout the spleen up to, and including, the follicular artery.

NSE, again demonstrable by all techniques and sensitive to E-600 and TEPP, is widely distributed through the spleen. Activity is present in the cells lining the sinusoids (Fig. 8), in cells scattered through the cords of Billroth, and in cells in the follicles. The last are evenly distributed through-

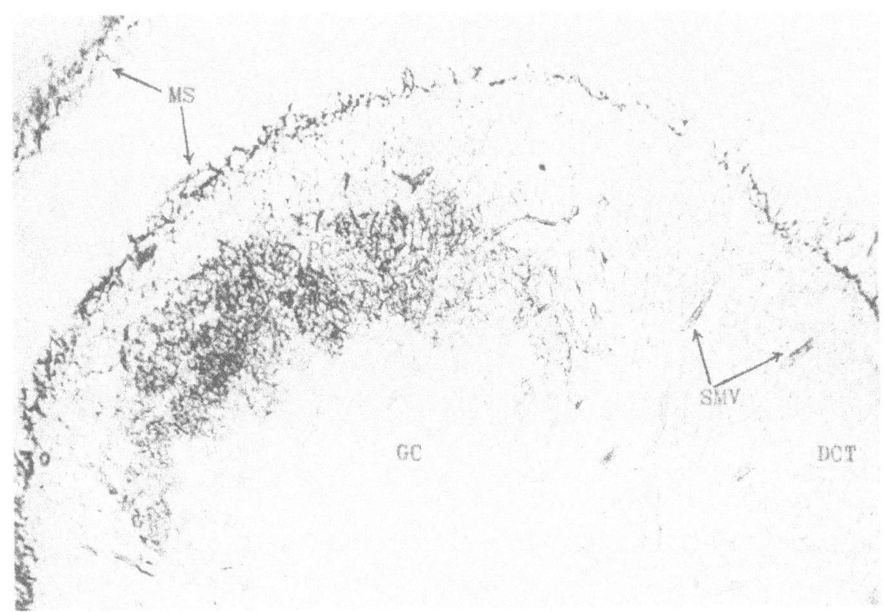

Fig. 3. AChE in a segment of lymph node cortex showing the typical distribution of the enzyme in marginal sinus (MS), submarginal vessels (SMV), outer diffuse tissue (DCT), and the submarginal cap (PC) to the nodule. The germinal center of the nodule (GC) is devoid of activity. Section thickness 16 μ; × 123.

out the follicle. An occasional faint reaction is shown by capillaries in the follicles, but this is exceptional. The NSE in the cells lining the sinusoids is inhibited by $1 \cdot 10^{-5}$ M E-600, but that in the follicles and cords of Billroth only by $1 \cdot 10^{-2}$ M E-600. The NSE activity at all sites in the spleen is sensitive to $1 \cdot 10^{-6}$ M TEPP.

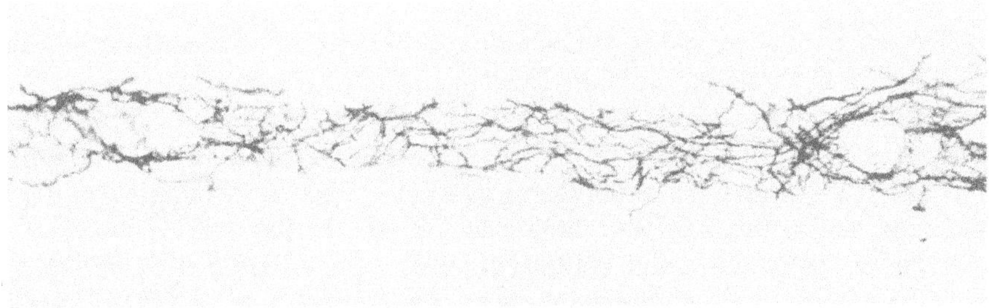

Fig. 4. BChE in nerve fibers which are arranged as a perivascular plexus around a medullary artery. The surrounding tissue of the medulla is devoid of activity. Section thickness 16 μ; × 135.

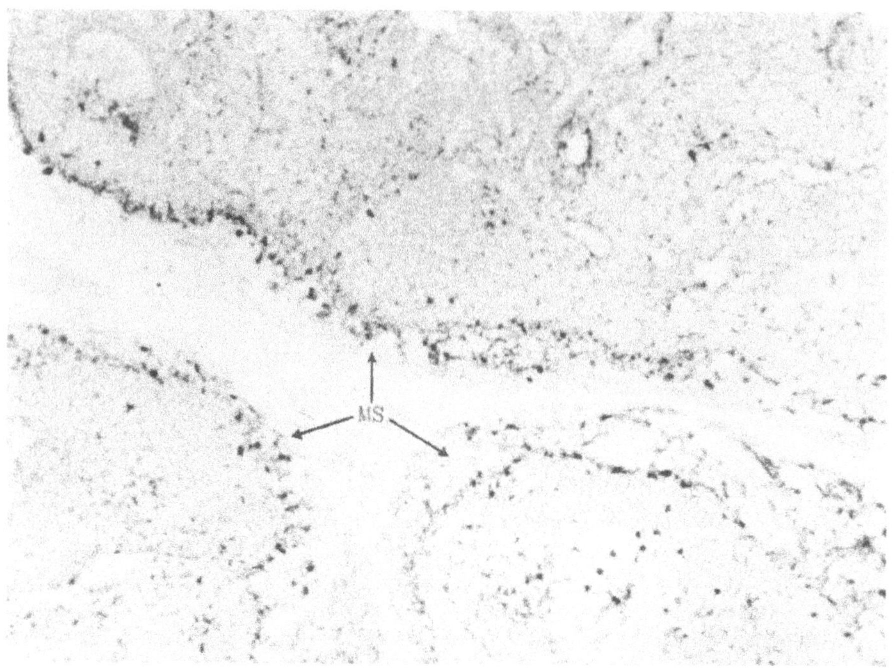

Fig. 5. Distribution of NSE in the marginal sinus (MS) of three opposed portions of cortical lymphoid tissue. Activity can also be seen in cells scattered through the submarginal cortex. α-Naphthyl acetate technique. Section thickness 20 μ; × 55.

AChE in the liver is present only in cells lining the sinusoids of (hexagonal) lobules. The cells showing this reaction are centri- and midlobular in position (Fig. 9). It can be demonstrated by experiments involving the use of intravitam India ink [7, 15] that the enzyme is present in phagocytic RE cells. Such preparations show that enzyme activity is closely related to colloidal particles in the phagocytic cells lining the sinusoids. These cells appear negative for BChE and NSE.

DISCUSSION

The vascular, probably endothelial, localization of the esterases is readily seen in those animals injected with Berlin Blue intravascularly. It has been suggested that esterases in endothelium are derived from blood plasma [16], but this seems unlikely, since the enzymes are not ubiquitously present throughout the endothelial system. They are found only in certain areas of lymphoid tissue, localized regions of the central nervous system [17], placenta [16], and hypophysis [16]. In addition, although the endothelial cholinesterase of lymphoid tissue in the rabbit is principally AChE, the main plasma enzyme in this animal is propionylcholinesterase [18]. Hence, it seems reasonable to consider that the vascular esterases are

Fig. 6. NSE in the medulla of a lymph node. Activity is present in cells which are arranged mainly on the outer surfaces of the medullary cords. α-Naphthyl acetate technique; section thickness 20 μ; × 52.

formed in situ. Similarly, it is believed that the esterases in the marginal sinuses are synthesized by the cells containing the enzymes and are not derived from afferent lymph, since some tissues draining into first regional nodes with high marginal sinus activity have themselves little cholinesterase [4]. The enzymes in the marginal sinus are not considered to be present in reticular fibers [2, 16], but are located in the cytoplasmic processes of cells which have been demonstrated by electron microscopy to cover the reticular fibers in the sinus [19]. Similarly, it is believed that the AChE in the outer diffuse cortical tissue of lymph nodes and in the follicles of spleen is also present in the cytoplasm of cells with attenuated, elongated processes, and is not present in reticular fibers. The sinusoidal and phagocytic nature of the AChE-containing cells in liver has been clearly shown. Although these hepatic RE cells do not appear to contain histochemically detectable amounts of BChE and NSE, low levels of activity cannot be excluded because of the overshadowing high concentrations of these enzymes in adjacent hepatocytes. Experiments are to be undertaken to fractionate the hepatic RE element [20] and quantitatively determine its enzyme content.

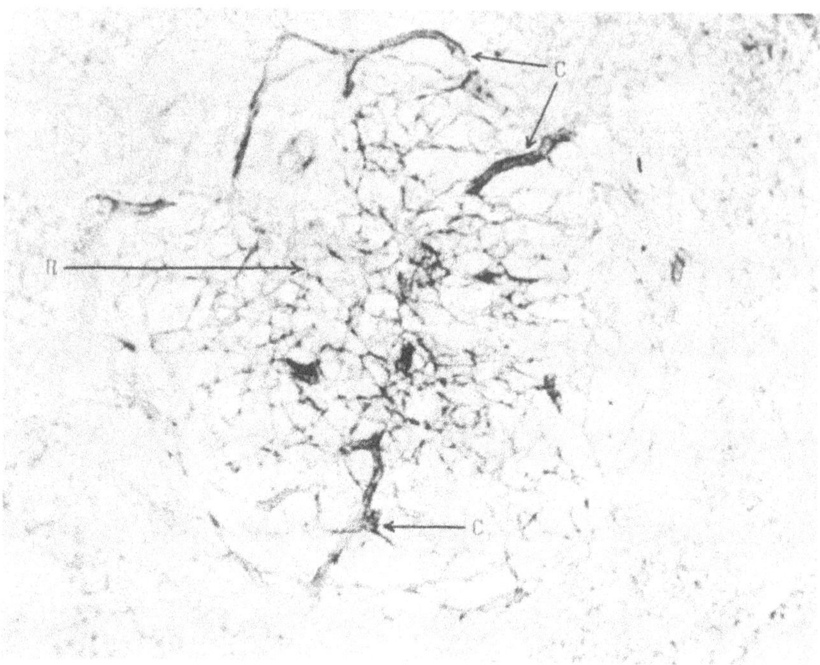

Fig. 7. AChE in a follicle of the spleen. Activity is present in capillaries (C) and the cytoplasmic processes (R) of cells which pervade the whole follicle. Section thickness 16 μ ; $\times$ 185.

In interpreting the results obtained from lymph nodes, attention has been paid to the observation that there exists a correlation between the mitotic activity of differentiated tissues and their degrees of lymphatic drainage [21]. In view of this, some potentially toxic esters which have been produced as a result of lipid metabolism during mitosis in a tissue may be passing in the afferent lymphatics from the tissue to its first regional node [4, 22]. A large number of such toxic choline- and noncholine-containing esters could be inactivated by the enzymes in the marginal sinus or submarginal vessels, since it is now clear that the esterase group of enzymes can act on a wide spectrum of substrates [23]. The cholinesterases in cortical nodules could have a similar function in respect to esters produced in the germinal centers.

Although the above concept could hold for tissues which drain directly into regional lymph nodes, the means by which toxic products released into the circulation from myeloid tissue are inactivated requires a different interpretation. In this case the esterase activity in serum, splenic sinusoids, follicular capillaries, or the hepatic RE cells could perform this function.

A further possibility is that the esterase fraction of the spleen is concerned in the detoxification of bacterial toxins. In vitro [24, 25] and in vivo

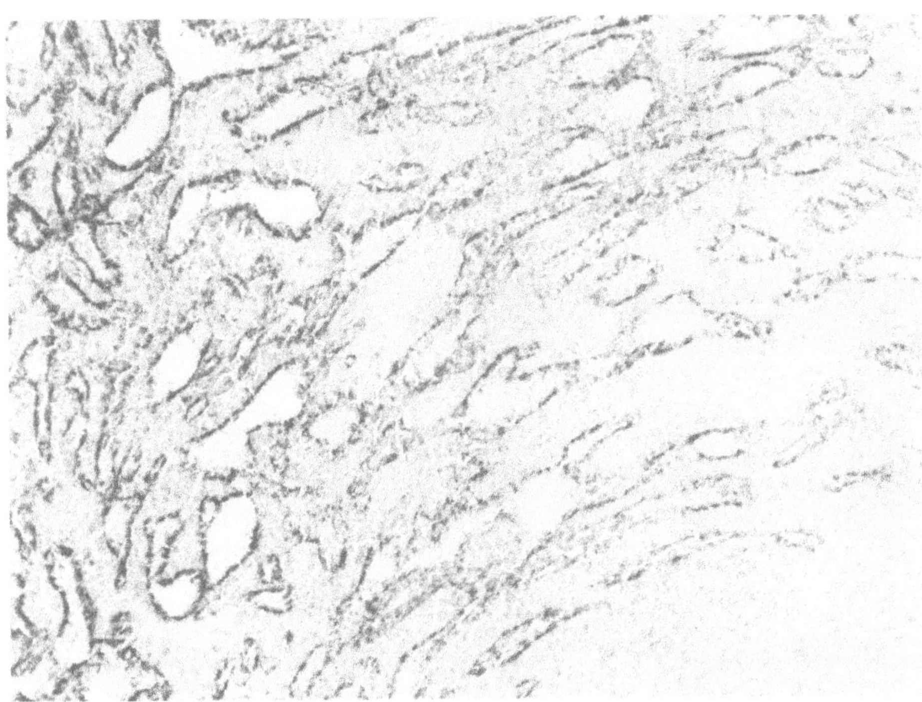

Fig. 8. NSE in cells lining the sinusoids of the spleen. α-Naphthyl acetate technique; section thickness 20 μ; $\times$ 111.

[26] studies have demonstrated the presence of an endotoxin-detoxifying factor in the spleen. A protein fraction capable of detoxifying bacterial endotoxin has been extracted from the spleen. This fraction has the properties of an esterase type of enzyme and is sensitive to TEPP [25]. Both the AChE and NSE activities detected histochemically in the spleen are sensitive to TEPP and are strategically situated to play a part in the inactivation of bacterial toxins. The TEPP-sensitive esterase fractions of lymph nodes and liver may also be concerned in bacterial detoxification, since endotoxin-detoxifying fractions have also been shown to exist in these tissues [24, 27].

Hepatic RE AChE may be concerned in the inactivation of endogenous or bacterial toxins, and possibly the hydrolysis of any acetylcholine released into the portal venous drainage area [8], yet it is also conceivable that the enzyme plays some general role in lipid and ester metabolism. In support of this suggestion are the observations that variations in hepatic RE function can be induced by simple lipids [28] and choline [29]. It has also been demonstrated that macrophages have the ability to take up fatty acids, possibly by phagocytosis [30], and incorporate them into triglycerides, phospholipids, and cholesterol esters [31]. Besides, in vitro experiments

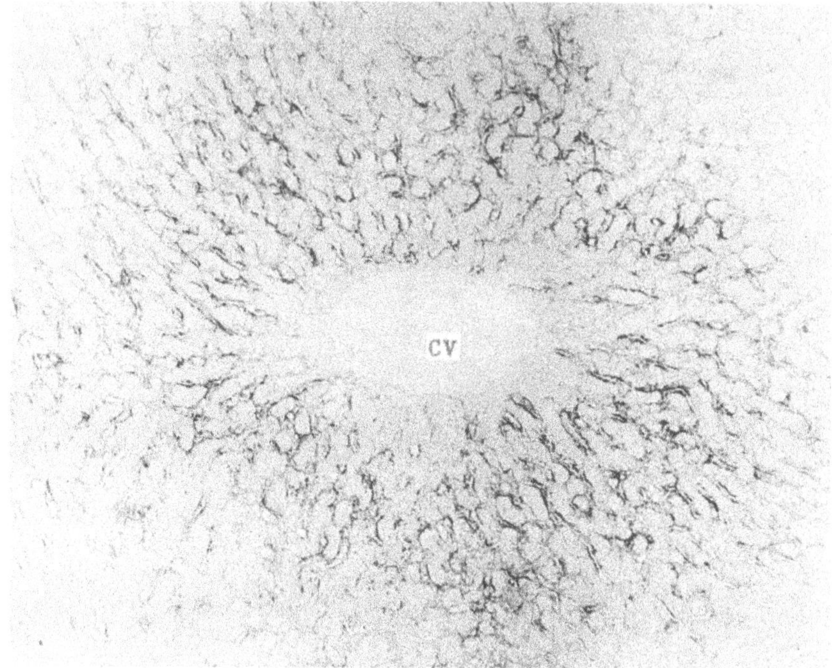

Fig. 9. Distribution of AChE in a liver lobule. The activity is present in centri- and midlobular cells lining the sinusoids. The wall of the centrilobular vein is devoid of activity. Section thickness 20 μ; × 113.

have shown that macrophages have the ability to synthesize lipids [32].

The observations that choline induces transformation of fibroblasts into macrophages [33], and that this substance also stimulates RE activity [29], suggests that wide variations in ester metabolism can be dealt with by flexible RE cellular systems with inherent properties for equilibration.

The suggestion of a role for RE esterases in lipid metabolism and detoxification is in keeping with the localization of cholinesterases and nonspecific esterases in other tissues where such processes occur. In hepatocytes, for example, the high concentrations of BChE are believed to be concerned in the hydrolysis of potentially toxic esters produced during fatty acid metabolism in these cells [15, 34]. AChE and NSE are present in the secretory cells of sebaceous glands, where they are believed to be concerned in lipid metabolism leading to the production of sebum [35]. The detection of esterases in the cytoplasm of fat cells provides convincing evidence for a direct role of these enzymes in lipid metabolism [36]. The hydrolysis of acetylcholine by AChE, and hence the prevention of prolonged depolarization at cholinergic synapses and neuroeffector endings, may be regarded as a further example of the role of esterases in detoxification.

REFERENCES

1. N. D'Agostini and B. Rossatti, J.Anat., 93:354, 1959.
2. R.F. Dorfman, Nature, 190:1021, 1961; L. Dumont, Compt. Rend. Soc.Biol., 149:960, 1955; C.E. Smith and B.K. Henon, Anat.Rec., 135:207, 1959.
3. G. Rogister and M.A. Gerebtzoff, Acta Anat., 32:39, 1958.
4. B. Ballantyne and R.G. Burwell, Nature, 206:1123, 1965.
5. B. Ballantyne and G.A. Bunch, J.Comp.Neurol., 127:471, 1966.
6. G.B. Koelle, J.Pharmacol.Exp.Therap., 100:158, 1958.
7. T. Williams, J.Histochem.Cytochem., 10:435, 1962.
8. B. Ballantyne, Experientia, 22:25, 1966.
9. M.S. Burstone, Enzyme Histochemistry, New York, Academic Press, 1962, p. 293.
10. P.C. Diegenbach, Nature, 207:308, 1965.
11. C.W.M. Adams, E.A. Marples, and J.R. Trounce, Clin.Sci., 19:473, 1960.
12. A.G.E. Pearse, Histochemistry, London, Churchill, 1960, p. 886.
13. S.J. Holt and R.F.J. Withers, Nature, 170:1012, 1958.
14. B.J. Davis and L. Ornstein, J.Histochem.Cytochem., 7:297, 1959; B.J. Davis, Proc.Soc.Exptl.Biol.Med., 101:90, 1959.
15. B. Ballantyne, J.Anat., 100:704, 1966.
16. M.A. Gerebtzoff, Cholinesterases, London, Pergamon, 1959.
17. J.C. Crooke, Nature, 199:41, 1963; G.B. Koelle, J.Comp.Neurol., 100:211, 1954; A.C. Palmer and A.R. Ellerker, Quart.J.Exptl. Physiol., 46:344, 1961.
18. K.-B. Augustinsson, in: G.B. Koelle, Ed., Handbuch der Experimentellen Pharmakologie, Vol. 15, Cholinesterases and Anticholinesterase Agents, Berlin, Springer-Verlag, 1963, p. 97.
19. R.E. Moe, Am.J.Anat., 112:311, 1963.
20. S.St.George, in: J.H.Heller, Ed., Reticuloendothelial Structure and Function, New York, Ronald Press, 1960, pp. 449-461.
21. R.G. Burwell, Lancet, ii:69, 1963.
22. B. Ballantyne, J.Anat., 98:689, 1964.
23. R.D. Chessick, J.Histochem.Cytochem., 2: 258, 1954; M. Dixon and E.C. Webb, Enzymes, London, Longmans, 1964, p. 192; D.F. Heath, Organophosphorus Poisons, Oxford, Pergamon, 1961, p. 103; L.D. Mounter and R.M. Cheatham, Enzymologia, 25:215, 1963; D. Nachmansohn and I.B. Wilson, in: F.F. Nord, Ed., Advances in Enzymology, New York, Interscience Publishers, 1951, Vol. 12, p. 259.
24. W.R. Keene, J.Lab.Clin.Med., 60:433, 1962.
25. E.E. Smith, S.H. Rutenberg, A.M. Rutenberg, and J.Fine, Proc. Soc.Exptl.Biol.Med., 113:781, 1963.
26. T. Wiznitzer, N. Better, W. Rachlin, N. Atkins, E.D. Frank, and J. Fine, J.Exptl.Med., 112:1157, 1960.

27. R.-J. Trapani, V.S. Waravdekar, M. Landy, and M.J. Shear, J. Infect. Diseases, 110:135, 1962.
28. A.E. Stuart, G. Biozzi, C. Stiffel, B.N. Halpern, and D. Mouton, Brit. J. Exptl. Pathol., 41:599, 1960.
29. J.H. Heller, Science, 118:353, 1953.
30. P. Elsbach, Nature, 195:383, 1962.
31. A.J. Day and N.H. Fidge, J. Lipid Res., 3:333, 1962.
32. A.J. Day and N.H. Fidge, J. Lipid Res., 5:163, 1964.
33. M. Chevremont, Exptl. Cell Res., Suppl., 1:560, 1949.
34. J.W. Clitherow, M. Mitchard, and N.J. Harper, Nature, 199:1000, 1963.
35. B. Ballantyne and G.A. Bunch, Dermatologia, 134:51, 1967.
36. B. Ballantyne, J. Anat., 100:931, 1966.

Comparative Cytology of Alveolar and Peritoneal Macrophages from Germfree Rats*

Eva S. Leake and Eugene R. Heise†

Department of Microbiology, The Bowman Gray School of Medicine
Wake Forest University
Winston-Salem, North Carolina

INTRODUCTION

Differences between alveolar macrophages (AM) and peritoneal macrophages (PM) have been reported by several investigators. Myrvik et al. [1], Dannenberg et al. [2], Cohn and Wiener [3], and Leake et al. [4], found that rabbit AM contained higher levels of hydrolases than oil-induced PM, and that AM exhibited a higher rate of endogenous oxygen consumption than oil-induced PM [4]. Oren et al. [5] studied the phagocytic process in guinea pig AM and casein-induced PM and reported that AM depend to a considerable degree upon oxidative phosphorylation as a source of energy for phagocytosis. In contrast, PM apparently depend only on glycolysis as the source of energy for that function.

Pavillard [6] compared AM and PM (noninduced) obtained from pathogen-free rats in their ability to kill *Escherichia coli* and *Staphylococcus aureus*. He found that the PM were more efficient than AM in killing these bacteria.

The above observations tend to indicate that marked differences exist in the physiological properties between lung and peritoneal macrophages. The relationship of these properties to their potential immunologic capabilities is as yet unknown.

This report is concerned with a study of the ultrastructure of AM and PM from germfree rats. The data to be presented further support the concept that AM and PM represent two distinct cell populations.

* This study was supported by research grant AI-05663 from the National Institutes of Health, USPHS, Bethesda, Maryland.

† Trainee on USPHS Training Grant T1 AI 268. Present address: Department of Microbiology, University of Washington School of Medicine, Seattle, Washington.

MATERIALS AND METHODS

Animals

Germfree Wistar rats* weighing 225-250 gm were killed by injection of air into one of the tail veins.

Peritoneal Macrophages

Ten to 15 ml of chilled Hanks' balanced salt solution (BSS) containing 0.2% EDTA [6] adjusted to a final pH of 7.2 were deposited into the opened peritoneal cavity. After a gentle massage, the fluid was transferred to a centrifuge tube. This procedure was repeated a second time and the fluid recovered was added to the first wash. The cell suspension was centrifuged in the cold at 800 rpm for 5 min.

Alveolar Macrophages

The lungs were removed from the thoracic cavity with the trachea closed by means of a small hemostat according to a technique described elsewhere [7]. The lungs were insufflated with 2-3 ml chilled Hanks' BSS containing 0.2% EDTA (pH 7.2). The fluid was drained into a centrifuge tube by keeping the lungs in an inverted position. This procedure was repeated three times. All washings were pooled and the cell suspension was centrifuged in the cold at 800 rpm for 5 min.

Light Microscopy

Smears were prepared from the sedimented cells and were stained with Wright's stain.

Electron Microscopy

The cell pellets obtained after centrifugation were immediately fixed in cold Palade's fixative [8] for 1 hr. After fixation, the cells were dehydrated in increasing gradient concentrations of ethyl alcohol and two changes of propylene oxide followed by embedment in maraglas [9]. Thin sections were made with a Porter–Blum ultramicrotome, mounted on bare copper grids and stained with lead citrate. The stained sections were examined with an RCA-EMU-3G electron microscope employing an accelerating voltage of 100 kV. Thick sections (1-2 μ) were stained with toluidine blue [10] and were observed with the light microscope.

Quantization of Acid Phosphatase, Cathepsin, and Lysozyme

AM and PM were harvested according to the techniques described above. The cell suspensions in Hanks' BSS were centrifuged at 1000 rpm for 10 min at 4°C. The cells were washed once with physiological saline, centrifuged at the same speed, and resuspended in saline. Cell counts were made using

---

*Germfree rats purchased from Manor Farms, Staatsburg, N. Y.

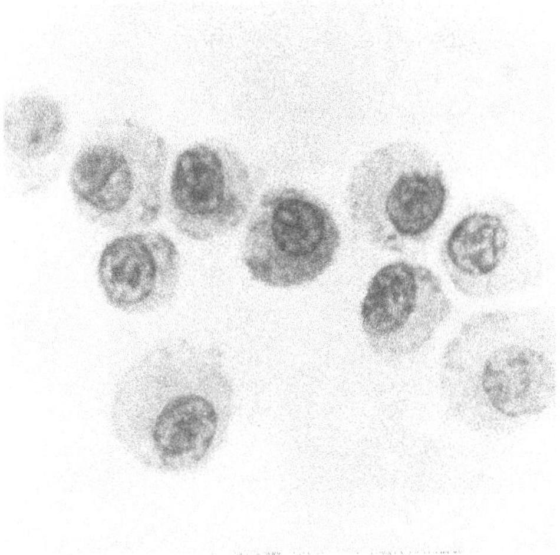

Fig. 1. Smear of alveolar macrophages obtained from germ-free Wistar rats. Wright's stain. Note the round nuclei and large cytoplasmic volume. × 1200, reduced 25% for reproduction.

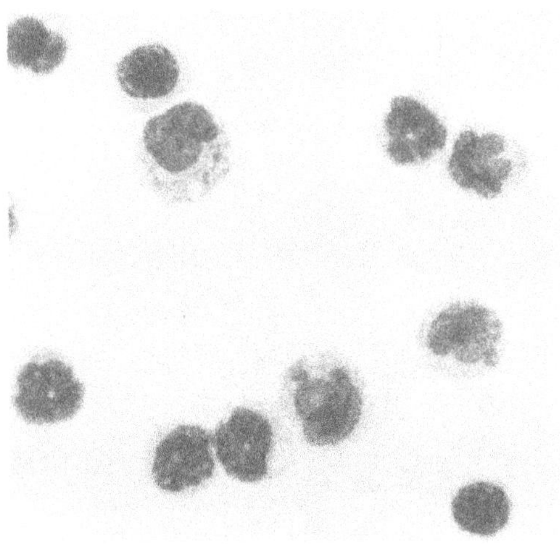

Fig. 2. Smear of peritoneal macrophages obtained from germ-free Wistar rats. Wright's stain. The irregularity of the nuclei and the lower cytoplasm-to-nucleus ratio are apparent when compared with AM in Fig. 1. × 1200, reduced 25% for reproduction.

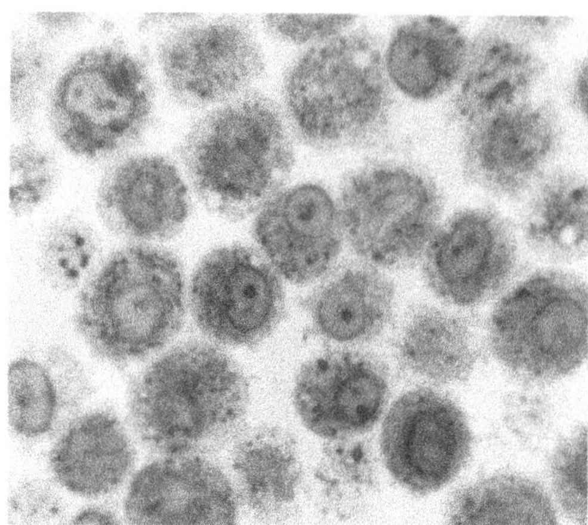

Fig. 3. Section of alveolar macrophages embedded in maraglas and stained with toluidine blue. The nuclei appear round or oval, and some show indentations of the nuclear membrane. Nucleoli are clearly visible. The cytoplasm shows large numbers of granules. × 1200, reduced 25% for reproduction.

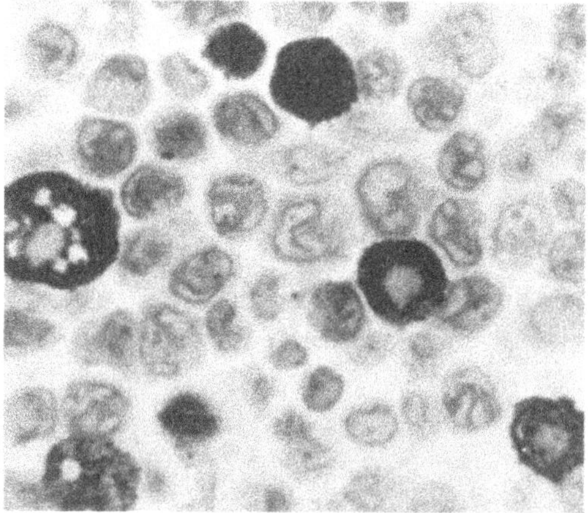

Fig. 4. Section of peritoneal macrophages embedded in maraglas and stained with toluidine blue. The diversity in nuclear outline is marked. Nucleoli are less numerous than in sections of AM. The cytoplasm does not show granular structures similar to those seen in AM. × 1200, reduced 25% for reproduction.

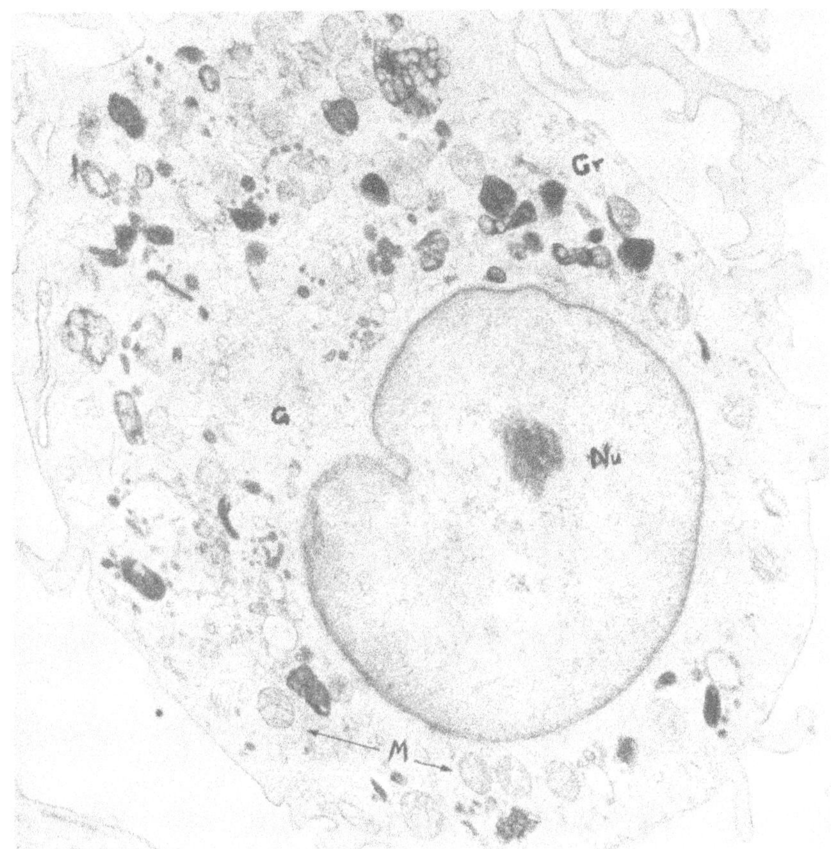

Fig. 5. Electron micrograph of an alveolar macrophage, procured from a germfree rat, demonstrates a slightly indented oval nucleus and its nucleolus (Nu). Round mitochondria (M), moderately developed Golgi apparatus (G), and a variety of electron opaque structures (Gr) in the cytoplasm are evident. Note the relative absence of ER. x 11,250, reduced 25% for reproduction.

Table I. Hydrolase Content of Alveolar and Peritoneal Macrophages from Germfree Rats

Enzymes	Range (activities per 10^6 cells)		Ratio of the mean values PM/AM
	Alveolar macrophages	Peritoneal macrophages	
Acid phosphatase (units)	4.3 - 7.7	0.35-0.95	1:9
Cathepsin (units)	0.69 - 1.19	0.08-0.13	1:9
Lysozyme (μg)	11.5 - 18.5	0.03-0.13	1:150

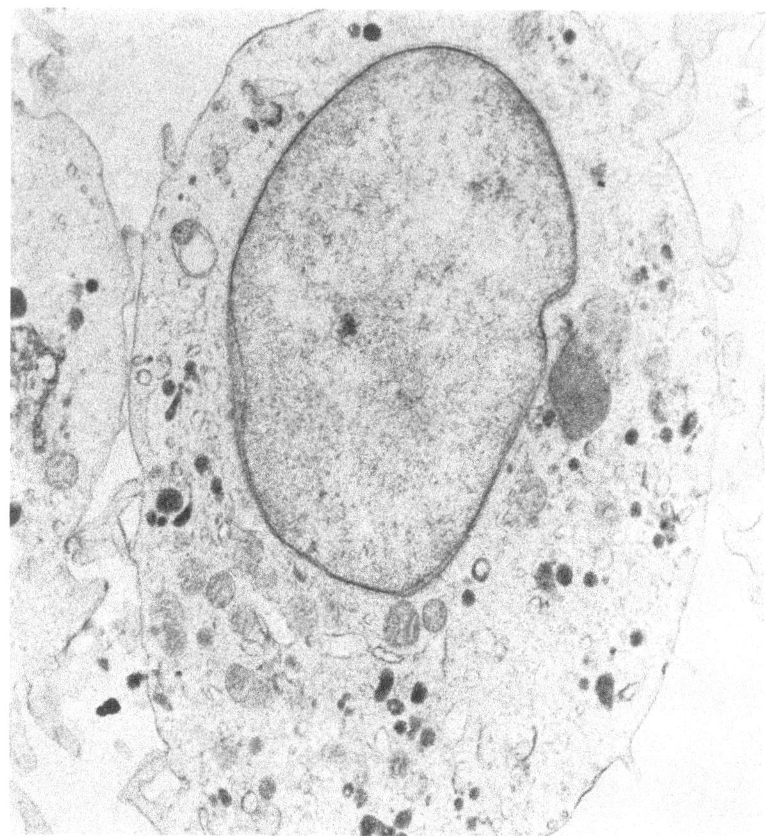

Fig. 6. Alveolar macrophage with an oval nucleus frequently seen in these cells. Round mitochondria, scant Golgi apparatus, and electron opaque cytoplasmic structures resemble those in Fig. 5. × 11,250, reduced 25% for reproduction.

a standard hemocytometer. Cell extracts were prepared by freezing and thawing the cell suspension for five consecutive cycles. Cellular debris was removed by centrifugation at 2500 rpm for 10 min at 4°C (International centrifuge, Model CS). Acid phosphatase was measured by the method of Hofstee [11]. Cathepsin was determined by a modification of Anson's method as described in a previous publication [12]. Lysozyme was assayed according to the method described by Myrvik et al. [1].

RESULTS

Light Microscopy

The homogeneity of the AM recovered from germfree rats is similar to that described for AM procured from conventionally reared rabbits [7]. The cell populations obtained from the peritoneal cavity consisted of approximately 90-95% mononuclear cells. The remainder of the cells included mast cells and occasional polymorphonuclear cells (less than 3%). Figures 1 and 2 correspond, respectively, to smears of AM and PM stained with Wright's stain. It was observed that AM tend to assume a spherical shape and contain a round eccentric nucleus. In comparison, PM exhibited an elongated and lobulated nucleus which appeared to produce distension of the cell membrane in some instances resulting in an irregular cell outline. The cytoplasm-to-nucleus ratio was observed to be higher in AM than in PM. In general, AM appeared to be larger than PM. These features are further demonstrated in Figs. 3 and 4, which correspond to sections of AM and PM embedded in maraglas and stained with toluidine blue.

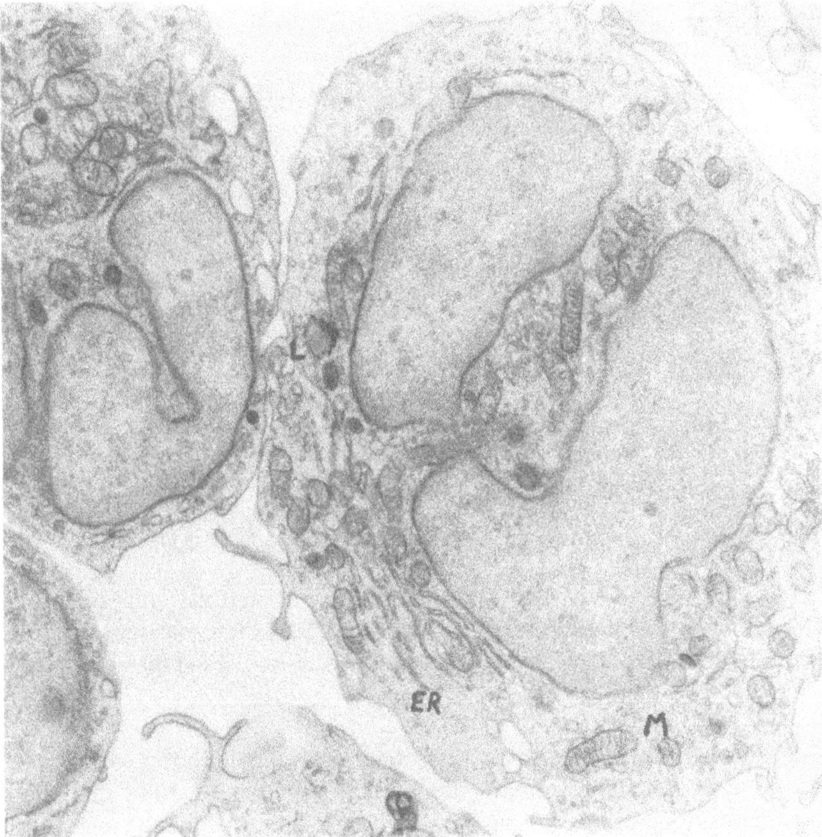

Fig. 7. Electron micrograph of a peritoneal macrophage from a germfree rat. Note the lobulated nucleus, elongated mitochondria (M), well-developed profiles of rough ER, and the paucity of electron-dense granules in the cytoplasm. L-lipid. × 11,250, reduced 25% for reproduction.

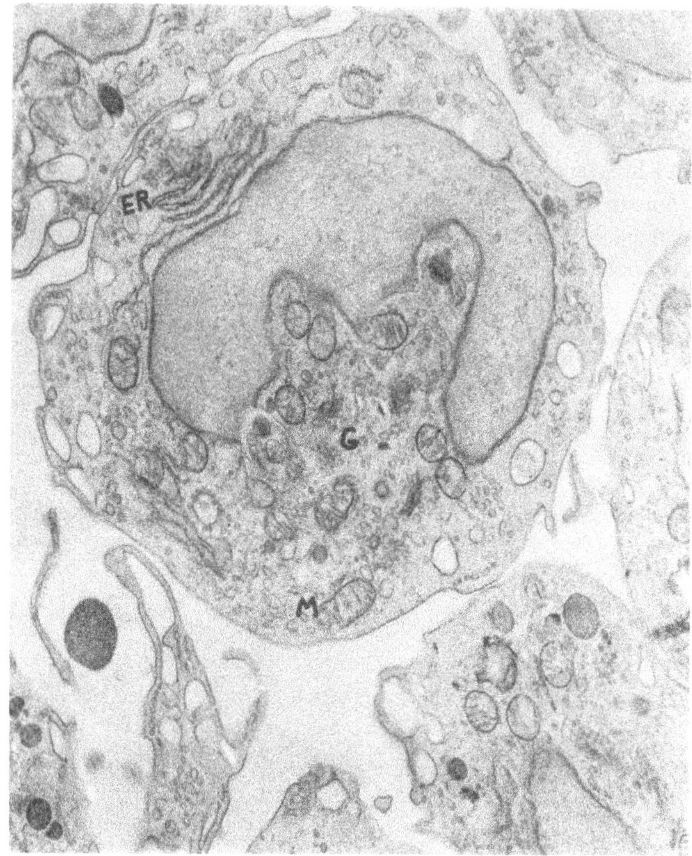

Fig. 8. Peritoneal macrophage exhibiting structures similar to those described in Fig. 7. × 11,250, reduced 25% for reproduction.

Electron Microscopy

This study was designed to compare a few structural components that might be considered unique to either AM or PM. Five main morphologic differences were observed in thin sections, and are illustrated in Figs. 5-10.

(1) Nuclear Shape

AM showed a circular-to-oval nuclear outline which in several instances contained indentations of the nuclear membrane. The nucleus of PM never assumed a similar shape. Instead, it showed lobulations and deep clefts, depending on the plane of section. In addition, nucleoli were more frequently observed in AM than in PM.

(2) Endoplasmic Reticulum

Well-defined profiles of rough endoplasmic reticulum (ER) were commonly seen in PM. In contrast, rough ER was essentially absent in AM.

(3) Golgi Complex

This structure was usually more developed in PM than in AM.

(4) Cytoplasmic Granules

A large number of highly dense granules with varied sizes and shapes was a constant component of the cytoplasm of AM. On the other hand, PM were essentially devoid of such structures.

(5) Mitochondria

These organelles appeared to be larger in size and more elongated in PM than in AM, although the total number could possibly be larger in AM than in PM as the result of a larger cell volume in AM.

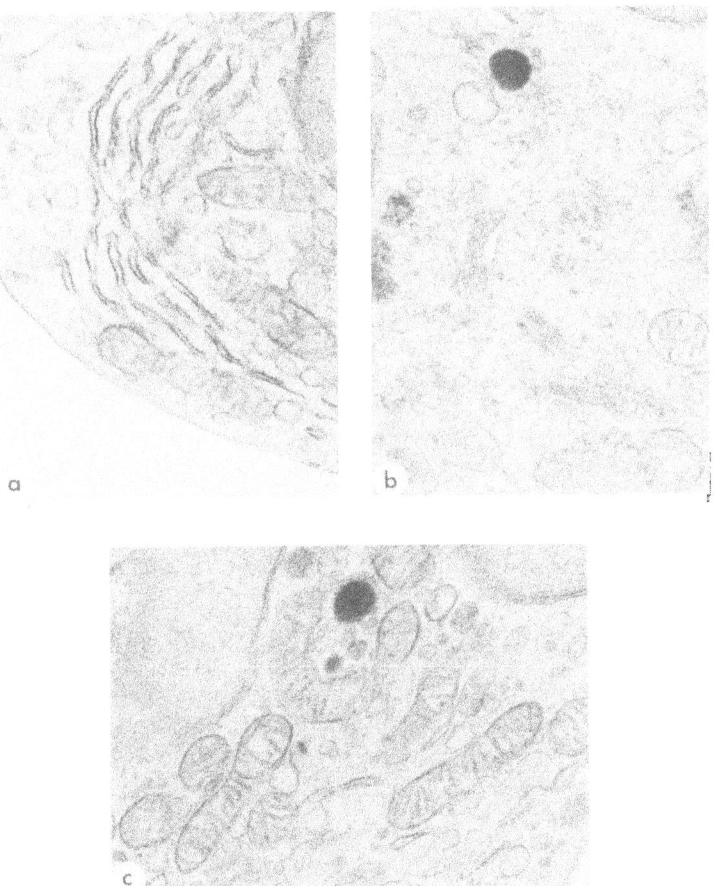

Fig. 9. Three outstanding structures observed in peritoneal macrophages from germfree rats: (a) well-developed rough ER; (b) well-developed Golgi apparatus; (c) elongated mitochondria. × 22,000, reduced 25% for reproduction.

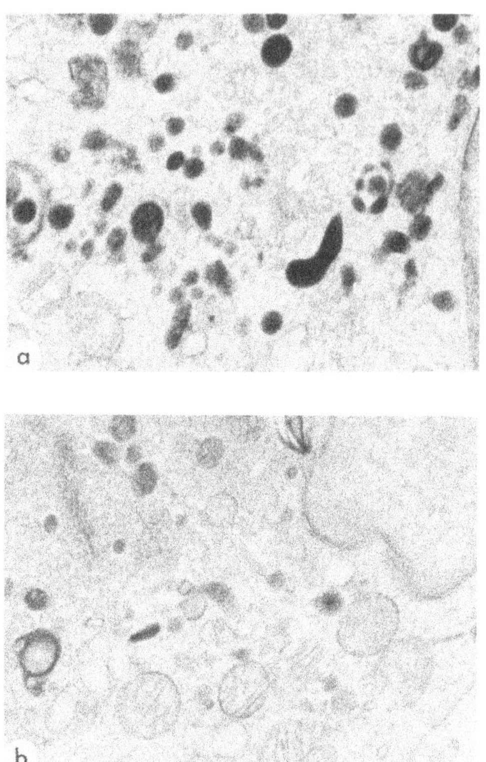

Fig. 10. Electron micrograph illustrating two structures routinely observed in alveolar macrophages from germfree rats: (a) varied electron-opaque cytoplasmic granules, and (b) round-to-oval mitochondria. ×15,000, reduced 25% for reproduction.

Lipid deposits were present in some PM but they were generally absent in AM. The electron micrographs confirmed that AM are slightly larger in size than PM. The average diameter of AM was approximately 1.5 times the average diameter of PM.

Quantity of Enzymes in Cell Extracts

Table I summarizes the data obtained from biochemical determinations of acid phosphatase, cathepsin, and lysozyme in cell extracts of AM and PM procured from germfree rats. It can be noted that acid phosphatase and cathepsin levels in AM were 9-fold that in PM. Lysozyme levels in AM were over 100-fold that in PM.

DISCUSSION

Recent studies of Bauer and collaborators [13] on macrophages from germfree and conventional mice have indicated that there is a great similarity in number, distribution, histologic and histochemical characteristics of macrophages in lymph nodes and spleens of these two groups of mice. The macrophages from conventional mice showed a greater digestive capacity than macrophages from germfree mice, although no difference was recorded in their phagocytic ability. The above authors believe that this enhancement in digestive ability could be the result of continuous exposure to the immunologic effects of the microbial flora.

The comparatively higher content of acid hydrolases present in AM as compared to PM has also been interpreted as the result of constant stimulation by bacteria entering the respiratory tract. By comparison, PM would be expected to encounter bacteria only sporadically. In an attempt to clarify this difference, Heise and Myrvik [14] studied the content of acid phosphatase, cathepsin, and lysozyme in AM and PM from germfree and conventional rats. The levels of these three enzymes were consistently higher in AM than in PM independently of the presence or absence of microbial flora. Accordingly, the high levels of acid hydrolases found in AM from germfree rats did not seem to be related to the presence of living microorganisms. However, the effect of inhaled bacterial residues and particulate organic material on hydrolase levels of AM remains to be determined. These particulates undoubtedly are present in food and bedding in the environment of germfree rats.

The great variety of cytoplasmic granules observed in AM could possibly represent phagosomes containing residues of phagocytosed material and/or cell components undergoing turnover in AM. Undoubtedly, AM are constantly engaging particulates which gain access to the respiratory tract even in the germfree environment. PM probably very seldom engage foreign material in the peritoneum. This could explain the lack of equivalent numbers of such structures in their cytoplasm. If the electron-dense granules in AM contained large amounts of lysosomal hydrolases, an explanation would be available to account for the higher levels of these enzymes in AM as compared to PM.

The differences in metabolic activities of AM and PM described by several investigators [4, 5] might be expected to correlate with differences in the mitochondrial content in these two populations of cells. However, AM and PM from germfree rats did not show a marked difference in the relative numbers of mitochondria present. The majority of the mitochondria in PM were elongated, whereas mitochondria in AM exhibited an oval-to-round appearance. These differences in mitochondrial morphology cannot readily explain the preferential aerobic metabolism of AM as compared with the glycolytic metabolism favored by PM.

Peritoneal macrophages frequently contained well-developed rough ER that appeared as long channels at the periphery of the cell. In contrast to the PM, long profiles of rough ER were rare in AM from germfree rats.

Free ribosomes were not abundant in either cell population although nucleoli were more often observed in AM than in PM. The high levels of hydrolases in AM are presumably the result of active synthesis by these cells, coupled with storage in the Golgi complex and lysosomes. The paucity of both a well-developed rough ER and free ribosomes in the cytoplasm of AM fail to account for the marked differences in hydrolase content of AM and PM.

The relatively well-developed ER in PM tends to suggest that PM may be more actively engaged in protein biosynthesis than AM. Further clarification of these points would be highly desirable.

It has been proposed by Cohn and Wiener [3] that AM and PM may originate from common monocytic stem cells. According to this concept, the stem cells would differentiate under the influence of their environments into their respective cell populations. In a subsequent study, Cohn and Benson [15] reported that BCG-stimulated alveolar macrophages represented fully mature cells incapable of further differentiation. In later studies, Cohn et al. [16] presented specific criteria for evaluating levels of differentiation of mouse peritoneal macrophages which included: (1) increase in cell size, (2) increase in numbers of electron opaque granules, (3) hypertrophy of the Golgi apparatus, and (4) increase in apparent number and length of mitochondria. No change in nuclear size or structure was noted. According to these criteria they considered that the peritoneal macrophage is more "mature" than the blood monocyte.

Extending these basic criteria to the AM, it logically follows that AM are more "mature" than PM, based on size and numbers of electron-opaque granules. However, when the Golgi complex and the number and size of mitochondria were compared in AM and PM, the above criteria were not fulfilled.

The comparatively extensive rough ER in PM compared to AM may further support this contradiction. If AM is the mature counterpart of PM, the nuclei of stimulated PM might be expected to transform to an oval or round nucleus analogous to the nucleus in AM. This transformation has not been documented to the authors' knowledge, even though many experiments have been conducted in which PM have been intensively stimulated both in vivo and in vitro.

Collectively, the data presented in this study further support the idea that AM and PM represent distinct and different cell populations. In this regard, it is possible that they may originate from a common stem cell and that their respective environments induce two specialized forms of differentiation.

SUMMARY

The morphology of alveolar (AM) and peritoneal (PM) macrophages obtained from germfree rats was studied with light and electron microscopes. Smears and thick sections of maraglas-embedded cells demonstrated that AM are larger in size and have a larger cytoplasm-to-nucleus ratio than PM. AM showed a round-to-oval nucleus, whereas PM showed an elongated and lobulated nucleus. Observations with the electron microscope revealed that, in general, AM possessed round mitochondria, poorly developed rough ER and Golgi apparatus, and contained large numbers of electron-dense granules in their cytoplasm. PM exhibited elongated mitochondria and relatively well-developed rough ER and Golgi apparatus. In comparison to AM, PM contained fewer electron-dense granules.

ACKNOWLEDGMENT

We wish to thank Mrs. Brigitte Reiff for her valuable assistance.

REFERENCES

1. Q.N. Myrvik, E.S. Leake, and B. Fariss, "Lysozyme content of alveolar and peritoneal macrophages from the rabbit." J.Immunol., 86:133, 1961.
2. A.M. Dannenberg, Jr., M.S. Burstone, P.C. Walter, and J.W. Kinsley, "A histochemical study of phagocytic and enzymatic functions of rabbit mononuclear and polymorphonuclear exudate cells and alveolar macrophages. I. Survey and quantitation of enzymes, and states of cellular activation." J. Cell Biol., 17:465, 1963.
3. Z.A. Cohn and E. Wiener, "The particulate hydrolases of macrophases. I. Comparative enzymology, isolation, and properties." J. Exptl. Med., 118:991, 1963.
4. E.S. Leake, D. Gonzalez-Ojeda, and Q.N. Myrvik, "Enzymatic differences between normal alveolar macrophages and oil-induced peritoneal macrophages obtained from rabbits." Exptl. Cell Res., 33:553, 1964.
5. R. Oren, A.E. Farnham, K. Saito, E. Milofsky, and M.L. Karnovsky, "Metabolic patterns in three types of phagocytizing cells." J. Cell Biol., 17:487, 1963.
6. E.R.J. Pavillard, "In vitro phagocytic and bactericidal ability of alveolar and peritoneal macrophages of normal rats." Australian J. Exptl. Biol. Med. Sci., 41:265, 1963.
7. Q.N. Myrvik, E.S. Leake, and B. Fariss, "Studies on pulmonary alveolar macrophages from the normal rabbit: A technique to procure them in a high state of purity." J. Immunol., 86:128, 1961.
8. G.E. Palade, "A study of fixation for electron microscopy." J. Exptl. Med., 95:285, 1952.

9. J.A. Freeman and B.O. Spurlock, "A new epoxy embedment for electron microscopy." J. Cell Biol., 13: 437, 1962.
10. B. Trump, E. Smuckler, and E. Benditt, "A method for staining epoxy sections for light microscopy." J. Ultrastruct. Res., 5: 343, 1961.
11. B.H.J. Hofstee, "Direct and continuous spectrophotometric assay of phosphomonesterases." Arch. Biochem. Biophys., 51: 139, 1954.
12. E.S. Leake and Q.N. Myrvik, "Differential release of lysozyme and acid phosphatase from subcellular granules of normal rabbit alveolar macrophages." Brit. J. Exptl. Pathol., 45: 384, 1964.
13. H. Bauer, F. Paronetto, W.A. Burns, and A. Einheber, "The enhancing effect of the microbial flora on macrophage function and the immune response. A study in germfree mice." J. Exptl. Med., 123: 1013, 1966.
14. E.R. Heise and Q.N. Myrvik, "Levels of lysosomal hydrolases in alveolar and peritoneal macrophages from conventional and germfree rats." Federation Proc., 25: 439, 1966.
15. Z.A. Cohn and B. Benson, "The differentiation of mononuclear phagocytes. Morphology, cytochemistry, and biochemistry." J. Exptl. Med., 121: 153, 1965.
16. Z.A. Cohn, J.G. Hirsch, and M.E. Fedorko, "The in vitro differentiation of mononuclear phagocytes. IV. The ultrastructure of macrophage differentiation in the peritoneal cavity and in culture." J. Exptl. Med., 123: 747, 1966.

The Role of the Environment in Determining the Discriminatory Activity of the Human Phagocytic Cell

A. E. Stuart

Department of Pathology
University of Edinburgh
Edinburgh, Scotland

A basic attribute of the reticuloendothelial system of cells is the capacity for discrimination – discrimination between old and new, living and dead, indigenous and foreign material. Some examples from pathology follow. They are all well known and each touches on the question of discriminatory activity.

Figure 1 is a tissue section from the lung of a man who died from Goodpasture's syndrome. It shows multiple pulmonary hemorrhages, and the alveolar phagocytes have ingested red cells and converted many of them to hemosiderin. How do phagocytes discriminate between normal and effete red cells?

Jenkin and Karthigasu [1] working with an experimental system of liver perfusion, showed that opsonins were required for the phagocytosis of autologous effete red cells. On the other hand, Vaughan and Boyden [2],using an elegant in vitro technique, suggested that opsonization might not be important after all. Contrary opinions are reflected by the use of different techniques but clearly there remains a great deal to be learned about this type of discriminatory activity.

Figure 2 shows the tissue response in a case of avian tuberculosis and the vigorous phagocytic response to this infectious agent is evident. Figure 3 is from a thyroid nodule in which macrophages have ingested colloid. Colloidophagy in the thyroid gland is a well-recognized phenomenon, but what change in the colloid is necessary before phagocytosis can occur? Both the colloid and the macrophage are indigenous and the homeostatic mechanisms which prevent macrophages from ingesting colloid in a normal gland remain unknown.

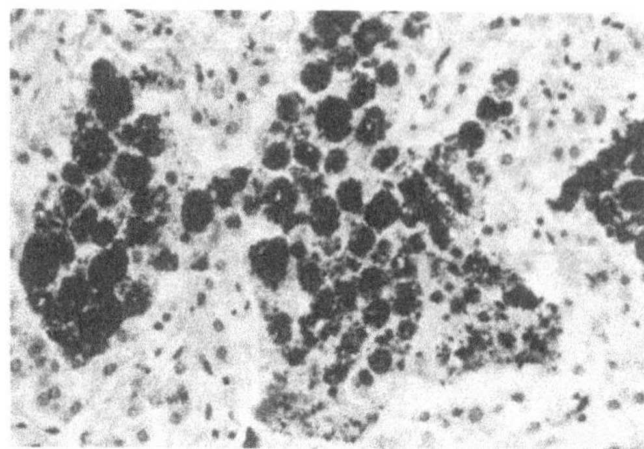

Fig. 1. Hemosiderin-laden macrophages in lung from a case of Goodpasture's syndrome. P. B. R. and hematoxylin. × 290, reduced 25% for reproduction.

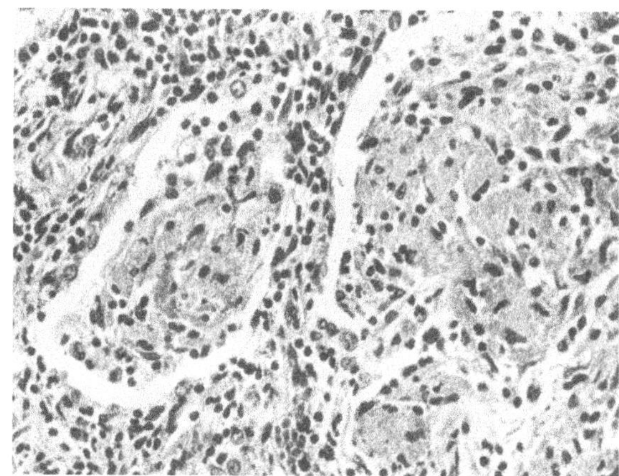

Fig. 2. Macrophage reaction to avian tuberculosis of lung. H. and E. × 350, reduced 25% for reproduction.

Figure 4 shows the uptake of lipid droplets by phagocytes in an atheromatous plaque situated near the arch of the aorta. Homologous chylomicrons are poorly phagocytosed, but here there has been ready ingestion of fatty material. What is the basis for this type of discrimination? Particle size, surface charge, and the nature of the fatty acids will enter into the problem, but none alone can give a wholly satisfactory answer. The next two examples are electron micrographs from the neighborhood of a granuloma in the liver of a mouse infected with Salmonella typhimurium. Here is a large histiocyte (Fig. 5) burrowing into the depths of a liver cell. So far, attempts to demonstrate any chemotactic response of mononuclear cells in vitro have been disappointing (McCutcheon [3], Harris [4]).

Figure 6 shows a macrophage which has entered the cytoplasm of a liver cell. Its pseudopodia have engulfed some injured mitochondria. These mitochondria are swollen and the cristae have become indistinct, but whether the cell is alive or dead one cannot say. The exquisite precision of this process must depend on the ability to distinguish between normal and injured tissue. Boyden [5] suggests that phagocytic discrimination is dependent upon differences in structure between "familiar" macromolecules normally exposed to body fluids and "unfamiliar" macromolecules of foreign matter and of injured cells.

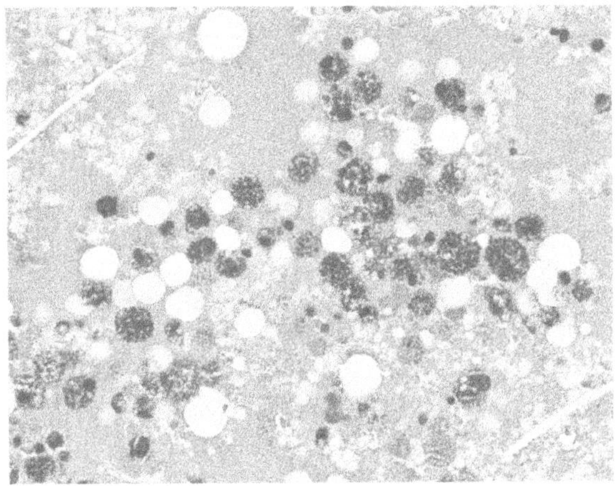

Fig. 3. Colloidophagy within large follicle of a thyroid adenoma. P. A. S. × 350, reduced 25% for reproduction.

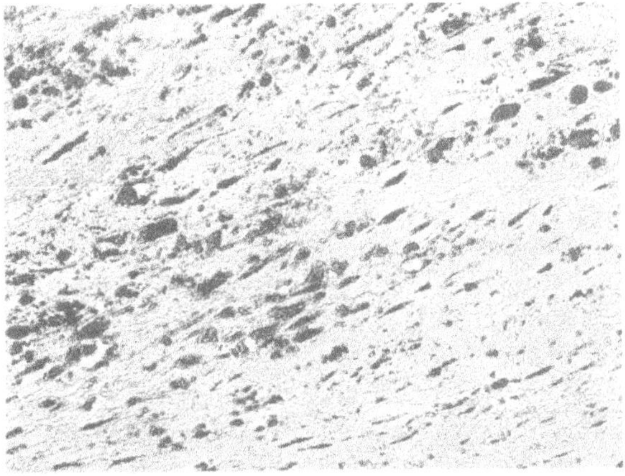

Fig. 4. Lipophages in atheromatous plaque of aorta. Sudan. × 130, reduced 25% for reproduction.

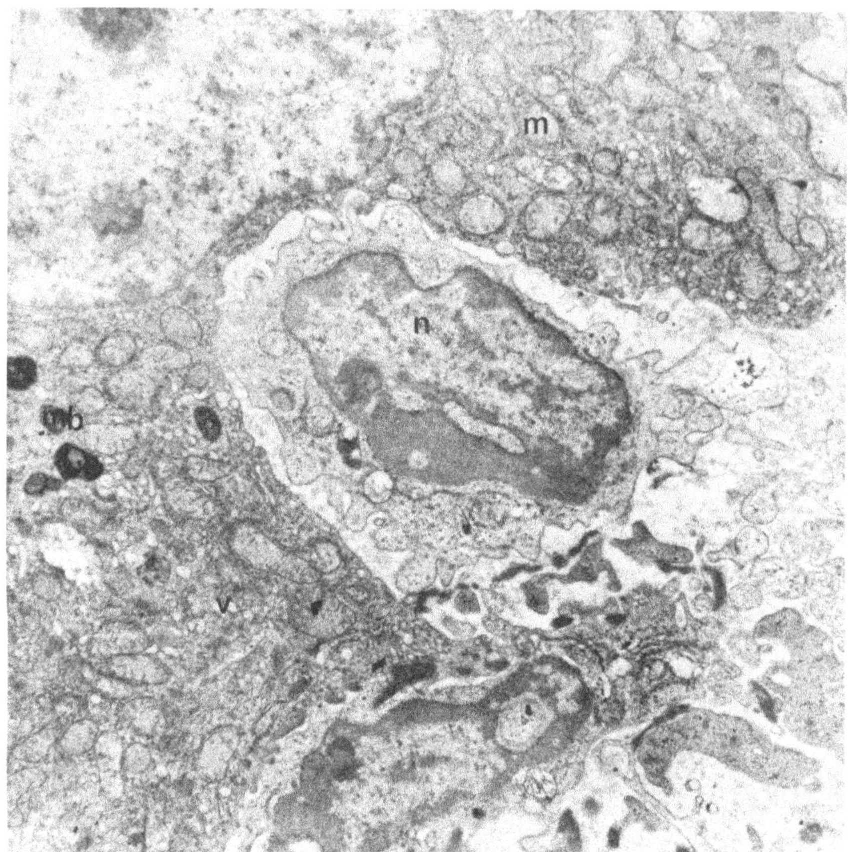

Fig. 5. Liver 48 hr after infection with S. typhimurium. A histiocyte h has burrowed into the cytoplasm of a liver cell and borders on its nucleus n. The invaded liver cell shows early but reversible degenerative changes, e.g., flocculation of mitochondrial matrices m, vesiculation of smooth-surfaced endoplasmic reticulum v, and increased number of electron-dense microbodies mb. × 10,000, reduced 25% for reproduction.

Although phagocytic recognition of injured liver tissue may depend on opsonic factors reactive with unfamiliar macromolecules, the possibility of direct contactual "recognition" between the surface of the macrophage and superficial or deep receptors in injured cells cannot be ruled out. Phagocytosis of particles is facilitated and accelerated by their coating with specific antibodies but it is important to realize that invertebrates also possess some capacity for the recognition of foreign particles. Figure 7 shows the gland of Faussek which is situated behind the eye of the octopus and which elaborates leucocytes (Fig. 8) of the monocytic type. Injection of colloidal carbon by the intravenous route has revealed an extensive reticulo-endothelial apparatus which has no difficulty in recognizing the carbon particles as foreign and does so without the benefit of a lymphoid-plasma cell system.

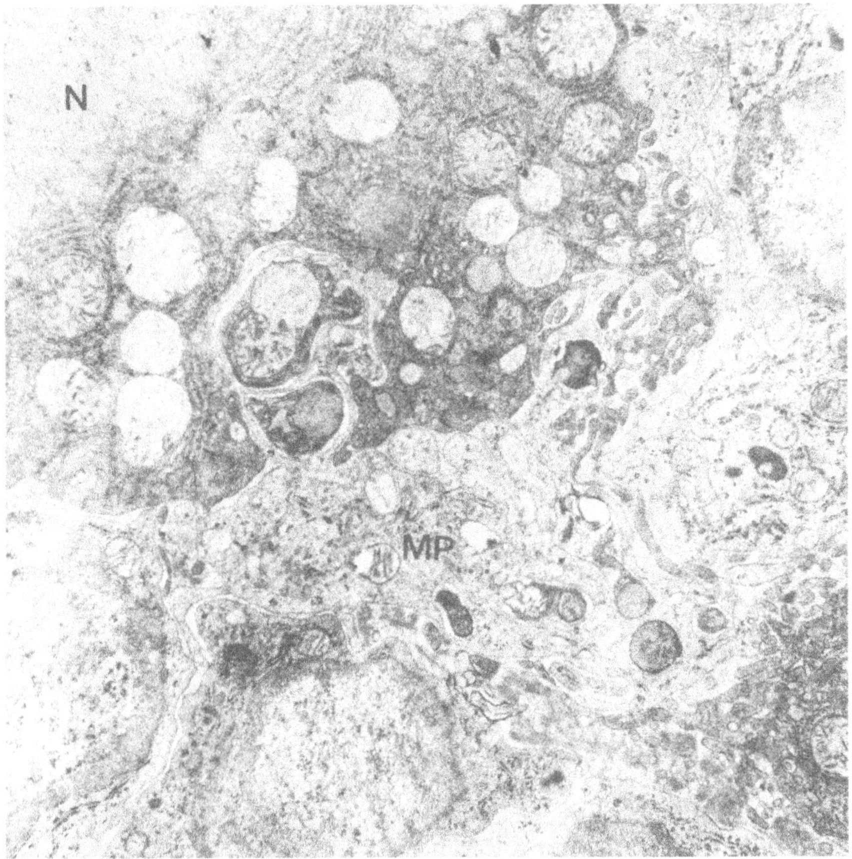

Fig. 6. Liver 48 hr after infection with S. typhimurium. Pseudopodia from a macrophage MP have extended into the substance of a liver cell with nucleus N and phagocytosed a mitochondrion and a piece of cytoplasm. × 13,000, reduced 25% for reproduction.

The present work is concerned with whether macrophages will distinguish between autologous, homologous, and heterologous red cells in tissue culture, and investigates the opsonizing potency of different kinds of antiserum.

The general plan of the experiments has been to incubate human macrophages in AB serum. Red cells of a variety of known blood groups were added and after a suitable interval the preparations were examined. The effect of the natural isoagglutinins A and B, isoimmune anti A, Rhesus anti (D+), and a hemolysin were studied by incubating red cells in appropriate dilutions of these different antisera, which were then added to the cultures of macrophages.

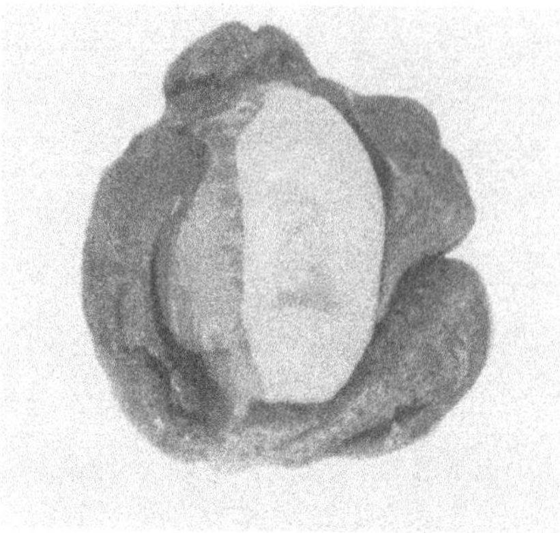

Fig. 7. Gland of Faussek showing the three lobes, dark after carbon injection, surrounding the optic ganglion. × 3.

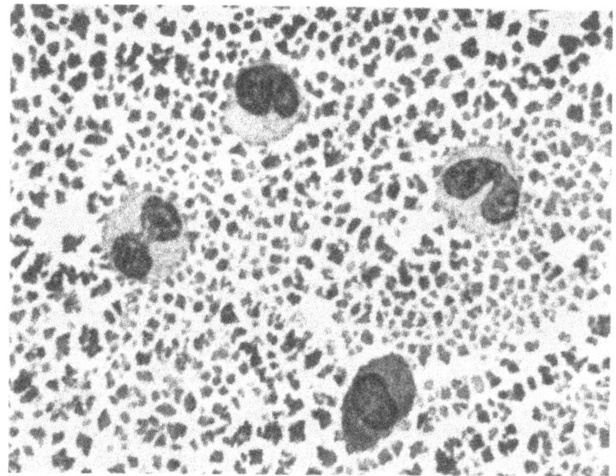

Fig. 8. Peripheral blood of Eledone cirrosa showing monocytoid cells. Leishman's stain. × 1000, reduced 25% for reproduction.

MATERIALS AND METHODS

Preparation of Human Macrophages

Cadaveric Macrophages

The subject should be not more than 2 hr dead and free from abdominal disease; the young or middle aged are more suitable than the elderly. The skin over the iliac fossa was cleaned with 70% alcohol, and a large needle or small trocar pushed through skin, muscle, and peritoneum, taking care to avoid the bladder and the bowel (Fig. 9). The trocar was connected by plastic tubing to a 6-liter reservoir of physiological saline situated 10-12 ft above the body; 3-5 liters of saline were then introduced into the peritoneal sac, and the abdomen pressed repeatedly up and down while the saline was running. This takes 15-20 min.

Then an incision 2.5 cm long was made in the right iliac fossa, after which a small hole 1 cm in diameter was made in the peritoneum. Plastic tubing 2 cm in diameter was pushed through the hole for a distance of 16-23 cm (Fig. 10). The terminal 12 cm of this tube contained multiple perforations 0.5 cm in diameter. The abdominal fluid was then aspirated by suction into flasks. Bloodstained fluids are to be avoided, and if the holes of the intraperitoneal part of the tube become blocked by fat, then the vacuum should be closed and the tube rotated.

Macrophages from Peritoneal Dialysis

The fluid from patients treated by peritoneal dialysis is a convenient and reliable source of macrophages. The fluid should be clear and straw-colored. A tinge of pink is acceptable but heavily bloodstained fluid cannot be recommended. All apparatus used in these procedures should be sterile.

Treatment of the Peritoneal Fluid. The fluid was centrifuged at 300 g in 500-ml containers for 15 min at 10°C. The supernatants were discarded and the deposits pooled in Glaxo tissue culture medium 199 containing both penicillin and streptomycin. The cells were gently centrifuged once more and resuspended in tissue culture medium containing 10% human AB serum. Human serum from other blood groups is equally satisfactory for growth purposes. The nucleated cell count should be between 1.5 and 2 million cells per milliliter. The optimal volume for seeding coverslips in test tubes containing coverslips (19 × 6 mm) is 1.5 ml; hexagonal Pyrex baby feeding bottles require 10 ml and large Roux flasks require 50 ml. The cultures were incubated at 37°C for 24-28 hr, when debris was removed by gently flicking the tube with the forefinger and rinsing with medium 199. The tubes were replenished with fresh medium containing 10% serum. They were incubated at an angle of 5° from the horizontal.

Reaction of Macrophages with Homologous Erythrocytes

Red cells from blood donors were obtained. These consisted of 9 Group A donors, 10 Group O, and 2 Group AB. The majority were Rh(D+). The cells were used within 24 hr of venepuncture and were washed twice in an excess of saline before making to a 5% suspension. Volumes of 0.1 were added to the macrophage monolayers, shaken, and incubated at 37°C for 2 hr.

Reaction of Macrophages with Heterologous Erythrocytes

Fowl and mouse red cells were obtained fresh, washed twice, and made to a 5% suspension. Volumes of 0.1 ml were than added to the monolayers.

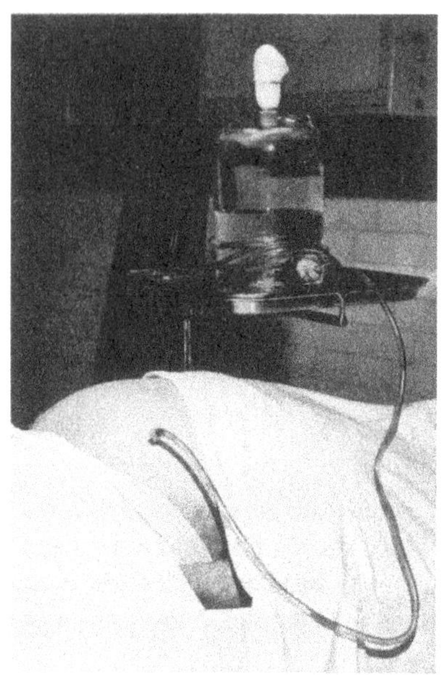

Fig. 9. Trocar in position in abdominal cavity of cadaver. The peritoneal sac has been filled with saline from the flask.

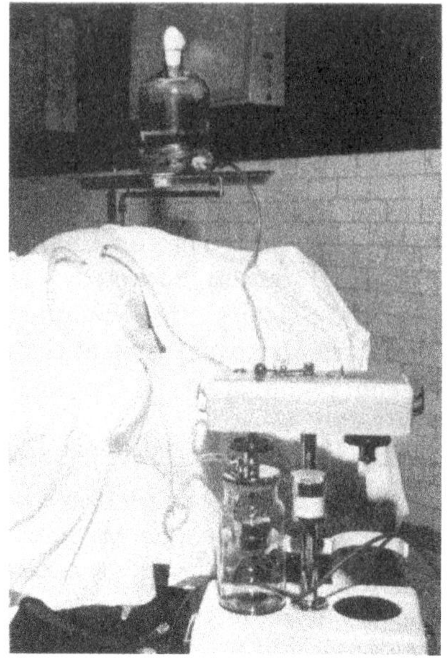

Fig. 10. Removal of peritoneal fluid into a sterile flask.

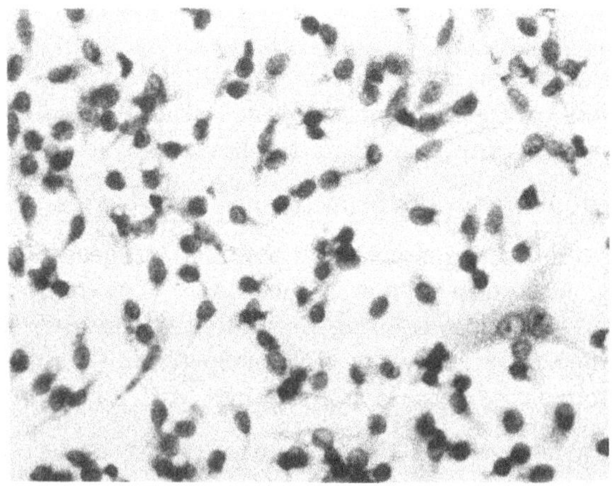

Fig. 11. Normal pattern. 48-hr culture. × 350, reduced 25% for reproduction.

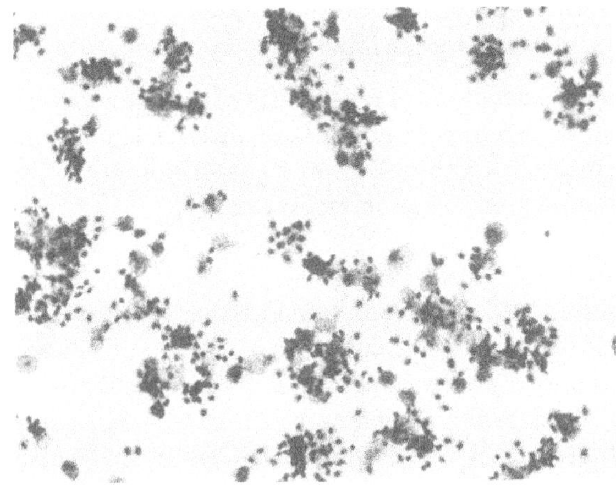

Fig. 12. Patternal adherence. 48-hr culture. × 350, reduced 25% for reproduction.

Fig. 13. Pattern of phagocytosis. 48-hr culture. × 350, reduced 25% for reproduction.

Reaction of Macrophages to Red Cells Treated with Natural and Immune Agglutinins

Ten-percent suspensions of fresh cells of the appropriate blood group were made in neat human AB serum and mixed with an equal volume of anti-serum suitably diluted. The cells were sensitized at 37°C for 2 hr; 0.1 ml volumes were then added to the monolayers.

Source of Antisera

Isoagglutinins A and B were obtained from single sources. They were not hemolytic and had an agglutination titer of $1/2$-$1/4$. The isoimmune anti-A serum showed only a trace of hemolysis when incubated neat with A1 red cells at 37°C for 1 hr in the presence of excess human complement. It gave an agglutination titer of $1/32$. Doubling dilutions of this serum were prepared in AB serum and mixed with equal volumes of a 10% suspension of A1 cells also in AB serum. After sensitization for 2 hr at 37°C, 0.1 ml volumes were added to the monolayers for a titration by erythrophagocytosis. The Rhesus anti-D sera were both pooled preparations with titers of $1/40$ and $1/128$ by the antiglobulin test.

The rabbit hemolysin was a pooled antiserum prepared in rabbits by the injection of washed human red cells. The hemolytic titer was $1/4$ and the agglutination titer $1/128$.

Staining Methods

At the end of the incubation with macrophages the tubes were shaken, the supernatant removed, and the coverslips washed thoroughly in saline. They were fixed in methanol and diluted Leishman's stain was added for 15-30 mins. The control cultures always included one or two coverslips to which starch granules had been added. These were stained by P.A.S.

Assessment of Results

Coverslips were examined microscopically and graded as negative (Fig. 11), adherence (Fig. 12), and phagocytosis (Fig. 13). In some cases 600 macrophages were counted and the number of macrophages containing one or more red cells expressed as a percentage.

The results of the experiments on macrophage—red cell interactions are based on eight primary cultures obtained from different individuals and a total of 453 coverslip preparations derived from these cultures.

RESULTS

Morphology of the Cultures

Most of the cells (Fig. 14) had adhered to coverslips within 48-72 hr, and their cytoplasm was spread out on the glass. Their shape was variable; many had numerous and short processes, some cells were round, and others

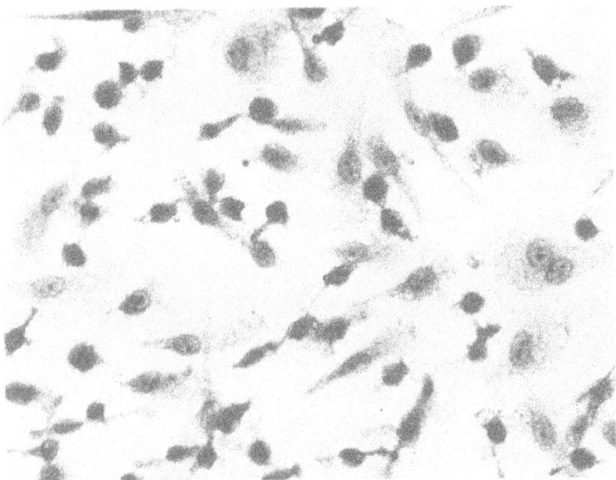

Fig. 14. Five-day culture of human cells. x 350, reduced 25% for reproduction.

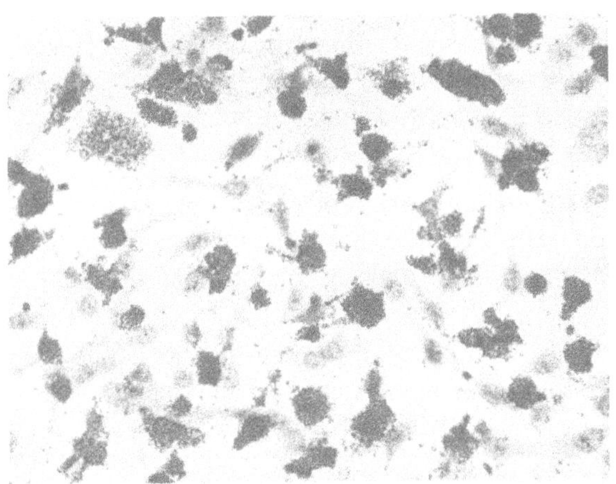

Fig. 15. Phagocytosis of starch granules, x 350, reduced 25% for reproduction.

were spindle shaped. The nucleus was oval or indented, the nuclear membrane clearly defined, and nucleoli were absent. These cells readily phagocytosed starch granules (Fig. 15).

There was a much smaller population of cells, between 5 and 10% of the total number, which did not phagocytose. They were often large and elongated although pleomorphic and triangular forms could be found. Their cytoplasm was deep blue with Leishman's stain and contained minute fenestrations (Fig. 16). Longitudinal striae were present in the thicker parts of the cytoplasm. These cells never contained leucocytic granules. The pro-

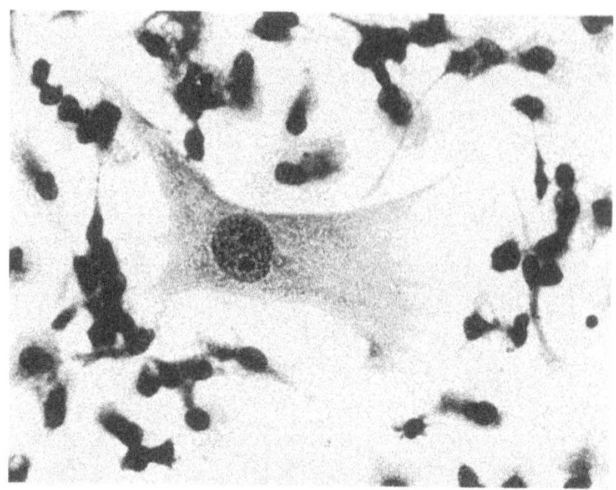

Fig. 16. Large serosal cell in a 13-day culture. × 350, reduced 25% for reproduction.

cesses were often long and tenuous. The nucleus was very large and characteristic. It was round or oval, finely granular, and never indented or lobed. The nuclear membrane was rather irregular and poorly defined. The nucleus was much less basophilic than the surrounding cytoplasm although the intranuclear chromatin was intensely basophilic.

These chromatin bodies were distinctive, variable in shape but often round or Y-shaped with irregular borders. There were between two and five per cell. Between the fifth and tenth day of culture the cells visibly in-

Table I. Reactivity of Human Macrophages from a Single Group A Donor to Erythrocytes of Different Blood Groups

Type of red cell	Number of red cell donors	Result
Group A	9	Negative
Group B	3	Negative
Group O	10	Negative
Group AB	2	Negative

Table II. Reactivity of Human Macrophages Grown in AB Serum to Red Cells Treated with Natural and Immune Agglutinins

Nature of antiserum	Number of primary cultures	Number of individual tests	Result
Isoagglutinins A or B	4	8	Adherence-phagocytosis
Isoimmune anti-A	2	16	Phagocytosis
Rhesus anti-D	6	12	Negative
Rabbit hemolysin	5	10	Phagocytosis

Table III. Effect of Complement on Erythrophagocytosis with Rabbit Anti-Human Red Cell Serum

Source of serum	Dilution of serum	Percentage phagocytosis
Normal rabbit serum with complement	100	<1
	200	<1
	400	<1
Normal rabbit serum inactivated by heat	100	<1
	200	<1
	400	<1
Immune rabbit serum with complement	100	Uncountable
	200	24
	400	2
Immune rabbit serum without complement	100	60
	200	15
	400	1

Table IV. Protocol of a Typical Experiment. Macrophages from M. R. (Group O Rh+) Grown in AB Serum

Cells added to culture	Result
M. R. red cells	Negative
Mouse red cells	Negative
Fowl red cells	Adherence
M. R. cells in AB serum	Negative
A cells in AB serum	Negative
B cells in AB serum	Negative
A cells in B serum	Adherence
A cells in M. R. serum	Adherence
B cells in M. R. serum	Adherence
M. R. cells + rhesus anti(D+)	Negative
M. R. cells + rabbit hemolysin	Phagocytosis
A1 cells + isoimmune anti-A	Phagocytosis

creased in number and the macrophages became relatively fewer. Mitotic figures were sometimes seen. Between the 15th and 30th day of culture the large nonphagocytic cells predominated.

Effect of Adding Erythrocytes of Different Blood Groups

These experiments (Table I) gave consistently negative results, provided that the macrophages were incubated in human AB serum. There were no signs of adherence and phagocytosis was never observed.

Reactivity of Macrophages to Red Cells Treated with Antibodies

Isoagglutinins A and B caused adherence of red cells to macrophages. Phagocytosis was also present but to a variable and often low degree. Positive results were obtained only with high serum concentrations of the order of $1/2$ or $1/4$ and any effect was rapidly lost on dilution.

Immune anti-A serum gave massive phagocytosis and the macrophages were so filled with red cells that it was difficult to see the nucleus. The titer by erythrophagocytosis was $1/8$. The anti-D (Rh+) sera gave consistently negative results and neither adherence nor phagocytosis was noted (Table II).

Rabbit hemolysin gave a marked degree of phagocytosis up to a dilution of $1/200$. The absence of heat labile factors did not markedly affect the titer obtained by erythrophagocytosis (Table III). The protocol of a typical experiment is shown in Table IV. The macrophages derived from a single donor failed to recognize blood cells of different groups and neither adherence nor phagocytosis was observed. Mouse cells were also negative although some adherence was noted with fowl cells. The appropriate isoagglutinin caused adherence, whereas both the immune anti-A serum and rabbit hemolysin strongly promoted phagocytosis. The anti-D serum had no effect.

DISCUSSION

These experiments show that human macrophages are unable to distinguish between normal red cells of different ABO blood groups. It would appear that any changes produced on the cell surface by these antigens are not of a sufficient degree to be recognized as foreign on contact with the cytoplasm of homologous macrophages in culture. The addition of an appropriate isoagglutinin caused marked adherence of red cells to macrophages but relatively little phagocytosis occurred.

A criticism is that many of the red cells were agglutinated in the tissue culture tubes and these may have been too large for phagocytosis. On the other hand, agglutinates of a similar size prepared by the action of a hemolysin showed massive phagocytosis. Loutit and Millison (1946) found that red cell agglutinates produced in vitro by anti-A serum appeared largely to disperse in the circulation of Group A subjects, in that the survival of these pre-agglutinated cells was relatively normal. These in vivo findings are comparable to the present in vitro work which revealed adherence of isoagglutinin-treated cells to macrophages.

The action of the "hemolytic" antibodies was strikingly different. Both the immune anti-A serum and the rabbit hemolysin promoted clear and indubitable ingestion of erythrocytes. The serological titration of the anti-A serum showed only a trace of hemolysis, whereas the titer by erythrophagocytosis was $1/8$. This suggests that the discriminatory activity of the human macrophage is not without a moderate degree of sensitivity. It is tempting to suggest that the macrophage can discriminate between hemagglutinating and hemolytic antibodies. The response to the former could be mainly adherence and to the latter phagocytosis. However, the hemagglutinating sera were low in titer and the observed differences may reflect the number of globulin molecules bound to the red cell surface and need not imply any intrinsic difference in the quality of the antibody.

Cutbush and Mollison [6] found lytic antibodies were especially capable of bringing about destruction of injected red cells in vivo, and this is consistent with our hypothesis that lytic antibodies promote ingestion rather than adherence of red cells. The failure to demonstrate any effect of anti-D was surprising, especially in the light of the detailed studies of Jandl, Jones, and Castle [7], who found that red cells sensitized by incomplete anti-D antibodies were filtered off by the spleen. Mollison and Paterson [8], however, found a normal survival time of cells sensitized in vitro, after initial destruction of a small number. Bonnin and Schwartz (1954) also did not detect erythrophagocytosis when they mixed anti-D coated cells with leucocytes from the buffy coat of blood. The situation is complicated by the fact that mouse macrophages grown in AB serum will readily detect incomplete anti-D antibodies (Stuart and Cumming [9] and perhaps one ought to consider the possibility that human macrophages from the peritoneum differ in their responses from those of the liver and spleen. The work of Nelson and Buras [10] has produced experimental data to support the view that macrophages may vary in different organs and it would be of interest to know if macrophages from the human spleen differed from those elsewhere.

In the case of heterologous cells, the erythrocytes of the mouse did not interact with human macrophages, whereas those from the fowl gave some adherence. This was probably due to traces of natural antibodies present in human serum and need not detract from the view that even wide species differences do not result in contactual recognition between red cells and macrophage.

The main conclusions reached in this work are that human macrophages in tissue culture are unable to recognize major blood group differences in red cells and fail to interact with red cells from some other species. When the appropriate isoagglutinin is present, adherence occurs. The human macrophage is extremely sensitive to hemolytic antibody, either isoimmune or heteroimmune, to which it responds by phagocytosis. It seems that the reaction of human macrophages to red cells is determined entirely by the presence of opsonins either in the environment or on the cell surface.

SUMMARY

Human macrophages have been isolated and cultured from the peritoneal sac. The cells were grown in human AB serum and erythrocytes from different blood groups added. No interaction occurred. Similar results were obtained with red cells from other species, provided natural opsonins were absent, from the culture medium. It seems that blood group differences are not sufficiently distinctive to permit direct contactual recognition by the macrophage. The addition of isoagglutinins promoted mainly adherence. Isoimmune anti-A serum and hemolysins caused intense phagocytosis. The findings support the view that the discriminatory activity of the human macrophage is opsonin-dependent.

ACKNOWLEDGMENTS

The author is indebted to the Wellcome Trust for a research grant, and to Dr. R.A. Cumming for advice and the supply of antisera and blood samples without which this work could not have been done. The invaluable help of Mrs. J. Lowther and Miss E.A. Davidson is gratefully acknowledged.

REFERENCES

1. C.R. Jenkin and K. Karthigasu, Compt. Rend. Soc. Biol., 156 : 1006, 1962.
2. R.B. Vaughan and S.V. Boyden, Immunology, 7(2) : 118, 1964.
3. M. McCutcheon, Physiol. Rev., 26 : 319, 1946.
4. H. Harris, Physiol. Rev., 34 : 529, 1954.
5. S. Boyden, Intern. Rev. Exptl. Pathol., 2 : 311-351, 1963.
6. M. Cutbush and P. L. Mollison, Brit. J. Hematol., 4 :115-137, 1958.
7. J.H. Jandl, A.R. Jones, and W.B. Castle, J. Clin. Invest., 36 : 1428, 1957.
8. P.L. Mollison and J.C.S. Paterson, J. Clin. Pathol., 2 : 109, 1949.
9. A.E. Stuart and R.A. Cumming, Vox Sanguinis. In press.
10. E.L. Nelson and N.S. Buras, J. Immunol., 90 : 412, 1962.

Some Effects of Divalent Cations on In Vitro Phagocytosis*

G. V. Metzger and L. J. Casarett

Department of Radiation Biology and Biophysics
University of Rochester Medical Center
Rochester, New York

ABSTRACT. An in vitro investigation of phagocytosis by rat peritoneal macrophages is reported. Some effects of divalent cations on binding and engulfment of several metal oxides and carbon particles are described.

Calcium and magnesium concentrations were varied by the treatment of protein-free Tyrodes medium with EDTA or ion-exchange resin in preliminary studies, and by the addition to 0.145 M NaCl. Removal of Ca^{++} resulted in a consistent decrease of the phagocytic index (expressed as percentage of cells containing particles). Conversely, addition of Ca^{++}, within limits, enhanced the phagocytic index with a peak effect at 10^{-4} M for metal oxide particles studied. In all cases, Mg^{++} did not significantly change the phagocytic index from control levels (with 0.145 M NaCl and no divalent ions). Unlike the metal oxides, Ca^{++} did not significantly change the phagocytic index from control levels for the carbon particles.

Additional experiments on the variation of the phagocytic index as a function of time, incubating medium, particle-concentration, and type, are described. These experiments were carried out to determine whether Ca^{++} increased the "rate" of phagocytosis, or the total number of cells phagocytizing. The binding of cells to various surfaces was also investigated as a function of divalent ion concentrations.

The possible mechanisms of the actions of Ca^{++} in the phagocytic process are discussed in the light of the data presented.

* This work was performed under AEC Contract W-7401-ENG-49.

INTRODUCTION

Studies on the in vitro requirements of phagocytosis have been investigated and reviewed by many authors in recent years (Gordon and King [1], Carpenter [2], Cohn [3], Rowley [4]).

One of the earliest investigations on the ion requirements associated with phagocytosis was that of Hamburger [5], whose work, along with other early studies, has been reviewed by Mudd, McCutcheon, and Lucké [6]. Among the studies of Hamburger which are pertinent here is his finding of enhanced phagocytosis of several types of particles, including carbon, by polymorphonuclear leucocytes upon addition of $CaCl_2$ to both protein-free and protein-containing media. He found no such enhancement with $MgCl_2$.

The effects of addition of the cations of aluminum, iron (ferric), thorium, and chromium on the phagocytosis of bacteria, in the absence of serum, have been investigated by Neufield and Etinger-Tulcyznika [7] and Gordon and Thompson [9].

A more recent study of the effects of divalent cations on in vitro phagocytosis by polymorphonuclear leucocytes has been carried out by Wilkins and Bangham [10]. These authors demonstrated the phagocytic-enhancing properties of calcium ions as an increase in the phagocytosis of PSL (polystyrene latex) and starch particles by addition of $CaCl_2$ up to 10^{-3} M in 0.145 M NaCl, with greatest enhancement at this concentration. As for the effects of added calcium ions in serum, they found enhancement of the phagocytosis of the PSL particles, but none for the starch grains. In contrast to Hamburger's work, these authors also reported an enhancement of phagocytosis of PSL particles in serum with addition of $MgCl_2$.

Most investigations of the role of cations on the engulfment process have used polymorphonuclear leucocytes as the phagocytic cells, and have, more often than not, involved the use of protein-containing media, based on reports that phagocytosis by such cells requires the presence of serum proteins (Fenn [11], cited by Carpenter [12]; Boyden [11]). Also, many of the particles used in these experiments (PSL, starch, bacteria, etc.) often have ionogenic groups on their surfaces, permitting the possibility of divalent or trivalent cations forming electrostatic bonds between anionic groups on the cell membrane and test particles or proteins covering the particles (Wilkins and Bangham [10]). Consequently, few experimental data have been accumulated on the effects of divalent cations on in vitro phagocytosis by non-PMN phagocytes in protein-free media, using particles void of ionogenic groups on their surfaces. Thus, while hypotheses have been put forward to explain the enhancing role of calcium ions in the presence of proteins (Wilkins and Bangham [10]), less attention has been given to explaining the role of calcium or magnesium ions in protein-free media.

The present work is concerned with an investigation of the effects of two divalent cations, calcium and magnesium, in a protein-free medium consisting of 0.145 M NaCl, on the phagocytosis by peritoneal macrophages of nonionogenic insoluble metal oxide and carbon particles.

MATERIALS AND METHODS

Cell Suspensions

Mononuclear, phagocytic cells (peritoneal macrophages) were obtained as follows. Adult rats of the Rochester strain (Wistar-derived) were injected intraperitoneally with 10 cc of 0.1% glycogen in physiological saline ("priming"). Four to five days later, the rats were sacrificed by cervical dislocation and the exudate was harvested immediately by washing the peritoneum with 20 cc of 0.145 M NaCl. This time interval (4-5 days) was selected on the basis of a peak collection of predominantly mononuclear cells (see "Results").

The exudate thus obtained from each rat was collected in 15-cc siliconized centrifuge tubes, centrifuged for 5-10 min at about 70 g and resuspended in fresh 0.145 M NaCl. The exudate obtained usually contained 80-90% of the desired mononuclear cells, the remaining cell types being made up of mostly PMN, some mast cells, and, occasionally, a few red blood cells. The concentration of exudate obtained was almost always higher than $1 \cdot 10^6$ cells/cc exudate.

Final stock suspensions of mononuclear cells were obtained by pooling individual resuspended samples. The concentrations of the final suspensions were determined by use of the Coulter Counter Model B.

Incubating Medium

The final incubating medium consisted of the following to give a total volume of 2 cc per incubating flask: 1.0 cc stock cell suspension in 0.145 M NaCl; 0.5 cc stock particle suspension in 0.145 M NaCl; and 0.5 cc appropriate concentrations of $CaCl_2$ or $MgCl_2$ (in 0.145 M NaCl) to give desired final concentrations.

Unless otherwise stated, all incubations were carried out in 10-cc siliconized Erlenmeyer flasks for a period of 15 min at 37°C, with gentle shaking in a Dubnoff incubator. Total volumes were increased in the time course experiments.

Determination of Phagocytic Index

Immediately after incubation, the flasks were removed and smears quickly made of the contents of each incubating flask. The smears were stained with Wright's stain and mounted. The phagocytic index was determined under oil immersion in the manner used by Hamburger [5] and Wilkens and Bangham [10], i.e., by determining the percentage of phagocytes which had engulfed test particles during the incubation period. This index was selected largely because of the ease and accuracy with which it could be measured. Other indices are currently being considered for extension of the work reported here.

Two to four separate determinations of the phagocytic index were made for each flask, each determination consisting of a count of 100 cells. Thus, a total of 200-400 cells were counted per flask, from which a mean was calculated and plotted.

Particle Suspensions

The particle suspensions were prepared by adding known amounts of the particles to 200 cc of 0.145 M NaCl, followed by violent shaking for a minute. The suspensions were left for an hour to allow large particles to settle. The supernate was then used as a stock particle suspension. Concentrations of the stock-particle suspensions were obtained with a hemocytometer.

All particles were obtained in the dry powdered form free of any emulsifiers or stabilizers. The Al_2O_3 and Cr_2O_3 particles were obtained from Buehler, Ltd.* Particle sizes were estimated from dried smears under oil immersion, and indicated a size range of about 0.5-1.5 μ, with the dominant particle dimension being about 0.9 μ for the particles used.

RESULTS

The method of obtaining suspensions of the peritoneal macrophages has already been described. Collections on the fourth and fifth days contained the largest percentage of cells of the mononuclear variety. Exudate obtained after the first and second days usually contains large numbers of PMN-leucocytes with the mononuclear cells making up only a small fraction of the total number. Figure 1 is a bar graph representation of a typical differential analysis of the exudate for two rats as a function of the number of days after priming injection, beginning with Day 0, at which time the cells were harvested without any previous priming injections.

Preliminary studies of the phagocytosis of the test particles by these peritoneal macrophages were carried out in Tyrode's solution, a protein-free, balanced salt solution with glucose, containing Ca^{++} and Mg^{++}. It was found that treatment of the Tyrode's incubating medium with either 0.1% EDTA or Na-cationic exchange resin always resulted in a significant decrease in the phagocytic index from that obtained with an untreated but otherwise equivalent incubating medium. These results led the authors to pro-

---

*Buehler Ltd., Illinois.

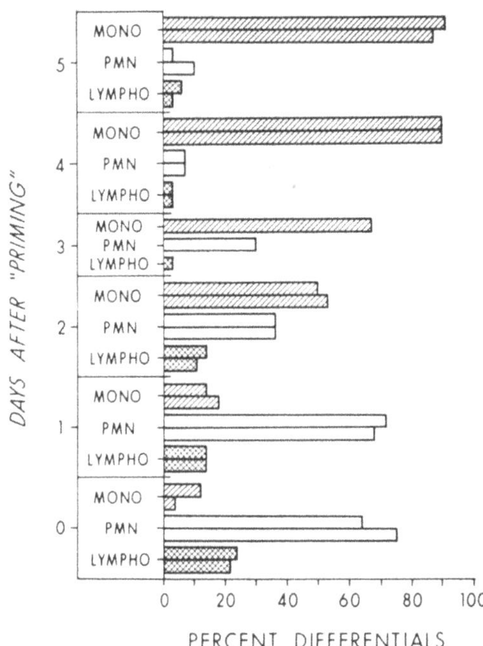

Fig. 1. Percentage differential of cell types found in peritoneal exudate as a function of days after priming with 0.1% glycogen in physiological saline. The zero-day refers to exudate harvested without such priming.

ceed with an investigation of Ca^{++} and Mg^{++} on the process of phagocytosis, since presumably these ions were removed upon treatment of the medium with the EDTA or the cationic exchange resin.

Ca^{++} vs Mg^{++} in Phagocytosis of Several Metal Oxides

A study was made of the relative enhancing effects of varying concentrations of added $CaCl_2$ or $MgCl_2$ in 0.145 M NaCl on the in vitro phagocytosis of chromic oxide (Cr_2O_3), manganese dioxide (MnO_2), ferric oxide (Fe_2O_3), and aluminum oxide (Al_2O_3) particles. Figure 2 shows some typical data for the variation of the phagocytic index as a function of the log-molar concentration of added $CaCl_2$ or $MgCl_2$. Each point in the figure represents a mean of two to three determinations, each of which was a random count of 100 cells. Control values of the index obtained with neither divalent cation in the incubating medium (0.145 M NaCl) are plotted on the ordinate.

With the exception of the Fe_2O_3 particles, $CaCl_2$ addition caused significant enhancement of the phagocytic index, whereas $MgCl_2$ was without effect

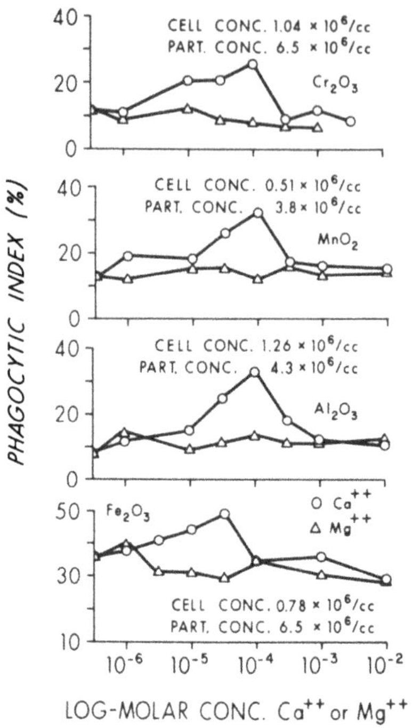

Fig. 2. Significance of calcium enhancement given by plus or minus two standard deviations at control and 10^{-4} M $CaCl_2$: ±1% control and ± 1% 10^{-4} M Ca^{++}, for Cr_2O_3; ± 0% control and ± 3% 10^{-4} M Ca^{++}, for MnO_2; ± 3% control and ± 3% 10^{-4} M Ca^{++} for Al_2O_3; ±1% control and ± 10% 10^{-4} M Ca^{++} for Fe_2O_3.

and did not change the index significantly from control levels.* The enhancing effects with addition of $CaCl_2$ increased up to 10^{-4} M, beyond which the index rapidly fell back to control levels.

Each of these experiments has been repeated several times at different values of cell and particle concentrations, and similar enhancement of phagocytosis by calcium ions has been obtained in all cases. High control levels and only slight enhancement with addition of $CaCl_2$ (of borderline significance) have been obtained on all experiments with Fe_2O_3 particles.

Ca^{++} vs Mg^{++} in the Phagocytosis of Carbon Particles

Experiments similar to those for the metal oxides were carried out for carbon particles, to see whether a nonmetal oxide, also void of any iono-

* Enhancement was considered significant only if the phagocytic index at 10^{-4} M $CaCl_2$, plus or minus two standard deviations, did not overlap with the control values, plus or minus two standard deviations.

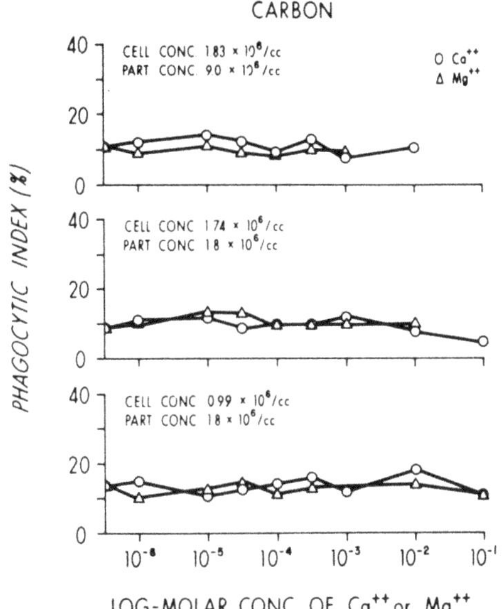

Fig. 3. Ca^{++} vs Mg^{++} for the phagocytosis of carbon particles.

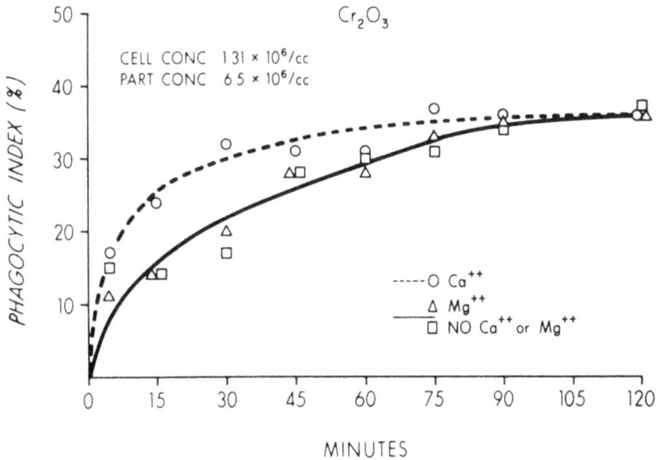

Fig. 4. Phagocytic index for Cr_2O_3 particles as a function of time for three incubating media: 10^{-4} M $CaCl_2$ and 10^{-4} M $MgCl_2$ in 0.145 M NaCl, and just 0.145 M NaCl alone.

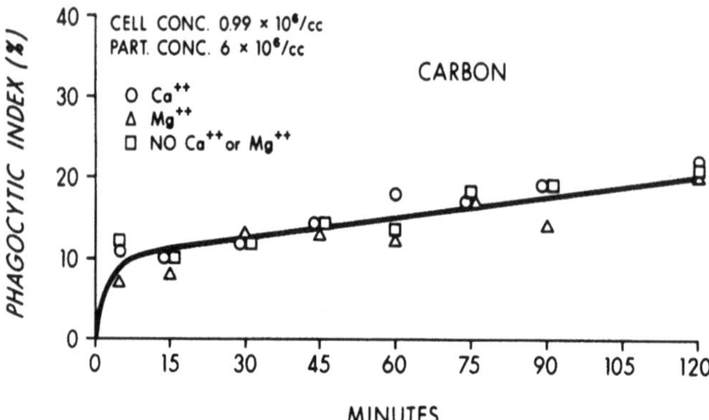

Fig. 5. Phagocytic index for carbon particles as a function of time for three incubating media: 10^{-4} M $CaCl_2$ and 10^{-4} M $MgCl_2$ in 0.145 M NaCl, and just 0.145 M NaCl alone.

genic groups, would behave similarly to the metal oxides upon addition of $CaCl_2$. Figure 3 shows a typical response of the phagocytic index as a function of the log-molar concentrations of either added $CaCl_2$ or $MgCl_2$, for several concentrations of carbon particles. All results (from $1 \cdot 10^6$ to $9 \cdot 10^6$/cc particle concentration) indicate that neither Ca^{++} nor Mg^{++} significantly changes the phagocytic index from control levels.

Phagocytic Index as a Function of Time of Incubation

A time course experiment was carried out to determine whether the enhancing effects of added $CaCl_2$ were due to an increasing rate of phagocytosis of the metal oxides or to an increasing number of cells capable of phagocytizing. Figure 4 shows a typical response of the phagocytic index as a function of time of incubation for Cr_2O_3 particles in 0.145 M NaCl alone, or with added 10^{-4} M $CaCl_2$ or $MgCl_2$. The effect of added $CaCl_2$ is to increase the rate of phagocytosis, since the final percentage of cells participating (at 2 hr) is about the same for all three incubating media. Again, added $MgCl_2$ caused little if any change in the phagocytic index from control levels without divalent cations present. The figure illustrates the usual enhanced phagocytic index of the $CaCl_2$ medium compared to that of the other two at 15 min incubation, and also suggests that such differences are greatest at about 30 min incubation of cells and particles.

Similar time course experiments were carried out for the carbon particles; Figure 5 illustrates the results of such an experiment. It is readily apparent that the values at any particular time are not significantly different from one another (for any of the three incubating media) and a single curve can be drawn through all the points. Thus, neither Ca^{++} nor Mg^{++} shows any significant enhancement of the phagocytic index for any period of incubation up to 2 hr, at which time the index has reached a maximal level.

DISCUSSION

Three general mechanisms have suggested themselves as possible modes of action of calcium ions in enhancing phagocytosis. The first involves calcium ions activating some enzyme, or enzymes, related to, and perhaps necessary for, the engulfment process (Allison [21]). The second mechanism pictures calcium ions modifying the three-dimensional structure (stereochemistry) of the membrane components, somehow making the engulfment process easier. The last involves calcium ions changing the physical nature of the cell surface by chelation to anionic groups, making the cell surface more attractive (or less repulsive) to certain types of particles.

In the present experiments, a fourth mechanism, involving divalent cations bridging anionic groups between cell and particle surfaces, was thought to have been eliminated by using insoluble metallic oxide and carbon particles, void of any ionogenic groups to which calcium or any other ions could bind. The use of carbon represented a check to see if the peritoneal macrophages would respond similarly, upon addition of $CaCl_2$ to the incubating medium, to particles different in chemical and physical properties from the metal oxides.

With the exception of the results for carbon, and possibly of Fe_2O_3, the enhancement of phagocytosis with calcium ions suggests the possibility of these ions' playing an enzyme-activating role. However, one would assume such a mechanism to be independent of the particle being engulfed. Although in the light of the data with carbon this first mechanism now looks less attractive, it may still be a possibility in a modified form (i.e., a surface enzyme sensitive to the type of particle being engulfed).

At present, no simple mechanism has suggested itself as to how the binding of calcium ions to the membrane, and the possible structural (stereochemical) modifications caused by such binding, might bring about an enhancement of the engulfment process.

The apparent dependence of calcium enhancement of phagocytosis on the nature of the particle being engulfed suggests that the role of calcium ions may be to modify the surface properties of the cells (or perhaps even the particles). The chelation of calcium ions to anionic groups on the cell surface may decrease the repulsion or increase the attraction between cell and certain particle surfaces.

In relation to this third mechanism, the technique of electrophoresis has provided information on some of the surface properties of both cells and particles (Bangham [13], Mehrishi [14], Bangham [15]). For example, it has been shown by this technique that most mammalian cells possess a net negative charge at their surfaces, apparently due to an excess of anionic surface groups. Investigation of the types of ionic groups which contribute to such electrophoretic mobility of cells are underway by several investigators (Cook [16], Granzer [17]).

It has also been known for some time that certain particles (quartz, Fe_2O_3, glass, etc.) possess an electrophoretic mobility, even though these particles, in a protein-free medium, are supposedly void of ionogenic groups (carboxyl, phosphate, sulfate, etc.) (Abramson [18], Mehrishi [14]). Among the metal oxides used in the present experiments only the Fe_2O_3 is known to exhibit a positive electrophoretic mobility, the remaining metal oxides having negative electrophoretic mobilities (Glasstone [19]). Thus, with the exception of Fe_2O_3, the metal oxides apparently possess negatively charged surfaces, which may induce a hydration layer with the negative ends of the water dipoles facing the outside. Questions still remain as to the genesis of these surface charges, and whether they are due to actual ions on the surfaces of the particles (hydroxyl ions and others), representing full charges, or only partial negative charges due to polarity of the molecules at the surfaces.

Calcium ions present in the medium may decrease the electrostatic repulsive forces between the negative cell and the negative particle surfaces, and allow for greater cell—particle contact. Also, the possibility exists of chelation of calcium ions to the particle surfaces, in the event that there does exist fully charged anions on these particles. Thus, the role of electrostatic forces between (hydrated) anionic groups of the cell membrane and the (partial or full) negative charges on the surfaces of certain particles, and how various cations may affect such forces, need further investigation as possible factors determining the rate of phagocytosis.

The existence of positively charged Fe_2O_3 particles may explain the unusually high control values of the phagocytic index obtained with this particle, as well as the slight enhancement of its phagocytosis upon addition of $CaCl_2$. In this case, the positively charged Fe_2O_3 particles would be attracted rather than repelled by the negatively charged cell surface, and the binding of calcium ions to anionic groups of the membrane would not be expected to increase the rate of engulfment. Thus, the high control values attained in the absence of calcium ions may be explained by electrostatic attraction between the cell and Fe_2O_3 particles.

Although the surface properties of carbon particles in aqueous media have not been well defined, it is possible that carbon does not possess either a positively or negatively charged surface, or at least one that is very strong. That is, the carbon surface may be neutral, and because of the absence of a negative charge its engulfment would be insensitive to the decrease of the negative charge of the cell membrane by calcium ions. It should be noted that the present findings with carbon, as well as those of Fenn [11], are in contradiction to those of Hamburger [5], who found enhancement of phagocytosis of carbon upon addition of $CaCl_2$ to an apparently protein-free medium.

The greater chelating powers of calcium over magnesium ions may explain the enhancing results with calcium and the lack of such results with magnesium for most of the metal oxides. Bangham [13] has found the electrophoretic mobility of blood cells to be more readily reduced with calcium than magnesium ions, apparently due to greater binding of calcium to the anionic groups of the membrane. However, Wilkins and Bangham [10] failed to show a decrease in the electrophoretic mobility of polymorphonuclear leucocytes with added $CaCl_2$. Katchalsky [20] has illustrated the greater binding powers of calcium to synthetic polyglutamic acid over that found from magnesium ions.

Recently, work by Allison [21] and Garvin [22], as well as preliminary work of the present authors, has indicated that calcium ions do not affect the adhesiveness of cells to glass surfaces. Whether such experiments actually relate to the role of calcium ions in increasing cell-particle contact before engulfment remains to be further studied. Currently, methods are being tried to measure any changes in cell-particle contact as a function of $CaCl_2$ concentration.

In view of the data that exist at present, much work remains to be done to elucidate the nature and roles of both cell and particle surfaces (as well as particle shape and size), in the engulfment phase of phagocytosis. Such knowledge is essential to an understanding of the initial phases of this physiological process, and may also have value in an understanding of the physiopathologic responses to insoluble particulate material.

REFERENCES

1. G.B. Gordon and D.W. King, "Phagocytosis," Am.J. Pathol., 37:279-292, 1960.
2. P.L. Carpenter, Immunology and Serology, Philadelphia, Saunders, 1965, pp. 296-316.
3. Z.A. Cohn, "The metabolism and physiology of the mononuclear phagocytes," in: B.W. Zweifach, L. Grant, and R.T. McCluskey (Eds.), The Inflammatory Process, New York, Academic Press, 1965, pp. 323-353.
4. D. Rowley, "Phagocytosis," Adv.Immunol., 2:241-264, 1962.
5. H.J. Hamburger, Physikalisch-chemische untersuchungen über phagozyten, Wiesbaden, 1912.
6. S. Mudd, M. McCutcheon, and B. Lucké, "Phagocytosis," Physiol.Rev., 14: 210-275, 1934.
7. F. Neufield and R. Etinger-Tulcyznska, "Beitrag zur Wirkungsweise der phagozytosserregenden immunkörper," Zentr. Bakteriol. Parasitenk. Abt.I. Orig., 114:252-263, 1929.
8. W.J. Nungester and A.M. Ames, "Effect of selected chemical substances on phagocytosis," J.Infect.Diseases, 90:51-60, 1952.
9. J. Gordon and F.C. Thompson, "The artificial opsonization of bacteria," Brit.J.Exptl.Pathol., 17:159-163, 1936.

10. D.J. Wilkins and A.D. Bangham, "The effect of some metal ions on in vitro phagocytosis," J. Reticuloendothelial Soc., 1:233-242, 1964.
11. W.O. Fenn, "The phagocytosis of solid particles. II. Carbon," J. Gen. Physiol., 3:465-482, 1920-21.
12. S. Boyden, "Cellular recognition of foreign matter," Intern. Rev. Exptl. Pathol., 2:311-356, 1963.
13. A.D. Bangham, B.A. Pethica, and G.V.F. Seaman, "The charged groups at the interface of some blood cells," Biochem. J., 69:12-19, 1958.
14. J.N. Mehrishi and G.V.F. Seaman, "Temperature dependence of the electrophoretic mobility of cells and quartz particles," Biochim. Biophys. Acta, 112:154-159, 1966.
15. A.D. Bangham and B.A. Pethica, "The adhesiveness of cells and the nature of the chemical groups at their surfaces," Proc. Roy. Soc. Edinburgh, Sect. A, 28:43-50, 1959.
16. G.M.W. Cook, "Sialic acids and the electrokinetic charge of the human erythrocytes," Nature, 191:44-45, 1961.
17. E. Granzer, G.F. Fuhrman, and G. Ruhenstroth-Bauer, "Untersuchungen über die mit Neuraminidase abspaltbaren Neuraminsäurederivate aus Oberflackenmenbranen normaler Leberzellen und Asciteshepatomzellen von Ratten, 'Hoppe-Seylers Z. Phisol. Chem., 337:52-56, 1964.
18. H.A. Abramson, "Electrokinetic phenomena. I. Adsorption of serum by quartz and paraffin oil," J. Gen. Physiol., 13:169-177, 1929.
19. S. Glasstone, Textbook of Physical Chemistry, New York, D. Van Nostrand Co., Inc., 1946, pp. 1238-1243.
20. A. Katchalsky, "Polyelectrolytes and their biological interactions," Biophys. J., 4:9-41, 1964.
21. F. Allison, Jr., M.G. Lancaster, and J.L. Crosthwaite, "Studies on the pathogenesis of acute inflammation. V. An assessment of factors that influence in vitro the phagocytic and adhesive properties of leucocytes obtained from rabbit peritoneal exudate," Am. J. Pathol., 43:775-795, 1963.
22. J.E. Garvin, "Factors affecting the adhesiveness of human leucocytes and platelets in vitro," J. Exp. Med., 114:51-73, 1961.

The Engulfing Potential of Peritoneal Phagocytes of Conventional and Germfree Mice*

E. H. Perkins, P. Nettesheim, T. Morita, and H. E. Walburg, Jr.

Biology Division
Oak Ridge National Laboratory
Oak Ridge, Tennessee

It is not known what role naturally occurring microbial flora play in the development of the phagocytic capacity of peritoneal phagocytes. A quantitative comparative study of phagocytes from conventional and germfree animals is therefore desirable. With the development of a simple quantitative method, we have been able to measure the in vitro engulfing potential of peritoneal cells from different strains of mice raised in conventional or germfree environments. In the work to be presented we found no difference in the engulfing potential of peritoneal phagocytes from conventional and germfree mice. The importance of a defined population of cells and quantitative techniques are stressed, and the in vitro functional maturation of peritoneal phagocytes is reported.

QUANTITATIVE CONSIDERATIONS

Differences observed in the engulfing capacity of populations of peritoneal exudate cells harvested from different strains of normal or stimulated mice raised in conventional or germfree environments can result from differences in the number of phagocytic cells in the exudate, or from differences in the engulfing efficiency of these cells. It was therefore mandatory to consider both quantitative and qualitative differences in the present study. For this reason we have utilized a simple, quantitative method to measure the in vitro engulfing potential of peritoneal phagocytes. Peritoneal exudate cells were harvested from mice, mixed with opsonized sheep erythrocytes (RBC) in 25-ml siliconized Erlenmeyer flasks, and in-

*Research sponsored by the U.S. Atomic Energy Commission under contract with the Union Carbide Corporation.

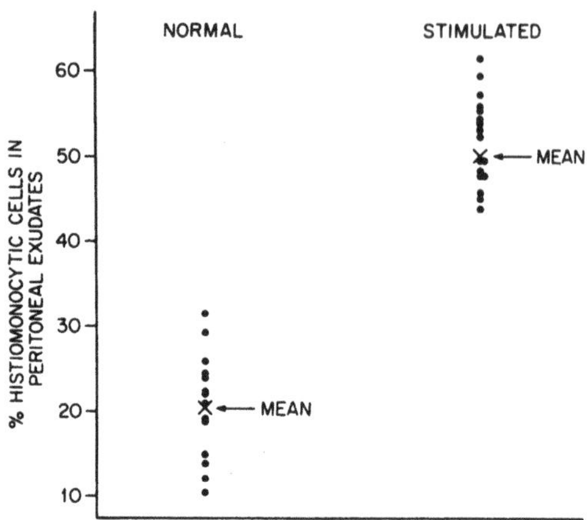

Fig. 1. Percent histiomonocytic cells in peritoneal exudates harvested from normal and stimulated conventional $1C3F_1$ mice. Stimulated mice received 2 ml 4% gelatin 48 hr prior to being killed. Differential counts made from smears of pooled peritoneal exudate cells from 25-150 mice, 12-20 weeks of age. Each point represents a separate experiment.

cubated at 37°C on an oscillatory shaker. At 15- to 30-min intervals, 1-ml aliquots of this cell suspension, which consisted of phagocytic cells engorged with RBC, unengulfed extracellular RBC, and the nonphagocytic elements of the exudate, were exposed to a brief, 40-sec, hypotonic shock which resulted in complete lysis of the extracellular RBC, while peritoneal phagocytes and the intracellular RBC were undamaged. The amount of hemoglobin liberated was a direct measurement of the number of unengulfed extracellular RBC. Knowing the number initially added to this closed system, one can calculate the percent engulfment and the average number of RBC engulfed per histiomonocytic cell. The details of the method have been published previously [1].

It is generally recognized that 90-95% of the cells in the peritoneal cavity of the normal, unstimulated mouse are mononuclear cells, and it is not uncommon for investigators to equate these mononuclear cells to phagocytic elements. However, the majority of these cells are medium and small lymphocytes. In general, in the normal, unstimulated mouse, only about 20% of peritoneal cells are identifiable in smears as histiomonocytic cells – the classical phagocytic elements (Fig. 1). The percentage of histiomonocytic cells is more than doubled as a result of the injection of gelatin which is a sterile irritant (Fig. 1), and, usually, the total number of cells that can be harvested from the peritoneal cavity is also increased.

We have previously demonstrated [1] that in this in vitro system the engulfing index (k)* is dependent upon the initial RBC–histiomonocytic cell ratio. Hence, meaningful comparative studies can be carried out only among different peritoneal cell populations when the RBC : histiomonocytic cell ratio is kept constant. Because not all cells in the exudate are phagocytes, and because the number of histiomonocytic cells is always less in unstimulated mice, differential cell counts of the exudate must be made, and then an appropriate number of RBC added.

ENHANCEMENT OF THE ENGULFING POTENTIAL (QUALITATIVE CHANGE)

From the data presented in Fig. 2, we see that exudate cells from stimulated mice have a markedly enhanced phagocytic capacity. However, this enhanced phagocytic capacity is related not only to an increased number of histiomonocytic cells in the exudate population, but also to an enhanced phagocytic efficiency of the histiomonocytic cell population. This can be established by inspection of the table at the bottom of Fig. 2. In the first instance, the RBC : histiomonocytic cell ratio was 4 : 1 for both stimulated and nonstimulated exudate cells. The RBC inoculum for stimulated exudate cells was $17.4 \cdot 10^6$ [$(4.4 \cdot 10^6) \cdot 4$], of which 90% were engulfed within 1 hr. The average number of RBC engulfed per histiomonocytic cell was 3.57 (see column 4, Fig. 2), whereas, with nonstimulated exudate cells the RBC inoculum was $6.0 \cdot 10^6$; 38% were engulfed within 1 hr to yield an average number of 1.62 RBC engulfed per histiomonocytic cell. The enhanced phagocytic efficiency of the stimulated cell population was correlated with increase in both the number of histiomonocytic cells engulfing RBC and the number of RBC engulfed per active phagocyte. This same pattern is observed at a 20 : 1 RBC:histiomonocytic cell ratio. The percent RBC engulfed was smaller because the RBC inoculum per histiomonocytic cell was much larger. However, the absolute number of RBC engulfed was increased and, therefore, the average number of RBC per histiomonocytic cell was larger.

An exploration of the types of stimuli that might produce a highly efficient histiomonocytic cell population is presented in Tables I-III. Both particulate and soluble, antigenic and nonantigenic material, specifically related or unrelated to the target particle (sheep and rat erythrocytes, $5 \cdot 10^8$; gelatin, 4%; S. typhi lipopolysaccharide, 20 μg) were injected into donor mice (Table I). Differential counts demonstrated that while different stimuli resulted in quantitative differences in the histiomonocytic cell population, the relative engulfing efficiency of the different populations appeared comparable, regardless of the inducing stimulus.

*k is derived from the equation $n/n_0 = e^{-kt}$, where k is the engulfing index, n_0 is the number of extracellular RBC at time zero, and n is the number of extracellular RBC at time t when t is ≤ 1 hr.

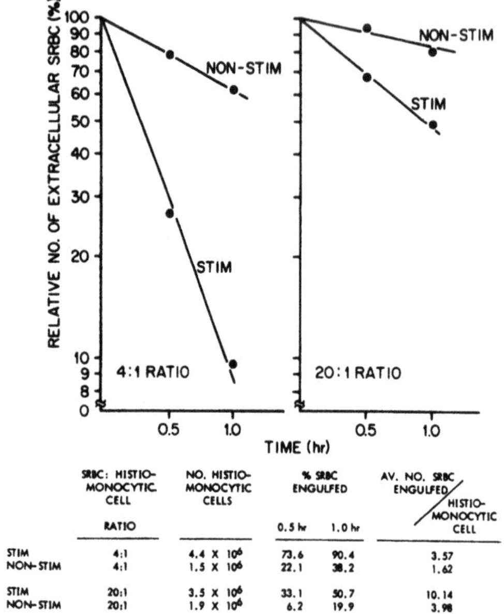

	SRBC: HISTIO-MONOCYTIC CELL RATIO	NO. HISTIO-MONOCYTIC CELLS	% SRBC ENGULFED		AV. NO. SRBC ENGULFED / HISTIO-MONOCYTIC CELL
			0.5 hr	1.0 hr	
STIM	4:1	4.4×10^6	73.6	90.4	3.57
NON-STIM	4:1	1.5×10^6	22.1	38.2	1.62
STIM	20:1	3.5×10^6	33.1	50.7	10.14
NON-STIM	20:1	1.9×10^6	6.2	19.9	3.98

Fig. 2. Differences in the engulfing potential of peritoneal phagocytes from normal (nonstimulated) and stimulated conventional $1C3F_1$ mice. Stimulated mice received 2 ml 4% gelatin 48 hr prior to being killed.

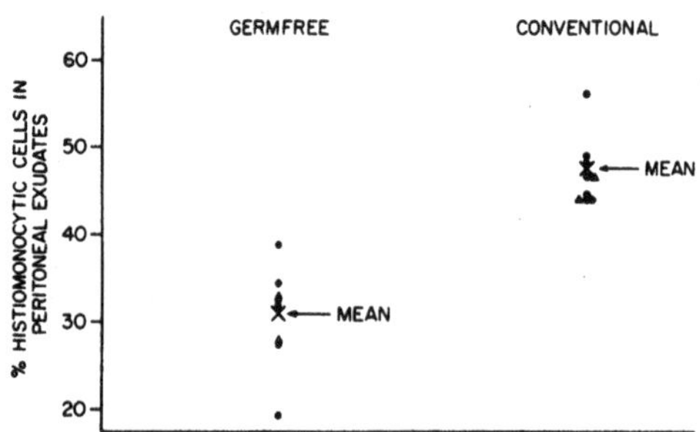

Fig. 3. Percent histiomonocytic cells in peritoneal exudates harvested from conventional and germfree mice that received 2 ml 4% gelatin 48 hr prior to being killed. Differential counts made from smears of pooled peritoneal exudate cells from 15 to 50, 12-16-week-old mice. ●, CF1; Δ, C3H. Each point represents a separate experiment.

Table I. The Effect of Various Stimuli on the Engulfing Efficiency of Peritoneal Phagocytes Harvested from Conventional $1C3F_1$ Mice

Stimulus	No. histiomonocytic cells/ml	No. RBC/ml	% RBC engulfed	No. RBC engulfed / No. histiomonocytic cells	Av. No. RBC engulfed per histiomonocytic cell
		RBC : Histiomonocytic Cell Ratio 3.9 : 1			
Sheep RBC	$5.1 \cdot 10^6$	$20.0 \cdot 10^6$	91.1	$\frac{18.2 \cdot 10^6}{5.1 \cdot 10^6}$	3.57
Rat RBC	$4.2 \cdot 10^6$	$16.4 \cdot 10^6$	85.6	$\frac{14.0 \cdot 10^6}{4.2 \cdot 10^6}$	3.33
Gelatin	$3.8 \cdot 10^6$	$14.7 \cdot 10^6$	87.0	$\frac{12.9 \cdot 10^6}{3.8 \cdot 10^6}$	3.39
LPS	$3.0 \cdot 10^6$	$11.7 \cdot 10^6$	91.0	$\frac{10.7 \cdot 10^6}{3.0 \cdot 10^6}$	3.57
		RBC : Histiomonocytic Cell Ratio 19.5 : 1			
Sheep RBC	$5.1 \cdot 10^6$	$100.0 \cdot 10^6$	49.9	$\frac{49.9 \cdot 10^6}{5.1 \cdot 10^6}$	9.78
Rat RBC	$4.2 \cdot 10^6$	$82.0 \cdot 10^6$	42.1	$\frac{34.5 \cdot 10^6}{4.2 \cdot 10^6}$	8.20
Gelatin	$3.8 \cdot 10^6$	$73.8 \cdot 10^6$	40.7	$\frac{30.0 \cdot 10^6}{3.8 \cdot 10^6}$	7.89
LPS	$3.0 \cdot 10^6$	$58.6 \cdot 10^6$	49.0	$\frac{28.7 \cdot 10^6}{3.0 \cdot 10^6}$	9.57

A commercial preparation of sterile, pyrogen-free saline, which was used routinely in these experiments as the diluent, was then used as a sterile irritant. Although saline injection did not significantly increase the number of histiomonocytic cells in the exudate, their engulfing efficiency was equal to that of the gelatin-induced population, indicating that the two populations were qualitatively identical (Table II).

In order to determine if an injection of exogenous material or fluid was a necessary requisite for the enhancement of the engulfing efficiency of the histiomonocytic cell population, or if mobilization of endogenous cells and fluid movement was sufficient, a sterile needle was inserted intraperitoneally in a simulated injection. It can be seen from Table III that, again, quantitatively, the response was not greatly enhanced, but the resulting histiomonocytic cell population was nearly comparable with that of the positive control (gelatin stimulation), thereby furnishing evidence that the resulting inflammatory response was sufficient to induce a highly efficient histiomonocytic cell population in the absence of exogenous fluid.

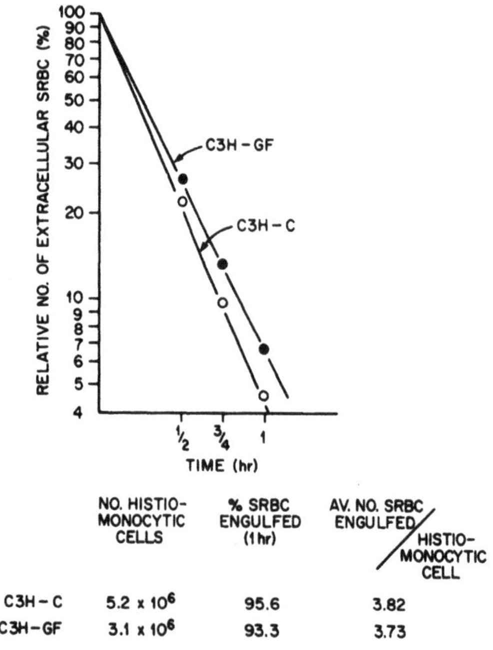

Fig. 4. Engulfing potential of peritoneal phagocytes from stimulated, conventional (C), and germfree (GF) C3H mice. RBC: histiomonocytic cell ratio 4 : 1. Stimulus, 2 ml 4% gelatin 48 hr prior to being killed.

Table II. The Effect of Sterile Pyrogen-Free Saline on the Engulfing Efficiency of Peritoneal Phagocytes Harvested from Conventional $1C3F_1$ Mice

	No. histiomonocytic cells/ml	No. RBC/ml	% RBC engulfed	$\frac{\text{No. RBC engulfed}}{\text{No. histiomonocytic cells}}$	Av. No. RBC engulfed per histiomonocytic cell
		RBC : Histiomonocytic Cell Ratio 4 : 1			
Gelatin	$3.5 \cdot 10^6$	$13.8 \cdot 10^6$	95.1	$\frac{13.2 \cdot 10^6}{3.5 \cdot 10^6}$	3.80
Saline	$1.5 \cdot 10^6$	$6.0 \cdot 10^6$	98.0	$\frac{5.9 \cdot 10^6}{1.5 \cdot 10^6}$	3.93
		RBC : Histiomonocytic Cell Ratio 20 : 1			
Gelatin	$3.5 \cdot 10^6$	$69.2 \cdot 10^6$	50.7	$\frac{35.1 \cdot 10^6}{3.5 \cdot 10^6}$	10.03
Saline	$1.5 \cdot 10^6$	$30.0 \cdot 10^6$	51.4	$\frac{15.4 \cdot 10^6}{1.5 \cdot 10^6}$	10.26

Table III. The Effect of Needle Insertion on the Engulfing Efficiency of Peritoneal Phagocytes Harvested from Conventional $1C3F_1$ Mice

Stimulus	No. of histiomonocytic cells/ml	No. RBC/ml	% RBC engulfed	$\frac{\text{No. RBC engulfed}}{\text{No. histiomonocytic cells}}$	Av. No. RBC engulfed per histiomonocytic cell
		RBC : Histiomonocytic Cell Ratio 4 : 1			
Gelatin	$5.9 \cdot 10^6$	$23.7 \cdot 10^6$	95.8	$\frac{22.7 \cdot 10^6}{5.9 \cdot 10^6}$	3.84
Needle Insertion	$2.6 \cdot 10^6$	$10.5 \cdot 10^6$	82.0	$\frac{8.6 \cdot 10^6}{2.6 \cdot 10^6}$	3.31
No Treatment	$1.4 \cdot 10^6$	$5.5 \cdot 10^6$	12.0	$\frac{0.7 \cdot 10^6}{1.4 \cdot 10^6}$	0.50

ENGULFING POTENTIAL OF PERITONEAL CELLS OF CONVENTIONAL AND GERMFREE MICE

Experiments were then conducted to determine if the engulfing potential of peritoneal phagocytes from conventional mice was superior to that of germfree mice. We initially observed that 48 hr after gelatin injection the percentage of identifiable histiomonocytic cells in peritoneal fluid was always greater in mice raised in a conventional environment than in germfree mice (Fig. 3). However, apart from this distinction, we could detect no difference in the engulfing potential of peritoneal phagocytes from conventional and germfree mice. In Table IV the engulfing efficiency of CF1 conventional and germfree mice is compared. It can be seen that there is a difference in the number of histiomonocytic cells in the exudate depending on their origin and previous treatment. CF1 conventional mice, stimulated 48 hr earlier with gelatin, yielded the largest number of histiomonocytic cells, and CF1 germfree mice without stimulation, the least. However, no difference was seen between gelatin-stimulated CF1 conventional and germfree mice in terms of either the percent RBC engulfed within 1 hr or the average number of RBC engulfed per histiomonocytic cell. Similarly, no difference was seen in these two indices between nonstimulated CF1 conventional and germfree mice.

In a similar manner, no difference was seen in the engulfing efficiency of peritoneal phagocytes from conventional and germfree C3H mice that were stimulated with gelatin 48 hr earlier (Fig. 4). It is apparent that a strain difference exists between CF1 and C3H or $1C3F_1$ mice. The engulfing potential of CF1 mice has constantly been significantly less than either C3H or $1C3F_1$ mice. This lower engulfing potential is related to a decreased engulfing efficiency of the peritoneal phagocytes of this strain, instead of differences in number of phagocytic cells.

IN VITRO MATURATION OF THE ENGULFING POTENTIAL

To determine if the observed enhanced phagocytic efficiency of the stimulated histiomonocytic cell population could be ascribed to transformation of nonphagocytosing histiomonocytic cells into functional phagocytosing cells, or whether it represents the mobilization of fully functional elements into the peritoneal cavity, or a joint contribution of both, the following experiments were conducted.

Peritoneal cells harvested from normal, nonstimulated, conventional $1C3F_1$ mice were cultured in vitro [1]. Representative aliquots were then removed at 1 min and at 12, 24, 48, and 72 hr and tested for their engulfing capacity. The RBC : histiomonocytic cell ratio was 4 : 1. The results presented in Fig. 5 clearly demonstrate that increasing functional capacity is an inherent characteristic of the existing histiomonocytic cell population. Differential counts made at the time each aliquot was removed demonstrated that the number of identifiable histiomonocytic cells did not in-

Table IV. The Engulfing Efficiency of Stimulated* and Nonstimulated Conventional and Germfree CF1 Mice (RBC : Histiomonocytic Cell Ratio 4.3 : 1)

	No. histiomonocytic cells/ml	No. RBC/ml	% RBC engulfed	No. RBC engulfed / No. histiomonocytic cells	Av. No. RBC engulfed per histiomonocytic cell
Conventional (Stim)	$4.8 \cdot 10^6$	$20.0 \cdot 10^6$	72.8	$\frac{14.6 \cdot 10^6}{4.8 \cdot 10^6}$	3.04
Germfree (Stim)	$3.2 \cdot 10^6$	$14.0 \cdot 10^6$	73.3	$\frac{10.3 \cdot 10^6}{3.2 \cdot 10^6}$	3.22
Conventional (Nonstim)	$1.7 \cdot 10^6$	$8.4 \cdot 10^6$	14.0	$\frac{1.6 \cdot 10^6}{1.7 \cdot 10^6}$	0.65
Germfree (Nonstim)	$1.5 \cdot 10^6$	$6.4 \cdot 10^6$	15.0	$\frac{1.0 \cdot 10^6}{1.5 \cdot 10^6}$	0.67

*Stimulated mice received 2 ml 4% gelatin 48 hr prior to being killed.

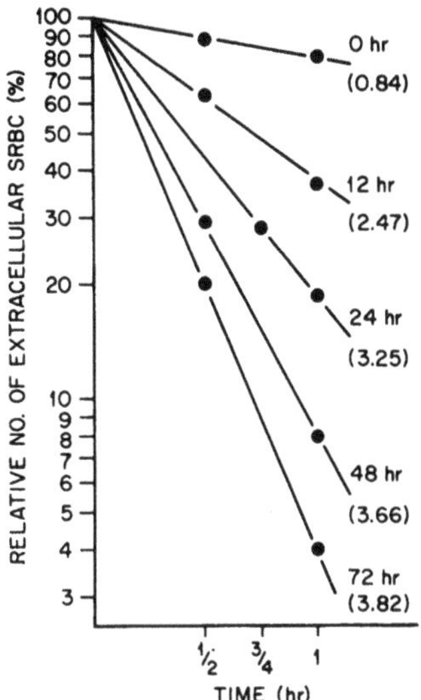

Fig. 5. Enhanced engulfing potential of normal, nonstimulated, peritoneal phagocytes harvested from conventional $1C3F_1$ mice as a function of length of time of culture. Numbers in parentheses: average number of RBC engulfed per histiomonocytic cells.

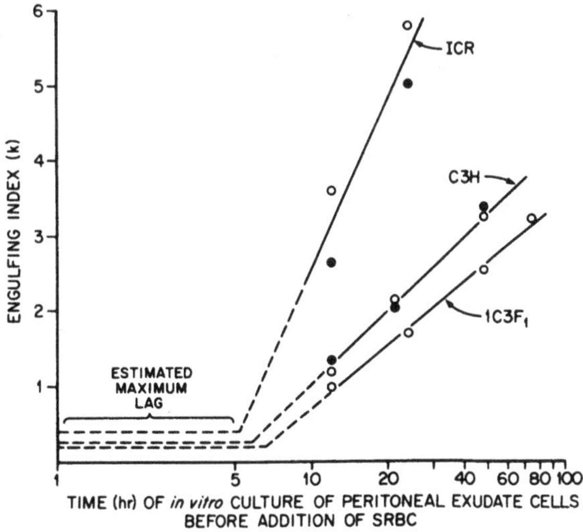

Fig. 6. Change in engulfing index of peritoneal exudate cells as a function of in vitro culture time. O Conventional; ● germfree.

crease. Furthermore, although the total number of cellular elements decreased with increase in the in vitro culture time, the absolute number of histiomonocytic cells remained constant. This indicates that transformation of nonhistiomonocytic cells into functional histiomonocytic elements is unlikely. Therefore, we can conclude that during in vitro culture preexisting, nonfunctional histiomonocytic cells matured into phagocytic cells.

MATURATION OF THE ENGULFING POTENTIAL OF PERITONEAL CELLS OF CONVENTIONAL AND GERMFREE MICE

A comparison of this enhanced engulfing potential as a function of in vitro culture time was then made between populations of peritoneal exudate cells harvested from normal, nonstimulated, conventional and germfree mice to determine if the histiomonocytic cells of germfree animals were comparable to their conventional counterparts.

The results of these experiments are shown in Fig. 6. The engulfing index (k), which represents the rate at which RBC were engulfed, has been plotted for peritoneal exudate cell populations from conventional and germfree ICR and C3H mice, and for the conventional $1C3F_1$ mice. It can be seen that no difference exists between the conventional and germfree mice of a given strain, although strain differences are apparent. The significant observation is that populations of peritoneal exudate cells from both conventional and germfree mice responded in a similar manner. A prominent lag phase exists, which may reflect a period of adaptation, after which there is an increase in the engulfing efficiency of the population typical of a standard growth curve. Although there is a marked difference in the rate at which the engulfing efficiency increased for the three strains of mice, interestingly enough there was a characteristic and distinct lag phase which did not differ. Indeed, it would be expected, although not shown in this figure, that a plateau level would be reached as the engulfing efficiency reached a maximum, where all histiomonocytic cells would be participating in the removal of RBC from the culture.

CONCLUSIONS

The enhanced phagocytic capacity of peritoneal exudate cells of stimulated mice was correlated with both a higher percentage of histiomonocytic cells in the peritoneal exudate and, perhaps of greater significance, an enhanced phagocytic efficiency of the induced histiomonocytic cell population. In an in vitro system, this enhanced phagocytic efficiency of the populations was shown to result from a functional maturation of preexisting histiomonocytic cells present in the exudate. Cohn and associates [2-7], in describing the in vitro differentiation of mononuclear phagocytes, noted increases in cell size and protein content, accumulations of phase-dense granules, and increased production of certain hydrolytic enzymes. Stimulus for this functional maturation is as yet unknown. In vivo, it may be related to the dramatic shift and mobilization of fluid and cellular elements into and out of the peritoneal cavity, whereas in vitro it may related to properties of the medium or endogenous cellular material liberated from injured and dying cells.

Peritoneal exudate cells harvested from both conventional and germfree mice which had received a prior intraperitoneal injection of a sterile irritant possessed markedly enhanced engulfing capacities. The percentage of identifiable histiomonocytic cells in these stimulated exudates was greater in mice raised in a conventional environment. Although strain differences were apparent, no difference could be detected in the engulfing potential of the phagocytic cells from conventional and germfree mice of the same strain. Peritoneal phagocytes from ICR had a greater phagocytic potential than C3H mice which, in turn, had a greater potential than CF1 mice. This enhanced phagocytic potential was shown to be due to the functional maturation of histiomonocytic cells, and not to transformation of nonhistiomonocytic cells into phagocytic elements. Histiomonocytic cells from germfree mice were as competent as their conventional counterparts in undergoing in vitro maturation. These results show that naturally occurring microbial flora is unimportant in the development of the engulfing potential of peritoneal phagocytes.

REFERENCES

1. T. Morita and E.H. Perkins, "A simple quantitative method to assess the in vitro engulfing and degradative potential of mouse peritoneal exudate cells," J. Reticuloendothelial Soc., 2:406-419, 1965.
2. Z.A. Cohn and B. Benson, "The differentiation of mononuclear phagocytes," J. Exptl. Med., 121:153-170, 1965.
3. Z.A. Cohn and B. Benson, "The in vitro differentiation of mononuclear phagocytes. I. The influence of inhibitors and the results of autoradiography," J. Exptl. Med., 121:279-287, 1965.
4. Z.A. Cohn and B. Benson, "The in vitro differentiation of mononuclear phagocytes. II. The influence of serum on granule formation, hydrolose production, and pinocytosis," J. Exptl. Med., 121:835-848, 1965.
5. Z.A. Cohn and B. Benson, "The in vitro differentiation of mononuclear phagocytes. III. The reversibility of granule and hydrolytic enzyme formation and the turnover of granule constituents," J. Exptl. Med., 122:455-466, 1965.
6. Z.A. Cohn, J.G. Hirsch, and M.E. Fedorko, "The in vitro differentiation of mononuclear phagocytes. IV. The ultrastructure of macrophage differentiation in the peritoneal cavity and in culture," J. Exptl. Med., 123:747-756, 1966.
7. W.E. Bennett and Z.A. Cohn, "The isolation and selected properties of blood monocytes," J. Exptl. Med., 123:145-159, 1966.

Pharmacological Stimulation and Depression of the Phagocytic Function of the RES

Kurt B. P. Flemming

Department of Radiobiology and Pharmacology
Heiligenberg Institute
Baden, Germany

The pharmacological influence of the phagocytic activity of the RES has been worked upon to a great extent in recent years. I do not intend to give a summary of the important results of this work, but to report on some of the experiments in this field which I and my coworkers have made. The experiments were made mainly on mice, but also on rats. We used here the carbon clearance test [1] because it appears to be the best method of examining the phagocytic function of RES in the whole animal.

In the first series of experiments I have been able to confirm the effect of intravenous injections of simple fats on mice found by Stuart and his coworkers [2] and by Cooper [3]. Olive oil and triglycerides (triolein, tricaprin, tripalmitin, tristearin, 2-oleodistearin) stimulated phagocytosis, whereas alkylic esters of fat (ethyl palmitate, ethyl stearate, ethyl oleate, cholesterol oleate) decreased it [4]. Furthermore, we found that these substances had the same effect on rats [5]. However, it is curious that the destructive effect of ethyl palmitate on mice as found by Stuart, and proved by us, does not occur in the case of rats. The spleen of rats showed in like manner histological signs of injury after ethyl palmitate; these were localized in the red pulp and made themselves noticeable in a disappearance of lymphocytes and in a formation of vacuoles. The white pulp was however not changed for certain, because no necroses were found.

Second, a report is given of a series of experiments in which several substances of botanical origin were tested. The starting point was DiCarlo's statement [6] that the leaves of a Venezuelan plant, *Maytenus laevis*, stimulated the phagocytic activity of RES in mice when injected intravenously as a suspension. This could be confirmed after an injection of 50–100 mg of leaf substance per kilogram body weight [7]. Moreover, it was found that smaller amounts, as low as 0.5 mg/kg, still stimulated phagocytosis (Fig. 1). The stimulating effect of *M. laevis* leaves on phagocytosis could also be proved in rats.

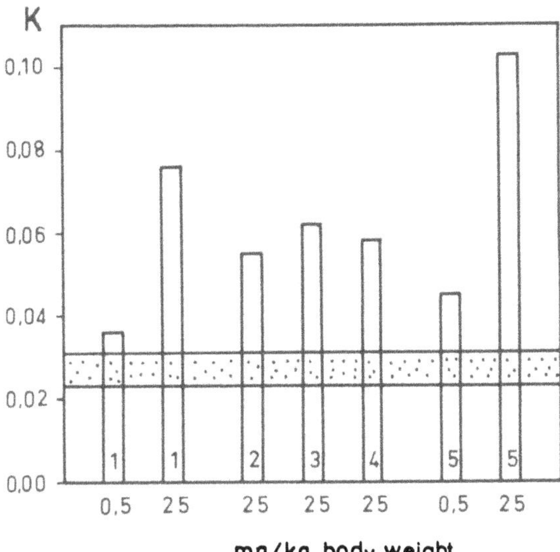

Fig. 1. Phagocytic stimulation by substances of plant origin. Mice, phagocytic index K 24 hr after injection. ⁚⁚⁚ Control. (1) *Maytenus laevis* leaves; (2) cellulose; (3) starch; (4) chlorophyll; (5) Scholler lignin.

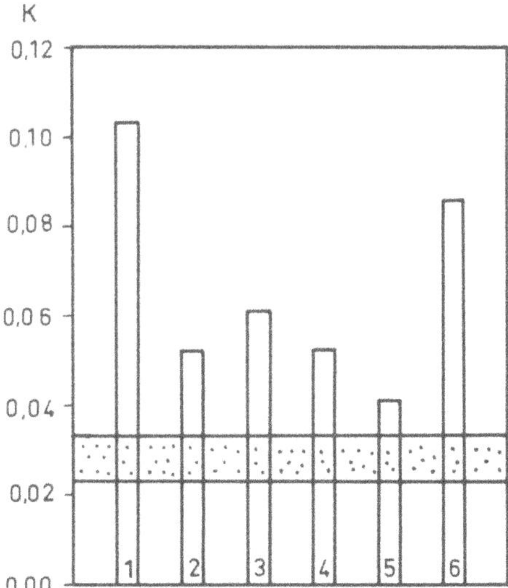

Fig. 2. Strong stimulating effect of Scholler lignin on phagocytosis (mice). (1) Scholler lignin; (2) Björkman lignin; (3) Cuproxam lignin; (4) catechin; (5) phlobaphenes; (6) methanol extract of Scholler lignin. 25 mg/kg body weight of each substance.

In order to acquire information on the drug present in the M. laevis leaves, some botanical products were tested (Fig. 1). Cellulose, starch, and chlorophyll stimulated phagocytosis, too, but their effect was considerably weaker than that of M. laevis leaves. A particular lignin preparation, Scholler lignin, which is produced by the effect of acids and heat from spruce wood, increased the phagocytic index to values of more than three times normal (25 mg/kg body weight). Its effect was stronger than that of M. laevis leaves. A dose as low as 0.5 mg/kg was still effective. Doses larger than 25 mg/kg hardly increased the effect. The climax of the effect was 24 hr after the injection; after four days the effect was over. The substance was also effective in rats.

The stimulating effect of Scholler lignin was surprising, for DiCarlo found no increase in phagocytosis when using bark which contains more lignin than the leaves. Therefore, Scholler lignin was compared with three other lignin preparations. These were Cuproxam lignin, which is produced chemically like Scholler lignin, and Björkman lignin. This preparation is obtained mechanically from the wood without using any chemical methods. The comparative examination showed that all these lignins increased the phagocytic index somewhat, but to much less degree than Scholler lignin (Fig. 2). The large increase in phagocytosis using Scholler lignin cannot be due, therefore, to the lignin alone. Apparently it contains another substance with a stronger effect than lignin.

Further experiments on this substance stimulating phagocytosis stemmed from the fact that in the dried leaves and in wood, tannins such as catechin are to be found. These tannins become, by means of self-condensation, high molecular so-called phlobaphenes, which are chemically similar to lignin from which they are derived, and which appear in the production of Scholler lignin. Using chemical methods, three different phlobaphenes were obtained from Scholler lignin, Björkman lignin, and catechin. Like pure catechin, these phlobaphenes had only a weak stimulating effect on phagocytosis (Fig. 2). A methanol extract from Scholler lignin had a stronger effect. Lignins are supposed to be insoluble in methanol. Therefore, one is obliged to conclude that there is an active substance contained in Scholler lignin which enters the methanol.

We cannot give any details yet concerning the origin and the chemical nature of this active substance. Perhaps it is already to be found in spruce wood, the original material for the production of Scholler lignin. Since Cuproxam and Björkman lignin, both with a weak effect, are also obtained from spruce wood, this supposition is not very likely. One possibility may be that the active substances stimulating phagocytosis are lost in the production of Cuproxam and Björkman lignin, but remain in the production of Scholler lignin. Another possible explanation of the effect of Scholler lignin could be that the active substance is not present in the original material, but has been produced from the wood by the chemical procedures of Scholler's method.

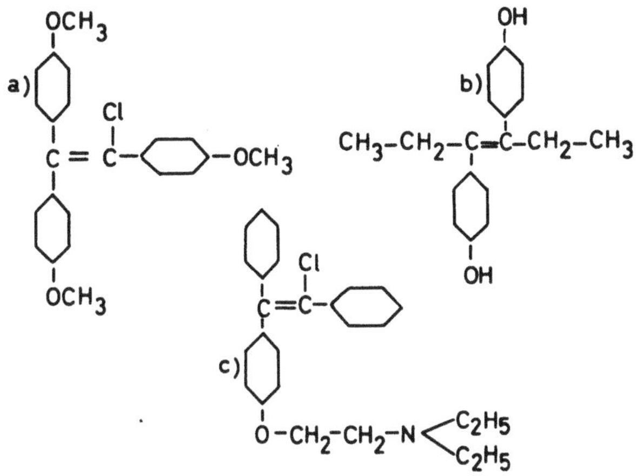

Fig. 3. (a) Chlortrianisene (Tri-anisyl-chloro-ethylene = TACE); (b) diethylstilbestrol; (c) clomiphene.

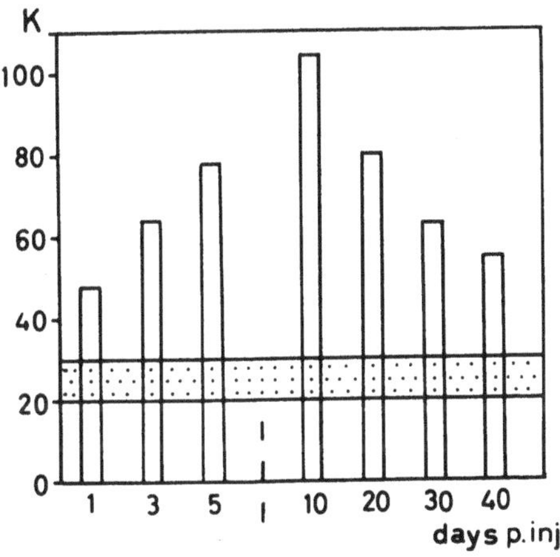

Fig. 4. Long-lasting phagocytic stimulation by TACE (male mice). Phagocytic index K on different days after s.c. injection of 2 mg TACE.

In a third series of experiments, estrogenic substances were used. Nicol and coworkers discovered the stimulating effect of the estrogens on phagocytosis [8, 9]. They found that it is coupled with an increase of γ-globulin content in the serum and with a higher production of antibodies and agglutinins. Therefore, they believe that the estrogens play an important part in resistance to infection.

Among the substances tested by Nicol is also to be found tri-anisyl-chloro-ethylene, or TACE. This pro-estrogen has a chemical structure similar to diethylstilbestrol (Fig. 3) and is stored in the fat tissues.

Then it slowly enters the blood, and in the liver it is changed into an estrogenic substance whose chemical structure is unknown. Nicol has found that TACE stimulated the phagocytic activity when given repeatedly every day subcutaneously or orally. He stated that perhaps TACE could be a RES stimulant to be used clinically because its estrogenic effect is weak and the side effects on the liver, spleen, and adrenal glands are less than those caused by other natural and synthetic estrogens.

We confirmed Nicol's results and found further that 24 hr after a single injection of 2 mg of TACE the phagocytic index was significantly increased (Table I). At this time the effect of TACE was just as strong as that of estradiol and rather stronger than that of diethylstilbestrol. The effect of these substances continued to increase after three days, as Nicol found out after repeated use, too; estradiol and diethylstilbestrol had reached or already passed their climax three days after the injection. Ten days after the injection their effect was only weak; the TACE effect, on the contrary, had still increased and produced a high K value at this point. This strong effect of 2 mg could not be increased by a dose ten times as high (20 mg). On the other hand, the low dose of 0.2 mg was still significantly effective ten days after a single injection. Considering the possible practical use mentioned by Nicol, it is particularly remarkable that the stimulating effect of TACE on phagocytosis could still be clearly seen as long as 40 days after one single injection of 2 mg (Fig. 4). This long effective period of TACE can be explained by the fact that it passes very slowly from the fat to the blood.

As previously mentioned, the chemical nature of the substance stimulating phagocytosis coming from TACE is still unknown. One hint perhaps can be taken from a comparison of results Nicol obtained in the examination of diethylstilbestrol derivatives. He found that the stimulating effect on phagocytosis of diethylstilbestrol is connected with the double bond between

Table I. Phagocytic Stimulation by Different Estrogens. Male Mice. K Values on Different Days After Injection. 2 mg of Each Substance in 0.4 ml Olive Oil Subcutaneously

Substance	Days after injection		
	1	3	10
Olive oil (control)	0.023 ± 0.005	=	=
TACE	0.048	0.061	0.102
Estradiol benzoate	0.055	0.077	0.039
Diethylstilbestrol	0.039	0.048	0.031

the two C atoms and with the p-hydroxy phenyl groups. Perhaps the three p-methoxy phenyl groups of TACE are demethylated in the liver to p-hydroxy phenyl groups.

From this viewpoint our finding is of interest that a TACE derivative, Clomiphene® (Fig. 3) also stimulates phagocytosis; its effect is, however, much weaker than that of TACE. Clomiphene, just like TACE, contains a C=C double bond. But, differing from TACE, it has only one substituted benzol ring on which a hydroxyphenyl group could occur by means of an enzymatic change. Perhaps the weaker effect of Clomiphene must be explained by this slight difference.

Until now there were shown possibilities of influencing the phagocytic activity of the RES by special pharmacologic substances. We also conducted experiments in which the mentioned substances were used in order to deal with a radiobiological problem. Since X-irradiated animals are more sensitive to bacterial infection than nonirradiated animals [10], it was supposed that the resistance to irradiation depends upon the activity of the RES [11, 12].

This supposition was supported by the fact that bacterial endotoxins have a protective effect against irradiation [12-14]. This radiation protection effect should be causally connected with the stimulating effect of the endotoxin on phagocytosis. Accordingly, an organism with an increased phagocytic activity should be more resistant in general to irradiation than an organism with a normal phagocytic activity.

In order to test this hypothesis experimentally, mice were injected with substances which influence the phagocytic activity of the RES. At the time of the phagocytic change, the phagocytic index K of some of the experimental animals was determined. At the same time, others were X-irradiated and the survival rate was measured after 30 days. The changes in the phagocytic activity and the survival rate could then be compared. The results are schematically summarized in Fig. 5.

First, I tested Pyrexal®, an endotoxin from *Salmonella abortus equi*, and TACE. Both substances had, besides the stimulating effect on phagocytosis, a strong radiation protection effect [14, 15]. This supported the hypothesis concerning the existence of causal connections between phagocytic activity and resistance to irradiation. It must however be considered that the tested substances influence not only phagocytosis but also, more or less, the liver, spleen, and bone marrow. If their phagocytic effect alone was responsible for the increased resistance to irradiation, then the effect of doses of different strengths on phagocytic activity and the survival rate should agree. This was, however, not the case. The climax of the phagocytic increase was reached after only slight doses of Pyrexal (0.01 μg). For a maximum radioprotective effect, on the contrary, a dose

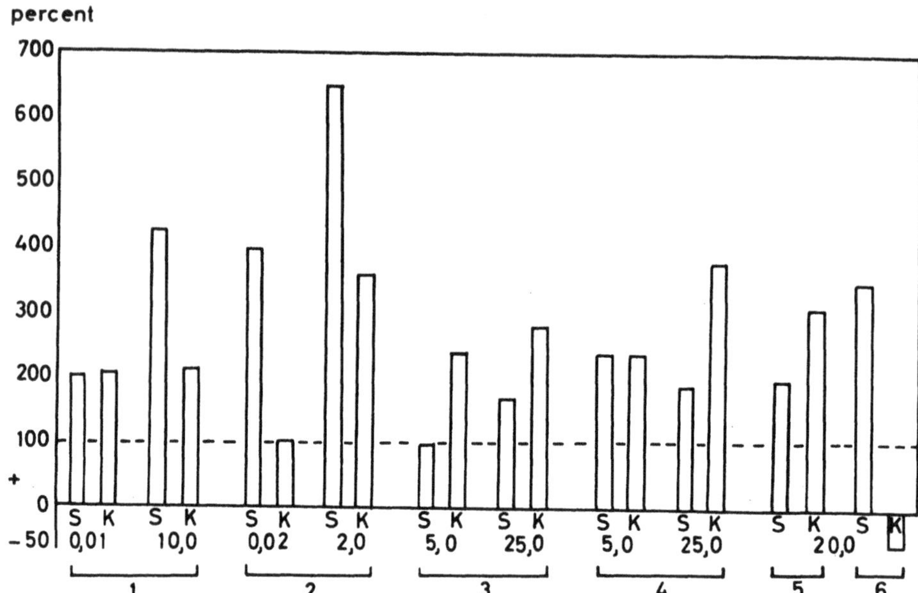

Fig. 5. Comparison between radiation protection and influence on phagocytosis schematically (mice). S = survival rate 30 days after x-irradiation (640 to 750 r); K = phagocytic index K on the day of irradiation. Control = 100%. TACE was injected 10 days before irradiation and the carbon clearance test. The other substances were injected 24 hr before irradiation and the carbon clearance test. (1) Pyrexal, 0.01 and 10.0 μg; (2) TACE, 0.02, and 2.0 mg; (3) Maytenus laevis leaves, 5.0 and 25.0 mg; (4) Scholler lignin, 5.0 and 25.0 mg; (5) tricaprin, 20 mg; (6) ethyl stearate, 20 mg.

of Pyrexal 10-100 times larger was necessary. Similar proportions were found in the case of TACE, 0.02 mg of which did not influence phagocytosis at all. Instead, it increased the survival rate to a certain extent. This disagreement contradicts the view that there is a connection between phagocytic stimulation and radiation protection.

One might raise the objection that in consideration of the complex effects of Pyrexal and TACE mentioned, other substances which mainly influence phagocytosis and have at the same time only slight other effects on the organism, would be more suitable for experiments of this kind. Therefore, M. laevis leaves and Scholler lignin were used in such experiments. These phagocytic-stimulating substances also had a noticeable radioprotective effect. A comparison between doses of different strength showed in this case also that there is no agreement between radiation protection and phagocytic stimulation.

The lack of such an agreement could be seen more clearly in a comparison between phagocytic-stimulating and phagocytic-inhibiting fat substances. Substances of both these groups, as tricaprin or ethyl stearate, influenced survival rate in the same way concerning the protective effect against irradiation, although their effect on phagocytic activity was the opposite. The results of the experiments show that a pharmacologically increased phagocytic activity is not necessarily coupled with an increased survival rate against x rays. The protective effect of RES stimulants against irradiation cannot therefore be due simply to their phagocytic-stimulating effect.

SUMMARY

The RES stimulating and depressing effects of simple fat substances in mice were confirmed. Ethyl palmitate depressed phagocytic activity in rats, but did not lead to a necrosis of the spleen as it did in mice.

Some well-known botanical products such as starch or chlorophyll exert a mild stimulating phagocytic activity, although the leaves from *Maytenus laevis* and lignin prepared by Scholler's method had a much stronger effect. The active components of these substances are still unknown but seem to be soluble in methanol.

The stimulating effect of the pro-estrogen TACE (chloro-tri-anisene) on phagocytic activity was investigated in detail and compared with the effect of some other estrogens.

The influences of the mentioned substances and of the endotoxin Pyrexal on phagocytic activity and survival rate after X-irradiation were compared. There was no strict relation between these two parameters.

ACKNOWLEDGMENTS

The research on this subject has been supported by Grant Str.Sch.186 from the Bundesminister für wissenschaftliche Forschung. I am much indebted to Mrs. Sandra Schneider for the translation of the German text into English.

REFERENCES

1. G. Biozzi, B. Benacerraf, and B.N. Halpern, Brit.J.Exptl.Pathol., 34:441, 1953.
2. A.E. Stuart, G. Biozzi, C. Stiffel, B.N. Halpern, and D. Mouton, Brit.J.Exptl.Pathol., 41:599, 1960; A.E. Stuart and G.N. Cooper, J.Pathol.Bacteriol., 83:245, 1962; A.E. Stuart, Lancet, 2:896, 1960; J.Pathol.Bacteriol., 84:193, 1962.
3. G.N. Cooper, J.Reticuloendothelial Soc., 1:50, 1964.
4. K. Flemming, Nature, 200:1117, 1963.
5. K. Flemming, C. Flemming, and E. Kroma, in preparation; E. Kroma, Inaugural Dissertation, Universität Freiburg, 1965.

6. F.J. DiCarlo, L.J. Haynes, N.J. Silver, and G.E. Phillips, J. Reticuloendothelial Soc., 1:224, 1964.
7. K. Flemming, Naturwissenschaften, 52:346, 1965; B. Graack and K. Flemming, Naunyn-Schmiedebergs Arch. Exptl. Pathol. Pharmakol., 253:32, 1966.
8. T. Nicol, D.L.J. Bilbey, and C.G. Druce, Nature, 190:418, 1961; T. Nicol, D.L.J. Bilbey, L.M. Charles, J.L. Cordingley, and B. Vernon-Roberts, J. Endocrinology, 30:277, 1964.
9. C.C. Ware and T. Nicol, Nature, 186:974, 1960.
10. C.P. Miller, Ann. N.Y. Acad. Sci., 66: 280, 1956; Ch.B. Rosoff, J. Exptl. Med., 118:935, 1963.
11. G.V. Taplin, C. Finnegan, P. Noyes, and G. Sprague, Am. J. Roentgenol. Radium Therapy and Nucl. Med., 71:294, 1954.
12. B.W. Zweifach and L. Thomas, J. Exptl. Med., 106:385, 1957.
13. W.W. Smith, J.M. Alderman, and R.E. Gillespie, Am. J. Physiol., 191:124, 1957; E.J. Ainsworth and H.B. Chase, Proc. Soc. Exptl. Biol. Med., 102:483, 1959; H. Balner, L.J. Old, and D.A. Clarke, Radiation Res., 15:836, 1961.
14. K. Flemming and Ch. Flemming, Strahlentherapie, 131:150, 1966.
15. K. Flemming, Naturwissenschaften, 51:59, 1964; K. Flemming, Progr. Biochem. Pharmacol., 1:564, 1965; K. Flemming and M. Langendorff, Strahlentherapie, 128:109, 1965.

The Action of Some Natural Substances on the RES

L. Bolis and R. W. I. Kessel*

Institute of General Physiology
University of Rome, Italy

and

G. Petti

Istituto Superiore di Sanità
Biology Laboratory, Rome, Italy

INTRODUCTION

Work by a number of investigators (Heller [1, 2], Biozzi [3], DiLuzio [4], and Bolis [5]) has shown that a variety of lipids, including those that are normal constituents of cell membranes, may affect the activity of the RES. It was of interest to investigate the activity of some of these membrane lipids not only on the phagocytic activity of the animal as a whole, but also on the isolated phagocytic cell, and upon subcellular membrane-bound structures including the phagocytic vacuole and lysosome. This investigation was expected to increase our understanding of the phagocytic and post-phagocytic activities of the cell, as well as to study the relationship between the lipid structure of biological membranes and their function.

MATERIALS AND METHODS

The compounds tested for biological activity were: (1) phosphatide–peptide fraction, isolated from rat liver cell membrane (Tria and Barnabei [6, 7]); (2) cholesterol, washed and recrystallized; (3) lecithin (General Biochemicals, Lot No. 58612, from egg, chromatographically pure); (4) α-lysolecithin (General Biochemicals, Lot No. 59164, chromatographically pure).

Three techniques have been employed to assess the interaction of membrane compounds with the RES.

* Permanent address: Department of Microbiology, University of Massachusetts, Amherst, Mass.

(1) Clearance of Colloidal Carbon

The technique of Halpern and Biozzi [8] was used, employing Gunther–Wagner carbon and Swiss albino mice.

For each animal there was then calculated: the phagocytic index (K), i.e., the constant of the equation of disappearance of carbon from blood, and the corrected phagocytic index (α), which measures the phagocytic activity per unit weight of liver and spleen.

(2) Action on Isolated Macrophages

Guinea pig macrophages with or without phagocytosed brucellae (Brucella abortus SA-s) were exposed to the test compounds, as described by Kessel [9]. Peritoneal macrophages were harvested from a guinea pig and suspended in 10% serum in a balanced salt solution (Hanks). Brucellae were added and the mixture placed into culture tubes at 37°C. After 1 hr, when phagocytosis of brucellae had occurred, the cultures were washed free of extracellular bacteria.

The medium was replaced with streptomycin plus or minus the compounds whose activity was to be examined. Appropriate controls were employed to demonstrate that the presence of streptomycin did not kill the intracellular brucellae, and that neither did the compounds alone.

A typical test will thus include cultures (macrophages containing living brucellae) exposed to:

1. Hanks alone.
2. Hanks + streptomycin.
3. Hanks + compound to be tested.
4. Hanks + streptomycin + compound.

The number of living intracellular brucellae were counted at the end of the phagocytosis period (i.e., before exposure to streptomycin), and again 4-6 hr later, using colony dilution counts.

(3) Action on Isolated Lysosomes

Lysosomes were obtained from the livers of Sprague-Dawley rats by DeDuve's method [10]. By homogenization of liver from rats and successive ultracentrifugation of the homogenates, a subcellular fraction rich in lysosomes was obtained corresponding substantially to the M + L fraction, described by DeDuve. This was suspended in 0.25 M sucrose. The compounds tested were added directly to the fraction. One part of the particle suspension was mixed with one hundredth its volume of concentrated solution of the test compounds dissolved in sucrose. The release of acid phosphatase was investigated at different times during the preliminary incubation of the fraction, at pH 5 at 37°C. These conditions are osmotically satisfactory ones, and correspond to possible situations in vivo.

RESULTS

(1) Clearance of Colloidal Carbon

The effects of membrane compounds on the ability of mice to clear colloidal carbon from the vascular compartment are shown in Figs. 1 and 2. It may be seen that lecithin, lysolecithin, and the phosphatide–peptide fraction (each at 0.05 mg/g for three and seven days) all led to an increased rate of clearance, while cholesterol (at the same dose) has no significant effect at either the third or the seventh day.

(2) Action on Macrophage Permeability

Prior to testing the ability of these compounds to enhance the penetration of macrophages by streptomycin, their toxicity for the isolated macrophage was assessed. In the absence of added serum (i.e., a macrophage monolayer with a Hanks BSS (balanced salt solution) supernatant, the following observations were made.

Lecithin, at 100 μg/ml, caused no morphological alteration of the cells within a 6-hr test period. α-Lysolecithin and the phosphatide–peptide fraction, each at 100 μg/ml, caused severe morphological damage within 20 min. Neither compound, however, caused damage at 10 μg. Cholesterol, at 100 μg/ml, appeared to cause no morphological change, although the presence of crystals made assessment difficult. It had no effect at 10 μg/ml.

These compounds were then tested for their ability to alter macrophage permeability to streptomycin (as assessed by the intracellular killing of brucellae) at 10 and 20 μg/ml. However, as shown in Table I, at these concentrations no effect was noted with any of the compounds. (Chlorpromazine, which is known to augment streptomycin preparation, served as a positive control.) Although α-lysolecithin was not employed in this particular experiment, it likewise did not lead to enhanced penetration of streptomycin in other experiments.

(3) Action on Isolated Lysosomes

The effects of lecithin, α-lysolecithin, and phosphatide–peptide fraction on the release of acid hydrolases from isolated rat liver lysosomes is shown in Fig. 3. Cholesterol, in 0.25 sucrose, at 125 μg/ml, had no effect, confirming the previous findings of DeDuve [12], Bolis and Petti [13]. Chromatographically pure egg lecithin acts in a manner similar to that previously reported by Bolis and Petti [13] for relatively impure lecithin preparations from brain and egg. Chromatographically pure α-lysolecithin and the phosphatide–peptide fraction promote the release of acid hydrolase.

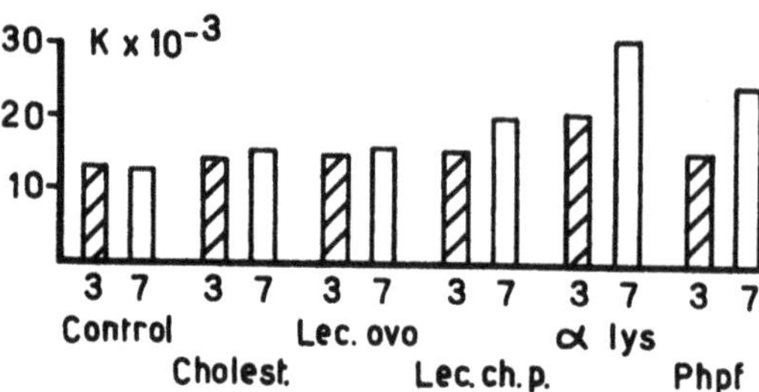

Fig. 1. Carbon clearance in normal and treated mice.

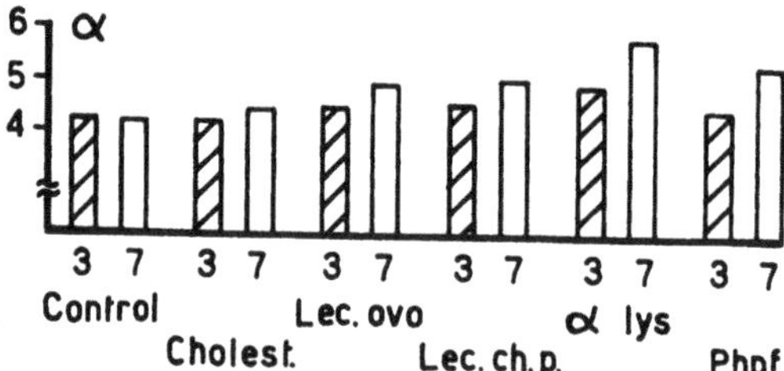

Fig. 2. Carbon clearance in normal and treated mice.

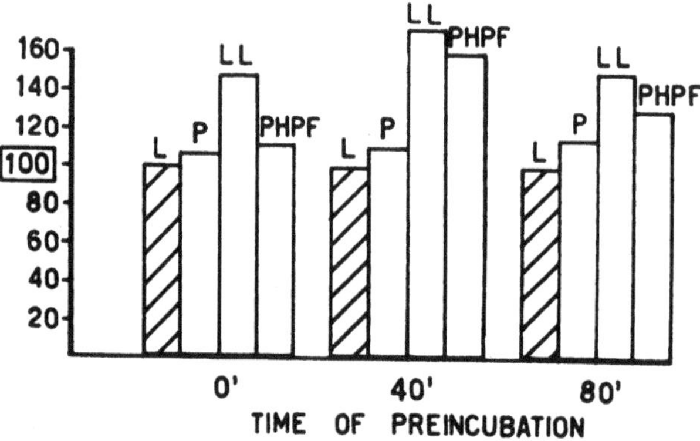

Fig. 3. Acid phosphatase activity after preincubation during 0, 40, and 80 min at 37° and pH 5, in purified fraction M + L, added with different agents. (% of free activity with control.) L = free activity, P = lecithin chromatographically pure, LL = α-lysolecithin, PHPF = phosphatide peptide fraction.

Table I. The Effect of Membrane Compounds (at 20 μg/ml) on the Penetration of Isolated Macrophages by Streptomycin (at 10μg/ml)

	Surviving Intracellular Brucellae (× 10^5) After 5 hr Incubation
Controls	
Hanks alone	2.90
Streptomycin	1.85
Phosphatide–peptide	2.65
Cholesterol	2.60
Lecithin	2.10
Chlorpromazine (2.5μg/ml)	2.35
Experimentals	
Phosphatide–peptide + streptomycin	2.60
Cholesterol + streptomycin	2.50
Lecithin + streptomycin	2.35
Chlorpromazine + streptomycin	1.20

DISCUSSION

The results presented above, using three different biological systems, are in qualitative agreement with each other. Thus, α-lysolecithin and phosphatide–peptide fraction, which have a marked and early effect on the RES function in the whole animal, also have an early effect on the isolated phagocytic cell and on the lysosomal particle. Lecithin has a less dramatic effect on the RES and on the lysosomal particle. Cholesterol has little or no effect on any of these biological systems. These findings are in agreement with the hypothesis that the administration of lipids affects a variety of membrane functions. The inability to demonstrate an effect upon the subcellular phagocytic vacuole may be due to the relatively severe effect upon other membranous structures – either the external limiting membrane or the internal lysosomal membrane – i.e., "toxicity," is observed before an effect on the phagocytic vacuole.

It may be supposed that the presence of exogenous lipids may strongly influence the function of biological membranes. In addition, lipid molecules or lipid and protein compounds, as well as lipid solvents or enzymes that affect lipids, especially phospholipases, can deeply alter transport phenomena [14, 15]. Marro and Coll demonstrated that a lysolecithin affects sodium transport in cardiac muscle [15] and Tria and Barnabei [16] that a phosphatide–peptide fraction enhances the penetration of labeled amino acids.

REFERENCES

1. J.H. Heller, in: J.H. Heller, Ed., Reticuloendothelial Structure and Function. New York, Ronald Press, 1960, p. 189.
2. J.H. Heller, Ann.N.Y.Acad. Sci., 88:116, 1960.
3. G. Biozzi, Brit.J.Exptl.Pathol., 41:599, 1960.
4. N.R. DiLuzio, Ann.N.Y.Acad.Sci., 88:244, 1960.
5. L. Bolis, Atti Accad.Med.Lombarda, 16:494, 1961.
6. E. Tria and O. Barnabei, Ric. Sci., 27:1546, 1957.
7. E. Tria and O. Barnabei, Ric.Sci., 30:2212, 1960.
8. B. Halpern and G. Biozzi, Ann.Inst.Pasteur, 80:582, 1951.
9. R.W.I. Kessel, in: L. Hobby, Ed., Antimicrobial Agents and Chemotherapy, 1966.
10. F. Appelmans and C. DeDuve, Biochem.J., 59:426, 1955.
11. C. DeDuve et al., Biochem.Pharmacol., 9:97, 1962.
12. C. DeDuve et al., Biochem. Pharmacol., 9:97, 1962.
13. L. Bolis and G. Petti, Proc.Symp.Biophys.Physiol.Biol.Transport. Protoplasma, In Press. 1967.
14. J.H. Quastel, in: Kleinzeller and A. Kotyk, Eds., Membrane Transport and Metabolism. New York, Academic Press, 1961, p.512.
15. F. Marro et al., Boll.Soc.Ital.Biol.Sper., 35:1813, 1959.
16. E. Tria and O. Barnabei, Proc.Symp.Biophys.Physiol.Biol.Transport Protoplasma, In Press. 1967.

Effect of Bacillus Calmette Guerin on the Metabolism of Alveolar Macrophages*

Quentin N. Myrvik and Dolores G. Evans†

Department of Microbiology, The Bowman Gray School of Medicine
Wake Forest University
Winston-Salem, North Carolina

Numerous investigations have been carried out employing in vitro studies to characterize the change in biochemical activities of phagocytes subsequent to particle uptake. Sbarra and Karnovsky [1] reported that following ingestion of polystyrene spherules, polymorphonuclear cells (PMN) doubled their rate of oxygen uptake during a 60-min incubation period. Oren et al. [2] reported that guinea pig peritoneal macrophages (PM) exhibited a tripling of their rate of oxygen uptake in a similar experiment. In contrast, they also observed that guinea pig alveolar macrophages (AM) did not appreciably demonstrate an increased rate of oxygen uptake 60 min after phagocytizing polystyrene spherules.

On the other hand, Ouchi et al. [3] reported that rabbit AM exhibited almost a 50% increase in oxygen uptake 60 min after phagocytizing heat-killed Staphylococcus albus in vitro when the macrophage : bacteria ratio exceeded 1 : 64. A void in our knowledge exists regarding long-term experiments involving different types of bacteria and their effect on metabolism of phagocytic cells.

The present study involves introducing bacteria by way of the intratracheal route into rabbits and monitoring in vitro the metabolic status of AM for up to 10 days following the injection of the microorganisms.

Results will be presented which indicate that the pattern and duration of the stimulation of alveolar macrophages varies with the microorganism ingested.

* This study was supported by research grant AI-05667 from the National Institutes of Health, USPHS, Bethesda, Maryland.
† Trainee on USPHS Training Grant T1 AI 268.

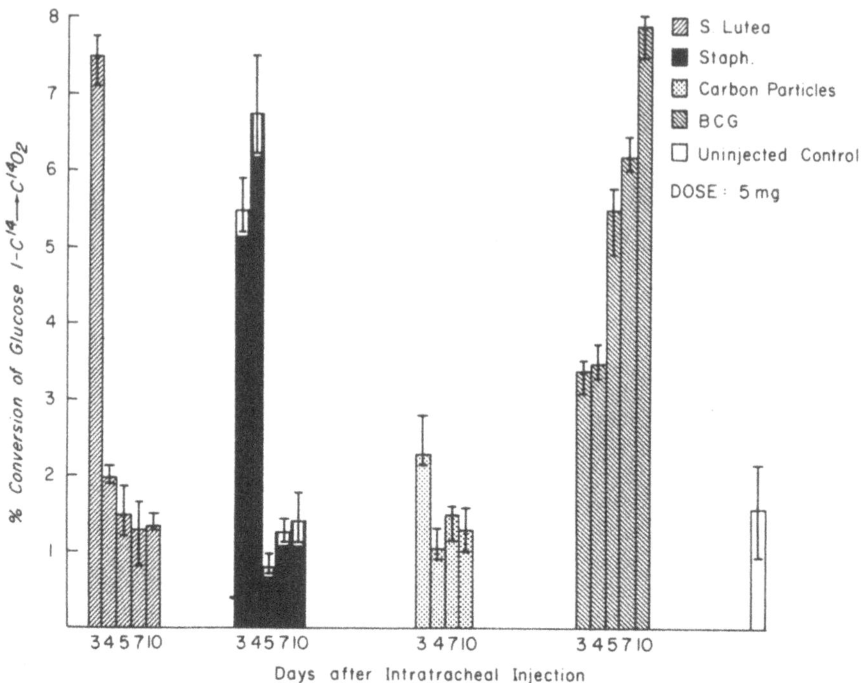

Fig. 1. Comparative effect of bacteria on metabolism of alveolar macrophages.

MATERIALS AND METHODS

Animals

New Zealand White rabbits weighing between 2 and 2.5 kg were used.

Microorganisms

The BCG strain of *Mycobacterium bovis* was grown on Proskauer and Beck's broth. *Sarcina lutea* and *Staphylococcus aureus* were grown on trypticase soy broth. The cultures were autoclaved, harvested, washed in sterile distilled water, and lyophilized.

Metabolic Studies

Macrophages were harvested from lungs according to a technique previously described [4]. Viability was monitored by employing the trypan blue exclusion technique [5]. The cells were washed once in Hanks' BSS and distributed in 50-ml Erlenmeyer flasks (8×10^6 cells/flask) which contained 5.0 ml of medium 199 without serum or glucose. One-tenth ml of glucose 1-C^{14} (446,850 CPM/ 0.1 ml) or glucose 6-C^{14} (409,700 CPM/ 0.1 ml) was added to the flasks. Carbon dioxide was trapped in 0.5 ml of hy-

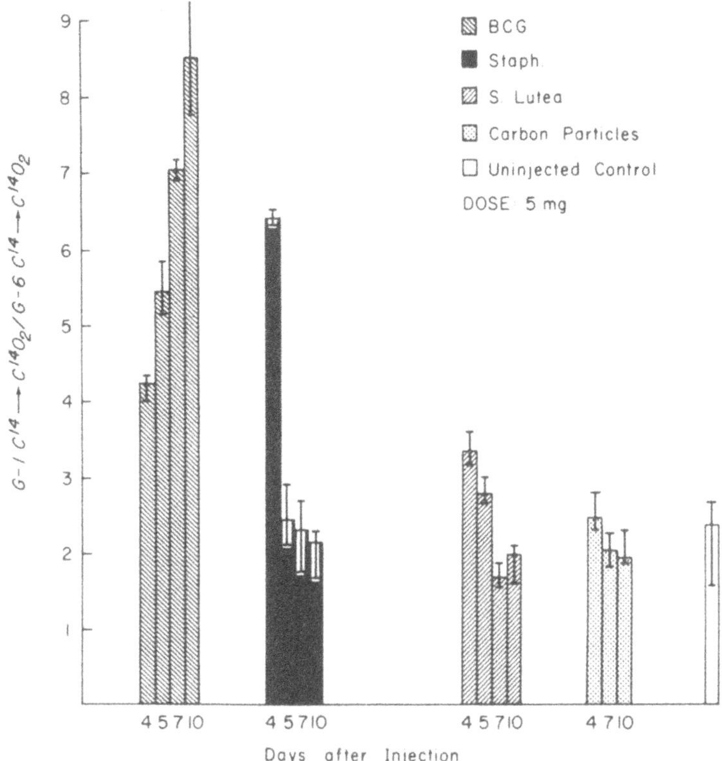

Fig. 2. Ratio of $C^{14}O_2$ from glucose 1-C^{14}-glucose 6-C^{14}.

mine hydroxide.* After 1 hr incubation with the labeled glucose, the reaction was stopped with 0.5 ml of concentrated sulfuric acid. Three ml liquid scintillation solution was added to the hymine hydroxide vials. Counts were determined with a Packard liquid scintillation counter. The reliability of the procedure was monitored by assaying known amounts of $NaHC^{14}O_3$ under the experimental conditions described.

Electron Microscopy

An aliquot of the cells suspended in chilled Hanks' BSS was centrifuged at 4°C at 800 rpm for 5 min. The supernate was removed with a capillary pipette. The remaining cell pellet was fixed in Palade's 1% osmium tetroxide [6] for 1 hr. The cells were dehydrated in increasing concentrations of ethyl alcohol and two changes of propylene oxide followed by embedding in maraglas [7]. Sections were cut on a Porter–Blum ultramicrotome and mounted on bare copper grids. The sections were stained either with lead

*Packard, Inc., Downers Grove, Illinois.

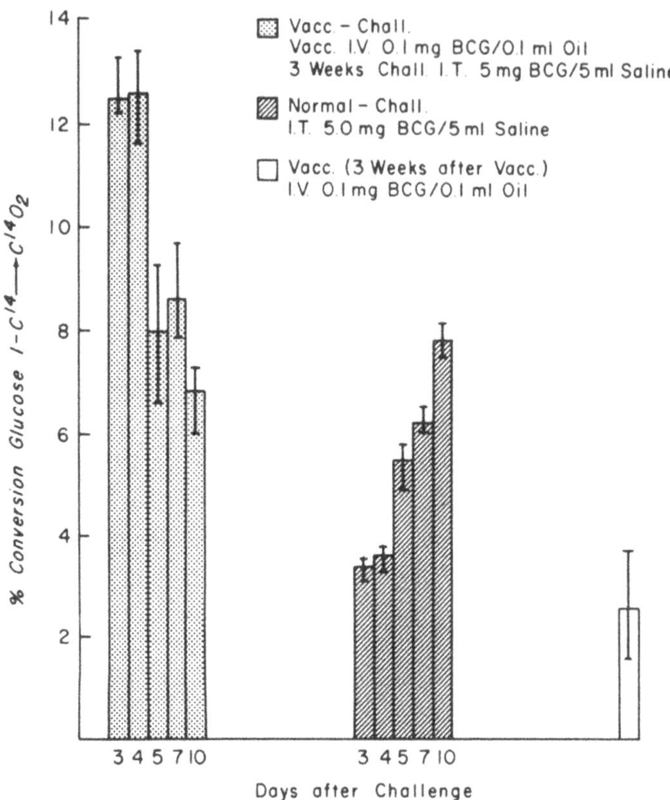

Fig. 3. Effect of BCG vaccination and challenge on glucose metabolism of alveolar macrophages.

citrate or double-stained with uranyl acetate and lead citrate. The stained sections were examined with an RCA-EMU-3G electron microscope employing an accelerating voltage of 100 kv.

RESULTS

Comparative Effect of Bacteria on Metabolism of Alveolar Macrophages

Four series of rabbits were inoculated intratracheally with 5 mg of BCG, S. aureus, S. lutea, and carbon (India ink) suspended in 5 ml of saline. The rabbits in each series were divided into five groups and sacrificed at 3, 4, 5, 7, and 10 days after intratracheal injection. It can be noted in Fig. 1 that the pattern of metabolic stimulation as measured by the percent conversion of glucose 1-C^{14} to $C^{14}O_2$ is notably delayed in the case of the BCG-injected animals when compared with the S. aureus- and S. lutea-injected animals. Colloidal carbon produced only a slight stimulation at the three-day interval.

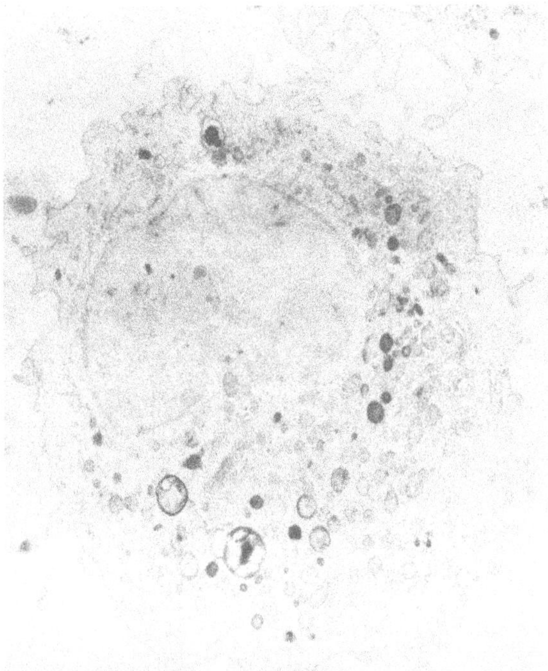

Fig. 4. Electron micrograph of a typical normal rabbit alveolar macrophage. Note oval and round mitochondria dispersed in cytoplasm. A moderately developed Golgi apparatus is evident. The number of electron-opaque granules is typical of that seen in normal alveolar macrophages. A sparse distribution of ER is present. Lead citrate. × 8250.

These results indicate that BCG produces a relatively long-term chronic-type of metabolic stimulation. Only slight reduction of the maximum rate of metabolism (10 days) occurred 16 days after injection of BCG.

Ratio of $C^{14}O_2$ from Glucose 1-C^{14} to Glucose 6-C^{14}

A second set of rabbits was divided into four series and inoculated by the intratracheal route with 5 mg of BCG, S. aureus, S. lutea, and carbon (India ink) suspended in 5 ml saline. Groups of rabbits were sacrificed at 4, 5, 7, and 10 days after intratracheal inoculation. The macrophages were harvested and their metabolic activities estimated. The ratios of $C^{14}O_2$ derived from glucose 1-C^{14}/glucose 6-C^{14} were then calculated.

These results are summarized in Fig. 2. Note that the change in ratios roughly approximates the changes in conversion of glucose 1-C^{14} to $C^{14}O_2$ depicted in Fig. 1.

The results clearly show that the hexose monophosphate shunt pathway is preferentially stimulated following the ingestion of the microorganisms

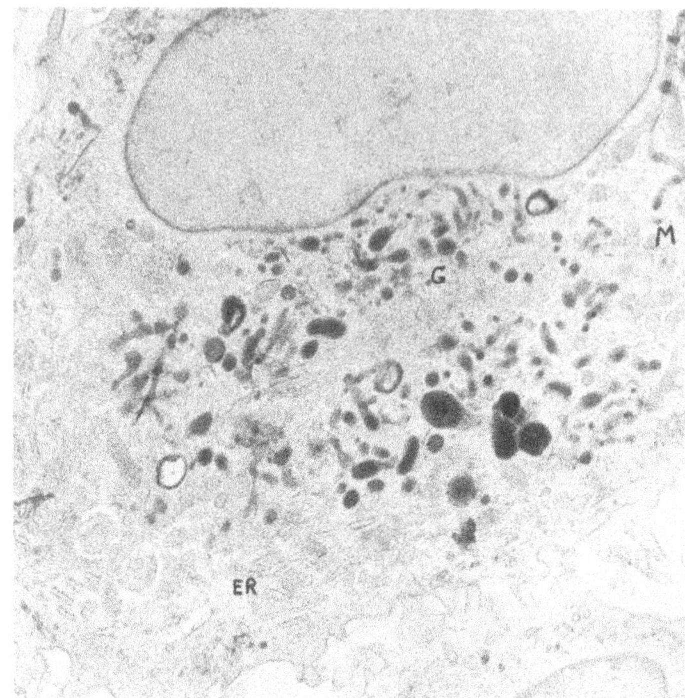

Fig. 5. Alveolar macrophage obtained from a rabbit 5 days after intratracheal injection of killed BCG. Note the scattered ER, the moderately developed Golgi apparatus (G), and the moderate numbers of mitochondria (M). The most striking feature in this cell is the large number of electron-opaque structures in the cytoplasm. Uranyl acetate-lead citrate. x 11,250.

employed. Again it can be noted that BCG produces a delayed response with a maximal ratio occurring about 10 days after injection. In contrast, S. aureus and S. lutea produced elevated ratios on Day 4, which returned to normal on Day 5. Carbon produced an insignificant change in the ratio under the conditions of these experiments.

Effect of BCG Vaccination and Challenge on Glucose Metabolism of Alveolar Macrophages

A series of rabbits were divided into three groups which were given the following injections:

(1) Normal-Challenged. Fifteen rabbits were given 5 mg of BCG by the intratracheal route. At 3, 4, 5, 7, and 10 days groups of three rabbits were sacrificed. Alveolar macrophages were collected and the percent conversion of glucose 1-C^{14} to $C^{14}O_2$ was determined.

(2) Vaccinated – Not Challenged. Fifteen rabbits were given 0.1 mg of BCG in 0.1 ml Bayol F by the intravenous route. After three weeks these

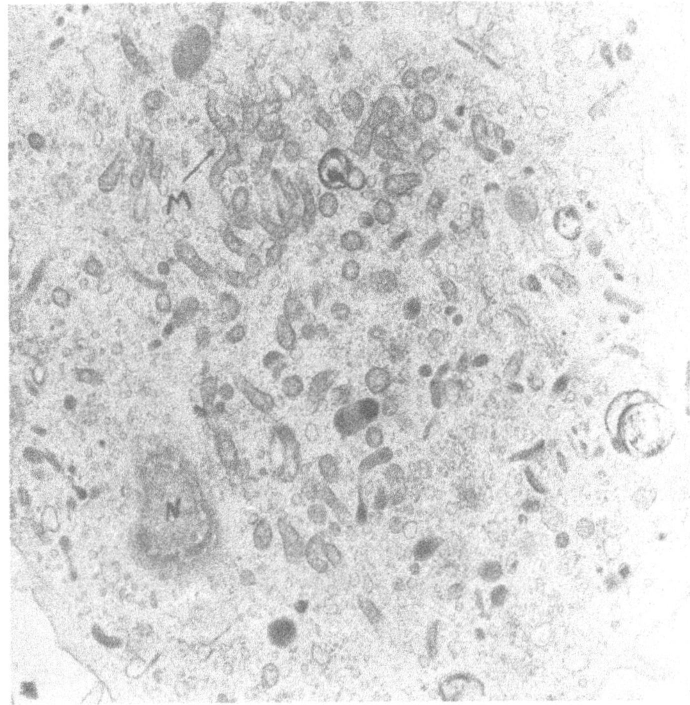

Fig. 6. Section of an alveolar macrophage at the 10-day interval after intratracheal injection of killed BCG demonstrating the increase in size and number of mitochondria (M). At the lower left corner of the picture appears a portion of the nucleus (N). Branching of mitochondria was frequently seen (arrow). Lead citrate. × 11,250.

animals were sacrificed in groups of three as companion controls to the vaccinated–challenged animals. Alveolar macrophages were collected and the percent conversion of glucose 1-C^{14} to $C^{14}O_2$ was determined.

(3) Vaccinated–Challenged. Fifteen rabbits were given 0.1 mg of BCG in 0.1 ml Bayol F by the intravenous route. All animals were challenged three weeks after vaccination by injecting 5 mg BCG by the intratracheal route. Groups of three rabbits were sacrificed 3, 4, 5, 7, and 10 days after the challenge dose was given. Alveolar macrophages were collected and the percent of conversion of glucose 1-C^{14} to $C^{14}O_2$ was determined.

A summary of these results is presented in Fig. 3. Note that the vaccinated–challenged animals demonstrated a peak in their rate of glucose metabolism on the third and fourth day after challenge, whereas the normal-challenged group showed a peak in metabolic activity at the 10-day interval. In addition, it can be noted that the total activity is higher in the vaccinated–challenged group. The alveolar macrophages obtained from the nonchal-

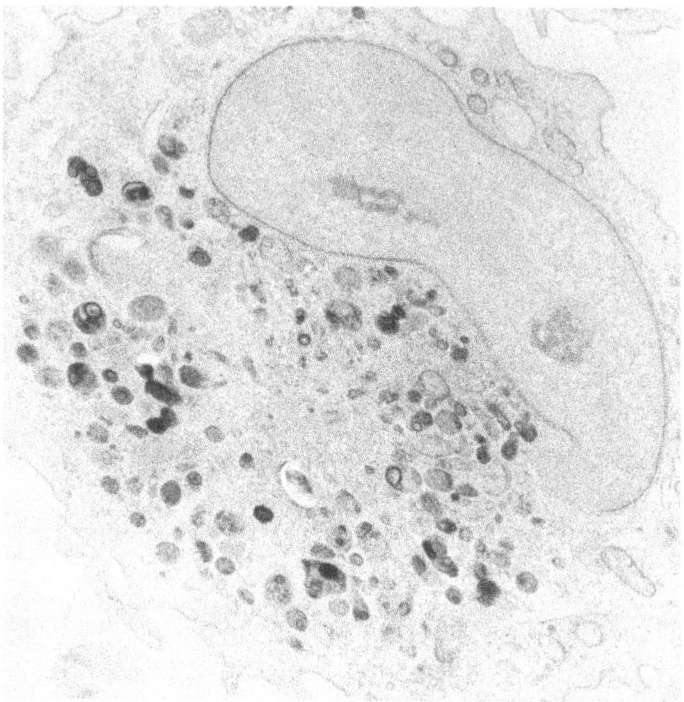

Fig. 7. Alveolar macrophage obtained from a rabbit 10 days after intratracheal injection of killed BCG. Electron-opaque granules are abundant in the cytoplasm. Lead citrate. × 11,250.

lenged vaccinated control group showed only an apparent slight stimulation in metabolic activity.

Ultrastructure of BCG-Stimulated Alveolar Macrophages

The ultrastructure of alveolar macrophages removed from the lungs 10 days after intratracheal injection of BCG was studied in an attempt to correlate morphologic changes with the elevated metabolic activity found at this interval. Samples were prepared and examined for the presence of increased numbers of electron-opaque granules, increased quantity of endoplasmic reticulum, increased numbers of mitochondria, and increased cell size.

A section of a typical normal alveolar macrophage is depicted in Fig. 4. Note that endoplasmic reticulum (ER) is poorly developed although a moderate number of electron-opaque granules are present. As a rule, mitochondria were present in relatively small numbers and usually assumed an oval-to-round form in macrophages from normal unstimulated rabbits.

Figure 5 illustrates a typical alveolar macrophage obtained from a rabbit five days after intratracheal injection of BCG. The changes noted at this interval indicate that the electron-opaque granules are increased in number coupled with an increase in ER. However, the mitochondria appeared to be similar in number to those seen in normal macrophages. Occasionally, the mitochondria exhibited an apparent increase in size.

Figure 6 illustrates a representative section of an alveolar macrophage obtained from a rabbit 10 days after intratracheal injection of BCG. The most striking feature noted was a marked increase in the number and size of mitochondria. The number of electron-opaque granules (Fig. 7) was approximately equivalent to the number seen in cells obtained at the 5-day interval. In general, during the course of BCG stimulation, an increase in the size of alveolar macrophages was also a prominent feature. However, increases in the development of ER were not commonly observed in cells at this interval.

DISCUSSION

The data presented in this study indicate that heat-killed BCG produce a different time course of metabolic stimulation of alveolar macrophages than that produced by *Staphylococcus aureus* and *Sarcina lutea*. An explanation of this difference is not readily apparent on the basis of these studies. Previous observations in this laboratory have revealed that heat-killed BCG can persist in stainable form in macrophages for up to 30 days in vivo. However, the mere persistence of BCG cannot explain the chronic nature of the enhanced metabolic activity because colloidal carbon failed to produce a similar pattern of stimulation. On the other hand, it is possible that some slowly metabolizable biochemical component in BCG is responsible for the chronic type metabolic stimulation observed. Accordingly, an organism like *S. lutea* which is catabolized much more rapidly than BCG, might be expected to produce an early short-term stimulation pattern. Both *S. aureus* and *S. lutea* produced such patterns. A search is in progress for the microbial product which is capable of stimulating glucose metabolism in alveolar macrophages.

The studies concerned with the effect of BCG vaccination and challenge on glucose metabolism of alveolar macrophages revealed a marked acceleration in the peak of the metabolic response curve as compared to normal-challenged rabbits. These observations suggest that metabolic enhancement might be under the influence of some form of hypersensitivity mechanism. This possibility could have important implications in so-called acquired cellular immunity, because metabolic stimulation could lead to increased rates of phagocytosis, hydrolase synthesis, as well as cellular proliferation. In this regard, the investigations of Mackaness [8] with *Brucella*, *Listeria*, and *Mycobacterium* suggest that mobilization of immune macrophages is a specific response, whereas the final expression of cellular immunity on the intracellular level is nonspecific.

It is equally possible that BCG was phagocytized and catabolized faster in alveolar macrophages from vaccinated rabbits. This, in turn, could release microbial products at a faster rate resulting in an accelerated metabolic stimulation pattern. Experiments involving "immune" alveolar macrophages that are challenged in vitro with BCG might help elucidate this aspect of the response.

In the companion morphologic study, it was observed that a marked increase in the number and size of mitochondria coincided with the peak in the metabolic rate of alveolar macrophages procured 10 days after intratracheal injection of BCG. Paradoxically, an increase in ER and electron-opaque granules was seen around the fifth day after injection of BCG. It is of interest that this interval coincides with the peak in the hydrolase response curve investigated by Heise et al. [9]. The functional utility of the enhanced metabolic activity at the 10-day interval awaits further study.

A detailed study of the metabolic and morphologic modulations of alveolar macrophages as a consequence of primary and secondary encounters with microorganisms may provide an insight into the mechanisms of conversion of these phagocytic cells from the normal to the immune state. Alveolar macrophages appear to be well suited for such a study.

SUMMARY

The intratracheal injection of 5 mg heat-killed BCG produced a stimulation in the rate of glucose metabolism of alveolar macrophages which reached its peak 10 days after injection. In contrast, equivalent amounts of either _Staphylococcus aureus_ or _Sarcina lutea_ produced a peak in the rate of metabolism three to four days after injection. Carbon failed to produce comparable significant increases in metabolism during these intervals. BCG-vaccinated (i.v.) rabbits were challenged after three weeks with 5 mg BCG. In this case, the peak in the rate of glucose metabolism of alveolar macrophages occurred three to four days after injection. In addition, the peak was higher than that reached in normal-challenged animals. A companion morphologic study of alveolar macrophages obtained from rabbits at various intervals following a single 5-mg dose of BCG revealed that a marked increase in number and size of mitochondria was associated with the peak (10-day) in metabolic activity.

REFERENCES

1. A.J. Sbarra and M.L. Karnovsky, "The biochemical basis of phagocytosis. I. Metabolic changes during the ingestion of particles by polymorphonuclear leukocytes," J.Biol.Chem., 234:1355, 1959.

2. R. Oren, A.E. Farnham, K. Saito, E. Milofsky, and M.L. Karnovsky, "Metabolic patterns in three types of phagocytizing cells," J. Cell Biol., 17:487, 1963.
3. E. Ouchi, R.J. Selvaraj, and A.J. Sbarra, "The biochemical activities of rabbit alveolar macrophages during phagocytosis," Exptl. Cell Res., 40:456, 1965.
4. Q.N. Myrvik, E.S. Leake, and B. Fariss, "Studies on pulmonary alveolar macrophages from the normal rabbit: A technique to procure them in a high state of purity," J.Immunol., 86:128, 1961.
5. W.F. McLimans, E.V. Davis, F.L. Glover, and G.W. Rake, "The submerged culture of mammalian cells: The spinner culture," J.Immunol., 79:428, 1957.
6. G.E. Palade, "A study of fixation for electron microscopy," J.Exptl. Med., 95:285, 1952.
7. J.A. Freeman and B.O. Spurlock, "A new epoxy embedment for electron microscopy," J.Cell Biol., 13:437, 1962.
8. G.B. Mackaness, "The immunological basis of acquired cellular resistance," J.Exptl.Med., 120:105, 1964.
9. E.R. Heise, Q.N. Myrvik, and E.S. Leake, "Effect of Bacillus Calmette-Guerin on the levels of acid phosphatase, lysozyme, and cathepsin in rabbit alveolar macrophages," J.Immunol., 95:125, 1965.

Reticuloendothelial System Stimulation by Estrogens and Thorium Dioxide Retention in Rat Liver*

Giuseppe Grampa

Istituto di Anatomia e Istologia Patologica
dell'Università di Milano
Milano, Italy

For a better understanding of the pathogenesis of malignant liver tumors related to Thorotrast in man [1], an experimental study was undertaken, with the aim of obtaining thorium dioxide-induced tumors in rat liver. Preliminary results have been reported [2, 3].

Castration and estrogen administration in male rats were used in order to increase thorium dioxide retention in the liver, due to the stimulating effect of estrogens on the reticuloendothelial system (RES), as shown, among others, by Nicol et al. [4, 5].

It is the purpose of this paper to present morphological evidence, at light and at electron microscope (EM) levels, that the liver of castrated estrogen-treated rats does contain more thorium dioxide than the liver of control animals.

MATERIALS AND METHODS

Male rats of the Wistar and Sprague-Dawley strains, aged 2 months (average weight 170 g) were castrated and injected with estradiol valerate† (10 mg, intramuscularly) and with Thorotrast‡ (1 cc in the femoral vein), 10 and 17 days, respectively, after castration.

Animals were sacrificed in triplets, for short-term and long-term observations, 1, 5, and 15 min, 1 and 12 hr, 1, 3, 5, 11, and 15 days, every 2 months, and from 3 up to 21 months, after thorium dioxide injection. A

*Work supported in part by contract 343/RB with the International Atomic Energy Agency in Vienna.

† Progynon Depot, Farmaceutici Schering, Milano (Italy).

‡ Fellows-Testagar Inc., Detroit, Michigan (USA).

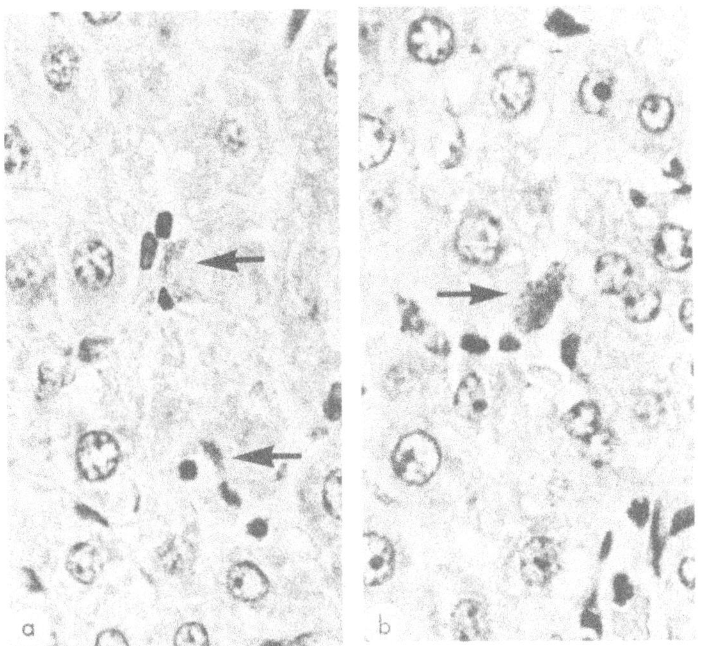

Fig. 1. Histological picture of Thorotrast aggregates (arrows) in the liver 1 hr after injection. H.E. 800 ×, reduced 10% for reproduction. (a) Control (rat 9D/64). Thorotrast attached to Kupffer cells in sinusoids; (b) estrogen-treated animal (rat 5D/64). Thorotrast in the cytoplasm of an enlarged Kupffer cell.

comparable group of rats was injected only with Thorotrast and sacrificed at the same time intervals.

Fragments of liver were fixed in 10% buffered formalin and embedded in paraffin for histology. Histological sections were stained with hematoxylin and eosin and with PAS hematoxylin.

Small pieces of liver were fixed in Palade's fluid, in buffered glutaraldehyde, and embedded in Epon 812 for EM. Silver sections were examined with an RCA 3F EM, after staining by Watson's and Karnovsky's methods.

OBSERVATIONS

Under the light microscope, Thorotrast retention in Kupffer cells may be followed beginning 1 hr after injection. Earlier findings are scanty and not reliable.

In control animals, thorium dioxide aggregates are mostly stuck to the cell membrane, toward the sinusoid, while in estrogen-treated animals they fill the enlarged cytoplasm of Kupffer cells (Figs. 1a and 1b).

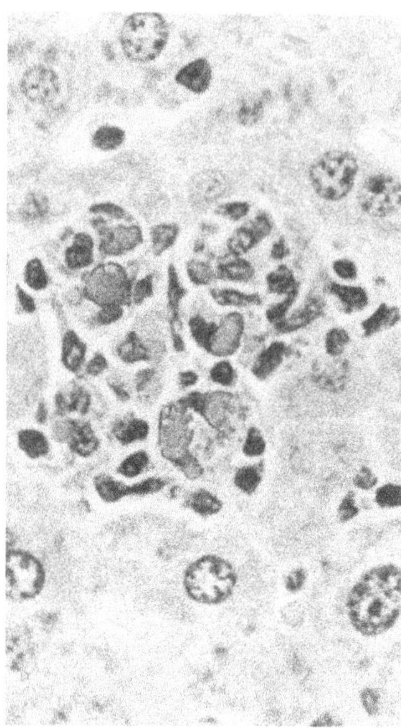

Fig. 2. Small clusters of histiocytes around coarse thorium dioxide aggregates 6 months after Thorotrast injection. Estrogen-treated animal (rat 411C/64). H.E. 800 x, reduced 10% for reproduction.

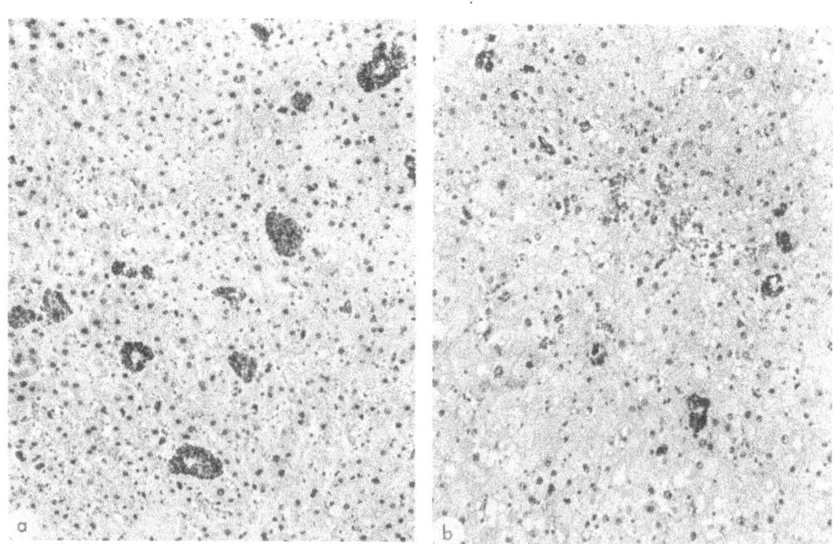

Fig. 3. Thorium dioxide distribution 21 months after injection. H.E. 180 x, reduced 10% for reproduction. (a) Control (rat 44C/64); (b) estrogen-treated animal (rat 33C/64).

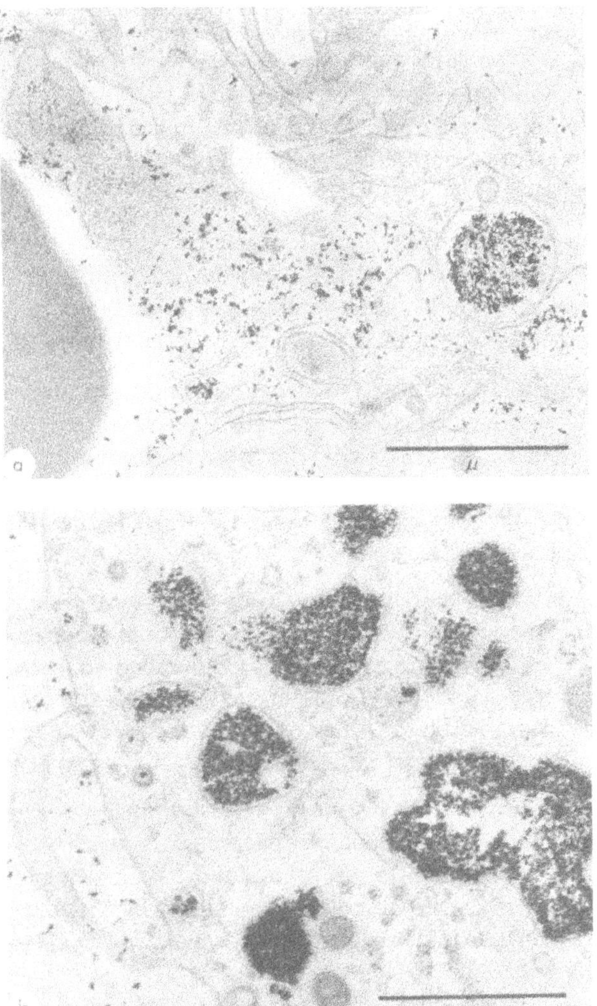

Fig. 4. EM picture of thorium dioxide absorption in the liver 15 min after injection. (a) Control (rat 10D/64). Granules in a sinusoid and in the cytoplasm of a Kupffer cell. (b) Castrated, estrogen-treated animal (rat 11D/64). Closely packed granules are contained in cytoplasmic vacuoles of various size, some with a clear central portion. Few granules are present in the sinusoid.

Thorium dioxide deposition increases with time and large aggregates are seen close to the periportal spaces, in accordance with the findings of Guimaraes and Lamerton in mice [6].

After several months, nodular histiocytic proliferation, more marked in castrated estrogen-treated rats, is observed around thorium dioxide aggregates (Fig. 2).

Higher content of thorium dioxide in the liver of estrogen-treated rats, in comparison with control animals, is evidenced by counting the number of large aggregates (30 μ or more in diameter) per mm^2 of histological sections. Values in castrated estrogen-treated rats are over 40% higher than in comparable control rats. The pattern of thorium dioxide aggregates 21 months after injection is shown in Fig. 3 (a – control, and b – castrated estrogen-treated rat).

EM observations allow one to follow thorium dioxide absorption by Kupffer cells, as soon as 1 min after injection. The difference between intact and castrated estrogen-treated animals is clearly demonstrated by observations performed 15 and 60 min after Thorotrast injection.

After 15 min, control animals show Thorotrast granules in the sinusoids, close to the cell membrane and finely dispersed in cytoplasmic vacuoles of Kupffer cells (Fig. 4a). Estrogen-treated animals show numerous cytoplasmic vacuoles filled with closely packed Thorotrast granules, while the number of Thorotrast granules free in the sinusoidal space is smaller than in control animals (Fig. 4b).

Sixty minutes after Thorotrast injection, intact animals show many thorium dioxide aggregates in the sinusoids, close to Kupffer cell membranes. Kupffer cells contain few cytoplasmic vacuoles, with thorium dioxide granules in the peripheral portion, leaving a clear center. In castrated estrogen-treated animals, most of the thorium dioxide is intracellular and many vacuoles are completely filled with dense aggregates.

Three days or more after injection, both in estrogen-treated and control animals, thorium dioxide deposits become larger and denser, confluence of single vesicles takes place, and Kupffer cells appear extremely swollen. Their cytoplasm is completely occupied by thorium dioxide deposits. Focal cytoplasmic degeneration is a frequent finding, but no nuclear damage has been observed.

DISCUSSION

Thorotrast particles enter the cells by a mechanism of pinocytosis*; the cell membrane synthesis and flow incorporate Thorotrast granules,

---

* The uptake of colloidal particles with the dispersion medium is referred as phagocytosis or pinocytosis, which are similar processes, differing primarily in relation to the quantities of liquid of the suspending dispersion medium that are absorbed [7].

physicochemically adsorbed to the cell surface membrane, into vesicles and vacuoles derived from the surface membrane [7]. Small vesicles rapidly form large vesicles [8, 9], which occur much more in the endothelial cells than in the parenchymal cells [10], even if a large amount of thorium dioxide in hepatocytes has been observed in rabbits [11].

The stimulating effect of estrogens on the RES has been extensively studied with the carbon clearance technique [4, 5] and estradiol is the most effective estrogen in this respect. The mechanism of estrogen action on the RES is not known; increased cell membrane permeability may be involved, perhaps as the result of binding of estrogen molecules with proteins at the cell membrane [5]. Light and EM observations here reported offer morphological evidence that castration and estrogens increase Thorotrast uptake in the liver by Kupffer cells and are in accordance with the hypothesis of a modified cell membrane permeability.

CONCLUSIONS

Estrogen treatment does increase phagocytic activity of the RES and enhances Thorotrast absorption in the liver; light microscope and EM observations fit a suggested mechanism of modified cell membrane permeability.

Increased thorium dioxide retention in the liver may offer an experimental model for a better understanding of liver tumors induced by Thorotrast, provided that estrogen effect per se on proliferative processes in the liver is properly evaluated. It seems appropriate, in this respect, to consider the possibility that hormonal factors may play a role in some cases of human liver tumors related to Thorotrast. It may be more than coincidental that over two thirds of liver hemangioendotheliomas associated with Thorotrast in the literature [12] are in males, some of which have long-standing hepatic insufficiency.

REFERENCES

1. G. Grampa and A. Tommasini Degna, Recenti Progr.Med., 26:290, 1959.
2. G. Grampa and A. Severini, Boll.Soc.Ital.Patol., 8:12, 1963.
3. G. Grampa, Atti Soc.Ital.Patol., 9:717, 1965.
4. T. Nicol and D.L.J. Bilbey, in: J.H. Heller, Ed., Reticuloendothelial Structure and Function, New York, Ronald Press, 1960, p. 301.
5. T. Nicol, B. Vernon-Roberts, and D.C. Quantock, J.Endocrinol., 34:163, 1966.

6. J.P. Guimaraes and L.F. Lamerton, Brit.J.Cancer, 10:527, 1956.
7. J. Wiener, D. Spiro, and W. Margaretten, Am.J.Pathol., 45:783, 1964.
8. R.N. Baillif, Ann.N.Y.Acad.Sci., 88:3, 1960.
9. J.C. Hampton, Acta Anat., 32:262, 1958.
10. J.R. Casley-Smith and P.C. Reade, Brit.J.Exptl.Pathol., 46:473, 1965.
11. M. Capocaccia and A. Vallebona, Radiol.Med., 23:389, 1936.
12. Bibliography on Thorotrast. Vienna, International Atomic Energy Agency, 1964, 1965.

The Effects of Steroid Hormones on Local and General Reticuloendothelial Activity: Relation of Steroid Structure to Function

T. Nicol, D. C. Quantock, and B. Vernon-Roberts

Department of Anatomy
King's College, University of London
London, England

ABSTRACT. The effects of various steroid hormones on phagocytosis and on the cellular and fluid phases of the local inflammatory response have been studied using the carbon clearance technique and a modified cotton pellet implantation technique in intact mice. Preliminary investigations showed that changes in the dry weight of the pellets removed on the fifth day after implantation could be completely accounted for by changes in fluid exudate (protein) content and were not significantly affected at this time by alterations in cell content (assessed histologically).

It was found that: (1) cortisone, hydrocortisone, and prednisone depressed phagocytic activity and inhibited both fluid and cellular phases of the inflammatory response; (2) DOCA and progesterone were slight stimulants of phagocytic activity and increased both fluid and cellular phases of the inflammatory response; (3) 17β-estradiol, estrone, estriol, ethinylestradiol, and estradiol monobenzoate, which are strong stimulants of phagocytic activity, reduced the amount of fluid exudate but increased the number of cells at the inflammatory site; (4) testosterone and methyltestosterone had no effect on phagocytic activity, but increased both fluid and cellular phases of the inflammatory response; and, (5) hydrocortisone, DOCA, 17β-estradiol, ethinylestradiol, testosterone, and progesterone have the same overall effects on the fluid and cellular phases of the inflammatory response when administered by subcutaneous injection or by local impregnation into the pellets. These findings show that the steroid hormones have profound effects on the inflammatory response, and that estrogens have the unique property of being "anti-inflammatory" with respect to the fluid exudate response but "inflammatory" with respect to cellular response.

It was found that anti-inflammatory and inflammatory action could be related to specific features of the steroid molecule.

INTRODUCTION

We have previously shown that stimulation of the reticuloendothelial system (RES) leads to raised body defense indicated by increased phagocytic activity, and increased protection of experimental animals against virulent infections, and that the strongest RE stimulants are the estrogens. We also showed that cyclical variations in RE activity occur during the estrus cycle and during pregnancy in the rat and mouse, and that RE activity falls after ovariectomy. These findings coincided with the variations in plasma estrogen levels known to occur in the human subject, and led us to suggest that estrogen – especially 17β-estradiol – is the principal natural stimulant of body defense in both the male and the female (Nicol, Bilbey, Charles, Cordingley, and Vernon-Roberts [1], Nicol and Vernon-Roberts [2]). Further, we have established that the estrogen molecule has two biological activities, one acting on the RES and the other on the reproductive tract, and that they act independently although contained in the same molecule (Nicol, Vernon-Roberts, and Quantock [3-5]).

Invading microorganisms are rapidly removed from the circulation by the "fixed" RE phagocytes lying along the endothelium of the blood sinusoids and capillaries, whereas in the connective tissues they are removed by "free" phagocytes which actively accumulate in the inflamed area. Our previous researches have dealt chiefly with the influence of hormones on the "fixed" RE phagocytes. The present investigation was designed to study the effects of various steroid hormones on both the "fixed" and "free" cells of the RES simultaneously in the same animal.

MATERIALS AND METHODS

We have continued to assess the activity of the "fixed" RE cells by using the carbon clearance test, since nonspecific body defense is predominantly due to the phagocytic activity of the RES. The essential details of the test have been described previously (Nicol et al. [6]), and our complete technique has also been reported (Vernon-Roberts [7]). As in our previous communications, the index of total body phagocytic activity or phagocytic index is denoted by the symbol K. The K value indicates the rate of removal of the carbon from the blood stream by the RE cells. Although useful for comparison with other published work, it is not a linear index and it is more correct to express phagocytic activity as the reciprocal of K, since this gives a linear dose–response relationship ($Kr = 1/K \cdot 10^3$) and allows statistical analysis of the results.

The activity of the "free" RE cells was assessed by measuring the local inflammatory response, using a modified cotton pellet granuloma assay based on the technique first described by Meier, Schueler, and Desaulles [8]. Our complete technique has been reported elsewhere (Quantock [9]). The essential details are as follows. Cotton dental pellets (Johnson & Johnson) were dried, individually weighed, steam-autoclaved, and redried in a dry-sterilizing oven. Two pellets were then implanted subcutaneously into each animal, one in each flank, through a dorsal midline incision under ether anesthesia using sterile technique. The animals of each dose response group received pellets of identical weight. On the fifth day of implantation, the pellets, containing inflammatory exudate and cells (granuloma) were removed. No attempt was made to dissect out the surrounding granulomatous reaction, since this procedure reduces the quantitative efficiency of the assay. The pellets were then dried at 60°C for 48 hr and weighed again. The differences between the initial and final dry weight of each pellet is the dry granuloma weight; this is a measure of the local inflammatory response and consists of the protein content of the fluid part of the exudate plus the cellular ingrowth. The fifth day was chosen as the optimum time to remove the pellets, since preliminary experiments in untreated animals showed the least scatter about the mean weight gain of the pellets at this time.

We measured the cellular ingrowth into the pellet by a cell-counting technique at the fifth day of implantation. Pellets complete with body wall and overlying skin were fixed in formol-saline and embedded in gelatin. Sections were cut 10 μ thick with a freezing microtome and stained with hematoxylin and eosin. Differential cell counts were made using a graticule eyepiece containing 40 squares arranged in a rectangle ($4 \cdot 10$ squares). The narrow edge of the rectangle was aligned along the edge of the pellet and a differential cell count was made in an area of pellet 0.08 mm $\times$ 0.2 mm. Six of these fields were counted in each section, three on the superficial (skin) surface, and three on the deep surface. The number of cells in the six areas counted in each section were added together so that the final cell count represented the number seen in an area of 0.096 mm^2. Previous anti-inflammatory assay techniques have tended to assess separately either the fluid exudate phase or the cellular phase of the inflammatory response, but little attempt was made to correlate these two phases in the same investigation. In the present research we have found that changes in the dry weight of the cotton pellet at the fifth day of implantation are due chiefly to alterations in the protein content of the fluid part of the exudate. They are not significantly affected at this time by alterations in the cellular content.

Intact (nonadrenalectomized) male mice (T.O. Swiss strain) weighing 20-25 g were used for these investigations. Groups of ten animals were used to assess the effect of each dose of steroid on carbon clearance and the local inflammatory response, and ten animals were used as controls for each dose-response investigation. The animals received the steroid in 0.1

Table I. Effect of Various Doses of Cortisone Acetate, Hydrocortisone, Prednisone, and Desoxycorticosterone Acetate (DOCA) on the Phagocytic Activity of the RES and on Granuloma Formation in Intact Male Mice

Daily dose for 4 days, mg	Cortisone Acetate			Hydrocortisone			Prednisone			DOCA		
	K	Kr ± S. E.	Granuloma wt., mg ± S. E.	K	Kr ± S. E.	Granuloma wt., mg ± S. E.	K	Kr ± S. E.	Granuloma wt., mg ± S. E.	K	Kr ± S. E.	Granuloma wt., mg ± S. E.
0.01	23	43 ± 2.10 *	5.8 ± 0.2*	18	56 ± 1.27	5.2 ± 0.1	18	57 ± 3.63	4.5 ± 0.1*	19	54 ± 2.16 *	5.5 ± 0.1*
0.1	22	46 ± 1.78 *	5.4 ± 0.1*	14	68 ± 2.01 *	4.9 ± 0.1*	13	84 ± 5.49 *	4.1 ± 0.1*	22	49 ± 1.63 *	5.8 ± 0.2*
1.0	18	55 ± 2.00	4.5 ± 0.1*	6	182 ± 6.89 *	4.7 ± 0.1*	8	147 ± 9.86 *	3.9 ± 0.1*	19	51 ± 2.03 *	6.4 ± 0.2*
10.0	10	102 ± 5.12 *	4.0 ± 0.1*	6	175 ± 7.21 *	4.4 ± 0.1*	9	124 ± 6.88 *	3.7 ± 0.1*	20	50 ± 1.65 *	6.6 ± 0.2*
Controls	18	57 ± 2.16	5.1 ± 0.1	18	56 ± 2.57	5.2 ± 0.1	18	55 ± 2.45	5.2 ± 0.2	16	64 ± 2.28	5.2 ± 0.1

*P < 0.05

Table II. Effect of Various Doses of 17β-Estradiol, Estrone, and Estriol on the Phagocytic Activity of the RES and on Granuloma Formation in Intact Male Mice

Daily dose for 4 days, mg	17β-Estradiol			Estrone			Estriol		
	K	Kr ± S. E.	Granuloma wt., mg ± S. E.	K	Kr ± S. E.	Granuloma wt., mg ± S. E.	K	Kr ± S. E.	Granuloma wt., mg ± S. E.
0.01	30	34 ± 1.04 *	5.2 ± 0.1	22	45 ± 2.86 *	5.0 ± 0.1	16	59 ± 3.21	5.1 ± 0.1
0.1	40	26 ± 1.19 *	4.8 ± 0.1 *	42	25 ± 1.68 *	5.2 ± 0.1	29	33 ± 2.68*	5.1 ± 0.2
1.0	47	22 ± 1.29 *	4.0 ± 0.1 *	52	20 ± 1.12 *	4.1 ± 0.2 *	53	20 ± 1.01*	4.9 ± 0.1
10.0	33	32 ± 2.29 *	4.8 ± 0.1 *	75	14 ± 1.06 *	4.3 ± 0.1 *	36	27 ± 2.10*	4.8 ± 0.1 *
Controls	18	57 ± 2.16	5.1 ± 0.1	16	60 ± 2.16	5.1 ± 0.1	16	60 ± 2.16	5.1 ± 0.1

*P < 0.05

ml peanut oil once daily for four days. Controls received only 0.1 ml peanut oil once daily. Phagocytic activity was assessed on the fifth day of implantation, and immediately thereafter the animals were sacrificed and the pellets removed. All compounds were given by subcutaneous injection, except for methyltestosterone, which was administered by stomach tube.

RESULTS

Controls

Before implantation the dried pellets used weighed 8.0-10.0 mg. It can be seen from Tables I-VI that after implantation for five days the pellets gained about 5 mg dry weight in all the untreated animals.

Effect of Cortisone, Hydrocortisone, Prednisone, and Desoxycorticosterone Acetate (DOCA) (Table I)

Cortisone

Cortisone produced mild stimulation of phagocytic activity when given in daily doses of 0.01 and 0.1 mg, had no effect when the daily dose was 1.0 mg, and produced marked depression of phagocytic activity when the daily dose reached 10.0 mg. The two lower daily doses (0.01 and 0.1 mg) increased granuloma weight, but the two higher daily doses (1.0 and 10.0 mg) reduced granuloma weight compared with the controls.

Hydrocortisone

When given at a daily dose of 0.01 mg, hydrocortisone had no effect on phagocytic activity or granuloma weight. However, at a daily dose of 0.1 mg and above, there was marked depression of phagocytic activity and granuloma weight was reduced.

Prednisone

Prednisone had no effect on phagocytic activity when the daily dose was 0.01 mg, but produced marked depression in doses above this level. As the daily dose increased, a progressive reduction in granuloma weight was observed.

DOCA

DOCA produced mild stimulation of phagocytic activity and increased granuloma weight with all the daily doses used.

Effect of 17β-Estradiol, Estrone, and Estriol (Table II)

17β-Estradiol

17β-Estradiol stimulated phagocytic activity in all the doses used. The animals receiving 10.0 mg daily showed signs of toxicity; phagocytic activity, although still stimulated, was below the level observed with a daily dose

Table III. Effect of Various Doses of Estradiol Monobenzoate and 17β-Ethinylestradiol on the Phagocytic Activity of the RES and on Granuloma Formation in Intact Male Mice

Daily dose for 4 days, mg	Estradiol Monobenzoate			17α-Ethinylestradiol		
	K	Kr ± S. E.	Granuloma wt., mg ± S. E.	K	Kr ± S. E.	Granuloma wt., mg ± S. E.
0.01	23	40 ± 1.98*	5.1 ± 0.1	29	34 ± 1.00*	5.6 ± 0.1
0.1	28	34 ± 1.66*	5.2 ± 0.2	38	26 ± 1.00*	4.0 ± 0.1*
1.0	43	22 ± 1.33*	4.7 ± 0.1*	65	15 ± 0.99*	3.8 ± 0.1*
10.0	16	61 ± 3.26	4.5 ± 0.1*	21	48 ± 1.76*	5.2 ± 0.1
Controls	16	60 ± 2.16	5.1 ± 0.1	18	55 ± 2.45	5.2 ± 0.2

*P < 0.05

Table IV. Effect of Various Doses of Testosterone and Methyltestosterone on the Phagocytic Activity of the RES and on Granuloma Formation in Intact Male Mice

Daily dose for 4 days, mg	Testosterone			Methyltestosterone		
	K	Kr ± S. E.	Granuloma wt., mg ± S. E.	K	Kr ± S. E.	Granuloma wt., mg ± S. E.
0.01	18	59 ± 3.10	5.5 ± 0.1*	18	59 ± 4.17	5.0 ± 0.1
0.1	18	57 ± 2.33	5.7 ± 0.1*	18	57 ± 1.89	5.0 ± 0.2
1.0	17	60 ± 3.62	7.0 ± 0.2*	17	60 ± 3.78	5.5 ± 0.1*
10.0	8	122 ± 5.92*	5.9 ± 0.1*	19	54 ± 2.10	6.4 ± 0.2*
Controls	18	57 ± 2.62	5.2 ± 0.1	17	58 ± 1.34	5.1 ± 0.1

*P < 0.05

of 1.0 mg. Granuloma weight was reduced by 17β-estradiol given in daily doses of 1.0-10.0 mg, maximum reduction was observed when the daily dose was 1.0 mg.

Estrone

Estrone administration resulted in a progressive increase in phagocytic activity as the daily dose increased. The two higher doses of estrone (1.0 and 10.0 mg) reduced granuloma weight.

Estriol

Estriol stimulated phagocytic activity in all the doses used. The animals receiving 10.0 mg daily showed signs of toxicity; phagocytic activity, although still stimulated, was below the level observed with a daily dose of 1.0 mg. The highest daily dose (10.0 mg) slightly reduced granuloma weight but the doses below this level had no effect.

Effect of 17β-Estradiol-3-Monobenzoate and 17α-Ethinylestradiol (Table III)

Estradiol Monobenzoate

Estradiol monobenzoate stimulated phagocytic activity in the three lower doses given, but had no effect at the highest daily dose (10.0 mg) and the animals in this group showed signs of toxicity. The two higher doses of estradiol monobenzoate (1.0 and 10.0 mg) reduced granuloma weight.

Ethinylestradiol

Ethinylestradiol stimulated phagocytic activity in the three lower doses given, but had no effect at the highest daily dose (10.0 mg) and the animals in this group showed signs of toxicity. When given in daily doses of 0.1 and 1.0 mg, ethinylestradiol markedly reduced granuloma weight, but had no significant effect in doses above and below this level.

Effect of Testosterone and 17α-Methyltestosterone (Table IV)

Testosterone

Testosterone had no effect on phagocytic activity in the three lower doses given, but the highest daily dose (10.0 mg) markedly depressed phagocytic activity and the animals in this group showed marked signs of

Table V. Effect of Various Doses of Progesterone on the Phagocytic Activity of the RES and on Granuloma Formation in Intact Male Mice

Daily dose for 4 days, mg	K	Kr ± S. E.	Granuloma wt., mg ± S. E.
0.01	21	50 ± 1.89 *	5.3 ± 0.2
0.1	22	46 ± 2.12 *	5.0 ± 0.2
1.0	19	56 ± 2.14	6.2 ± 0.2*
10.0	19	55 ± 3.21	6.3 ± 0.1*
Controls	17	58 ± 1.34	5.1 ± 0.1

*$P < 0.05$

toxicity. All the doses of testosterone caused an increase in granuloma weight, the maximum weight being attained with 1.0 mg.

Methyltestosterone

Methyltestosterone had no effect on phagocytic activity in any of the doses used. The two higher doses (1.0 and 10.0 mg) of methyltestosterone caused an increase in granuloma weight.

Effect of Progesterone (Table V)

Progesterone produced mild stimulation of phagocytic activity in the two lower doses given but had no significant effect in daily doses of 1.0 mg and above. The two higher doses of progesterone caused a marked increase in granuloma weight, but it had no effect at daily doses of 0.1 mg and less.

Effect of Local Administration of Various Steroids (Table VI)

Since we found that the above steroids all acted on the inflammatory response when given systemically, it seemed rational to ascertain whether these steroids also acted when given locally. For this purpose the pellets were impregnated with some of the steroids before implantation. Each dose of steroid was dissolved in 0.15 ml of 2.5% ethanol. Each animal was then implanted in one flank with a pellet containing 0.001 mg of the compound under investigation, and in the other flank with a pellet containing 0.01 mg of the same compound. These two different doses were used so

Table VI. Effect of Impregnation of Cotton Pellets with Various Compounds on Granuloma

Compound used	Number of animals in group	Mean granuloma wt., mg ± S. E.	
		Pellets impregnated with 0.001 mg of compound	Pellets impregnated with 0.01 mg of compound
Cortisone	10	4.8 ± 0.1 *	4.3 ± 0.1 *
Hydrocortisone	10	4.3 ± 0.1 *	3.9 ± 0.1 *
Prednisone	10	4.2 ± 0.1 *	3.8 ± 0.1 *
Desoxycorticosterone acetate	10	6.0 ± 0.2 *	6.5 ± 0.2 *
17β-Estradiol	10	4.9 ± 0.1	4.5 ± 0.1 *
17α-Ethinylestradiol	10	4.7 ± 0.1 *	4.3 ± 0.1 *
Testosterone	10	5.7 ± 0.1 *	6.1 ± 0.1 *
Progesterone	10	6.0 ± 0.1 *	6.4 ± 0.2 *
Controls	10	5.2 ± 0.1	5.2 ± 0.1

*$P < 0.05$

Table VII. Effect of Subcutaneously Administered Steroids on Total and Differential Cell Counts in Cotton Pellet Granulomas in Intact Male Mice

Steroid (1.0 mg daily for 4 days)	Differential Cell Distribution						Total cells counted
	Polymorphonuclear leucocytes		Macrophages		Fibroblasts		
	Cells counted, ± S. E.	% of Total ± S. E.	Cells counted, ± S. E.	% of Total ± S. E.	Cells counted, ± S. E.	% of Total ± S. E.	
Hydrocortisone	4 ± 1.73 *	1.50 ± 0.58	236 ± 16.12*	91.27 ± 0.44*	19 ± 1.47 *	7.22 ± 0.20*	258 ± 18.65*
Desoxycorticosterone acetate	32 ± 3.16 *	1.78 ± 0.22	1650 ± 341.16*	88.83 ± 1.21*	168 ± 22.36	9.39 ± 1.18*	1850 ± 360.91*
17β-Estradiol	14 ± 4.36	1.47 ± 0.53	775 ± 58.48*	77.67 ± 1.16	207 ± 11.46	20.86 ± 0.92	996 ± 58.19*
17α-Ethinylestradiol	14 ± 3.70	1.14 ± 0.32 *	967 ± 60.00*	75.62 ± 2.22	295 ± 14.43 *	23.24 ± 1.92	1276 ± 42.60*
Testosterone	9 ± 1.73	0.59 ± 0.10 *	1321 ± 58.08*	84.10 ± 1.60	241 ± 25.57 *	15.32 ± 1.26	1571 ± 65.85*
Progesterone	24 ± 3.61	1.44 ± 0.27	1507 ± 139.41*	89.07 ± 0.76*	163 ± 30.42	9.49 ± 0.78*	1695 ± 169.76*
Controls	16 ± 1.53	2.53 ± 0.31	498 ± 28.10	77.42 ± 1.85	133 ± 26.73	20.05 ± 2.03	647 ± 76.01

*P < 0.05

Table VIII. Effect of Impregnation of Cotton Pellets with Various Steroids on Total and Differential Cell Counts in Cotton Pellet Granulomas in Intact Male Mice

Steroid (0.01 mg impregnated)	Differential Cell Distribution: Polymorphonuclear leucocytes		Macrophages		Fibroblasts		Total cells counted
	Cells counted, ± S. E.	% of Total, ± S. E.	Cells counted, ± S. E.	% of Total, ± S. E.	Cells counted, ± S. E.	% of Total, ± S. E.	
Hydrocortisone	2 ± 1.15	0.84 ± 0.45	242 ± 14.93 *	89.02 ± 1.25 *	28 ± 4.90 *	10.14 ± 1.64 *	272 ± 17.69 *
Desoxycorticosterone acetate	37 ± 14.19	2.04 ± 0.70	1445 ± 50.27 *	80.64 ± 0.78	310 ± 7.83 *	17.32 ± 0.51 *	1792 ± 65.75 *
17β-Estradiol	26 ± 10.21	1.17 ± 0.35	1707 ± 243.72 *	84.24 ± 1.59 *	302 ± 69.16	14.59 ± 1.41 *	2035 ± 315.96 *
17α-Ethinylestradiol	13 ± 2.00	0.79 ± 0.20	1446 ± 166.01 *	83.31 ± 0.60 *	279 ± 65.50	15.90 ± 0.80 *	1738 ± 210.55 *
Testosterone	10 ± 2.65	0.58 ± 0.27	1524 ± 103.28 *	85.45 ± 1.84 *	248 ± 26.98 *	13.97 ± 1.70 *	1782 ± 100.68 *
Progesterone	54 ± 7.57 *	2.91 ± 0.17	1463 ± 146.75 *	79.32 ± 1.27	334 ± 58.31 *	17.77 ± 1.26	1852 ± 211.81 *
Controls	12 ± 3.70	2.05 ± 0.86	484 ± 40.13	76.59 ± 1.68	138 ± 10.17	21.84 ± 0.76	631 ± 41.86

* $P < 0.05$

that any significant differences between the weights of the pellets in each flank could only be due to local action of the hormone. The control animals were implanted with pellets impregnated with 0.15 ml of 2.5% ethanol. The animals received no further treatment and the pellets were removed on the fifth day of implantation.

Cortisone, hydrocortisone, prednisone, 17β-estradiol, and ethinylestradiol reduced granuloma weight, while DOCA, testosterone, and progesterone increased granuloma weight. In all cases, the effect of the higher dose was greater than that of the lower dose. The results were similar to those obtained when these steroids were given subcutaneously.

Effect of Various Steroids on Total and Differential Cell Counts in Cotton Pellets (Tables VII and VIII)

When sections of the pellets were examined microscopically, it was found that the cell population consisted solely of macrophages, neutrophil polymorphonuclear leucocytes, and fibroblasts.

It can be seen from the tables that, when administered subcutaneously or by impregnation of the pellets, hydrocortisone reduced the total number of cells in the pellet, whereas DOCA, 17β-estradiol, ethinylestradiol, testerosterone, and progesterone increased the total number. The changes in the total cell counts were, in all cases, principally due to changes in the number of macrophages which formed 80-90% of the cells present.

The fact that estrogens increase cellular ingrowth into implanted cotton pellets and at the same time reduce the dry granuloma weight, suggest that the dry-weight changes at the fifth day of implantation are due chiefly to changes in the amount of protein in the pellet and are not significantly affected at this time by alterations in the cellular content. The changes in the protein content of the pellet are due to alterations in capillary permeability and reflect changes in the volume of the exudate or its protein concentration. Since, however, inflammatory fluid has the same protein concentration as serum, the changes in the protein content of the dry pellets are probably due to changes in the volume of exudate. For this reason we have interpreted changes in dry granuloma weight as indicating increase or decrease of fluid exudate.

DISCUSSION

Cortisone, Hydrocortisone, and Prednisone

We have shown that cortisone, hydrocortisone, and prednisone depress phagocytic activity and reduce inflammatory fluid exudate. The amount of exudate was reduced whether they were administered subcutaneously or by impregnation of the pellets before implantation. Hydrocortisone was selected to represent these compounds in the cell-count experiments, and was shown to reduce the number of cells at the inflammatory site both when given subcutaneously or locally.

Depression of phagocytic activity by cortisone, hydrocortisone, and prednisone is in agreement with the findings of Nicol and Bilbey [10, 11], Snell [12], and Nicol, Vernon-Roberts, and Quantock [6]. We also found that the administration of cortisone in doses of 0.01-0.1 mg produced mild stimulation of phagocytic activity and increase of inflammatory exudate. This is in contrast to the depression of phagocytic activity and the reduction of exudate produced by higher doses. This effect of low doses of cortisone on phagocytosis confirms our previous findings (Nicol et al. [6]) and those of Snell [12]. Robinson [13] and Crabbé [14] have also shown that small doses of cortisone enhance macrophage phagocytosis of bacteria and increase protection against infection. The mechanism by which these compounds depress phagocytosis is unknown, but factors affecting the protein binding of particles prior to phagocytosis and stabilization of cell membranes may be involved.

Reduction of inflammatory exudate by the glucocorticoids is said to be due to inhibition of increased capillary permeability (Ebert and Barclay [15]). Histamine is capable of producing all the microcirculatory changes which occur during the early phase of the inflammatory response, and the rate of occurrence of these changes is parallel to the rate of induced histamine synthesis (Schayer [16, 17]). In this connection it has been shown that the binding of induced histamine by the tissues is inhibited by administered cortisone (Goth et al. [18], Schayer, Smiley, and Davis [19]). The activation or release of proteases into tissues is a primary step in inflammation (Rocha e Silva[20]), and since lysosomes are believed to store enzymes and their precursors, glucocorticoids may inhibit inflammation by stabilization of lysosome envelopes (Weissmann and Thomas [21]), thus delaying the release or activation of proteolytic agents (Allison [22]).

The suppression by glucocorticoids of the cellular response during inflammation appears to be largely due to interference with margination and sticking of leucocytes to vascular endothelium (Ebert and Barclay [15], Allison, Smith, and Wood [23]), since hydrocortisone prevents the changes in the surface of endothelial cells and leucocytes caused by substances released from tissues after injury (Allison [22]). In the present research we have found that hydrocortisone caused a greater reduction in the percentage of fibroblasts than other cell types; and in this connection, it has been reported that glucocorticoids inhibit the mitosis and maturation of fibroblasts in vitro (Berliner [24]).

DOCA

DOCA stimulated phagocytic activity and increased both fluid and cellular components of the inflammatory response when given subcutaneously or locally. These findings may be related to the increase in capillary permeability to trypan blue and to increased wound healing after DOCA administration (Freed and Lindner [25], Pirani, Stepto, and Sutherland [26]).

17β-Estradiol, Estrone, Estriol, Estradiol Monobenzoate, and Ethinylestradiol

Stimulation of phagocytosis by the above estrogens confirms our previous findings (Nicol et al. [1], Nicol et al. [3, 6]). The mechanism by which estrogens stimulate phagocytosis is unknown, but it seems probable that both intracellular and extracellular factors are involved. Villee, Hagerman, and Joel [27] have shown that estrogen-sensitive tissues possess an estrogen-stimulable transhydrogenase located in the nonparticulate fraction of the cell and not present in other tissues. This transhydrogenase increases the rate of energy metabolism by oxidizing TPNH to TPN, and by increasing the yield of energy-rich phosphate. In this connection, it has been demonstrated that phagocytic cells have a very active pentose phosphate metabolic pathway. One consequence of this activity is an increased production of reduced pyridine nucleotides, particularly TPNH, during phagocytosis (Sbarra and Karnovsky [28]). It is also widely accepted that estrogens increase the binding effect of the plasma proteins (Roberts and Szego [29]), and this plays a vital part in the events leading to phagocytosis. In the present research we have also shown that the natural and synthetic estrogens reduce inflammatory exudate but increase the cellular response at the inflammatory site, whether administered subcutaneously or locally. Kitay [30] has demonstrated that estrogen increases the secretion of ACTH which, in turn, increases the output of adrenal corticosteroids. Estrogens may thus reduce capillary permeability indirectly by increasing plasma glucocorticoid levels. However, a direct effect of estrogen on capillaries cannot be excluded, since they inhibit the formation of inflammatory exudate in adrenalectomized animals, and ACTH has no direct effect (Glenn, Miller, and Schlagel [31]).

Despite the reduction in capillary permeability caused by estrogen, we found an increase in the number of cells at the inflammatory site. It is widely accepted that inflammatory cells migrate between the intercellular junctions of endothelial cells, but whether plasma proteins and fluid cross the capillary barrier via the interendothelial or transcytoplasmic route is uncertain. Our findings would support the concept that cells and fluid exudate cross the capillary barrier by different routes.

It has been established that the macrophages of inflammatory tissues are derived from circulating blood monocytes (Ebert and Florey [32], Paz and Spector [33]), and that monocytes actively divide in inflamed areas (Spector [34]). It has also been reported that estrogens stimulate mitosis (Bullough [35]). The increased number of macrophages we found after estrogen treatment may therefore be due to increased cell division. However, there is little doubt that estrogens also cause increased cell migration,

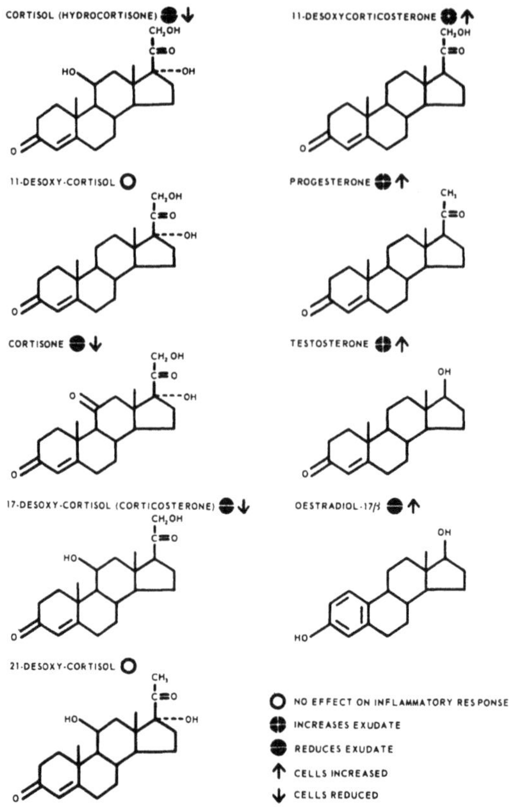

Fig. 1. Molecular configuration of various steroids and their effects on the inflammatory response.

since there is marked infiltration of the uterine endometrium by leucocytes and macrophages when blood estrogen levels are raised (Nicol and Vernon-Roberts [2]). Further, Spector and Storey [36] have demonstrated that extracts of estrogenized mouse uterus promote cellular migration in inflamed connective tissue.

Testosterone, Methyltestosterone, and Progesterone

Testosterone and methyltestosterone had no effect on phagocytic activity. Progesterone was a mild stimulant of phagocytosis in the lower dose range, but the effect disappeared as the dose was increased, confirming our previous findings (Nicol et al. [3-6]).

Testosterone, methyltestosterone, and progesterone increased both fluid and cellular components of the inflammatory response when given systematically or locally. It has been previously demonstrated that testosterone increases the formation of granulation tissue (Rubens-Duval and

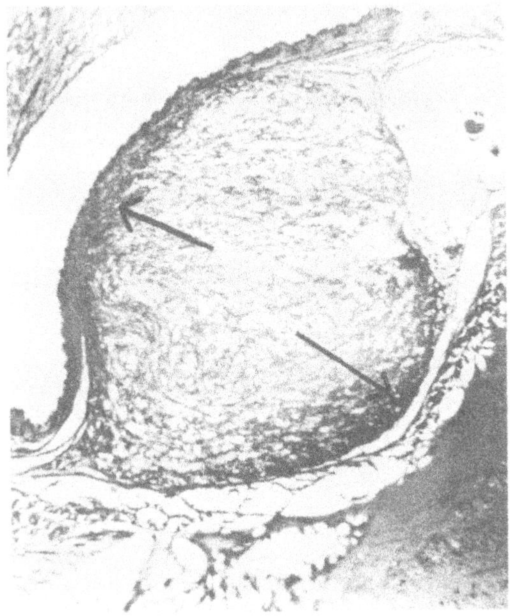

Fig. 2. Section of cotton pellet five days after subcutaneous implantation in the mouse. Control animal. Received peanut oil once daily for four days. Darkened areas (arrowed) indicate the extent of cellular infiltration. Hematoxylin and eosin. x 10.

Villiaumey [37]), and the tensile strength of healing wounds (DiGaddo and Fratta [38]), but the effects of androgens on capillary permeability have not previously been reported. Progesterone has been shown to increase capillary permeability to trypan blue (Freed et al. [25]), but its effect on the cellular response in inflammation has not previously been investigated.

Structure–Function Relationships

The structure–function relationships of the action of various steroids on the phagocytic activity of the fixed cells of the RES have been examined recently by Nicol, Vernon-Roberts, and Quantock [3, 4]. We postulated that all steroids act by occupying the same receptor, presumably the surface of an enzyme or the membrane of a cell or cell particle, and that differing effects of the steroids may be due to differences in their binding properties to cell membrane proteins in the target areas. It has been stated that steroid activity of any given type depends on chemical specificity (Solmssen [39], Schueler [40], Gordon [41], Höhn [42]). This suggests that these hormones function in metabolism by forming essential links with other substances, presumably proteins, and evidence has been produced showing that estrogens become more firmly bound to protein than other steroids (Szego and Roberts [43]). This provides a rational explanation for the greater

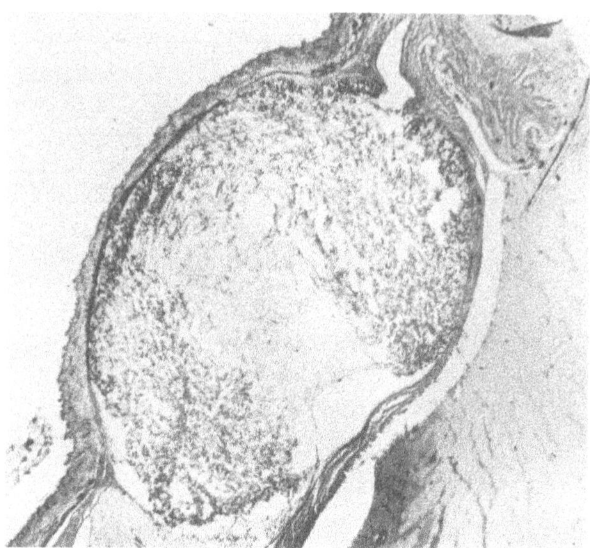

Fig. 3. Section of cotton pellet five days after subcutaneous implantation in the mouse. Animal received hydrocortisone 1.0 mg daily for four days. Shows absence of cellular infiltration around periphery of pellet. Hematoxylin and eosin. × 10.

activity of estrogenic substances if protein binding is a necessary preliminary to steroid hormone action. It follows that relatively larger doses of other steroids would be required to attach them to protein. In this connection, Schueler [40] noted that the dose of potent androgens needed to produce an androgenic effect in the rat is much greater than the amount of estrogen necessary to produce estrus. He postulated that this was due to the greater hydrogen bond-forming power of "estrogenic hydrogen" conferred by phenolic-OH groups. In the steroid estrogens ring A is aromatic with a phenolic-OH attached at C-3 (Fig. 1), whereas rings A of the other steroids are α,β -unsaturated ketones. Bush [44] has reviewed the evidence which suggests that it is the α-face of androgens, and the β-face of estrogens, corticosteroids, and gestogens which are primarily involved in the attachment of the molecule to the site of action. In this connection, we have shown in the steroid series that androgens are exceptional in having no effect on phagocytic activity.

The structure—function relationships of anti-inflammatory steroids have been reviewed by several authors during recent years. The results of the present investigation shed further light on the relationship of steroid structure to function in acting on inflammatory processes, since, in addition to the glucocorticoids, our results include the effects of desoxycorticosterone, estrogens, androgens, and progesterone.

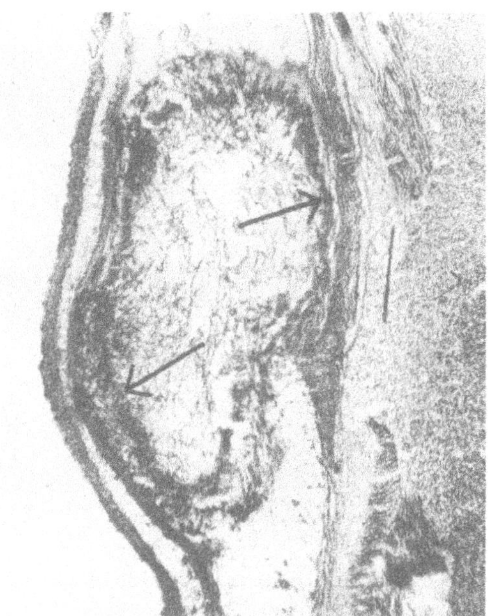

Fig. 4. Section of cotton pellet five days after subcutaneous implantation in the mouse. Animal received 17β-estradiol 1.0 mg daily for four days. Shows marked increase (arrowed) in cellular infiltration around periphery of pellet. Hematoxylin and eosin. × 10.

Although cortisone was the first steroid shown to have anti-inflammatory activity, it is more convenient from the standpoint of structure—function studies to consider cortisol (hydrocortisone) as the basic anti-inflammatory steroid. Cortisol, instead of cortisone, is the principal hormone produced by the adrenal cortex in most species (Bush [45]). The anti-inflammatory activity of cortisone appears to be largely due to its transformation in the body to cortisol (Peterson et al. [46]). Almost every part of the cortisol molecule appears to be important in determining anti-inflammatory activity. This can be illustrated by comparing the biological activity of cortisol with various analogs, each of which differs structurally in small respects (Fig.1).

Cortisol is the most potent naturally occurring anti-inflammatory corticosteroid. The crucial importance of the 11β-hydroxyl group is illustrated by a few comparisons. 11-Desoxy-cortisol (Reichstein's compound S) and the 11α-hydroxy epimer of cortisol are both devoid of anti-inflammatory activity (Polley and Mason [47], Peterson et al. [48]). Cortisone, which differs structurally from cortisol only in having an 11-keto in place of an 11β-hydroxyl group, has approximately 70% of the anti-inflammatory activity of cortisol.

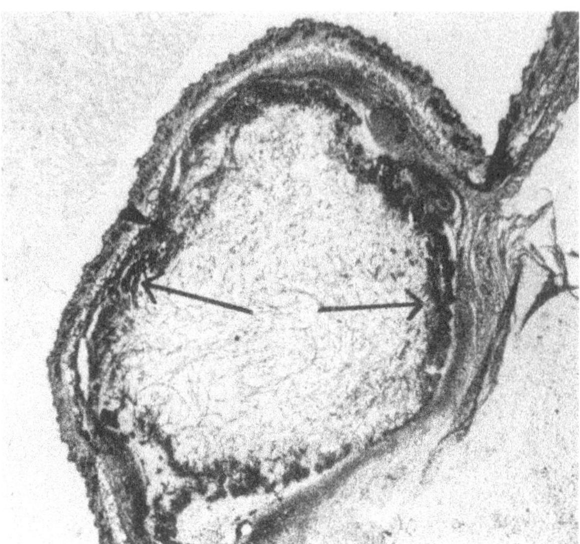

Fig. 5. Section of cotton pellet five days after subcutaneous implantation in the mouse. Animal received testosterone 1.0 mg daily for four days. Shows marked increase in cellular infiltration around periphery of pellet. Hematoxylin and eosin. x 10.

17-Desoxy-cortisol (corticosterone) has no anti-inflammatory activity in man, but has one-third of the potency of cortisol in the rat (Fried and Borman [49]), and is the principal steroid secreted by the adrenal in this species (Bush [45]). It thus appears that the 17α-hydroxyl group enhances anti-inflammatory activity but is not essential for this effect.

The importance of the 21-hydroxyl group in determining the biological activity of all the corticosteroids is illustrated by 21-desoxy-cortisol, which is devoid of anti-inflammatory, glucocorticoid, and mineralocorticoid activity (Goldfien et al. [50], Polley et al. [47]), although it possesses 11β-hydroxyl and 17α-hydroxyl groups.

In contrast, 11-desoxycorticosterone (DOC) is inflammatory, since it enhances both the cellular and fluid phases of the inflammatory process. Thus, corticosteroids devoid of hydroxyl groups at C-11 and C-17 are inflammatory and mineralocorticoid. Progesterone has the same inflammatory effect as DOC, but has no corticosteroid activity, since it is devoid of a hydroxyl group at C-21. Absence of the side-chain attached at C-17, as in testosterone, enhances inflammatory potency.

Since ring A and the 19-methyl group are the same in the corticosteroids, progesterone and testosterone, it would appear that the configuration of rings B, C, and D and the side-chain are responsible for the effects on the inflammatory process. In the estrogens, since rings B, C, and D are the same as in testosterone, an inflammatory effect might have been expected. We have shown that estrogens increase the cellular response, but the unexpected reduction in fluid exudate appears to be related to the changes in the molecule conferred by aromatic ring A and the absence of 19-methyl.

REFERENCES

1. T. Nicol, D. L. J. Bilbey, L. M. Charles, J. L. Cordingley, and B. Vernon-Roberts, "Oestrogen: the natural stimulant of body defence," J. Endocrinol., 30 : 277-291, 1964.
2. T. Nicol and B. Vernon-Roberts, "The influence of the estrus cycle, pregnancy, and ovariectomy on RES activity," J. Reticuloendothelial Soc., 2 : 15-29, 1965.
3. T. Nicol, B. Vernon-Roberts, and D. C. Quantock, "The effects of oestrogen : androgen interaction on the reticuloendothelial system and reproductive tract," J. Endocrinol., 34 : 163-178, 1966.
4. T. Nicol, B. Vernon-Roberts, and D. C. Quantock, "The effect of various anti-oestrogenic compounds on the reticuloendothelial system and reproductive tract in the ovariectomized mouse," J. Endocrinol., 34 : 377-386, 1966.
5. T. Nicol, B. Vernon-Roberts, and D. C. Quantock, "The effects of testosterone and progesterone on the response of the reticuloendothelial system and reproductive tract to oestrogen in the male mouse," J. Endocrinol., 37:17-21, 1967.
6. T. Nicol, B. Vernon-Roberts, and D. C. Quantock, "The influence of various hormones on the reticuloendothelial system: endocrine control of body defence," J. Endocrinol., 33 : 365-383, 1965.
7. B. Vernon-Roberts, "Hormone researches on the reticuloendothelial system," PhD Thesis, University of London, 1965.
8. R. Meier, W. Schueler, and P. Desaulles, "Zur Frage des Mechanismus der Hemmung des Bindegwebswachstums durch Cortisone," Experientia, 6 : 469-471, 1950.
9. D. C. Quantock, "The effect of various steroids on local and general body defence," PhD Thesis, University of London, 1966.
10. T. Nicol and D. L. J. Bilbey, "Substances depressing the phagocytic activity of the reticuloendothelial system," Nature, 182 : 606, 1958.
11. T. Nicol and D. L. J. Bilbey, "The effect of various steroids on the phagocytic activity of the reticuloendothelial system," in: J. H. Heller, Ed., Reticuloendothelial Structure and Function. New York, Ronald Press, 1960, pp. 301-320.
12. J. F. Snell, "Relationship of chromium phosphate clearance rates to resistance. I. The effects of some corticosteroids on blood clearance rates in mice," in: J. H. Heller, Ed., Reticuloendothelial Structure and Function. New York, Ronald Press, 1960, pp. 321-332.

13. H.J. Robinson, "The role of the adrenal glands in infection and intoxication," in: J.M. Yoffey, Ed., The Suprarenal Cortex. London, Butterworths, 1953, pp. 105-124.
14. J. Crabbé, "Enhancing action of small doses of cortisone on macrophage phagocytosis of staphylococci in rabbits," Acta Endocrinol., 21:41-46, 1956.
15. R.H. Ebert and W.R. Barclay, "Changes in connective tissue reaction induced by cortisone," Ann.Internal Med., 37:506-518, 1952.
16. R.W. Schayer, "Evidence that induced histamine is an intrinsic regulator of the microcirculatory system," Am.J.Physiol., 202:66-72, 1962.
17. R.W. Schayer, "Induced synthesis of histamine, microcirculatory regulation, and the mechanism of action of the adrenal glucocorticoid hormones," Progr.Allergy, 7:187-212, 1963.
18. A. Goth, R.M. Allman, B.C. Meritt, and J. Holman, "Effect of cortisone on histamine liberation by Tween in the dog," Proc.Soc. Exptl.Biol.Med., 78:848-852, 1951.
19. R.W. Schayer, R.L. Smiley, and K.J. Davis, "Inhibition by cortisone of the binding of new histamine in rat tissues," Proc.Soc.Exptl.Biol. Med., 87:590-592, 1954.
20. M. Rocha e Silva, "Bradykinin and histamine," Arch.Intern.Pharmacodyn., 103:212-220, 1955.
21. G. Weissmann and L. Thomas, "Studies on lysosomes. II. The effect of cortisone on the release of acid hydrolases from a large granule fraction of rabbit liver induced by an excess of vitamin A," J.Clin.Invest., 42:661-669, 1963.
22. F. Allison, "Anti-inflammatory agents," in: B.W. Zweifach, L.Grant, and R.T. McCluskey, Eds., Review of the Inflammatory Response. New York and London, Academic Press, 1965, pp. 559-576.
23. F. Allison, M.R. Smith, and W.B. Wood, "Studies on pathogenesis of acute inflammation; action of cortisone on inflammatory response to thermal injury," J.Exptl.Med., 102:669-676, 1955.
24. D.L. Berliner, "Biotransformation of corticosteroids as related to inflammation," Ann.N.Y.Acad.Sci., 116:1071-1083, 1964.
25. F.C. Freed and E. Lindner, "Effect of steroids of adrenal cortex and ovary on capillary permeability," Am.J.Physiol., 134:258-262, 1941.
26. C.L. Pirani, R.C. Stepto, and K. Sutherland, "Desoxycorticosterone acetate and wound healing," J.Exptl.Med., 93:217-228, 1951.
27. C.A. Villee, D.D. Hagerman, and P.B. Joel, "An enzymatic base for the physiologic functions of estrogens," Recent Progr.Hormone Res., 16:49-69, 1960.
28. A.J. Sbarra and M.L. Karnovsky, "The biochemical basis of phagocytosis. I. Metabolic changes during the ingestion of particles by polymorphonuclear leucocytes," J.Biol.Chem., 234:1355-1362, 1959.
29. S. Roberts and C.M. Szego, "Steroid interaction in the metabolism of reproductive target organs," Physiol.Rev., 33:593-629, 1953.

30. J.I. Kitay, "Effects of estradiol on pituitary—adrenal function in male and female rats," Endocrinology, 72:947-954, 1963.
31. E.M. Glenn, W.L. Miller, and C.A. Schlagel, "Metabolic effects of adrenocortical steroids in vivo and in vitro: relationship to anti-inflammatory effects," Recent Progr. Hormone Res., 19:107-199, 1963.
32. R.H. Ebert and H.W. Florey, "The extravascular development of the monocyte observed in vivo," Brit.J.Exptl.Pathol., 20:342-356, 1939.
33. R.A. Paz and W.G. Spector, "The mononuclear response to injury," J.Pathol.Bacteriol., 84:85-103, 1962.
34. W.G. Spector, Personal communication, 1966.
35. W.S. Bullough, "Hormones and mitotic activity," Vitamins Hormones, 13:261-292, 1955.
36. W.G. Spector and E. Storey, "A factor in oestrogen-treated uterus causing leucocyte emigration," J.Pathol.Bacteriol., 75:383-411, 1958.
37. A. Rubens-Duval and J. Villiaumey, "Effect of androgens on granulation tissue," Ann.Endocrinol.(Paris), 23:648-667, 1962.
38. M. DiGaddo and M. Fratta, "Influence of 4-chloro-testosterone acetate on wound-healing," Minerva Chir., 15:1227-1228, 1960.
39. U.V. Solmssen, "Synthetic estrogens and the relation between their structure and their activity," Chem.Rev., 37:481-598, 1945.
40. F.W. Schueler, "Sex hormonal action and chemical constitution," Science, 103:221-223, 1946.
41. E.S. Gordon, Ed., in: Symposium on Steroids. Madison, University of Wisconsin Press, 1950, pp. 212-217.
42. E.O. Höhn, "Steroids exerting a direct progestational effect on the rabbit endometrium," Nature, 169:844, 1952.
43. C.M. Szego and S. Roberts, "Steroid action and interaction in uterine metabolism," Recent Progr. Hormone Res., 8:419-470, 1953.
44. I.E. Bush, in: Currie et al., Eds., The Human Adrenal Cortex. Edinburgh, Livingstone, 1962, p. 138.
45. I.E. Bush, "Species differences in adrenocortical secretion," J.Endocrinol., 9:95-100, 1953.
46. R.E. Peterson, J.B. Wyngaarden, S.L. Guerra, B.B. Brodie, and J.J. Bunim, "The physiological disposition and metabolic fate of hydrocortisone in man," J.Clin.Invest., 34:1779-1794, 1955.
47. H.F. Polley and H.L. Mason, "Rheumatoid arthritis; effects of certain steroids other than cortisone and of some adrenal cortex extracts," J.Am.Med.Assoc., 143:1474-1481, 1950.
48. D.H. Peterson, S.H. Eppstein, P.D. Meister, B.J. Magerlein, H.C. Murray, H. Marian Leigh, A. Weintraub, and L.M. Reineke, "Microbiological transformation of steroids. IV. The 11 epimer of compound F and other new oxygenated derivatives of Reichstein's compound S. A new route to cortisone," J.Am.Chem.Soc., 75:412-415, 1953.
49. J. Fried and A. Borman, "Synthetic derivatives of cortical hormones," Vitamins Hormones, 16:303-374, 1958.

50. A. Goldfien, W.I. Morse, E.R. Froesch, W.F. Ganong, E.A. Renold, and G.W. Thorn, "Pharmacological studies in man of 11-, 17-, and 21-hydroxyl derivatives of progesterone and their fluorinated analogs," Ann. N. Y. Acad. Sci., 61:433-441, 1955.

The Quantitative Response of the Host Defense System after Stimulation*

John H. Heller and Emile G. Bliznakov

New England Institute for Medical Research
Ridgefield, Connecticut

Lack of understanding of the reticuloendothelial system (RES) has been fostered by the fact that too many specialists have been looking at segments of the system and too few generalists have looked at the system in toto. In an attempt to take a comprehensive view of the fundamental parameters involved in the defense of the host, we would use the term "host defense," which can include all physiologic parameters, instead of being limited by the restrictive nomenclature that is more conventional.

A series of papers from this Institute has suggested that certain non-toxic lipids derived from shark livers (Restim) can stimulate the host defense system and all of its presently measurable functions, including phagocytosis, intracellular destruction of phagocytosed organisms, specific antibody synthesis, efficacy of passive immunization, lysozyme production, survival time, and survivorship of animals or embryonated chicken eggs confronted with a lethal challenge [1-8].

It became apparent that the capacity of Restim to modify host resistance to experimental infections is wholly dependent upon a time–dose relationship. In extending this work it was observed that the curve of the dose–response relationship is W-shaped, with two peaks of protection, but not linear. The initial work was expanded to include additional model systems. This dose–response relationship was present in all systems in which the lipid Restim was tested.

This led to the idea that this dose–response relationship might be a function of the host defense mechanism and not of the type of stimulant used.

* This work was supported in part by research grants from The John A. Hartford Foundation, Inc., the Fannie E. Rippel Foundation, and the Reynolds Bagley Verney Foundation.

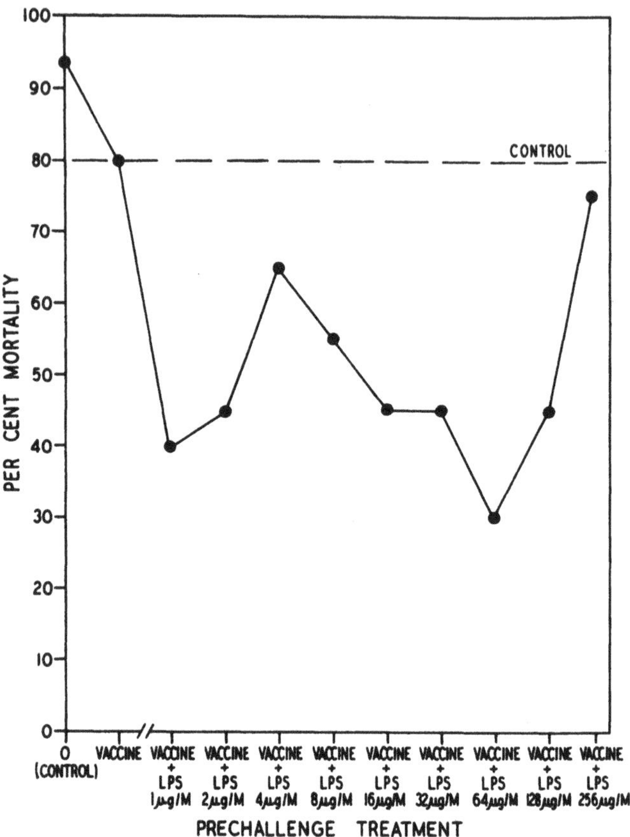

Fig. 1. Modification of the 20-day mortality by various doses of bacterial lipopolysaccharide (LPS) in mice vaccinated, and subsequently infected, with Salmonella typhimurium.

As a result, other materials known to stimulate the host defense mechanism were studied. These included simple lipids like triglycerides, bacterial lipopolysaccharide (LPS), and glucan. These substances were used in several model systems including studies of phagocytosis, antibody synthesis, protection of embryonated chicken eggs against lethal viral or bacterial infections, salmonella infection in mice, endotoxin shock in mice, Rous sarcoma in chicks, and Ehrlich ascites carcinoma in mice. Although all of the models have not been completely tested using multiple dose ranges, some of the studies are complete and others sufficiently advanced so that certain conclusions can be made concerning the type of response of the stimulated host-defense system.

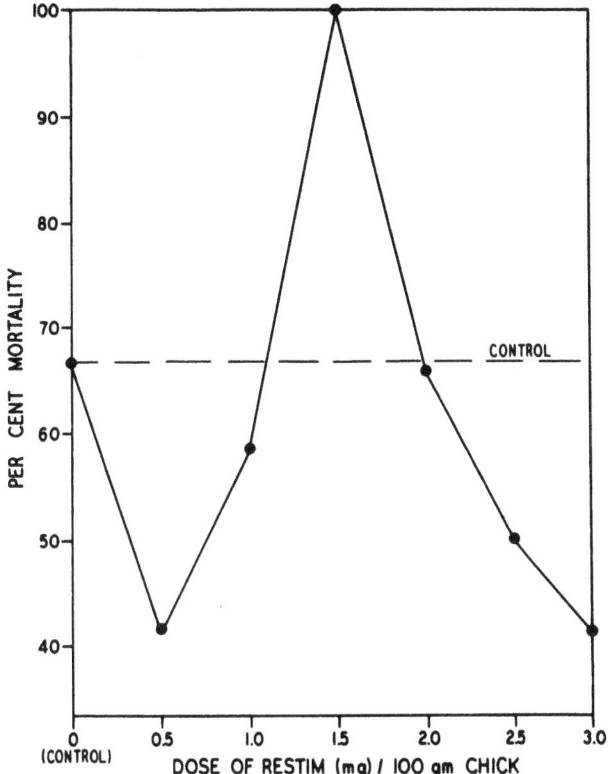

Fig. 2. Modification of the 90-day mortality by various doses of Restim in chicks infected previously with Rous sarcoma virus (RSV).

MATERIALS AND METHODS

Salmonella Typhimurium (ST) Infection in Vaccinated Mice

Male CF-1 mice (Carworth Farms, Inc., New City, New York) weighing 20 g were injected subcutaneously with 0.2 ml of an alcohol-treated ST-vaccine, diluted 1 : 250 in nonpyrogenic normal saline (Baxter Laboratories, Inc., Morton Grove, Illinois). After 19 days the mice were injected intravenously with 0.2 ml of varying dilutions of bacterial lipopolysaccharide (Escherichia coli 0126 : B8, Difco Laboratories, Detroit, Michigan), prepared in nonpyrogenic normal saline and kept in a 100°C water bath for 40 min. Two days later, the mice were infected intravenously with $6\text{-}8 \cdot 10^6$ viable ST cells* from an 18-hr culture. The cumulative mortality was re-

---

* Salmonella typhimurium, strain SR-11, was obtained through the courtesy of Smith, Kline and French Laboratories, Philadelphia, Pennsylvania.

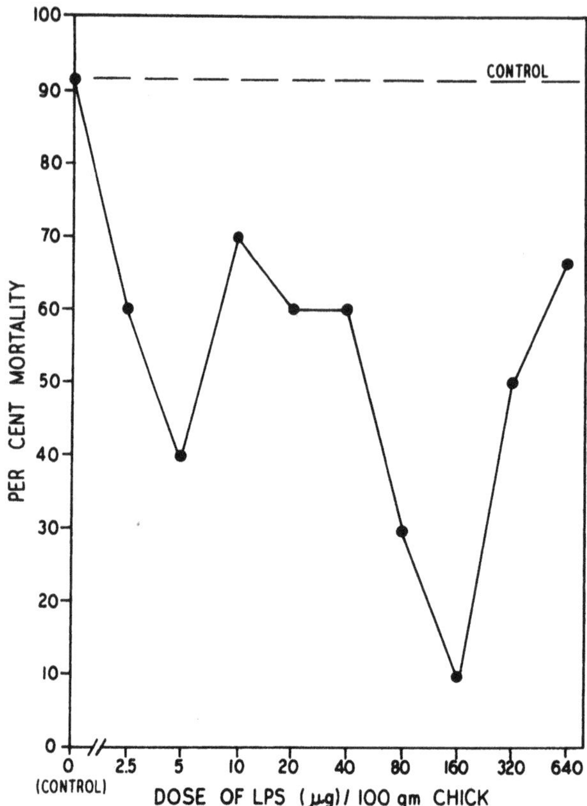

Fig. 3. Modification of the 90-day mortality by various doses of bacterial lipopolysaccharide (LPS) in chicks infected previously with Rous sarcoma virus (RSV).

corded daily for 20 days. In each experiment a minimum of 20 mice was used in each group. Each experiment was conducted twice.

Rous Sarcoma Virus (RSV) Infection in Chicks

Male and female White Leghorn chicks, hatched and raised in isolation at this Institute, were inoculated subcutaneously into the left wing web (0.2 ml for the experiments with Restim) or intraperitoneally (0.25 ml for the experiments with LPS) with undiluted RSV, * prepared at this Institute from pooled and rapidly growing tumors in young chicks. Seven days later the chicks were injected with shark-liver lipid, Restim, as an emulsion in 5% nonpyrogenic glucose (Baxter Laboratories, Inc., Morton Grove, Illinois), prepared by the use of procedures previously described [4], or with vary-

* Rous sarcoma virus was obtained from American Type Culture Collection, Washington, D. C.

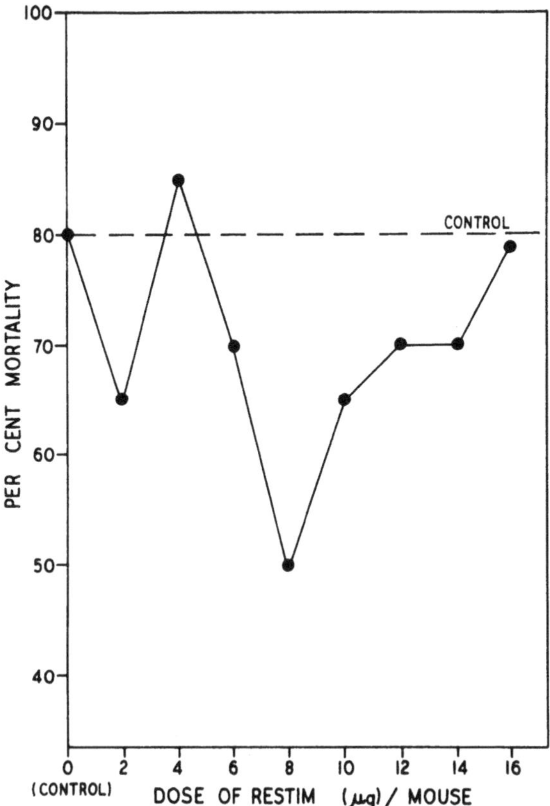

Fig. 4. Modification of three-day mortality by various doses of Restim in mice injected subsequently with bacterial lipopolysaccharide (LPS).

ing dilutions of bacterial lipopolysaccharides prepared as described above. The cumulative mortality in both group experiments was recorded daily for 90 days. In each experiment a minimum of 12 birds was used per group. Each experiment was conducted at least twice.

Endotoxin Shock in Mice

Male CF-1 mice (Carworth Farms, Inc., New City, New York) weighing 20 g were injected intravenously with varying amounts of shark-liver lipid, Restim, as an emulsion, or in the second group of experiments with varying dilutions of bacterial lipopolysaccharide, prepared as described above. Two days later, the mice were injected intravenously with 800 μg bacterial lipopolysaccharide per mouse, prepared as described above. The cumulative mortality was recorded daily for three days. In each experiment a minimum of 20 mice was used in each group. Each experiment was conducted at least twice.

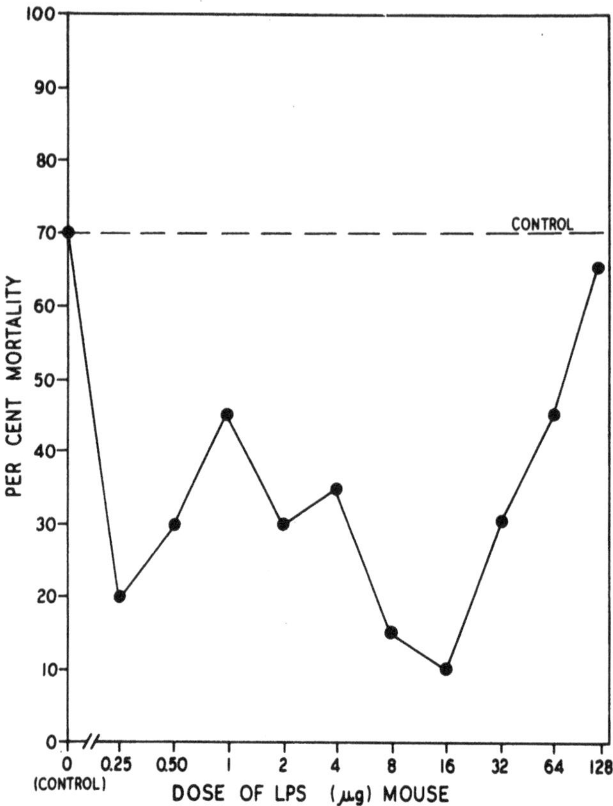

Fig. 5. Modification of three-day mortality by various doses of LPS in mice injected subsequently with bacterial lipopolysaccharide (LPS).

RESULTS

The data obtained using the models described above indicated that the response of the modified host-defense system is strongly dose-dependent, and that the response seems to be a characteristic of the systems involved and not of the stimulants used. When plotted, the data produced an irregular nonlinear curve that had two peaks of protection, thus forming a W-shaped curve. The protection peak that occurred at the low doses of stimulant was smaller than that produced by high doses of stimulant. The data shown in Fig. 1 were obtained using the ST-infection of vaccinated mice model and bacterial lipopolysaccharide as the stimulant. In Fig. 2 the data were obtained using the RSV-infected chicks model when the lipid Restim was the stimulant, while Fig. 3 was obtained using the same model with bacterial lipopolysaccharide as the stimulant. The endotoxin shock model was used to produce the data in Fig. 4 where the lipid Restim was the stimulant.

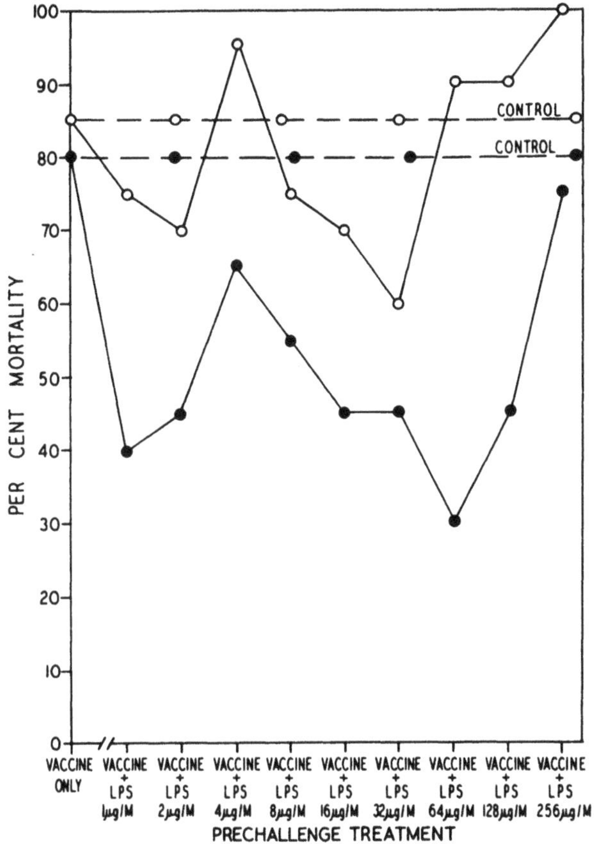

Fig. 6. Modification of the 20-day mortality by various doses of bacterial lipopolysaccharide (LPS) in mice vaccinated and subsequently infected with Salmonella typhimurium. The two curves represent two different experiments.

In Fig. 5, the endotoxin shock model was again used with bacterial lipopolysaccharide as the stimulant.

We conducted one group of experiments using glucan, and the W-shaped curve is again apparent. A second group of experiments involving an even larger number of animals is now in progress. The reproducibility of the W-shaped curve is shown in Fig. 6, where the model of Salmonella-vaccinated mice and lipopolysaccharide as a stimulant was used. The animals were infected with S. typhimurium. The two curves represent two different experiments done two months apart. Each point in both curves represents 20 animals. The similarity is obvious and is seen in all other systems used to date.

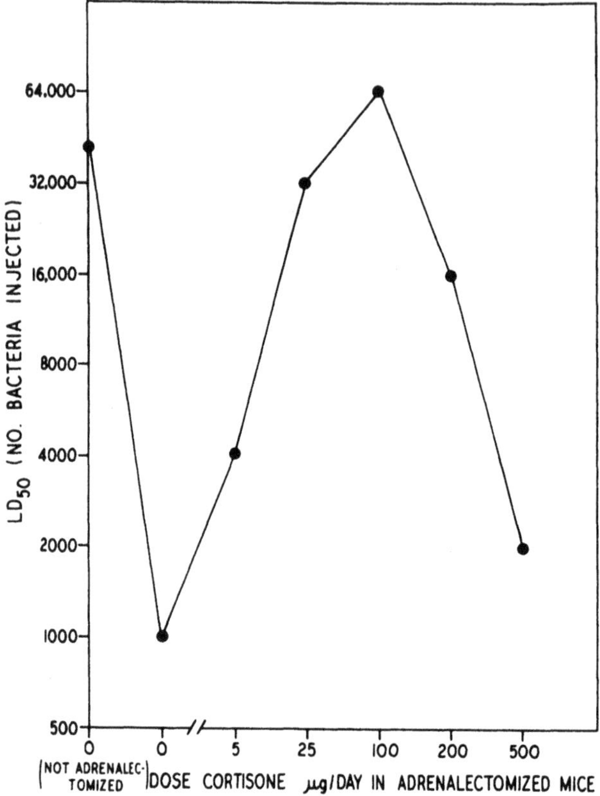

Fig. 7. Modification of LD_{50} by various doses of cortisone in adrenalectomized mice infected with pneumococci in the presence of specific antiserum. Based on data by Kass [21].

DISCUSSION

Data from other laboratories [9-23] indicate that investigators studying the experimental modification of the host-defense mechanism have apparently also observed different segments of the W-shaped dose-response relationship, but they have not adequately explored it in its entirety. This may explain the fact that different results have been obtained by some investigators, even when they have used the same stimulant.

We have used data from various authors' papers and put them in graphic form similar to the plots of our own data in order to demonstrate this point. For example, a paper by Kass [21] shows evidence of part of the W-shaped curve in a system where the LD_{50} from pneumococci is modified in adrenalectomized mice by different doses of cortisone in the presence of specific antiserum (Fig. 7).

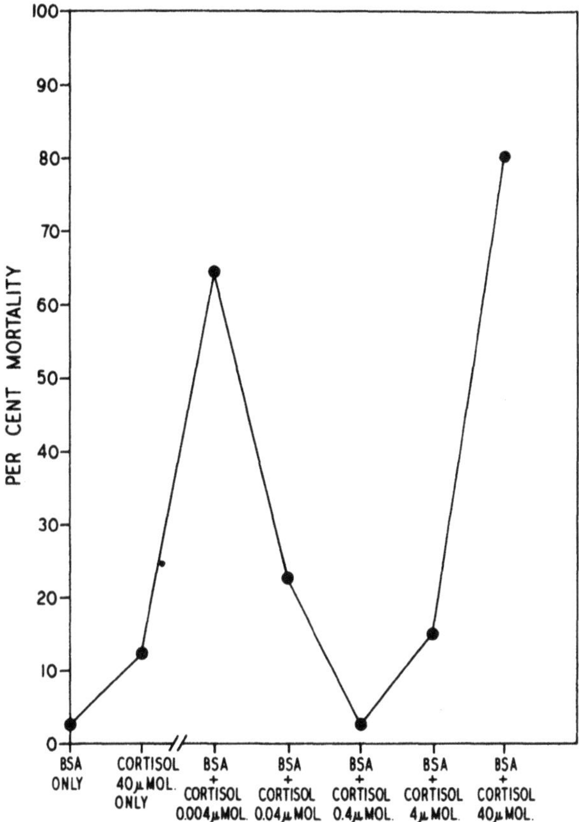

Fig. 8. Six-week mortality in mice injected at birth with various doses of cortisol mixed with bovine serum albumin (BSA). Based on data by Sorem et al. [22].

In another paper, by Sorem et al. [22], newborn mice were injected with a mixture of cortisol and bovine serum albumin. The amount of antigen was kept constant, but the amount of cortisol was varied. Figure 8 shows the mortality curve, which we believe is probably a portion of the W-shaped curve.

In a paper by Fox et al. [20], mice were infected with Salmonella enteritidis eight days after oral administration of an extract of Mycobacterium phlei. Figure 9 shows the W-shaped curve as a function of the dose of M. phlei.

A final example is included in some data from the paper of Landy et al. [23], where the level of bactericidal antibody titer in the secondary response is plotted as a function of a varying dose of antigen. The antigen used is the somatic antigen of S. enteritidis. These data were obtained in rabbits (Fig. 10).

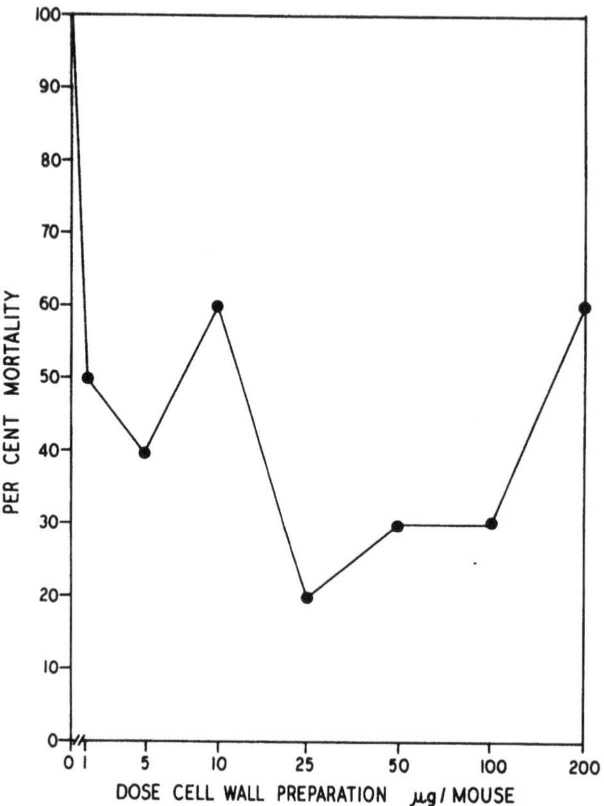

Fig. 9. Modification of the 10-day mortality by various doses of crude cell wall preparation from Mycobacterium phlei in mice infected with Salmonella enteritidis. Based on data by Fox et al. [20].

The characteristic dose dependency of the host's response suggested that it would appear logical to mathematically analyze portions of the dose-response curve and to derive a quantitative relationship which would indicate rate processes, and then attempt to fit biological events to the various segments of the curve. While such an attempt is a reasonable approach to use for a single-model system, it would appear to be of less value for multiple systems unless they all have a common mechanism. One might visualize that the first part of the curve represented some exponential process such as phagocytosis, while in the latter portions it represented a logarithmic curve such as one might expect to find in antibody synthesis. A W-shaped relationship curve appears when an experiment is designed so that it can be evaluated in 72 hr. An example is a lipopolysaccharide experiment where, after 72 hr, all the animals that will die are dead and those which are not will survive. However, essentially the same type of curve

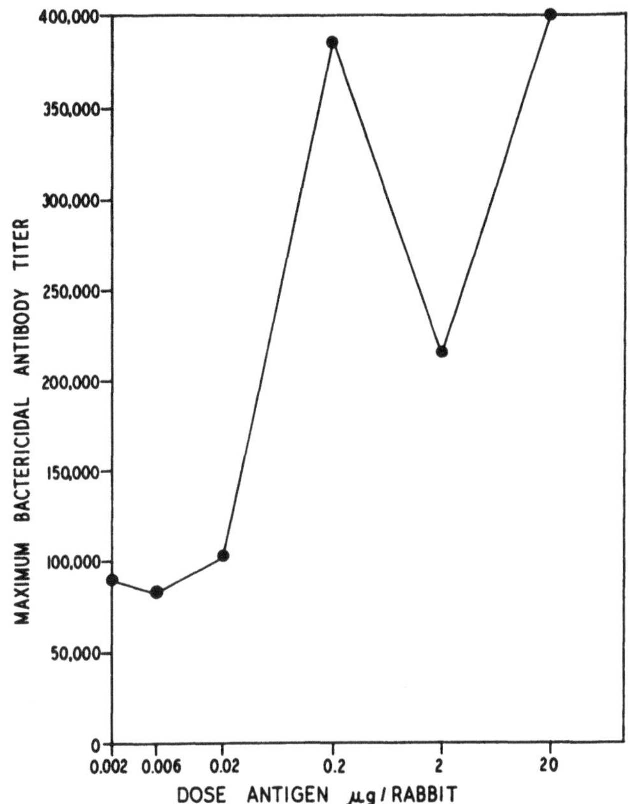

Fig. 10. Modification of the maximum secondary bactericidal antibody titer by various doses of somatic antigen of Salmonella enteritidis in rabbits. Based on data by Landy et al. [23].

appears in a model which extends over a 90-day period, such as the Rous sarcoma in chicks. It is difficult to believe that the same types of physiologic reactions are operating in a three-day period as operate over a 90-day period. Considerably more experimentation will have to be done before the causes of this dose-response relationship are at all clear. We feel that the best means to evaluate the dynamics of this process may be a detailed mathematical analysis of the data. It is clear, however, that the nature of the dose-response relationship is such that any hope of using a host-defense stimulant as a means of increasing the resistance to bacterial, viral, parasitic, or malignant disease must consider the critical narrow dose range that gives optimum results.

SUMMARY

Various single variables of host defense may be measured independently of others, but the total defense of the host is composed of a complex interconnected series of reactions. It is important, therefore, to study the overall effect of a substance having host defense modifying properties.

The results we have reported suggest that the response of the modified host-defense system is strongly dose-dependent and is characteristic of the system. If a wide range of doses is used, an irregular nonlinear curve is produced. The curve has two peaks of protection, forming a W-shaped curve, the peak occurring at lower doses being smaller than that occurring at higher doses.

The apparent characteristics of this relationship are such that multiple dose ranges must be used in further evaluation experiments in order to establish optimum doses for prophylactic or therapeutic use.

REFERENCES

1. J.P. Ransom, V.Z. Pasternak, and J.H. Heller, J.Bacteriol., 84:466-472, 1962.
2. J.P. Ransom, E. Bliznakov, V.Z. Pasternak, and J.H. Heller, Compt.Rend.Biol.(Paris), 156:1022, 1962.
3. J.H. Heller, J.P. Ransom, and V.Z. Pasternak, in: Rôle du système réticuloendothelial dans l'immunité antibactérienne et antitumorale, 1962. Paris, Colloques Internationaux du CNRS, 1963.
4. J.H. Heller, V.Z. Pasternak, J.P. Ransom, and M.S. Heller, Nature, 199:904-905, 1963.
5. J.H. Heller, E.G. Bliznakov, J.P. Ransom, D.J. Wilkins, and V.Z. Pasternak, in: The Reticuloendothelial System (Proc. IV Intern.Symp. on RES, Kyoto, 1964), 1965, pp. 375-388.
6. E.G. Bliznakov, J.Reticuloendothelial Soc., 1:360, 1964.
7. J.P. Ransom, E.G. Bliznakov, and L.S. Tuccio, Estratto Da III° Symposium Internazionale Sul Lisozima Di Fleming, Milano, 1964.
8. E.G. Bliznakov, submitted to Cancer Res., 1966.
9. J.B. Murphy, Monograph of the Rockefeller Institute, 21:1-168, 1926.
10. N. Kaliss, Cancer Res., 12:379-382, 1952.
11. A.G. Johnson, S. Gaines, and M. Landy, J.Exptl.Med., 103:225-246, 1956.
12. I.S. Johnson, L.A. Baker, and H.F. Wright, Ann.N.Y.Acad.Sci., 76:861-867, 1958.
13. J.L. Whitby, J.G. Michael, M.W. Woods, and M. Landy, Bacteriol. Rev., 25:437-446, 1961.
14. A.E. Stuart, in: Rôle du système réticuloendothelial dans l'immunité antibactérienne et antitumorale, 1962. Paris, Colloques Internationaux du CNRS, 1963, pp. 129-142.
15. G.N. Cooper, J.Reticuloendothelial Soc., 1:50-67, 1964.
16. A.E. Stuart and E. Davidson, J.Pathol.Bacteriol., 87:305-316, 1964.
17. J. Bubenik and P. Koldovsky, Folia Biol., 10:427-442, 1964.

18. D.S. Martin, P. Hayworth, R.A. Fugmann, R. English, and H.W. McNeill, Cancer Res., 24:652-654, 1964.
19. S.D. Chaparas and H. Baer, Proc.Soc.Exptl.Biol.Med., 120:260-262, 1965.
20. A.E. Fox, G.L. Evans, F.J. Turner, B.S. Schwartz, and A. Blaustein, J.Bacteriol., 92:1-5, 1966.
21. E.H. Kass, Ann.N.Y.Acad.Sci., 88:107-115, 1960.
22. G. Sorem and G. Terres, Nature, 209:1254-1255, 1966.
23. M. Landy, R.P. Sanderson, and A.L. Jackson, J.Exptl.Med., 122:483-504, 1965.

The Dissimilar Effects of Two RES Stimulants on Shock*

Gottfried Lemperle

New England Institute for Medical Research
Ridgefield, Connecticut

During the past decade, various agents have been found to stimulate some of the manifold functions of the RES. In animal experiments, an increased state of resistance to certain infections and transplantable tumors after the injection of these agents has often been demonstrated. On the other hand, host defense mechanisms may be adversely influenced by various diseases or injuries. There is evidence that at least some of the functions of the RES are significantly depressed during and after a period of severe traumatic shock. It seems logical that a rise in RES activity may prevent or equalize its depression. Paradoxically, most of the well-known stimulating agents such as BCG [1, 2], pertussis vaccine [3], zymosan [4, 5], triolein [6], and glucan (v. infra) render the animals increasingly susceptible to various forms of shock or endotoxin injections. Only pretreatment with endotoxin provides tolerance toward shock or otherwise lethal doses of endotoxin.

In opposition to the above-mentioned RES stimulants, restim, an "active" fraction of shark liver lipids [7], does not produce hyperplasia of the RES. It appears to exert its effect by alteration of the percentage of active RE cells and probably by increasing the functional state of the individual cells. It was therefore of considerable interest to us whether restim would produce similar effects on shock. Endotoxin injections in mice and severe burn trauma and postburn sepsis with gram-negative bacteria in rats have been used as shock models. In the reported experiments, the effect on shock mortality after pretreatment with restim or glucan, the polysaccharide fraction of zymosan [8], has been studied.

MATERIALS AND METHODS

The animals, a total of 524 male Swiss mice (Blue Spruce Farms, Altamont, New York) and 344 male CFN rats (Carworth Farms, New City, New

*This work was supported in part by grants from The John A. Hartford Foundation, Inc., The Fannie E. Rippel Foundation, and the Reynolds-Bagley-Verney Foundation.

York), were kept in rooms at 23°C and 50% humidity. Purina Lab Chow and water were allowed ad libitum.

Endotoxin Shock in mice was produced by intraperitoneal or intravenous injections of lipopolysaccharide S. typhosa 0.901 or E. coli 0.127:B8 (Difco Laboratories, Detroit, Michigan) in appropriate doses. The lipopolysaccharide was first suspended by boiling in pyrogen-free saline and then homogenized in a Virtis blender.

Standard Burns of 30% of the body surface were inflicted upon rats using a combination of the basket technique [9] and the plaster cast technique [10]. Five baskets were made for rats weighing 200, 225, 250, 275, and 300 g. Basket sizes accordingly were 30% of the surface area of the rats [11]. The anesthetized rats were placed in the appropriate baskets in an inverted position, and the shaved back was scalded for 10 sec in a waterbath kept at a constant temperature of 95°C. In this manner, full thickness, third-degree burns were produced.

Burn Infection. Pseudomonas aeruginosa could be cultivated from the feces of most rats. A pyocyanin-producing strain was isolated and a certain number of bacteria injected under the burned skin at different time intervals after the infliction of the burn.

RES Stimulation. Glucan (Fleischmann Laboratories, Stamford, Connecticut, Lot No. IF 5500) was suspended in pyrogen-free 5% glucose solution by boiling 1 hr and homogenizing in a Virtis blender. After centrifuging for 30 min at 4000 rpm, the supernatant was discarded and replaced by an equal volume of 5% glucose solution. Restim, a lipid fraction derived by column chromatography, was suspended in a 5% glucose solution by adding ninol (Stepan Chemical Company, Maywood, New Jersey) 5% by weight of lipid and treated for 1 min at 20,000 rpm in a Virtis homogenizer. The particle size in each suspension was found to be less than 2 μ. Colloidal carbon (No. C11/1431a, Günther-Wagner, Hanover, Germany), was used for

Table I. Modification of Endotoxin Lethality in Mice by RES Stimulation. Injection of Restim (5 mg/100 g) and Glucan (5 mg/100 g) Two Days Prior to Challenge

Pretreatment	LPS S. typhosa	Mortality	LD_{50} (mg)
Control	0.4 mg i.p.	0/20 = 0%	–
Restim	"	0/20 = 0%	–
Glucan	"	6/27 = 22%*	0.91
Control	0.75 mg i.p.	10/20 = 50%	0.75
Restim	"	6/20 = 30%	1.25
Glucan	"	17/20 = 85%*	0.44

*Significant at the 95% confidence level.

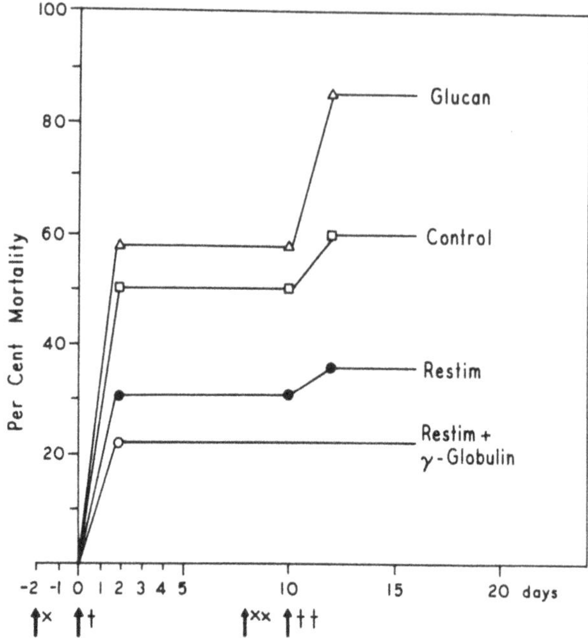

Fig. 1. Modification of endotoxin lethality by glucan and restim. × RES stimulation (restim 5 mg/100 g and glucan 5 mg/100 g). † Challenge with endotoxin (0.75 mg/mouse i.p.). ×× Second stimulating injections. †† Second challenge with 1.0 mg endotoxin. 20 mice/group.

Table II. The Effect of Restim in Combination with γ-Globulin (16.5 mg i. p. One Day Prior to Challenge or a Small Dose of Endotoxin (0.01 mg i. p. Ten Days Prior to Challenge) on Lethal Doses of Endotoxin

Pretreatment	LPS *E. coli*	Mortality	LD_{50} (mg)
Control	1.5 mg i.p.	17/17 = 100%	0.75
γ-Globulin	"	20/20 = 100%	0.75
Restim	"	16/20 = 80%	0.94
Restim + γ-globulin	"	15/20 = 75%*	1.00
Control	1.0 mg i.v.	20/20 = 100%	0.50
Restim	"	17/20 = 85%	0.60
Endotoxin 0.01 mg	"	15/20 = 75%*	0.75
Endotoxin + Restim	"	10/20 = 50%*	1.00

*Significant at the 95% confidence level.

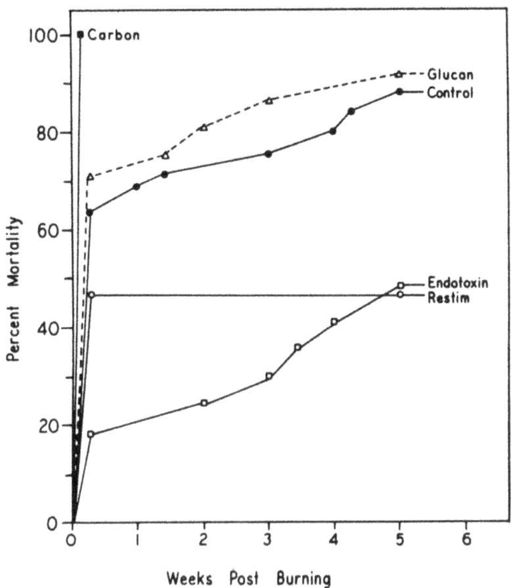

Fig. 2. Effect of RES stimulation on burn shock and postburn infection. Injections of restim (4 x 2 mg/100 g), glucan (4 x 2 mg/100 g), and endotoxin (4 x 0.1 mg/100 g) on alternate days before burning. 30 mg per 100 g of colloidal carbon injected 2 hr prior to burning (20 rats per group).

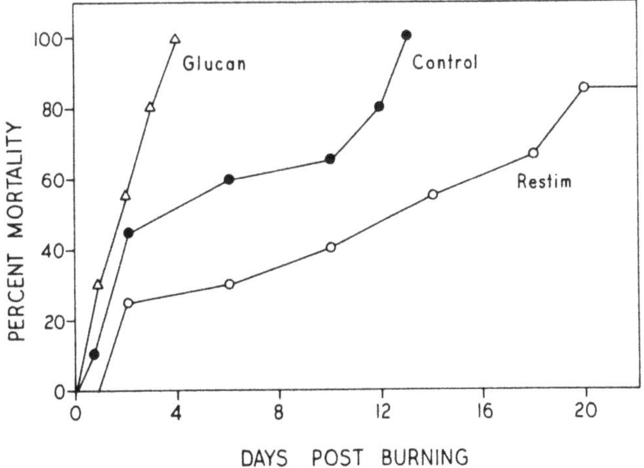

Fig. 3. Postburn mortality after infection with $1 \cdot 10^3$ P. aeruginosa s. c. immediately following burning. Injections of restim (5 mg/100 g) and glucan (10 mg/100 g) three days prior. Shock protection with saline i.p. equal to 10% of the body weight. 20 rats/group.

evaluation of the phagocytic function [4] and for partial RES blockade. Control animals were injected with equal amounts of the 5% glucose solution.

Anesthesia. The rats had to be slightly anesthetized with ether for injections into the femoral vein. Before burning, each untreated animal was given a dose of sodium pentobarbital (3.5 mg/100 g body weight). This dose, however, was an LD_{25} for glucan-stimulated rats, so that for this group a dose of 2.5 mg/100 g had to be used. Restim-stimulated rats generally needed a dose of 5.0 mg/100 g. This is an important finding in view of the detoxification of sodium pentobarbital after RES stimulation [12, 13].

RESULTS

(1) Endotoxin Shock in Mice. All animals were in obvious shock for 24-48 hr after the injection of an LD_{50} dose of endotoxin. Most deaths occurred in the control groups within 12-24 hr, in the glucan-treated groups within 6-24 hr, and in the restim-treated groups within 12-36 hr after challenge with endotoxin (Table I). After 10 days, the survivors of one experiment were given the same pretreatment and challenged with 1.0 mg LPS *S. typhosa* (Fig. 1). They showed the anticipated lower mortality, but again with the same relation to pretreatment. A third challenge with 1.5 mg endotoxin had no lethal effect. The LD_{50} for intraperitoneal injection of LPS *S. typhosa* into Swiss mice weighing 30 g was calculated from the data of five experiments, which significantly summarize the difference between these two RES stimulants (Table III).

Since it is now well established [14] that endotoxin administration evokes specific antibodies, and that restim increases existing antibody levels [15], a small amount of endotoxin (0.01 mg/mouse) was injected intravenously 10 days prior to challenge with an LD_{100} (Table II). From the experimental design, it cannot be concluded that the protective effect of restim toward endotoxin injection is mainly of an immunologic nature.

(2) Burn Shock in Rats. The most striking results of the four experiments were the opposing effects of the two RES stimulants – glucan and restim – on shock mortality and postburn infection (Fig. 2). The glucan-treated groups generally showed an earlier and higher mortality than the controls, whereas restim pretreatment always provided a certain protective effect on shock. Small doses of endotoxin induced the anticipated tolerance to burn shock, whereas carbon injections 2 hr before the burn procedure resulted in 100% mortality.

(3) P. aeruginosa Infection. Since late deaths in human burn patients are increasingly due to *P. aeruginosa* septicemia, burned rats were infected artificially with this gram-negative organism at different intervals. Constant differences in their effect on burn infection are shown, whether glucan and restim were given prior to (Fig. 3) or after the burn injury (Fig. 4).

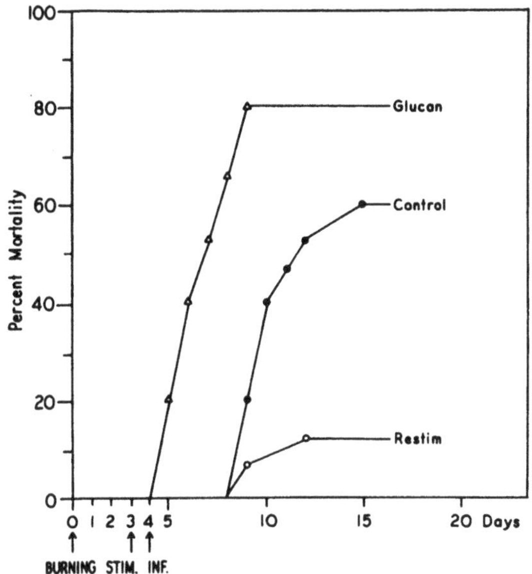

Fig. 4. Postburn mortality after infection with 1 · 10^2 P. aeruginosa s.c. on day 4 (INF). Injections of restim (5 mg/100 g) and glucan (10 mg/100 g) on day 3 (STIM). 20 rats /group.

DISCUSSION

Death from endotoxin injections, burn shock, and gram-negative infection is considered to be the result of toxemia in all cases. Hence, the mortality data in all reported experiments can be discussed from similar points of view, disregarding whether "burn toxin" [16] or endotoxin [17] play the major role in burn shock. Furthermore, it may be assumed that these probably different toxins are detoxified by similar intracellular mechanisms.

Table III. Average LD_{50} of i. p.-Injected Endotoxin from S. typhosa in 30-g Swiss Mice after Pretreatment with 5% Glucose (0.2 ml), Glucan (5 mg/ 100 g), or Restim (5 mg/ 100 g) Two Days Prior to Challenge (Total of 90 Animals per Group)

Summary of 6 experiments	LD_{50} of LPS S. typhosa i. p.
Controls	0.85 ± 0.04 mg
Glucan, 1.0 mg i. v.	0.64 ± 0.14 mg*
Restim, 1.0 mg i. v.	1.45 ± 0.16 mg*

*Significant at the 95% confidence level.

A prerequisite for a sufficient detoxification is a well-functioning RES. Ninety percent of the RE cells, the Kupffer cells, are located in the liver, and this organ is especially sensitive to a decreased blood flow such as occurs in shock. The manifold functions of both RE cells and parenchymal cells are depressed for a few days but soon recover in surviving animals [10, 18]. On the other hand, paralyzed phagocytic function, decreased antibody production, and the inability to detoxify endotoxin may be the cause of death in shock. The RE cells may be damaged (1) directly by endotoxin, which can alter the lysosomes into autophagic vacuoles [19], or (2) indirectly by the alteration of several neural endocrine and vascular mechanisms, which lead to tissue hypoxia and consequent changes in the permeability of the lysosomal membranes.

In an attempt to explain the different findings after restim and glucan injections, one has to consider all known differences between the two RE stimulants. Both increase phagocytic activity of the RES to a similar extent, and both have an enhancing effect on antibody production. Glucan, however, stimulates the RES by inducing hyperplasia, whereas restim causes no proliferation of the RE cells. Since little or nothing is known about a possible interference of RES stimulants with the ratio of blood lipids, blood clotting factors, catecholamines, glycogen metabolism, or corticosteroids, factors which all can play a decisive role in the outcome of shock, our considerations have to be confined to the cellular level. Recent investigations on the mechanisms of endotoxin action and of RES stimulation [2] suggest that both effects can be related to changes in the permeability of the lysosomal membranes of the RE cells. The point has been made [20] that tolerance to endotoxin is due to an increased stability of lysosomal membranes. Although the mechanism of endotoxin-detoxification has not yet been discovered, it appears that it does not involve hydrolytic splitting of the endotoxin molecule by lysosomal enzymes. It may be an oxidation of certain linkages [21] which would occur at other sites and other structures of the cell, instead of on the lysosomes. In any case, increased cellular injury can be expected when membrane disruptive agents such as endotoxin or "burn toxin" are phagocytosed by cells with labilized lysosomal membranes.

The gradual failure of the endotoxin-detoxifying mechanisms of the RE cells during the progression of endotoxin shock can be related to a release of their lysosomal contents. Lentz et al. [22] showed recently that the release of lysosomal enzymes during hemorrhagic shock was almost twice as much in glucan-pretreated rats as in the controls, in contrast to a 62% lower release after zymosan pretreatment, which had a shock-protective effect. In view of the latter, it has been suggested [23] that the lipid fraction of zymosan may be involved in the development of shock protection. Peritoneal macrophages showed no increased lysozyme content after intraperitoneal injection of restim [24], whereas intraperitoneal injection of BCG [25] was followed by a significant increase in intracellular acid phosphatase, β-glucuronidase, and cathepsin. If an increase in lysosomal hydrolases is the consequence of all hyperplasia-inducing stimulants, it is sufficient explanation for the increased susceptibility toward endotoxin and shock.

The decreased resistance toward endotoxin and shock in glucan-treated animals could also be due to an indirect action on lysosomes by interference with the level of adrenal hormones or glycogen storage in the liver. Cortisone probably stabilizes lysosomal membranes [20], counteracts loss of liver glycogen [26], and abolishes increased susceptibility to endotoxin after administration of zymosan [4]. Glucan injections cause increased conjugation of corticosteroids in the liver [27] and probably, like zymosan [12] and other stimulants [28], depletes liver glycogen. In case of shock or endotoxemia, this would mean that the increased need for corticosteroids cannot be satisfied or that the detoxifying mechanisms in the liver are already impaired.

Whether the protective action of restim on shock is due to an improvement in detoxification, an increase in antibody to endotoxin, or to a stabilization of the lysosomal membranes, has yet to be shown. It appears, however, from our present knowledge of restim, that its effect on endotoxin and shock is due to an increase in antibody in the presence of unaltered lysosomes.

SUMMARY

The effectiveness of the RES stimulants, glucan and restim, on endotoxin, burn, and septic shock in mice and rats was evaluated. Pretreatment with glucan, which causes a marked hyperplasia of the RES, increased susceptibility to endotoxin and shock significantly. Pretreatment with restim was always followed by a decreased mortality from shock. Restim appears to exert its stimulating effect by increasing the percentage of active cells or the capabilities of the individual RE cell, or both.

Since the mechanisms of both endotoxin action and RES stimulation can be related to changes in the permeability of the lysosomal membranes of the RE cells, it is suggested that the contrasting findings after glucan and restim stimulation are due to differences in the lysosomes within the stimulated RE cells.

REFERENCES

1. E. Suter, E.G. Ullmann, and R.G. Hoffman, "Sensitivity of mice to endotoxin after vaccination with BCG," Proc. Soc. Exptl. Biol. Med., 99:167, 1958.
2. K. Saito and E. Suter, "Lysosomal acid hydrolases and hyperreactivity to endotoxin in mice infected with BCG," J. Exptl. Med., 121:739, 1965.

3. S. Rutenberg and G. Michael, "Endotoxin-detoxifying capacity of RES in normal and pertussis-treated mice," Proc. Soc. Exptl. Biol. Med., 117:301, 1964.
4. B. Benacerraf, G.J. Thorbecke, and D. Jacoby, "Effect of zymosan on endotoxin toxicity in mice," Proc. Soc. Exptl. Biol. Med., 100 : 796, 1959.
5. H.H. Freedman and B.M. Sultzer, "Modification of lethality of endotoxin in mice by zymosan," Proc. Soc. Exptl. Biol. Med., 106 : 495, 1961.
6. A.E. Stuart and G.N. Cooper, "Susceptibility of mice to bacterial endotoxin after modification of RE function by simple lipids," J. Pathol. Bacteriol., 83: 245, 1962.
7. J.H. Heller, V.Z. Pasternak, J.P. Ransom, and M.S. Heller, "A new RES stimulating agent (restim) from shark livers," Nature, 199 : 904, 1963.
8. S.J. Riggi and N.R. DiLuzio, "Identification of a RE-stimulating agent in zymosan," Am. J. Physiol., 200 : 297, 1961.
9. S.R. Rosenthal, "Basket technique for producing standard thermal injuries in mice," J. Trauma, 1: 560, 1961.
10. G. Arturson, "The infliction and healing of a large standard burn in rats," Acta Path. Microbiol. Scand., 61:353, 1964.
11. M.O. Lee, "Determination of the surface area of the white rat with its application to the expression of metabolic results," Am. J. Physiol., 89:24, 1929.
12. W.R. Wooles and J.F. Borzelleca, "Prolongation of barbiturate sleeping time in mice by stimulation of the RES," J. Reticuloendothelial Soc., 1:354, 1964.
13. F.J. DiCarlo, L.J. Haynes, C.B. Coutinho, and G.E. Phillips, "Pentobarbital sleeping time and RES stimulation," J. Reticuloendothelial Soc., 2 : 367, 1965.
14. Y.B. Kim and D.W. Watson, "Modification of host responses to bacterial endotoxins. II. Passive transfer of immunity to bacterial endotoxin with fractions containing 19S-antibodies," J. Exptl. Med., 121: 751, 1965.
15. J.H. Heller, J.P. Ransom, and V.Z. Pasternak, "New advances in the stimulation of the RES," Colloq. Intern. Center Natl. Rech. Sci., 115: 89, 1963.
16. S.R. Rosenthal, "Pharmacologically active and lethal substances from skin," Arch. Environ. Health, 11:465, 1965.
17. J. Fine, "Current status of the problem of traumatic shock," Surg. Gynecol. Obstet., 120 : 537, 1965.
18. L.D. Hanback and M.S. Rittenbury, "Response of the RES in thermal injury," Surg. Forum, 16 : 47, 1965.
19. G. Weissmann and L. Thomas, "On a mechanism of tissue damage by bacterial endotoxins," in: Bacterial Endotoxins, New Brunswick, New Jersey, Rutgers University Press, 1964, p. 602.

20. A. Janoff, G. Weissmann, B.W. Zweifach, and L. Thomas, "Pathogenesis of experimental shock. IV. Studies on lysosomes in normal and tolerant animals subjected to lethal trauma and endotoxemia," J.Exptl.Med., 116 : 457, 1962.
21. W.E. Farrar, "Endotoxin detoxification by guinea pig tissue homogenates and possible significance of this reaction in vivo," Proc.Soc. Exptl.Biol.Med., 118 : 218, 1965.
22. P.E. Lentz, J.M. Lipo, and W.J. Stekiel, "Effect of hemorrhagic shock on rat plasma lysosomal hydrolase activity," Federation Proc., 24 : 587, 1965.
23. J.P. Filkins, J.M. Lubitz, and J.J. Smith, "The effect of zymosan and glucan on the RES and resistance to traumatic shock," Angiology, 15 : 465, 1964.
24. J.P. Ransom, E.G. Bliznakov, and L.S. Tuccio, "The role of lysozyme in resistance of mice to infections with gram-negative bacilli," in: Estratto da 3° Symposium Internazionale sul Lisozima di Fleming. Milan, Italy, Cesano Boscone, 1964, p. 1.
25. K. Saito and E. Suter, "Lysosomal acid hydrolases in mice infected with BCG," J.Exptl.Med., 121 : 727, 1965.
26. T. Fukuda, M. Okada, and T. Kobayashi, "On the mechanism of protection of endotoxin shock by glucocorticoids," Jap.J.Physiol., 14 : 560, 1964.
27. C.J. Nabors, D.L. Berliner, and T.F. Dougherty, "RE cell stimulation and steroid metabolism," J.Reticuloendothelial Soc., 1 : 353, 1964.
28. F.J. DiCarlo, B. Dubnick, J.M. Apgar, L.J. Haynes, N.J. Silver, and G.E. Phillips, "Effect of RES stimulants upon liver glycogen levels in mice," J.Reticuloendothelial Soc., 1 : 150, 1964.

Comparative Effect of Endotoxin and Reticuloendothelial "Blocking" Colloids on Selected Inducible Liver Enzymes*

L. Joe Berry, Manjul K. Agarwal,
and Irvin S. Snyder†

Department of Biology
Bryn Mawr College
Bryn Mawr, Pennsylvania

ABSTRACT. The LD_{50} of endotoxin lowers the activity of the hormonally inducible mouse liver enzyme tryptophan pyrrolase to less than one-half the control value and keeps it at a depressed level for about 24 hr. Endotoxin, by contrast, increases the activity of a similarly inducible liver enzyme, tyrosine-α-ketoglutarate transaminase. Endotoxin also prevents the induction of tryptophan pyrrolase by cortisone but does not prevent the induction of the transaminase. Either zymosan or glucan exerts an effect similar to endotoxin on both enzymes, except that the colloids do not prevent induction by cortisone. Both enzymes in mice made tolerant to endotoxin are less subject to change by endotoxin or zymosan than in normal mice. In animals given a series of injections of zymosan or saccharated iron oxide this does not occur.

INTRODUCTION

Since the classical work of Selye [1], the adrenal cortex has been recognized as essential in an animal's normal response to stress. In more recent years, the adrenal steroid hormones (hydrocortisone, cortisone, etc.)

* This work was supported by grants from the Department of Infectious Diseases, Smith Kline and French Laboratories, the National Science Foundation, and the Institute of Allergy and Infectious Diseases, National Institutes of Health.

† Recipient of the Faculty Research Professorship, 1966, University of Iowa College of Medicine. Present address: Department of Microbiology, University of Iowa College of Medicine, Iowa City, Iowa.

have been found to act as potent inducers of certain liver enzymes, especially tryptophan pyrrolase [2, 3, 4], tyrosine-α-ketoglutarate transaminase [5, 6], as well as others [7, 8, 9], possibly as a result of new synthesis of messenger RNA [10, 11, 12]. If one makes the obvious assumption that augmented levels of enzyme activity are important in maintaining homeostasis under conditions of stress, then procedures that sensitize to stress or protect against it might be found to alter the inducibility of key enzymes.

One way in which an animal's response to stress is subject to modification is through changes in function of the reticuloendothelial system (RES). Susceptibility to drum shock [13, 14], to hemorrhage and trauma [15], and to endotoxin [16, 17] is increased by "blockade" of the RES. Tolerance of acquired resistance to these stresses is reduced or reversed by blocking the RES [16, 18]. The question now to be explored is the extent to which RE blocking colloids influence the liver enzymes induced by adrenocorticoids in comparison with some of the established effects of endotoxin [18, 19, 20].

MATERIALS AND METHODS

Female Swiss-Webster albino mice were used when they weighed 22 ± 2 g. Weekly shipments from the breeder (Dierolf Farms, Boyertown, Pennsylvania) were received and they were housed in stainless steel cages with white pine shavings as bedding. Food and water were available ad libitum unless otherwise specified.

Tryptophan pyrrolase was assayed according to the method of Knox and Auerbach [2] as previously described [19]. Tyrosine-α-ketoglutarate transaminase was determined by the procedure of Rosen and Milholland [21].

Several RES blocking agents, saccharated iron oxide (Proferrin), zymosan, and glucan were used. Each was administered intravenously into a tail vein, and when a suspending agent had to be employed, nonpyrogenic isotonic sodium chloride solution (Baxter Laboratories, Morton Grove, Illinois) was used.

Carbon clearance was determined according to Benacerraf et al. [22] as a measure of RES activity.

A suspension of heat-killed Salmonella typhimurium, strain SR-11, prepared as previously described [19], served as endotoxin. This material yields values at the LD_{50} level similar to those derived with purified lipopolysaccharide. Injections were administered intraperitoneally in a volume of 0.5 ml.

RESULTS

An injection of the LD_{50} of endotoxin is followed by a decrease in tryptophan pyrrolase and by an increase in tyrosine-α-ketoglutarate transaminase.

Table I. Changes in Inducible Liver Enzymes with Time after an Injection of Either the LD_{50} of Endotoxin or 5 mg Cortisone Acetate

Each Value is the Mean Plus or Minus the Standard Error of the Mean for the Number of Determinations Shown in Parentheses

Time after injection, hr	Tryptophan pyrrolase activity* after		Tyrosine transaminase activity† after	
	LD_{50} endotoxin	5 mg cortisone	LD_{50} endotoxin	5 mg cortisone
0 - Control	18.8 ± 1.3 (15)	–	14.0 ± 1.1 (32)	–
6	7.6 ± 1.5 (6)	53.7 ± 3.5 (6)	28.9 ± 2.3 (12)	41.4 ± 3.1 (17)
17	7.3 ± 1.2 (7)	50.9 ± 3.8 (6)	45.5 ± 3.6 (9)	48.5 ± 3.4 (6)

*Expressed as μM kynurenine/g dry wt. liver/hr.
†Expressed as μg p-hydroxyphenylpyruvic acid/mg dry wt. liver/10 min.

Table II. Changes in Inducible Liver Enzymes with Time after a Concurrent Injection of the LD_{50} of Endotoxin and 5 mg Cortisone Acetate

Each Value is the Mean Plus or Minus the Standard Error of the Mean for the Number of Determinations Shown in Parentheses

Time after injection, hr	Enzyme activity after concurrent injection of endotoxin and cortisone	
	Tryptophan pyrrolase*	Tyrosine transaminase†
0 - Control	18.8 ± 1.3 (15)	14.0 ± 1.1 (32)
6	10.0 ± 0.7 (6)	45.7 ± 2.9 (11)
17	16.1 ± 3.8 (5)	41.1 ± 3.0 (8)

*Expressed as μM kynurenine/g dry wt. liver/hr.
†Expressed as μg p-hydroxyphenylpyruvic acid/mg dry wt. liver/10 min.

These observations are summarized in the data presented in Table I, columns 2 and 4, respectively. The changes at 6 hr are approximately the same as those at 17 hr. The rise that occurs in the transaminase is not seen in adrenalectomized mice [20]. The subcutaneous administration of 5 mg cortisone acetate is followed by similar increases in both of the enzymes. These results are given in columns 3 and 5 of Table I.

The reason why endotoxin has opposite effects on the two enzymes is not understood, but the basis for the rise in tyrosine transaminase is believed to be due to the release of endogenous corticoid.

The effect of concurrent injection of the LD_{50} of endotoxin and of 5 mg cortisone acetate on liver tryptophan pyrrolase and tyrosine transaminase is shown in the results presented in Table II. Note that endotoxin not only prevents the induction of tryptophan pyrrolase but actually lowers its activity at 6 hr. At 17 hr, however, activity is back to normal. Not shown by data in the table is the complete lack of induction of tryptophan pyrrolase when cortisone is given 4 hr after endotoxin [20]. Under these conditions, the activity of the enzyme is not significantly different at 6 and 17 hr from the values shown in Table I for endotoxin alone. With tyrosine transaminase, endotoxin has little influence on hormonal induction. This becomes especially obvious when the data of Table II are compared with those of the same enzyme in Table I.

When either zymosan or glucan are injected intravenously at a dose level of 2 mg, subsequent administration of an amount of endotoxin that kills 20% of control mice kills 90% to 95% of animals given the RES blocking agents. At this dose level, there is a decrease in tryptophan pyrrolase, as shown by the results summarized in Table III. There is no outstanding difference in the effect on the enzyme of these colloids and that of endotoxin (cf. Table I).

Tyrosine transaminase is seen to increase in activity 6 hr after administration of the colloids, as the data of Table III show. The change after zymosan is similar in magnitude to that resulting from endotoxin (Table I),

Table III. Change in Inducible Liver Enzymes with Time after an Injection of Either Zymosan or Glucan at a Dose Level (2 mg) Known to Sensitize to Endotoxin

Each Value is the Mean Plus or Minus the Standard Error for the Number of Determinations Shown in Parentheses

Time after injection, hr	Tryptophan pyrrolase activity* after		Tyrosine transaminase activity† after	
	Zymosan	Glucan	Zymosan	Glucan
0 - Control	22.3 ± 1.8 (14)	–	8.7 ± 0.4 (10)	–
6	5.3 ± 0.7 (7)	7.5 ± 0.6 (7)	39.1 ± 2.0 (9)	17.1 ± 2.3 (10)
17	12.2 ± 1.8 (7)	16.5 ± 2.4 (7)	19.0 ± 2.6 (9)	17.3 ± 2.3 (7)

* Expressed as μM kynurenine/g dry wt. liver/hr.

† Expressed as μg p-hydroxyphenylpyruvic acid/mg dry wt. liver/10 min.

Table IV. Change in Inducible Liver Enzymes when Cortisone (5 mg, subcut.) Is Given 4 hr after Either Zymosan or Glucan (2 mg, i.v.)

Each Value is the Mean Plus or Minus the Standard Error for the Number of Determinations Shown in Parentheses

Time after injection of colloid, hr	Enzyme activity when cortisone is given 4 hr after the colloid			
	Tryptophan pyrrolase* in mice given		Tyrosine transaminase† in mice given	
	Zymosan	Glucan	Zymosan	Glucan
0 - Control	20.0 ± 1.8 (11)	–	8.7 ± 0.4 (10)	–
6	7.4 ± 0.2 (7)	14.1 ± 3.0 (7)	40.9 ± 1.7 (7)	45.6 ± 2.7 (7)
17	31.7 ± 2.8 (7)	60.5 ± 4.3 (7)	35.3 ± 2.5 (7)	30.3 ± 1.2 (7)

* Expressed as μM kynurenine/g dry wt. liver/hr.

† Expressed as μg p-hydroxyphenylpyruvic acid/mg dry wt. liver/10 min.

Table V. Tryptophan Pyrrolase Activity Following Treatments Indicated in Normal Mice, Endotoxin-Tolerant Mice, and in Micé with the RES Activated by Five Daily Injections of 0.8 mg Saccharated Iron Oxide

Each Value is the Mean Plus or Minus the Standard Error of the Mean for the Number of Determinations Shown in Parentheses

Experimental treatment	Tryptophan pyrrolase activity* in		
	Control mice	Endotoxin-tolerant mice	Mice with RES activated by colloid
No treatment	25.1 ± 1.7 (15)	26.5 ± 1.4 (16)	19.4 ± 2.0 (12)
17 hr after LD_{50} endotoxin	5.8 ± 0.9 (10)	19.4 ± 1.2 (10)	5.0 ± 1.4† (13)
6 hr after 4 mg (i.v.) saccharated iron oxide	14.8 ± 1.3 (10)	27.4 ± 2.0 (10)	5.5 ± 2.0 (8)
6 hr after 4 mg (i.v.) saccharated iron oxide and 4 hr after 0.1 LD_{50} endotoxin (i.p.)	9.2 ± 0.6 (12)	15.2 ± 2.2 (12)	–

* Expressed as μM kynurenine/g dry wt. liver/hr.

† Only 1/8 LD_{50} of endotoxin injected in this group.

Table VI. Tyrosine-α-Ketoglutarate Transaminase Activity in Normal Mice, Endotoxin-Tolerant Mice, and in Mice with the RES Activated by Three Injections, on Alternate Days, of 1 mg Zymosan Following Treatment Indicated

Each Value is the Mean Plus or Minus the Standard Error of the Mean for the Number of Determinations Shown in Parentheses

Experimental treatment	Tyrosine transaminase activity* in		
	Control mice	Endotoxin-tolerant mice	Mice with RES activated by colloid
No treatment	12.0 ± 3.5 (10)	11.8 ± 2.0 (12)	14.1 ± 2.0 (18)
6 hr after LD_{50} endotoxin	48.6 ± 1.9 (10)	51.8 ± 2.7 (10)	29.6 ± 2.1† (12)
16 hr after LD_{50} endotoxin	55.6 ± 3.2 (10)	26.7 ± 2.2 (10)	65.0 ± 2.7 (10)

*Expressed as μg p-hydroxyphenylpyruvic acid/mg dry wt. liver/10 min.
† 4-hr value.

but it is less after glucan. The reason for this difference between the effect of zymosan and glucan is not known. The control value for the transaminase is less in Table III than in Tables I and II. This may be related to the time of day when animals were sacrificed. Fed mice have lower values than fasted animals, probably because of the role played by the release of endogenous corticoids in response to the stress of fasting.

Since an injection of endotoxin 4 hr prior to cortisone prevents hormonal induction of tryptophan pyrrolase (see above), under similar conditions the effect of zymosan and glucan was determined. The data are summarized in Table IV. Six hours after the colloid, and 2 hr after cortisone, tryptophan pyrrolase is below the control level of activity. Tyrosine transaminase, on the other hand, is fully induced. At 17 hr, 13 hr after cortisone, tryptophan pyrrolase activity is significantly elevated, especially when glucan was the colloid. The transaminase at this time was lower than at 6 hr. It is apparent, therefore, that the action of either zymosan or glucan is different from that of endotoxin in failing to prevent hormonal induction of tryptophan pyrrolase.

Mice made tolerant to bacterial endotoxin (by an injection on successive days with the following doses: 0.02, 0.02, 0.04, 0.04, 0.08, 0.08 LD_{50}) are more resistant to the lethal and other effects of endotoxin and show at the same time an activated RES. It was thus considered relevant to compare the behavior of the inducible liver enzymes in such animals along with those whose RES had been activated by a series of injections of colloid. The results with tryptophan pyrrolase are shown in Table V. It is apparent that 17 hr after the injection of the LD_{50} of endotoxin the enzyme is higher in tolerant mice than in the other two groups. The RES was more active, as judged by the "k" value for carbon clearance, in both mice treated with saccharated iron oxide (0.8 mg injected intravenously each day for five days) (k = 0.078), and in the endotoxin-tolerant group (k = 0.065), than in the controls (k = 0.044). Sequestration of endotoxin by phagocytic cells is not, therefore, an obvious explanation for these results. The greater activity of the enzyme under these conditions should not be attributed to the fact that endotoxin was employed for producing the activated RES. An injection of saccharated iron oxide also fails to lower tryptophan pyrrolase in tolerant mice but not in the other two groups. This can be seen also in Table V. There is something unique about tolerance not shared by mice given saccharated iron oxide (or zymosan or glucan, which yield similar results). Note, however, that an injection of saccharated iron oxide followed 2 hr later by the administration of 0.1 LD_{50} endotoxin results in a greater decrease in tryptophan pyrrolase activity in control and in tolerant animals than when either is given alone. Under these conditions, tolerance is broken and the enzyme is depressed.

The behavior of tyrosine-α-ketoglutarate transaminase in similar groups of animals is summarized in Table VI. The RES was activated in this series of experiments by the total of three intravenous injections of 1.0 mg zymosan contained in 0.2 ml, each on alternate days, rather than with saccharated iron oxide. (The specific type of colloid does not appear to exert significant influence on the nature of the results, as evidenced by unpublished observations.) In control mice, the LD_{50} of endotoxin elevates the transaminase and maintains it at a higher level for at least 16-17 hr. This may be seen in the second column of Table VI and the third column of Table II. In endotoxin-tolerant mice, the increase in this enzyme is not significantly different from that of controls at 6 hr, but at 16 hr postinjection it is only about one-half as active. If induction is the result of an endogenous release of adrenal steroids in response to the endotoxin, then the tolerant animal responds for a shorter period of time. This suggests that the endotoxin exerts less stress in these mice.

DISCUSSION

The foregoing results have shown that endotoxin, which is a colloid, and the commonly used RES blocking agents, saccharated iron oxide, zymosan, and glucan, all lower the activity of the inducible liver enzyme tryptophan pyrrolase following a single injection. The same materials increase the activity in intact mice of another inducible liver enzyme, tryosine-α-ketoglutarate transaminase. It is unlikely that these large particles exert their effect directly on the liver parenchymal cells, where the enzymes are believed to be located. Indeed, neither endotoxin nor zymosan alters the activity of either enzyme when added directly to the liver homogenate prior to the assay [20, 23]. This suggests that the action of the materials tested is mediated and the most obvious target cells are those that respond specifically to colloidal particles — the Kupffer cells of the liver and the other phagocytic cells of the RES. These are the cells known to ingest not only endotoxin but other colloids as well [24-26].

The initial effect of an injection of blocking colloid or of endotoxin cannot be distinguished on the basis of the reaction of the two inducible liver enzymes. The result is to lower tryptophan pyrrolase, to increase tyrosine transaminase, and to activate the RES (increase carbon clearance). There are differences, however, by means of which the action of endotoxin on these enzymes can be distinguished from those of the colloids. A series of injections of endotoxin results in the development of tolerance. Tryptophan pyrrolase is not lowered as much by an injection of the LD_{50} of endotoxin in tolerant mice compared to that in controls, while tyrosine transaminase is induced strongly in tolerant animals but for a shorter period of time than in normal mice. A series of injections of any one of several colloids makes the animals, by contrast, hyperreactive to endotoxin and depresses tryptophan pyrrolase in the liver.

Another important difference is the ability of endotoxin to prevent the cortisone induction of tryptophan pyrrolase, even when the two are given concurrently, but especially when the cortisone is administered 2 to 4 hr later. The transaminase responds normally. An injection of zymosan (or glucan) does not prevent the hormonal induction of tryptophan pyrrolase. Perhaps one might relate these effects to the dose of colloid used in relation to its toxicity, but even large doses of saccharated iron oxide capable of killing mice fail to prevent the induction of tryptophan pyrrolase by cortisone.

While a mediator of these effects must be sought, problems in identifying it can be foreseen. One must be aware of the possibility that mediation of endotoxin is different from mediation by a colloid, since the consequences are readily separable. Nevertheless, there are ample reasons from the work with endogenous pyrogens [27], with the link between endotoxin and interferon [28], and with endotoxin and its role as an "adjuvant" in the immune response [29] to accept as a tenable working hypothesis the concept of mediator in the metabolic response to endotoxin. Such a substance should become evident when properly sought experimentally.

The need for enzyme induction in an animal's response to stress is implied by the observations described in this report. Tryptophan pyrrolase is lowered by endotoxin but to a lesser extent in tolerant mice. RES "blocking" agents that sensitize to stress (endotoxin included) lower the enzyme and also permit it to be lowered in tolerant animals. The rapid and strong induction of tyrosine transaminase under the same conditions suggests that it is responding normally and hence is not to be implicated, at least on the basis of present data. How other inducible enzymes react to agents sensitizing to stress or to stress-inducing substances such as endotoxin remains for future work to elucidate.

REFERENCES

1. H. Selye, Stress, Montreal Acta, 1951.
2. W.E. Knox and V.H. Auerbach, J.Biol.Chem., 214:307, 1955.
3. P. Feigelson and O. Greengard, J.Biol.Chem., 237:1908, 1962.
4. R.T. Schimke, E.W. Sweeney, and C.M. Berlin, J.Biol.Chem., 240:322, 1965.
5. E.C.C. Lin and W.E. Knox, Biochim.Biophys.Acta, 26:85, 1957.
6. F.T. Kenney and R.W. Flora, J.Biol.Chem., 236:2699, 1961.
7. R.C. Nordlie, W.J. Arion, and E.A. Glende, Jr., J.Biol.Chem., 240:3484, 1965.
8. G. Weber, S.K. Srivastava, and R.L. Singhal, J.Biol.Chem., 240:750, 1965.
9. E. Shrago, H.A. Lardy, R.C. Nordlie, and D.O. Foster, J.Biol. Chem., 238:3188, 1963.
10. M. Feigelson, P.R. Gross, and P. Feigelson, Biochim.Biophys.Acta, 55:495, 1962.
11. F.T. Kenney and F.J. Kull, Proc.Natl.Acad.Sci. USA, 50:493, 1963.
12. O. Greengard, M.A. Smith, and G. Acs, J.Biol.Chem., 238:1548, 1963.
13. J.M. McKenna and B.W. Zweifach, Am.J.Physiol., 187:263, 1956.
14. S.M. Reichard, A.S. Gordon, and C.F. Tessmer, Ann.N.Y.Acad. Sci., 88:213, 1960.
15. B.W. Zweifach and L. Thomas, Reticuloendothelial Soc. Bull., 3:31, 1957.
16. P.B. Beeson, J.Exptl.Med., 86:39, 1947.
17. R.A. Good and L. Thomas, J.Exptl.Med., 96:625, 1952.
18. L.J. Berry and D.S. Smythe, J.Bacteriol., 90:970, 1965.
19. L.J. Berry and D.S. Smythe, J.Exptl.Med., 118:587, 1963.
20. L.J. Berry, D.S. Smythe, and L.S. Colwell, J.Bacteriol., 92:107, 1966.
21. F. Rosen and R.J. Milholland, J.Biol.Chem., 238:3725, 1963.
22. B. Benacerraf, G.J. Thorbecke, and D. Jacoby, Proc.Soc.Exptl. Biol.Med., 100:796, 1959.
23. M.K. Agarwal and L.J. Berry, J. Reticuloendothelial Soc. In press.
24. R.H. Rigdon and F.S. Schrantz, J.Lab.Clin.Med., 29:122, 1944.
25. J.P. Filkins, R.E. Chase, and J.J. Smith, J. Reticuloendothelial Soc., 2:287, 1965.
26. N. Cremer and D. Watson, Proc.Soc.Exptl.Biol.Med., 95:510, 1957.
27. R.D. Collins and W.B. Wood, Jr., J.Exptl.Med., 110:1005, 1959.
28. J.S. Youngner and W.R. Stinebring, Science, 144:1022, 1964.
29. H.H. Freedman, M. Nakano, and W. Braun, Proc.Soc.Exptl.Biol. Med., 121:1228, 1966.

On the Nature of Some Nonspecific Host Responses in Endotoxin-Induced Resistance to Infection*

Monique Parant, Francine Parant, and Louis Chedid

Centre National de la Recherche Scientifique, Paris, France

and Fernand Boyer

Institut Pasteur, Paris, France

"Tolerance" to endotoxins can be established by a previous injection of an unrelated O antigen which increases the host's resistance and his capacity for clearing the second dose of endotoxin. It has been shown that these responses are nonspecific, i.e., not mediated by antibodies, but are produced by degradation and detoxification of endotoxic lipopolysaccharides [1, 2, 3].

The present study concerns endotoxin-induced resistance to Klebsiella pneumoniae infection. It has been previously established with the aid of an extremely virulent strain of this gram-negative bacterium that mice treated with a minute amount of endotoxin can survive for several days even if they have been inoculated with one million lethal doses. Such protection is not abolished by hypophysectomy or adrenalectomy [4]. During this prolonged period of survival, the number of bacteria remains essentially at a stationary level in infected mice. This equilibrium – as experiments with sulfonamide have shown – is not related to a bacteriostatic effect but, instead, to a synchronism between the rate of division of the microorganism and the rate of its destruction by the host [5]. Finally, results obtained in conventional and germ-free newborn mice have indicated that this effect is unrelated to antibody formation [6]. The data presented here support the view that a nonspecific mechanism, independent of specific antibody formation and stimulated phagocytosis, are involved, and that, as a consequence of endotoxin treatment of the host, bacteria can be phenotypically modified in vivo, thus becoming less virulent.

---

* This paper is from the Service de Chimiothérapie Expérimentale et Endocrinologie, Institut Pasteur, Paris, France.

Table I. The Phagocytic Index "K" Following the Injection of Various Doses of ^{51}Cr–K. Pneumoniae in Both Immunized and Endotoxin-Treated Mice

Group	Amount injected, ml	Number of ^{51}Cr-labeled K. pneumoniae per 20 g		
		$4 \cdot 10^6$	$4 \cdot 10^7$	$4 \cdot 10^8$
Control	–	0.009 (5)*	0.007 (15)	0.009 (15)
Immune serum	0.01	–	0.114 (5)	–
Immune serum absorbed by		–		
SED	0.01	–	0.081 (5)	–
KpC	0.01	–	0.005 (5)	–
KpC	0.03	–	0.010 (10)	–
Immune serum	0.003	–	0.007 (5)	0.011 (5)
Immune serum	0.005	–	0.032 (5)	0.013 (5)
Immune serum	0.01	–	0.046 (10)	0.015 (5)
Immune serum	0.03	–	0.143 (5)	0.060 (5)
Endotoxin	1 μg	–	0.025 (15)	0.027 (15)

*The figures in parentheses indicate the number of mice.

Table II. A Comparison of the Effect of 10^9 Heated Homologous Bacteria on the Phagocytic Index "K" in Immunized and Endotoxin-Treated Mice Receiving Cr^{51}-Labeled K. Pneumoniae ($4 \cdot 10^7/20$ g)

Group	Phagocytic Index K
(a) Control	0.007 ± 0.0028*
(b) Immune serum	0.097 ± 0.021
(c) Immune serum + 10^9 bacteria	0.020 ± 0.006
(d) Endotoxin	0.031 ± 0.009
(e) Endotoxin + 10^9 bacteria	0.024 ± 0.002

*Standard deviation.

MATERIALS AND METHODS

Male mice of a Swiss albino strain (CNRS stock of Gif-sur-Yvette) weighing 20-25 g were used in all experiments. Endotoxin was extracted by Boivin's method [7] from the Danysz strain of Salmonella enteritidis and is hereafter referred to as "ASED." The Caroli strain of Klebsiella pneumoniae used in our experiments is cultured in nutrient broth to which serum is added and will be referred to as KpC. In some cases the germs were incubated in a synthetic medium containing glucose, nicotinic acid, and mineral salts [8].

Antiserum was obtained from mice that received intraperitoneal injections of 100, 200, and 300 million heat-killed klebsiellae during the first week, followed by three weekly injections of 1 billion germs during two weeks. The mice were bled eight days after the last immunization, and their heparinized plasma was pooled. In certain cases, this antiserum was absorbed by mixing it with bacteria so as to obtain a 10% suspension. The mixture was kept at 4°C for 30 min before being centrifuged at 3000 rpm for 20 min to remove the bacteria. This procedure was repeated twice.

Klebsiellae heated 1 hr at 60°C were labeled with Cr^{51}, according to the method described by Howard et al. [9]. Blood clearance of labeled bacteria was determined according to the method of Biozzi et al. [10], the radioactivity being measured in a well-type scintillating counter. The number of living bacteria was assayed by plating the blood and organ suspensions. The blood volume was estimated as described previously [11].

In certain experiments, bacteria were recovered from the blood and liver of donors and reinoculated into recipients. In such cases, erythrocytes in 1 ml of blood were lysed by adding 3 ml of distilled water before diluting in saline. The liver was ground in a Potter homogenizer and diluted in saline before being reinjected intravenously. In all cases (endotoxin, antiserum, bacteria, and cell suspensions) injections were made in the tail vein.

RESULTS

I. Rates of Clearance of ^{51}Cr-Labeled K. Pneumoniae in Endotoxin-Treated and Immunized Mice

It must be recalled that the survival of endotoxin-treated mice is only temporary whether they be infected with 10^7, 10^5, or even 10^2 viable bacteria. During the period of survival, the number of inoculated bacteria remains stationary, indicating that although the host can destroy several million organisms after each division of the bacteria, he is unable to kill all bacteria, even when as few as 10^2 klebsiellae are injected [5]. Preliminary experiments, employing passive immunization, showed that there is a relationship between the titer of antiserum and the size of the inoculum. Therefore, rates of blood-clearance were studied by comparing doses of isotopically labeled bacteria in mice treated either with 1 μg of endotoxin the day before* or with immune serum 1 hr before the experiment. In certain cases the antiserum was previously absorbed by K. pneumoniae or by S. enteritidis (SED).

The results given in Table I show that: (1) Antiserum at a dose of 0.01 ml increases the phagocytic index considerably. Moreover, this effect is specific as can be seen by homologous and heterologous absorption. (2) There is a strict relationship between the rate of blood clearance and the antigen/antibody ratio. Thus, for a given serum dilution, the smaller the inoculum, the steeper is the slope (K has a higher value). (3) In contrast to (2) above, the phagocytic index of the endotoxin-stimulated group is uniformly elevated, even when the inoculum increases ten times. (Experiments which will be published separately have shown that after endotoxin treatment mice can destroy 10^3 or 10^6 viable KpC with equal effectiveness). It must also be noted that the phagocytic index of the controls does not vary according to the dose of labeled bacteria, in contrast to the dose dependence seen in the case of carbon clearance [12].

II. Blockade of Phagocytosis by Heat-Killed Homologous Bacteria

The opsonizing effect of antiserum is suppressed by previous absorption (see Table I). Likewise, the influence of immune serum on phagocytosis and destruction of bacteria can be inhibited in vivo by "humoral blockade" if 10^9 heat-killed homologous bacteria are administered a few minutes after the antiserum.

In the following experiment (Table II), $4 \cdot 10^7$ ^{51}Cr-labeled KpC were injected to five groups of five mice each. A first group (a) served as controls; a second group (b) received 0.01 ml of antiserum 1 hr previously; a third group (c) received the same dose of serum and 10^9 heat-killed KpC; a fourth group (d) was injected with 1 μg of endotoxin the day before, and the fifth group (e) received the same treatment as (d) plus 10^9 heat-killed KpC 1 hr before challenge. The simultaneous injection of homologous heat-killed bacteria greatly diminished the phagocytic index of mice that received the immune serum, whereas it did not affect the rate of clearance of those which had been stimulated by endotoxin (the different values of K: 0.031 and 0.024 are not statistically significant.

The results were even clearer when similarly treated animals were sacrificed 24 hr after the inoculation of viable bacteria. In the following experiment four groups of five mice were treated like those of groups (b), (c), (d), and (e) before being infected with 10^5 living K. pneumoniae. Whereas the

*If the same dose is injected 48 or 72 hr before the tagged bacteria, its effect is slight or even nil.

Table III. A Comparison of the Effect of 10^9 Heated Homologous Bacteria on the Distribution of 10^5 Living Klebsiella Pneumoniae in Immunized and Endotoxin-Treated Mice

Group	Number of bacteria*			
	Total	Blood	Liver	Spleen
(b) Immune serum	145	10	95	40
(c) Immune serum + 10^9 bacteria	1,106,000	130,000	96,000	880,000
(d) Endotoxin	30,080	10,950	4,630	14,500
(e) Endotoxin + 10^9 bacteria	5,090	20	4,300	770

*Mice sacrificed 24 hr after inoculation.

Table IV. Distribution of Living Klebsiella Pneumoniae Injected into Normal and Endotoxin-Treated Mice

Group	No. of mice	Number of bacteria*				L/B†
		Total	Percentage in			
			Blood	Liver	Spleen	
Normal	15	111,720	72.2	12.6	15.2	0.19
Endotoxin-treated	15	86,090	34.3	36.4	29.3	1.22

*Mice sacrificed 1 hr after the inoculation of 10^5 K. pneumoniae.
†Ratio of bacteria recovered in 1 g of liver/1 g of blood.

simultaneous administration of homologous bacteria greatly inhibited the effect of the antiserum, it did not decrease the enhancement of phagocytosis produced by the endotoxin treatment (Table III).

III. Reinoculation into Normal Mice of Germs Recovered from Endotoxin-Treated Donors

Normal controls and endotoxin-treated (1 μg) mice were infected with 10^5 viable bacteria and sacrificed 1 hr later. The injection of antigen-stimulated phagocytosis and the following distributions were observed: Controls, 12.6% of the germs were recovered in the liver vs 72.2% in the blood (giving an L/B ratio of 0.19); endotoxin-stimulated, 36.4% vs 34.3% (L/B ratio of 1.2) (Table IV). The same distribution was obtained when mice were infected with 10^7 bacteria.

K. pneumoniae organisms recovered from the pooled blood of normal or of endotoxin-treated mice and those recovered from the liver homogenates of endotoxin-treated donors* were reinoculated into normal recipients in one of the following ways (Table V):

* Of the bacteria found in the liver, only 9% correspond to the blood con-

Table V. Distribution of Living Bacteria Recovered from the Blood and Liver of Mice and Reinjected into Normal Recipients

Dose of KpC injected to donors	Source of bacteria injected in recipients		No. of mice	Number of Bacteria* Total	Percentage in Blood	Liver	Spleen	L/B†
–	Control culture (a)		15	960	73	14	13	0.2
10^5	Normal	blood (b)	4	1615	77.5	7.5	15	0.09
10^5	Endotoxin-treated	blood (c)	10	1455	65.3	12	22.7	0.18
		liver (d)	20	585	36.8	52.1	11.1	1.4
		liver (e)‡	10	1240	68.5	18.6	12.9	0.27
10^7	Endotoxin-treated	blood (f)	5	1320	69.3	13	17.7	0.18
		liver (g)	5	560	33	56	11	1.7

*Mice sacrificed 1 hr after the inoculation of $5 \cdot 10^2$ K. pneumoniae.
†Ratio of bacteria recovered in 1 g of liver/1 g of blood.
‡After 2 hr incubation and redilution in a suspension of endotoxin-treated liver cells from noninfected mice.

The group of control (a) received about 500 bacteria that had been subcultured 2 hr in a synthetic medium before being injected.

The four following groups received bacteria transferred from donors sacrificed 1 hr after having been infected with 10^5 KpC. These bacteria were recovered from:

(1) The blood of normal mice (b).

(2) The blood of endotoxin-treated mice (c).

(3) The liver of endotoxin-treated mice (d).

(4) The same liver suspension was incubated for 2 hr at 37°C in a synthetic medium before being injected into the last group (e).

Since viable bacteria found in the liver undergo three divisions during incubation, livers of mice that had been treated with endotoxin but had not been infected were homogenized and added at the end of the incubation period. This procedure assured that the final 10-fold dilution injected into the recipients contained an amount of hepatic tissue equivalent to that in group (d).

---

tained in this organ in the endotoxin-treated group as against 36% in the controls. Therefore, the germs recovered in the liver of normal donors were not transferred.

The last groups received germs transferred from either the blood of endotoxin-treated donors inoculated with 10^7 KpC (f), or the liver of such mice (g). In the last two groups, the blood and liver were diluted 100 times more than in all other groups, proper care having been taken to reinoculate an average of 500 germs in a volume of 0.2 ml. Except in the case of group (e), bacterial division was avoided by keeping the blood and liver suspensions in an ice bath.

The recipients were sacrificed one hour after infection. Plating of their blood, liver, and spleen gave the results shown in Table V. The total bacterial count in groups (d) and (g), which received klebsiellae transferred from the liver of endotoxin-treated mice, showed no increase. Most of the bacteria (52.1% and 56%) were found in the liver, increasing the L/B ratio and indicating that these normal recipients phagocytosed as if they had been stimulated by endotoxin.

In all other cases, blood clearance was normal even when the germs were recovered from the liver but had been incubated for 2 hr. Thus, there is a reversal of the initial pattern if these bacteria were allowed to divide in vitro. The 10-fold increase of the klebsiellae during incubation could not explain such differences, since the same response was obtained when the donors had received 10^7 microorganisms instead of 10^5. Therefore, the results could not be due to the extent of dilution of blood or liver isolates.

DISCUSSION

A single injection of lipopolysaccharide increases the resistance to a variety of bacterial or viral infections as well as to a second challenge by endotoxins [13]. Natural antibodies have been held responsible for this effect [14, 15]. However, tolerance to endotoxins can be established in the mouse under conditions which exclude active antibody formation [1, 3]. Nevertheless, the possibility remains that endotoxin, because of its cytotoxic effects, could discharge preexisting antibodies or facilitate new protein synthesis through the stimulatory effect produced by DNA breakdown products [16] or by effect on cell permeability [17].

The data presented here concern the increased resistance to a *Klebsiella pneumoniae* infection, characterized by a greater capacity of the host to phagocytose and to destroy inoculated bacteria. The transfer experiments reported here show that the effects observed in this type of infection, which is greatly dependent in its outcome on phagocytosis, cannot be explained solely by a stimulation of the RES. Indeed, whereas bacteria recovered from a tolerant animal's blood are cleared normally, those that are transferred from the same donor's liver are phagocytosed very rapidly when they are reinoculated into a normal recipient. These results indicate that the bacteria found in the liver compartment represent a phenotypically unique population, and that these altered kelbsiellae can be ingested by normal RE cells. Such a phenotypic alteration does not appear to be related to opsonins, as seems to be the case in experimental Salmonella infections [18, 19]. There is no quantitative correlation between the stimulation produced by endotoxin and the number of klebsiellae inoculated, contrary to what is seen in immunized mice. This can be shown by measuring the phagocytic index of isotopically labeled bacteria or the distribution of viable bacteria in the host's blood and liver. Similarly, a prior injection of homologous bacteria inhibits the effects of antiserum but does not modify the phagocytosis of endotoxin-treated mice. All these results argue against an involvement of antigen–antibody reactions.

It is well established that virulent strains are cleared less rapidly than avirulent ones [18, 20]. If bacteria recovered from an endotoxin-treated mouse's liver are allowed to divide in vitro, they revert to their usual behavior, i.e., they are phagocytosed more slowly. Therefore, the resistant host seems to exert a short-term effect on microorganisms without modifying their genotype. This can explain why there is no colonial change or loss of virulence when the organisms are recovered from an infected animal's blood and are cultured in vitro before reinoculation.

How can such nonspecific alteration of the bacterial phenotype be visualized? Loss of virulence can be obtained if streptococci [21], brucellae [22], or klebsiellae [23] are pretreated with enzymes, affecting cell wall structure. In the case of klebsiellae, a phage-induced enzyme can strip the polysaccharide from the surface of the bacterium, thus reducing dramatically its virulence in vivo without affecting its viability in vitro. In the case of "tolerance" to endotoxin – which is a cell component – evidence indicates that the detoxifying ability acquired by the host is mediated by a nonspecific mechanism linked to "enzymatic" processes that can degrade [2, 24] or perhaps complex [25] the endotoxic polysaccharide molecule.

We suggest that in the endotoxin-stimulated animal a similar mechanism exists and that the cell wall antigen can be attacked in situ at a molecular level, without giving any detectable lasting alterations of the microorganism's viability, morphology, colonial aspect, or usual immunological reactions. Although this phenotypical change disappears after a few divisions, it could be sufficient to enable the host to clear such altered bacteria from his blood and destroy them. The probability of encounter between a given number of fixed targets (the Kupffer cells) and the modified bacteria could be strictly proportional to their concentration in the blood. Therefore, in contrast to what happens with humoral antibodies (which give a quantitative reaction), the percentage of trapped klebsiellae is always the same whatever the size of the inoculum. This mechanism may lead to a "pseudo-bacteriostatic" situation which, although of only a few days duration, can delay lethal effects and may thus permit immune responses to establish themselves.

SUMMARY

(1) A single injection of endotoxin can increase the resistance of mice to Klebsiella pneumoniae infections. Rates of clearance of ^{51}Cr-labeled bacteria and enumeration of the number of bacteria argue against the possibility that this effect is mediated by opsonins. In contrast to what is observed in specifically immunized mice, there is no relationship between the size of the inoculum and the degree of phagocytosis of endotoxin-treated animals. Moreover, the increased rate of blood clearance in endotoxin-treated animals is not inhibited by a simultaneous injection of heat-killed homologous bacteria.

(2) Experiments, in which bacteria recovered from the liver of endotoxin-treated donors have been reinoculated into normal recipients, indicate that a nonspecific mechanism capable of causing a temporary modification of the phenotype of the microorganisms plays a significant role. The nature of this modification in endotoxin-treated hosts appears to be an alteration of endotoxic cell wall constituents of the bacteria. This alteration enhances the bacteria's susceptibility to phagocytosis but is not maintained during subsequent multiplication in vitro. The results suggest also that RES stimulation is inadequate to explain completely the host's response or at least that it is not a prerequisite once the bacterium has been modified.

ACKNOWLEDGMENT

The authors express their sincere appreciation to Dr. W. Braun for his valuable remarks on editing this paper.

REFERENCES

1. L. Chedid, M. Parant, F. Boyer, and R.C. Skarnes, in: M. Landy and W. Braun, eds., Bacterial Endotoxins, New Brunswick, New Jersey, Rutgers University Press, 1964, p. 500.
2. R.C. Skarnes and L. Chedid, in: M. Landy and W. Braun, eds., Bacterial Endotoxins, New Brunswick, New Jersey, Rutgers University Press, 1964, p. 575.
3. F. Parant, M. Parant, H. Charlier, E. Sacquet, and L. Chedid, Ann. Inst. Pasteur, 110: Suppl. 3, 198, 1966.
4. M. Parant, F. Boyer, and L. Chedid, Compt. Rend. Acad. Sci. Paris, 260: 3218, 1965.
5. M. Parant, F. Boyer, and L. Chedid, Compt. Rend. Acad. Sci. Paris, 260:2630, 1965.
6. M. Parant and E. Sacquet, Compt. Rend. Acad. Sci. Paris, 262: 1914, 1966.
7. A. Boivin and L. Mesrobeanu, Rev. Immunol., 1: 553, 1935.
8. A. Lwoff, F. Nitti, and T. Trefouel, Ann. Inst. Pasteur, 67: 173, 1941.
9. J.G. Howard, G. Biozzi, B.N. Halpern, C. Stiffel, and D. Mouton, Brit. J. Exptl. Pathol., 40: 281, 1959.

10. G. Biozzi, B. Benacerraf, and B.N. Halpern, Brit.J.Exptl.Pathol., 34:441, 1953.
11. L. Chedid and M. Parant, Ann.Inst.Pasteur, 101:170, 1961.
12. G. Biozzi, B. Benacerraf, C. Stiffel, and B.N. Halpern, Compt.Rend. Soc.Biol., 148:431, 1954.
13. Symposium on bacterial endotoxins, in: M. Landy and W. Braun, eds., Bacterial Endotoxins, New Brunswick, New Jersey, Rutgers University Press, 1964.
14. M. Landy, J.G. Michael, and J.L. Whitby, J. Bacteriol., 83:631, 1962.
15. J.G. Michael, J.Exptl.Med., 123:205, 1966.
16. W. Braun and R.W.I. Kessel, In: M. Landy and W. Braun, eds., Bacterial Endotoxins, New Brunswick, New Jersey, Rutgers University Press, 1964, p. 397.
17. W. Braun, M. Nakano, and H. Freedman, Federation Proc., 25:370, 1966.
18. C.R. Jenkin and D. Rowley, J. Exptl.Med., 114:363, 1961.
19. C.R. Jenkin, Brit.J.Exptl.Pathol., 44:47, 1963.
20. W. Braun, Bacterial Genetics, 2nd ed., Philadelphia, Saunders, 1965.
21. G.G. Wiley and A.T. Wilson, J.Exptl.Med., 103:15, 1956.
22. S.S. Elberg, Bacteriol.Rev., 24:67, 1960.
23. M.H. Adams and B.H. Parks, Virology, 2:719, 1956.
24. R.C. Skarnes, Ann.N.Y.Acad.Sci., 133:644, 1966.
25. J.A. Rudbach, R.L. Anacker, W.T. Haskins, A.G. Johnson, K.C. Milner, and E. Ribi, Ann. N.Y.Acad.Sci., 133:629, 1966.

The Effect of Opsonized Colloids on the Enhancement of Endotoxin Lethality*

I. MacKay Murray

Department of Anatomy, State University of New York
Downstate Medical Center
Brooklyn, New York

The diverse physiologic functions which are altered following the intravenous injection of inert particles, have imposed, a priori, on the reticuloendothelial system (RES) a significance which belies its morphological appearance. This is exemplified by the striking increase in the sensitivity of several species of animals to the lethal effects of endotoxin when given within a definite interval of time after the intravenous injection of colloidal material [1]. Since the majority of these colloidal particles are phagocytized by the fixed reticuloendothelial cells of the liver and spleen, it has been suggested [2] that the functions of the RE cells are impaired for a variable period of time due to the presence of a mass of inert material contained within their cytoplasm. Blockaded RE cells would be temporarily unable to phagocytose additional foreign material such as endotoxins.

Support for this hypothesis was given by the observation that the clearance from the circulation of intravenously administered endotoxin was significantly delayed in those animals previously injected with the blockading colloid [3]. Presumably, the persistence of endotoxin within the circulation of the blockaded animals permitted either greater cellular damage or injury to other types of cells. More recently, evidence was presented which failed to show a reciprocal relationship between the RES and tolerance to endotoxin. Tolerance to endotoxin was produced without any alteration in the rate of colloid clearance from the circulation, and blockade of the RES failed to abolish tolerance [4]. The passive transfer of tolerance to endotoxin by serum [5] as well as a globulin fraction of serum [6] obtained from the tol-

* This study was supported by research grant AI-05913 from the National Institute of Allergy and Infectious Diseases, U. S. Public Health Service.

erant animal aroused suspicion as to whether or not the RES plays the primary role in the intravascular clearance of endotoxin.

Finally, the concept of blockade of the RES was challenged. The criterion used for the assessment of blockade was the quantitative reduction from the normal rate of clearance of a standard dose of colloid. Blockade by these standards was optimal if the surface properties of the blockading colloid and the testing colloid were identical but not if they were dissimilar particles [7].

There was increasing evidence that plasma factors or opsonins played a role in determining the rate of clearance of gelatin-stabilized colloids from the circulation. When identical particles were used for both blockade and testing, three laboratories reported that opsonization of the test dose in vitro resulted in normal rates of clearance [7, 8]. However, two laboratories [9] have reported negative results. In a system where antibody titers are more readily measured, the rate of clearance of foreign red blood cells was significantly higher in the rat as compared with the mouse, and was associated with a higher level of specific natural antibodies in the rat serum [2].

There is little controversy regarding opsonin-dependent clearance rates in immune systems. A direct relationship was found between the amount of antibody injected and the rate at which the homologous organisms were cleared from the circulation [10]. There is substantial evidence that serum factors, whether heat-labile or heat-stabile, are essential for the phagocytosis of inert particles [11]. The relative importance of antibody and complement in the phagocytic process may be best expressed by the experiments of Ward and Enders [12]. Although antibody was essential for phagocytosis, the addition of complement significantly increased the rate of phagocytosis.

The studies to be described were designed to answer a question posed by a rather tenuous hypothesis. If blockade of the RES results from the depletion of phagocytic stimulating factors from the circulation, is the increased sensitivity to endotoxin a result of this depletion? Would the supply of exogenous natural antibody against a gelatin-stabilized colloid modify the host's sensitivity to subsequent endotoxin?

PROPERTIES OF THE ANTIGEN AND ANTIBODY

When a suitable particle such as gold is suspended in a gelatin solution, it is enveloped by a layer of gelatin [13], and this particle now assumes the properties of gelatin as determined by electrophoresis and antigen–antibody reactions [14]. When the gelatin-stabilized particle, regardless of the type of particle used, is presented to the circulation, it appears to be recognized as gelatin and not carbon, gold, or chromium phosphate [7]. Therefore, the type of stabilizing material used seems to be of major importance. When

Table I. Agglutinin Titer Against Gelatin-Stabilized Chromium Phosphate in Rats Following Intravenous Injection of S. marcescens Endotoxin

Hours after injection	Saline	Endotoxin, μg/100 g		
		100	200	300
20	4	4	4	4
40	4	4	8	8
72	4	4	16	16
96	4	4	8	8

Table II. The Immediate Response to the Intravenous Injection of a Colloid–Antibody Complex

Antibody source	Cations added, μg /ml	Result
Serum	None	No effect
ACD serum	Ca^{++} 24, Mg^{++} 48	Anaphylactoid death
ACD plasma	None	No effect
Heparin plasma	None	No effect
Euglobulin	Ca^{++} 6, Mg^{++} 12	Anaphylactoid death
Euglobulin	None	No effect

increasing concentrations of gelatin are used to stabilize the colloid, there is a corresponding decrease in its rate of clearance from the circulation. Increasing the time of incubation of a gelatin–chromium phosphate mixture as shown by Dobson [15] enhances the gelatin effect. The degree of enhancement may possibly reflect quantitative differences in the completeness of coating. As the colloidal particles are gradually enveloped by gelatin, its surface area, and hence the number of its antigenic sites, would be increased. Theoretically, at least, the gelatin in this physical state would be capable of complexing more antibody. Zinsser [16] has shown that the amount of antibody adsorbed from serum was dependent on the surface area of the antigen presented.

The type of gelatin used to stabilize colloid may be critical. Maurer [17] has shown that there is a relationship between the molecular size and the amount of antibody complexed. Fish gelatin, which is used to stabilize a commonly used carbon colloid, does not have the same specificity as animal gelatin [7]. Exactly what happens when animal gelatin is used to stabilize carbon particles already stabilized by fish gelatin is speculative.

The gelatin used in these studies was P-20 salt-free gelatin obtained from the Knox Gelatin Company, Camden, New Jersey. Colloidal chromium phosphate was prepared according to a method described by Dobson [18], and was stabilized in 2% gelatin.

Natural antibodies against gelatin were found in the plasmas of various species of animal and from all available evidence appear to be specific for gelatin [19]. In common with other natural antibodies [20], its level remains remarkably constant within a particular strain for long periods. Depletion of gelatin antibody in the circulation was not observed following the intravenous injection of various nongelatin-stabilized colloidal materials [14]. The nonspecific stimulation of the RES following the administration of lipopolysaccharides derived from a variety of gram-negative organisms has been attributed by some to an increased phagocytic capacity of the RE cells [2], and by others to a humoral mechanism [21]. Natural antibodies against gelatin (Table I) were increased in the rat after intravenously administered endotoxin. The numbers refer to the reciprocals of the highest dilution at which visible agglutination occurred. The opsonin titer would be many times the agglutinin titer, but there does not appear to be direct linear relationship [10]. Antibody levels reached their highest values at a time which corresponds to maximal stimulation of the RES by endotoxin.

IN VITRO OPSONIZATION

Standardization experiments were done using various amounts of the colloid and followed at different time intervals by a standard dose of 150 μg per 100 g b.w. of Serratia marcescens endotoxin. The intravenous injection of 15 mg/100 g b.w. of gelatin-stabilized chromium phosphate resulted in maximal sensitivity to the standard dose of endotoxin injected intravenously 3 hr later. Unless otherwise stated, this schedule was followed throughout. The proportion of colloid to plasma, 15 mg/10 ml, was based on previously determined optimal ratios. After 1 hr in a shaking incubator at 37°C, the agglutinated colloid was separated by centrifugation, washed carefully several times with ice-cold isotonic sucrose, and resuspended in 2 ml of the sucrose. The resuspended complex was stable on standing with no evidence of increased aggregation when examined microscopically. Two of the preparations, as shown in Table II, when injected intravenously, were uniformly fatal within 2-4 min. At necropsy the lungs were distended with great dilatation of the pulmonary vessels. The remaining preparations, while similar in physical characteristics, had no visible effect on the rats. The lethal colloids had one feature in common, the addition of calcium and magnesium to the mixture. The known requirements of divalent cations for complement fixation and its inhibition by chelating agents and heparin suggested that the production of lethal opsonized colloids may be related to complement fixation. The ability of rat serum to generate anaphylatoxin in vitro by the addition of diverse substances [22], as well as antigen—antibody complexes, has been critically studied by Osler et al. [23]. There appears to be one feature in common: that fixation of complement is a prerequisite for anaphylatoxin

Table III. Modification of the Colloid-Induced Enhancement of Endotoxin Lethality by the Prior Injection of Isologous and Homologous Euglobulins

Euglobulin donor strain	Recipient strain	Dead/total, 24 hr after endotoxin
Lewis	Lewis	10/12
Lewis	Sprague–Dawley	1/12
Sprague–Dawley	Lewis	2/15
	Controls (euglobulin alone)	
Lewis	Lewis	0/10
Lewis	Sprague–Dawley	0/10
Sprague–Dawley	Lewis	0/10
	Controls (colloid alone)	
-------(Saline)	Lewis	18/20
-------(Saline)	Sprague–Dawley	9/9

Table IV. Modification of the Blood Clearance Rate of Gelatin-Stabilized Chromium Radio-Phosphate by the Prior Injection of Isologous and Homologous Euglobulins

Donor euglobulin strain	Number injected	Clearance rate (t/2 min)	0/0 injected radioactivity recovered	
			Liver	Spleen
Lewis	6	11.6 ± 0.45	78.4 ± 4.6	7.4 ± 1.2
Sprague–Dawley	6	27.6 ± 1.4	68.8 ± 4.9	9.6 ± 1.5
-----(Saline)	10	19.4 ± 0.90	74.1 ± 3.8	7.8 ± 0.9

production and those conditions which prevent complement fixation prevent the production of anaphylatoxin. The nonlethal opsonized colloids were as effective as nonopsonized colloid in enhancing the lethal effect of the subsequent endotoxin injection.

PRETREATMENT WITH OPSONINS

Euglobulin fractions were prepared from 20-ml volumes of serum obtained from both an inbred Lewis strain and the outbred Sprague-Dawley rats. The euglobulin fraction was injected 15 min before the colloid, which in turn was followed in 3 hr by the standard dose of endotoxin. As shown in Table III, a decrease in the sensitivity to endotoxin was apparent only when the host received the homologous fraction. Lewis rats pretreated with isologous euglobulin became prostrate 3-5 min after the colloid injection, whereas the homologous fractions produced a minor reaction.

Table V. The Effect of Excess Gelatin-Stabilized Colloid on Enhancement of Endotoxin Lethality

Donor strain euglobulin	Colloid (mg/100 g)	Recipient strain	Dead/total 24 hr after endotoxin
-------(Saline)	15	Lewis	22/24
-------(Saline	30	Lewis	4/20
Lewis	30	Lewis	8/10
Sprague-Dawley	30	Lewis	1/9

Clearance rates of tracer-labeled blockading doses of the colloid were also influenced by pretreatment with the euglobulin fractions (Table IV). The inhibiting effect of heterologous and homologous plasma fractions has been reported previously [24]. The amount of inhibition appears to be related to the relative degrees of antigenicity, i.e., greater for heterologous fractions. Fractions containing heterologous albumin had no inhibiting effect, whereas fractions containing alpha and beta globulins had the maximum effect. The mechanism by which the intravascular clearance rate of a gelatin-stabilized colloid is influenced by the introduction of a second dissimilar colloid, has been recently analyzed by Normann and Benditt [25]. They found that the degree of inhibition was not dependent on the amount of the second colloid injected, although the duration of inhibition was. A possible explanation might be that inhibition is the resultant of the competition for a nonspecific factor which is known to influence the rate of phagocytosis, e.g., complement.

Our studies would suggest that homologous euglobulins are recognized as foreign by the host. Although pretreatment with the euglobulin fractions influenced the host's sensitivity to endotoxin, as well as clearance rates, this was not reflected in the phagocytic capacity of the liver or spleen for the colloid.

When the standard dose of colloid was doubled (Table V), there was a significant decrease in the sensitivity of the control group of rats to the standard dose of endotoxin. This did not represent tolerance to endotoxin, for these rats were more sensitive than noncolloid-treated rats to larger doses of endotoxin. Pretreatment with isologous euglobulin in the appropriate host enhanced the lethality of the standard dose of endotoxin. Homologous euglobulins, however, were ineffective in altering the host's sensitivity.

The parenteral administration of immune antibodies, whether of heterologous or homologous origin, appear to opsonize as effectively as when introduced into the test tube. The many properties of natural antibodies have been clearly demonstrated in vitro, but there is meager information regarding its passive transfer. When properdin is taken as a representative sample of natural antibody [26], a similar situation is found. A significant rise in serum properdin levels in the rabbit did not occur following the injection of human properdin [27]. The protection of experimental animals against a bacterial challenge provided by purified human properdin was no more effective than heat-inactivated properdin [28]. This is in rather sharp contrast to the bactericidal effects of properdin as demonstrated in vitro. It might be of interest to test properdin in an isologous system. Perhaps maturation of natural antibodies as a result of constant stimulation alters their antigenicity. Finland and Sutliff [29] have reported that while children in the first decade of life had natural antibodies to pneumococci and their sera showed bactericidal and agglutinating titers as high as in the adult, there was no significant protection afforded to mice challenged with the homologous organism. Protection from adult serum was noticeably higher.

CONCLUSIONS

As a tentative hypothesis we have considered the likelihood of antigen–antibody complexes occurring in the bloodstream as a possible mechanism for enhancement of endotoxin lethality. Circulating gelatin–antibody complexes in the proper ratio may fix complement resulting not only in a more efficient removal of the colloid, but at the same time initiate the production of anaphylatoxin-like substances. The role of serotonin in anaphylaxis of the rat and the synergistic effect of serotonin and endotoxin on vascular damage may be pertinent to this study. Antigen excess or foreign materials which may compete with the antigen–antibody complex for complement may act to minimize the anaphylactic response in the host.

REFERENCES

1. P.B. Beeson, J.Exptl.Med., 86:29, 1947; R.A. Good and L. Thomas, J.Exptl.Med., 96:625, 1952.
2. B. Benacerraf, G. Biozzi, B.N. Halpern, and C. Stiffel, in: Physiopathology of the Reticuloendothelial System, Oxford, Blackwell Scientific Publications, 1957.
3. N. Cremer and D. Watson, Proc.Soc.Exptl.Biol.Med., 95: 510, 1957.
4. S.E. Greisman, F.A. Carozza, Jr., and J.D. Hills, J.Exptl.Med., 117: 663, 1963.
5. H.H. Freedman, J.Exptl.Med., 111:453, 1960.
6. Y.B. Kim and D.W. Watson, J.Exptl.Med., 121:751, 1965.
7. I.M. Murray, J.Exptl.Med., 117:139, 1963.
8. C.R. Jenkin and D. Rowley, J.Exptl.Med., 114:363, 1961; S.J. Normann and E.P. Benditt, J.Exptl.Med., 122:709, 1965.
9. G. Biozzi, C. Stiffel, B.N. Halpern, and D. Mouton, Proc.Soc.Exptl. Biol.Med., 112:1017, 1963; M.G. Koenig, R.M. Heyssel, M.A. Melly, and D.E. Rogers, J.Exptl.Med., 122:117, 1965.

10. G. Biozzi, C. Stiffel, B.N. Halpern, L. LeMinor, and D. Mouton, J.Immunol., 87:296, 1961.
11. W.O. Fenn, J.Gen.Physiol., 3:575, 1921; J.G. Hirsch and B. Strauss, J.Immunol., 92:145, 1964.
12. H.K. Ward and J.F. Enders, J.Exptl.Med., 57:527, 1933.
13. W. Reinders and W.M. Bendien, Rec.Trav.Chim., 47:977, 1928.
14. I.M. Murray, Am.J.Physiol., 204:655, 1963.
15. E.L. Dobson, in: Physiopathology of the Reticuloendothelial System, Oxford, Blackwell Scientific Publications, 1957.
16. H. Zinnser, J.Immunol., 18:483, 1930.
17. P.H. Maurer, J.Exptl.Med., 107:125, 1958.
18. E.L. Dobson and H.B. Jones, Acta Med.Scand., 144, Suppl. 273, 1952.
19. P.H. Maurer, J.Exptl.Med., 100:515, 1954.
20. M. Landy and W.P. Weidanz, in: Bacterial Endotoxins, New Brunswick, New Jersey, Rutgers University Press, 1964.
21. C. Jenkin and D.L. Palmer, J.Exptl.Med., 112:419, 1960.
22. F.G. Novy and P.H. DeKruif, J.Infect.Diseases, 20:589, 1917.
23. A.G. Osler, H.G. Randall, B.M. Hill, and Z. Ovary, J.Exptl.Med., 110:311, 1959.
24. I.M. Murray and M. Katz, J.Lab.Clin.Med., 46:263, 1955.
25. S.J. Normann and E.P. Benditt, J.Exptl.Med., 122:693, 1965.
26. R.A. Nelson, J.Exptl.Med., 108:515, 1958.
27. C.F. Hinz, Jr., R.J. Wedgwood, E.W. Todd, and L. Pillemer, J.Immunol., 85:547, 1960.
28. O.A. Ross, Am.J. Pathol., 34:471, 1958.
29. M. Finland and W.D. Sutliff, J.Exptl.Med., 57:95, 1933.

The Effect of a Reticuloendothelial-Depressing Substance on Survival From Shock*

Benjamin Blattberg and Matthew N. Levy

Research Laboratories
St. Vincent Charity Hospital
Cleveland, Ohio

Here is some evidence which has led us to postulate the formation of a reticuloendothelial-depressing substance (RDS) during shock.

Figure 1 is a diagram of the method used to autoperfuse the liver of the dog [1]. Blood from the femoral artery passed through a flowmeter and into the portal venous segment of the ligated splenic vein. The other femoral artery was used to bleed the dog to maintain arterial pressure automatically at 40 mm Hg for 90 min. Carbon clearances were determined at the start of the experiment K_1, and again after the reinfusion of the blood K_2 in the reservoir. Four groups of dogs were used. Two were control normotensive groups, one of which was perfused, and two were hypotensive groups, one of which was perfused. Figure 2 indicates the fall in the rate of carbon clearance ($K_1 - K_2$) of the four groups of experimental animals. The hemorrhaged group and the hemorrhaged-with-perfusion groups showed a very significant depression of the rate of carbon clearance when compared with the control and control-with-perfusion groups. We concluded that there is a depression in the ability of the RES of the hypotensive dog to clear carbon particles. Such depression is not primarily due to a decrease in the blood flow to the liver.

In a second experiment [2], shown in Fig. 3, carbon clearances were determined in a normotensive "assay" dog, before and after cross-transfusion with an "experimental" animal. The "assay" dog was placed on a balance and was maintained at constant weight by a solenoid valve activated by the balance. Portal venous blood from the "experimental" dog was directed into the portal vein of the "assay" dog via the ligated splenic vein. Blood was returned from a femoral artery to a femoral vein. There were three groups of experiments. The first served as a control. Both of the

* This investigation was supported by Public Health Service research grant HE 07403.

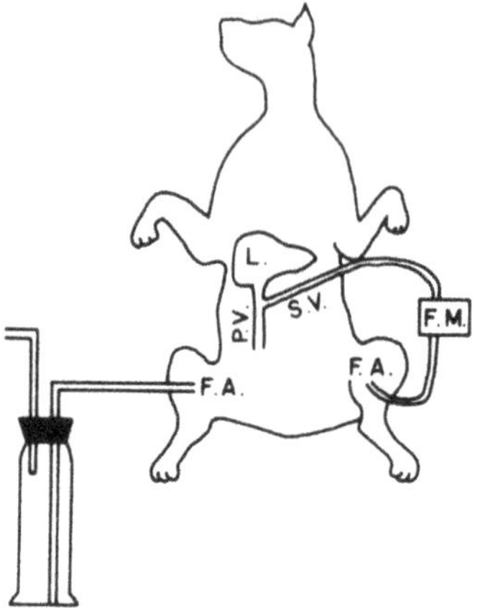

Fig. 1. Method of production of hypotension and perfusion of the liver.

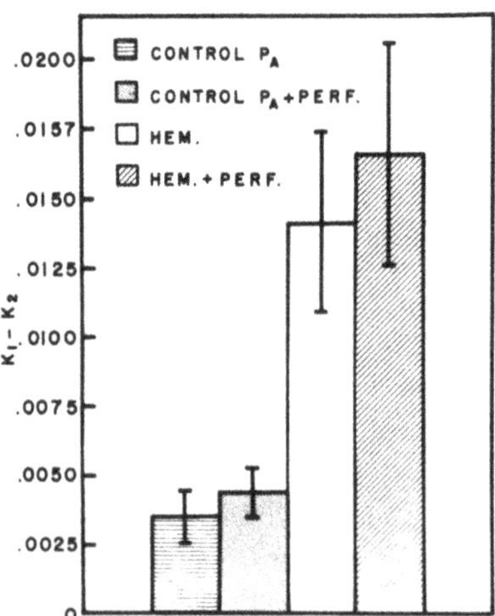

Fig. 2. Effects of hypotension and liver perfusion on the granulopectic activity of the RES.

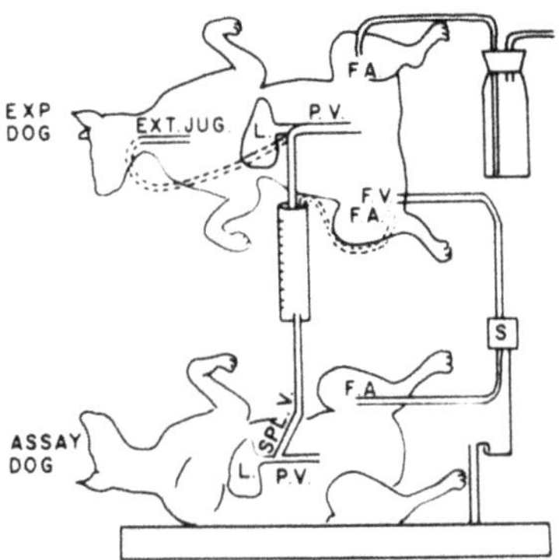

Fig. 3. Method for cross-transfusion of portal venous and of femoral arterial blood.

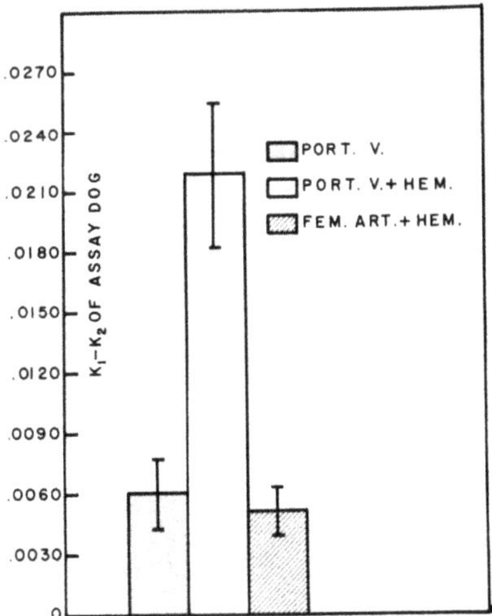

Fig. 4. Effect of cross-transfusion of blood from normotensive and hypotensive dogs on RES of normotensive animals.

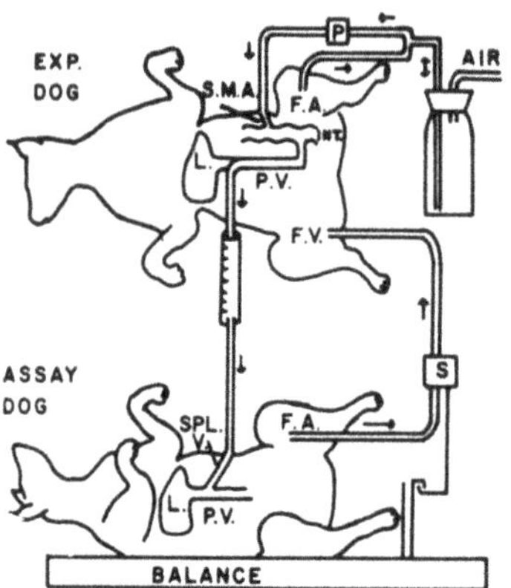

Fig. 5. Method for perfusion of superior mesenteric artery and of cross-transfusion of portal venous blood from hypotensive to normotensive dog.

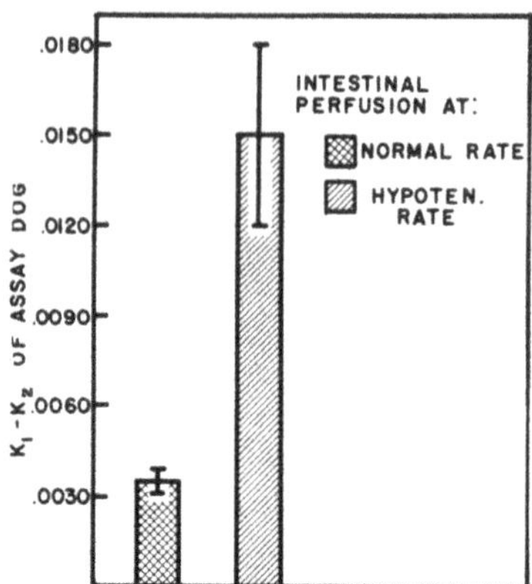

Fig. 6. Effect of rate of intestinal blood flow in hypotensive dogs on the granulopectic activity of normotensive dogs.

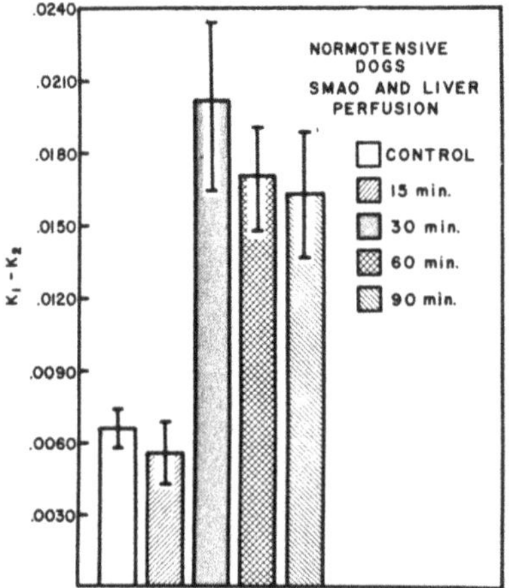

Fig. 7. Effect of duration of SMA occlusion on activity of the RES.

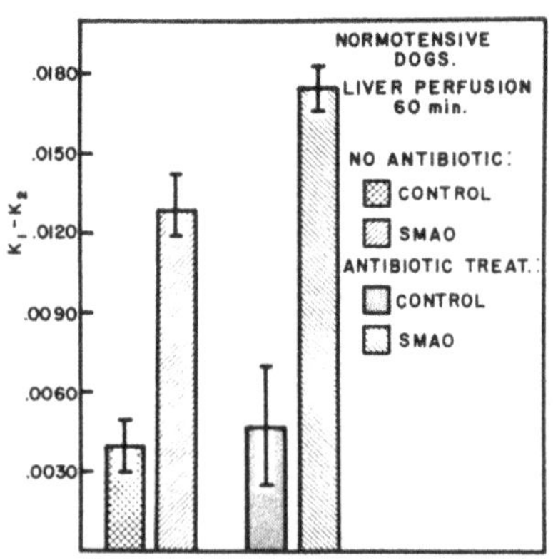

Fig. 8. Effect of previous treatment with antibiotics on the RES activity of normotensive dogs subjected to SMA occlusion.

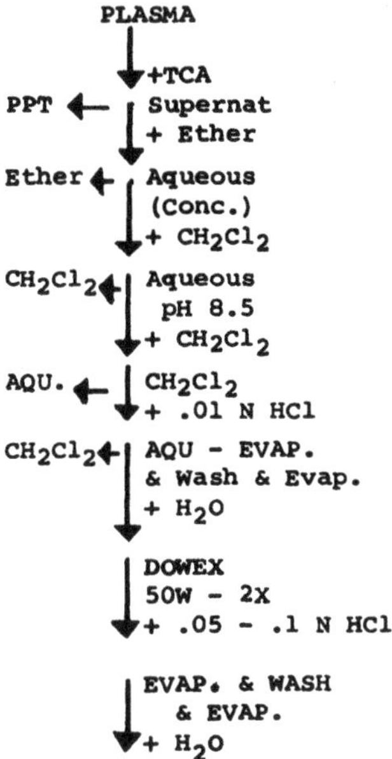

Fig. 9. Procedure for partial purification of RDS from shock plasma.

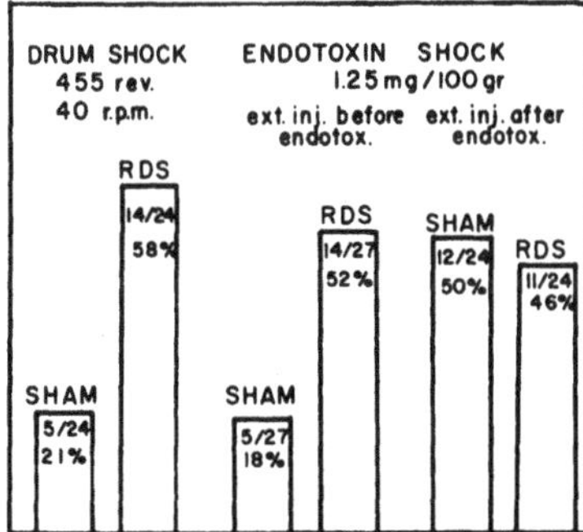

Fig. 10. Effect of extract of shock (RDS) and control (sham) plasmas on the mortality rate of rats subjected to drum shock and to endotoxin shock.

dogs remained normotensive. In the second group, the "experimental" animal was made hypotensive (40 mm Hg for 90 min), and was cross-transfused as described above during that time. In the third group, femoral arterial blood, instead of portal venous blood, was delivered to the "assay" dog from the hypotensive "experimental" one. The portal venous blood was shunted to the external jugular vein. In Fig. 4 are the values of $K_1 - K_2$ of the "assay" dogs. It may be seen that only in the second group, when portal venous blood from a hypotensive animal was cross-transfused, was there a significant depression of the RES of the assay animal. We concluded that RDS was present in the portal venous blood, but not detectable in the femoral arterial blood of the hypotensive "experimental" animals.

Using another cross-transfusion procedure [3], shown in Fig. 5, a pump was used to perfuse arterial blood through the superior mesenteric artery of the hypotensive "experimental" dog. The pump was adjusted so that intestinal blood flow would be at a normal rate (8-9 ml/kg/min) in one group and at a rate typically found in hemorrhagic hypotension (3-3.5 ml per kg/min) in the second group. In both groups the "experimental" dog was made hypotensive and perfused for 90 min. In Fig. 6, it is evident that there was a significant depression of the RES of the normotensive "assay" dog when the slow flow rate was used, as manifested by the large value of $(K_1 - K_2)$. These results suggest that a humoral RDS is formed only when the intestine of the hypotensive dog is made ischemic.

In a fourth experiment [4], ischemia of the intestine was produced in normotensive dogs by clamping the superior mesenteric artery (SMA) for various periods of time. Flow was maintained to the liver by autoperfusion of femoral arterial blood through a splenic vein. It was found, as shown in Fig. 7, that SMA occlusion of ½ hr was sufficient to depress the rate of clearance of carbon particles by the RES, thereby demonstrating that ischemia of the intestine in normotensive dogs produced RDS. This experiment was repeated in dogs pretreated with antibiotics (Fig. 8), so that gram-negative bacteria were no longer present in the fecal flora. RDS was produced in these animals when the SMA was occluded. This suggested that gram-negative bacterial products were not essential to the production of RDS.

Current attempts to devise more sensitive methods for the detection of RDS led to the use of the rat as the assay animal [5, 6]. Carbon is injected into a normal rat and K_1 is determined. An extract of plasma from a dog subjected to shock is then administered, a second injection of carbon is given, and K_2 is determined. The difference between the two carbon clearances $(K_1 - K_2)$ is considered to be a measure of the content of RDS. Plasma extract from sham-operated dogs is used as control.

The method for the chemical isolation of RDS, which we are presently using, is depicted in Fig. 9. Plasma from shocked dogs is precipitated with two volumes of trichloracetic acid. Ether is used to extract the acid from the supernatant solution, and the aqueous residue is concentrated by flash evaporation. The concentrate (acid pH) is extracted with methylene chloride, which is then discarded. The aqueous concentrate is made alkaline (pH 8.5), and again extracted with methylene chloride. To the organic extract is then added 0.01 N HCl, which is then flash-evaporated to dryness. The residue is taken up in water and again dried. The residue in water is applied to an aqueous Dowex (50W – 2X) column. The eluant, when 0.05-0.1 N HCl is applied to the column, is flash-evaporated and the residue washed with water and evaporated. The residue is taken up in 2 ml of water; on injection into the rat, it is found to contain RDS. Plasma from sham-operated dogs treated in this manner is without effect.

The next experiment on rats tested the effect of injection of RDS on drum and endotoxin shock [7]. In Fig. 10 is depicted the result of the injection of protein-free filtrate of shock plasma or sham plasma on survival of rats subjected to approximately an LD_{20}. It will be seen that a significantly increased number of animals died when given the shock extract after drumming. In endotoxin shock, when the extracts were injected before the endotoxin, the RDS had a lethal effect. However, when given after the endotoxin, there was no effect.

We concluded that RDS is formed in the ischemic intestine. It reduces the ability of the RES to clear toxic substances, thereby playing an important role in the shock syndrome.

REFERENCES

1. B. Blattberg and M.N. Levy, "Mechanism of depression of reticuloendothelial system in shock," Am.J.Physiol., 203: 111-112, 1962.
2. B. Blattberg and M.N. Levy, "A humoral reticuloendothelial-depressing substance in shock," Am.J.Physiol., 203 : 409-411, 1962.
3. B. Blattberg and M.N. Levy, "Formation of a reticuloendothelial-depressing substance in the ischemic intestine," Am.J.Physiol., 203: 867-869, 1962.
4. B. Blattberg and M.N. Levy, "Reticuloendothelial depression with superior mesenteric artery occlusion," Am.J.Physiol., 204 : 899-902, 1963.
5. B. Blattberg and M.N. Levy, "Detection of reticuloendothelial-depressing substance in shock," Am.J.Physiol., 209 : 71-74, 1965.
6. B. Blattberg and M.N. Levy, "Some properties of the reticuloendothelial-depressing substance of the dog," Am.J.Physiol., 210 : 312-314, 1966.
7. B. Blattberg, M.N. Levy, and I. Strong, "Effect of a reticuloendothelial-depressing substance on survival from shock," J. Reticuloendothelial Soc., 3:65–70, 1966.

Effect of Dextrans on Bacterial Infections in Mice

G. M. Fukui and M. Cardinale

Wallace Laboratories
Cranbury, New Jersey

The role of humoral and cellular factors in host resistance against bacterial infections has been well documented by others [6]. Selective suppression of the reticuloendothelial system (RES) has been utilized to elucidate the role of the RES in bacterial pathogenesis, i.e., carbon or saccharinated-iron (proferrin). In search for more appropriate material for selective suppression of the RES, studies were performed with highly purified and well-characterized dextrans currently available for "molecular sieving." Bonventre and Black-Schaffer [2] reported recently that high-molecular-weight dextran sulfate, but not the low-molecular-weight dextran sulfate or nonionic dextrans, affected the susceptibility of mice to infection with Staphylococcus aureus and Shigella flexneri. They were able to correlate their findings with the function of the RES.

The studies performed in our laboratories with ionic and nonionic dextrans indicated that the nonionic, as well as the ionic dextrans, were capable of either increasing or decreasing the susceptibility of mice to infection with Streptococcus mastitidis, Pseudomonas aeruginosa, Klebsiella pneumoniae, Salmonella typhimurium, and Salmonella typhosa (Ty2). The results of our studies, however, did not necessarily indicate a direct correlation of susceptibility of mice to RES function.

MATERIALS AND METHODS

Animals

Male Swiss-Webster mice weighing 20-25 g purchased from either Carworth Farms, Inc. or Charles River Breeding Laboratories, were utilized. All mice were acclimated to our laboratory conditions for at least three days prior to use. The mice were caged in units of 10 mice per cage and maintained in a well-ventilated animal room at 22-23°C with relative humidity at 40-50%. All animals had access to fresh water and Lab-Blox mouse feed (Wayne Allied Mills, Inc., Chicago) ad libitum.

Dextrans

All nonionic and ionic dextrans were purchased from Pharmacia Fine Chemicals, Inc. A 2% stock solution was prepared in physiological-saline solution and autoclaved (15 lb/15 min) to facilitate sterilization and solubilization. Appropriate dilutions were then made with sterile physiological saline.

Bacterial Pathogens

Klebsiella pneumoniae and *Pseudomonas aeruginosa* were grown on a modified nutrient agar slant. The cultures were incubated at 24°C for 18-20 hr and harvested. *K. pneumoniae* was washed off the agar with Difco brain-heart infusion (BHI) broth and *P. aeruginosa* in physiological saline to which tryptose and gelatin were added. Appropriate dilutions for virulence titrations were made in the solutions described above to maintain viability and virulence of the cultures.

Streptococcus mastitidis was grown on Difco BHI agar slants at 37°C for 18-20 hr and harvested by washing with physiological saline.

Salmonella typhimurium and *Salmonella typhosa* were grown for 18-20 hr on Difco tryptose agar and harvested with physiological saline.

Virulence Titrations

Four to five appropriate serial dilutions of the bacterial pathogens were prepared, and 0.2 ml was injected into mice either via the IP or IV route. A minimum of 10, and in most cases 20, mice were utilized for each challenge dose. The number of dead animals was recorded daily for the appropriate number of days depending upon the pathogen under study. Representative numbers of mice were autopsied and the pathogen isolated to ascertain the causative agent of death. The effect of dextrans on the susceptibility of mice was ascertained by comparing the number of viable pathogens required to kill 50% of the saline-treated and dextran-treated mice in terms of LD_{50}. The LD_{50} values were calculated by either the Reed and Muench [5] or Litchfield and Wilcoxon [4] methods, where confidence limits were desired.

Carbon Clearance

The assay was performed according to the methods described by Biozzi, Benacerraf, and Halpern [1] with Swiss-Webster mice weighing 20-25 g. Blood samples of 0.025 ml were obtained from the retroorbital sinus at 1, 4, 7, 10, and 13 min after the injection of 4 mg of carbon via IV route. The geometric mean values obtained from bleeding 5 mice in each test group were utilized to calculate the "K" values.

Phagocytic Studies

The effect of neutral and acidic dextran sulfates on the phagocytosis of S. typhimurium (ST_{19}) was studied by in vivo and in vitro assay methods. Either 2 mg of neutral dextran or 1 mg of acidic dextran was injected into the peritoneal cavity of separate groups of mice. Thirty minutes later, $3 \cdot 10^7$ cells S. typhimurium were injected IP. After allowing 10 min for phagocytosis, peritoneal exudate was harvested and smears prepared for microscopic examination. The slides were dried and stained by the method of Machiavello. The stained slides were examined microscopically with oil immersion objective (about 1000 ×) and scored for phagocytic activity by counting 100 macrophages at random and grouping the numbers of macrophages containing 0, 1-4, or 5-10 bacteria per monocyte.

The in vitro assay was performed by using a lucite ring (1.4 × 1.0 cm) sealed at one end with a coverslip. Approximately $5 \cdot 10^5$ mouse peritoneal macrophages in 1 ml of Hanks' balanced salt solution (HBSS) with 0.1% bovine serum albumin (BSA) were allowed to fix onto the coverslip for 2 hr at 37°C. The fixed monocytes were washed 5 times with HBSS. Then, 1 ml maintenance medium containing either 2 mg of neutral dextrans or 0.1 μg of dextran sulfate 500 was placed into the chamber. After 30 min incubation at 37°C, $1 \cdot 10^7$ S. typhimurium cells in 0.2 ml of tryptose broth was added. After 10 min incubation, the lucite rings were removed and the slides washed in HBSS. The slides were dried quickly by placing them in the path of air jets at 37°C for 10 min and were stained by the method of Machiavello (basic fuchsin, citric acid, methylene blue). Slides were examined by the method described previously.

In Vivo Growth Studies

The effect of dextrans on the growth of S. typhimurium, within diffusible chambers placed into the peritoneal cavity of a mouse, was studied. The chambers were made by sealing a 1 × 1.4 cm lucite plastic ring with a Millipore filter (0.45 μ pores). The chambers were sterilized by carboxyclaving and inoculated with approximately $2 \cdot 10^4$ S. typhimurium cells. Mice were anesthetized with nembutal, incision made to insert the chamber into the peritoneal cavity, and the incision was sutured. Three groups of 10 mice with chambers were treated via IP route with either saline, 2 mg Sephadex G-100 (fine), or 1 mg of dextran sulfate 500. Two chambers from each group were removed at 1, 4, 7, and 24 hr to ascertain the number of viable cells by plating on tryptose agar.

RESULTS

Toxicity of Dextrans

The cumulative results of several mouse toxicity titrations of the various dextrans administered by either the IP or IV route are presented in

Table I. The neutral dextrans (Sephadex series) were well tolerated by mice when injected via IP route.

Neutral dextrans, as well as acidic dextrans, were generally more toxic for mice when injected via the IV route. The dextran sulfates were more toxic than the neutral dextrans when administered via the IP route.

Susceptibility – P. aeruginosa and S. typhosa

The neutral and acidic dextrans administered to mice 30 min before challenge with P. aeruginosa or S. Typhosa increased the susceptibility of

Table I. Toxicity of Various Sephadex and Dextran-SO_4 for Swiss-Webster Mice

Sample	Type	LD_{50} (mg/mouse) IP	IV
Sephadex G-25	Coarse	>25	>25
	Fine	>25	2.6
	Superfine	>25	3.1
Sephadex G-50	Coarse	>25	1.6
	Fine	>25	0.82
	Superfine	>25	1.2
Sephadex G-100	Fine	>25	0.56
	Superfine	>25	0.70
Sephadex G-200	Fine	>25	0.37
	Superfine	>25	0.72
Dextran-SO_4	500	1.8	3.9
Dextran-SO_4	2000	2.8	1.7

Table II. Effect of Various Sephadex on Susceptibility of Mice to Pseudomonas aeruginosa Infection

Sephadex Treatment Designation	Type	Pseudomonas LD_{50} (cells)
Control	(Saline)	$1.7 \cdot 10^7$
G-25	Fine	$5.7 \cdot 10^6$
	Superfine	$4.7 \cdot 10^6$
G-50	Fine	$3.1 \cdot 10^6$
	Superfine	$1.9 \cdot 10^6$
G-100	Fine	$1.4 \cdot 10^6$
	Superfine	$1.1 \cdot 10^6$
G-200	Fine	$1.0 \cdot 10^6$
	Superfine	$4.6 \cdot 10^5$

mice to infection 2 to approximately 100-fold (Tables II, III, and IV). All the Sephadex was injected via the IP route at a dose of 2 mg per mouse and the dextran sulfates at 1 mg per mouse. One-tenth mg of dextran sulfate 500 injected via IV route increased the susceptibility of mice to Pseudomonas infection about four times and a similar dose of dextran sulfate 2000 increased susceptibility of mice to Pseudomonas infection more than 13 times.

Susceptibility – K. pneumoniae

All neutral dextrans tested increased the susceptibility of mice to K. pneumoniae infection when the dextrans were administered via the IP route 30 min before challenge (Table V). The G-200 type increased the susceptibility more than 130 times, whereas G-25 type increased susceptibility about 2-3 times. Other experiments utilizing fine types of G-25 and G-50 gave results comparable to those reported for coarse G-25 and G-50. Dextran sulfate 2000 administered either by the IP (1 mg) or IV (0.1 mg) route increased the susceptibility of mice to Klebsiella infection about 5-7 times (Table VI). Although dextran sulfate 500 injected via IV route (0.1 mg) re-

Table III. Effect of Various Dextran-SO_4 on Susceptibility of Mice to Pseudomonas aeruginosa Infection

Treatment				Pseudomonas LD_{50} (cells)
Designation	Type	Dose, mg/mouse	Route	
Control	(Saline)	–	IP or IV	$9 \cdot 10^6$
Dextran-SO_4	500	1	IP	$3.2 \cdot 10^5$
Dextran-SO_4	2000	1	IP	$<7 \cdot 10^5$
Dextran-SO_4	500	0.1	IV	$1.9 \cdot 10^6$
Dextran-SO_4	2000	0.1	IV	$<7 \cdot 10^5$

Table IV. Effect of Sephadex and Dextran-SO_4 on Susceptibility of Mice to Salmonella typhosa (Ty2) Infection

Treatment	LD_{50}
Control (Saline)	$1.0 \cdot 10^8$
G-25	$9.2 \cdot 10^6$
G-50	$1.7 \cdot 10^7$
G-100	$2.2 \cdot 10^7$
G-200	$1.7 \cdot 10^7$
Dextran-SO_4 500	$1.9 \cdot 10^6$
Dextran-SO_4 2000	$6.6 \cdot 10^6$

sulted in about a 10-fold increase in susceptibility of mice to Klebsiella infection, 1 mg of dextran sulfate 500 given via IP route resulted in marginal enhancement.

Susceptibility – S. typhimurium (ST_1)

Sephadex G-25, G-50, G-100, and G-200 increased the susceptibility of mice to S. typhimurium infection at a dose of 2 mg/ mouse via the IP route and at maximum tolerated doses via the IV route (Table VII). The fine grades of G-100 and G-200 types were more effective in enhancing sus-

Table V. Effect of Various Sephadex Administered via IP Route on Infectivity of Klebsiella pneumoniae for Mice

Sephadex Treatment			Klebsiella
Designation	Type	Dose (mg/mouse)	LD_{50} (cells)
Control	(Saline)	–	130
G-25	Coarse	2	42
		5	86
		10	43
G-50	Coarse	2	54
		5	37
		10	12
G-100	Fine	2	8
		5	3
		10	1
G-200	Fine	2	<1
		5	<1
		10	<1

Table VI. Effect of Various Dextran-SO_4 on Infectivity of Klebsiella pneumoniae for Mice

Dextran-SO_4 Treatment				Klebsiella
Designation	Type	Dose (mg/mouse)	Route	LD_{50} (cells)
Control	(Saline)	–	IP or IV	148
Dextran-SO_4	500	1	IP	130
Dextran-SO_4	500	0.1	IV	14
Dextran-SO_4	2000	1	IP	30
Dextran-SO_4	2000	0.1	IV	20

ceptibility thanthe coarse grades of G-25 or G-50 types. Also, the G-100 and G-200 neutral dextrans were found to be generally more effective when administered via the IP route for S. typhimurium infections.

Dextran sulfate 500 or 2000 administered via IP route at a dose of 1 mg/mouse resulted in about a 2-fold increase in susceptibility to infection. When the dextran sulfates were injected via the IV route at a dose of 0.1 mg/mouse, the 500 series reduced the susceptibility of mice to infection about 3-fold, whereas the 200 series elicited marginal enhancement of susceptibility (Table VIII). These effects observed 5 days after infection were still evident when deaths were observed at 14 days.

Susceptibility – S. mastitidis

All neutral dextrans tested increased the susceptibility of mice to infection with S. mastitidis when the dextrans were injected via the IP

Table VII. Effect of Various Sephadex Materials on Infectivity of Salmonella typhimurium for Mice

Sephadex Treatment				
Sephadex	Type	Dose (mg/mouse)	Route	Salmonella LD_{50} (cells)
Control	(Saline)	–	IP	$6.6 \cdot 10^5$
		–	IV	$1.9 \cdot 10^5$
G-25	Coarse	2	IP	$2.1 \cdot 10^5$
		2	IV	$4.0 \cdot 10^4$
G-50	Coarse	2	IP	$7.2 \cdot 10^4$
		0.5	IV	$6.4 \cdot 10^4$
G-100	Fine	2	IP	$<1 \cdot 10^5$
		0.25	IV	$6.6 \cdot 10^4$
G-200	Fine	2	IP	$<1 \cdot 10^5$
		0.1	IV	$5.0 \cdot 10^5$

Table VIII. Effect of Dextran-SO_4 on Susceptibility of Mice to Salmonella typhimurium Infection

Dextran-SO_4 Treatment				
Designation	Type	Dose (mg/mouse)	Route	Salmonella LD_{50} (cells)
Control	(Saline)	–	IP or IV	6,000
Dextran-SO_4	500	1	IP	2,700
	500	0.1	IV	17,000
Dextran-SO_4	2000	1	IP	2,000
	2000	0.1	IV	3,900

route 30 min before challenge (Table IX). Dextran sulfate 500 and 2000 increased the susceptibility of mice when administered at a dose of 1 mg per mouse via the IP route (Table X). However, when the dextran sulfates were injected via the IV route at a dose of 0.1 mg/mouse, the mice became less susceptible to infection. All animals in this test series were challenged with S. mastitidis via the IP route.

Time

Since previous studies with endotoxin indicated that the time interval between treatment and challenge with bacterial pathogens would dictate either an increased susceptibility or increased resistance to infection (Fukui [3]), experiments were performed to study this phenomenon with dextrans. Heretofore, all the results presented on the effect of dextrans were based on experiments where the dextran was injected 30 min before challenge. Several experiments were performed where the dextrans were injected 30 min, or 1, 2, 3, or 4 days before challenge. The results of a typical virulence titration are presented in Table XI. Sephadex G-100 fine and dextran sulfate 500 were found to increase the susceptibility of mice to Pseudomonas infection when administered to mice 30 min before challenge. However, when other groups of mice were treated 1, 2, 3, or 4 days before challenge, the mice appeared to become more resistant to Pseudomonas in-

Table IX. Effect of Various Sephadex on Susceptibility of Mice to Streptococcus mastitidis Infection

Treatment via IP Route at 1 mg/mouse		Streptococcus
Designation	Type	LD_{50} (cells)
Control	(Saline)	9.2
G-25	Coarse	4.0
G-50	Coarse	2.7
G-100	Fine	2.5
G-200	Fine	1.2

Table X. Effect of Dextran-SO_4 on Susceptibility of Mice to Streptococcus mastitidis Infection

Treatment				Streptococcus
Designation	Type	Dose (mg/mouse)	Route	LD_{50} (cells)
Control	(Saline)	–	IP or IV	12
Dextran-SO_4	500	1	IP	0.64
Dextran-SO_4	2000	1	IP	2.4
Dextran-SO_4	500	0.1	IV	19
Dextran-SO_4	2000	0.1	IV	42

fection. Similar results were obtained when mice were challenged with S. typhimurium.

Growth

In order to ascertain whether the increase in susceptibility of mice to infection by dextrans might be ascribed to increasing the susceptibility of the host instead of stimulating the growth and/or virulence of the pathogen, an experiment was performed to study the effect of dextrans on the growth of S. typhimurium within semipermeable chambers placed in the peritoneal cavity of mice. The Millipore filter (0.45 μ) used to seal the chamber was found to prevent the passage of S. typhimurium without restricting the passage of liquids. Separate groups of 10 mice, with chambers containing S. typhimurium, were treated with either saline, 2 mg of Sephadex G-100 (fine), or 1 mg of dextran sulfate 500 via the IP route 5-15 min after insertion of the chamber. At 1, 4, 7, and 24 hr after the insertion of the chamber, 2 mice from each group were sacrificed and the chambers removed

Table XI. Effect of Time of Dextran-SO_4 or Sephadex G-100 (Fine) Treatment on Susceptibility of Mice to Pseudomonas aeruginosa Infection

Time	LD_{50}	
	G-100 (2 mg/mouse)	Dex-SO_4 500 (1 mg/mouse)
Control (Saline)	$1.1 \cdot 10^7$	$1.1 \cdot 10^7$
0.5 hr	$1.0 \cdot 10^6$	$2.9 \cdot 10^6$
1 Day	$1.5 \cdot 10^7$	$5.0 \cdot 10^6$
2 Days	$1.4 \cdot 10^7$	$1.5 \cdot 10^7$
3 Days	$5.1 \cdot 10^7$	$1.0 \cdot 10^7$
4 Days	$5.1 \cdot 10^7$	$4.0 \cdot 10^7$

Table XII. Effect of Dextrans on Carbon Clearance

Dextrans	Clearance Rate "K"
Control (Saline)	0.0267
Sephadex	
G-25	0.0190
G-50	0.0289
G-100	0.0227
G-200	0.0279
Acidic	
Dex-SO_4 500	0.0607
Dex-SO_4 2000	0.0538

from the peritoneal cavity. The contents of the chambers were aspirated, washed thoroughly with 1.8 ml of tryptose broth, and viable assays made by agar plating technique. Sephadex G-100 or dextran sulfate 500 did not affect the growth rate of S. typhimurium placed in chambers.

Reticuloendothelial System (RES)

Carbon clearance assays performed on mice treated with dextrans, utilizing a regimen similar to those used to study their effect on susceptibility of mice to infection, indicated that neutral dextrans did not affect the clearance rates. However, dextran sulfate 500 and 2000 at a dose of 1 mg per mouse injected into the peritoneal cavity increased the rate of carbon clearance significantly (Table XII).

Similar results were also obtained by studying the effect of neutral dextrans on the phagocytosis of S. typhimurium (ST_{19}) by mouse peritoneal

Table XIII. Effect of Neutral Dextrans (Sephadex) on In Vivo Phagocytosis of S. typhimurium (ST_{19}) by Mouse Peritoneal Macrophages

Treatment	% Macrophage Containing 0, 1-4, or 5-10 Organisms		
	0	1-4	5-10
Saline (Control)	56	44	–
G-25	52	48	–
G-50	60	36	4
G-100	44	56	–
G-200	56	40	4

Table XIV. Effect of Sephadex and Dextran-SO_4 500 on In Vitro Phagocytosis of S. typhimurium (ST_{19}) by Mouse Peritoneal Macrophages

Treatment		% Macrophage Containing 0, 1-4, or 5-10 Organisms		
Sample	Concentration (mg/ml)	0	1-4	5-10
Saline (Control)	–	48	36	16
G-25	2	52	36	12
G-50	2	52	40	8
G-100	2	56	28	16
G-200	2	44	40	16
Dextran-SO_4 500	10^{-4}	44	44	12

Table XV. Effect of Sephadex and Dextran-SO_4 on Susceptibility of Mice to Endotoxemia

Treatment via IP Route			Endotoxin LD_{50} (μg/mouse)
Designation	Type	Dose (mg/mouse)	
Control	(Saline)	–	300
G-25	Fine	2	250
G-50	Fine	2	274
G-100	Fine	2	234
G-200	Fine	2	238
Dextran-SO_4	500	1	172
Dextran-SO_4	2000	1	78

Table XVI. Effect of Dextrans on Endotoxin-Induced Resistance of Mice to *Streptococcus mastitidis* Infection

Treatment via IP Route		Endotoxin PD_{50} (μg/kg)
Endotoxin	Dextran	
+ (Control)	–	2
+	Sephadex G-100 (Fine)	58
+	Dextran-SO_4 500	>1000
+	Dextran-SO_4 2000	2

Table XVII. Effect of Dextrans on Endotoxin-Induced Resistance of Mice to *Salmonella typhimurium* Infection

Treatment via IP Route		Endotoxin PD_{50} (μg/kg)
Endotoxin	Dextran	
+ (Control)	–	31
+	Sephadex G-100 (Fine)	130
+	Dextran-SO_4 500	84
+	Dextran-SO_4 2000	6

macrophages utilizing an in vivo and in vitro assay method (Tables XIII and XIV). The ST_{19} strain of S. typhimurium was used in these studies instead of the ST_1 strain, because the ST_{19} strain was found to be much more susceptible to phagocytosis. Dextran sulfate 500 at a concentration of $1 \cdot 10^{-4}$ mg/ml of the in vitro assay system did not show any effect on phagocytosis of S. typhimurium.

Antibody

Several experiments were performed to determine the effect of dextrans on the function of protective antibodies. Mice were immunized with either capsular material obtained from K. pneumoniae or heat-killed Klebsiella. Upon waiting seven days after the administration of the vaccine, the mice were treated with dextrans and challenged with K. pneumoniae. The results of the titrations indicated that the dextrans did not interfere with the protective action of the antibodies.

Endotoxin – Toxemia

Various Sephadex materials injected into the peritoneal cavity of mice prior to the injection of endotoxin (Difco E. coli LPS) elicited marginal increase in susceptibility to the lethal effects of endotoxin. The dextran sulfates increased the susceptibility of mice to endotoxin more effectively (Table XV).

Endotoxin – Protection

When Sephadex G-100 or dextran sulfate 500 was injected into mice 15-30 min before challenging mice pretreated with endotoxin, greater amounts of endotoxin were required to protect the mice against S. mastitidis or S. typhimurium infections (Tables XVI and XVII). In contrast to the above results, dextran sulfate 2000 did not minimize the protective effects of endotoxin against S. mastitidis infection. Furthermore, dextran sulfate 2000 appears to reinforce the protective effects of endotoxin against S. typhimurium infections.

DISCUSSION

Neutral or nonionic dextrans were generally well tolerated by mice when injected into the peritoneal cavity, whereas neutral dextrans were found to be toxic when injected into the veins of mice. The acidic dextrans were found to be equally toxic for mice when injected IP or IV. The neutral dextrans, as well as the high-molecular-weight acidic dextran sulfates, generally increased the susceptibility of mice to infection with the various bacterial pathogens tested. Depending upon the pathogen under study, the effect on increasing susceptibility was greater when the dextran was injected IV. These results confirm the observations reported by Bonventre and Black-Schaffer [2] in regard to the effect of dextran sulfates when studying infections with S. aureus and S. flexneri. However, in our studies utilizing other bacterial pathogens the neutral dextrans have been found also to influence the susceptibility of mice to infection.

The fact that the neutral dextrans were found to increase susceptibility of mice to infections with P. aeruginosa, K. pneumoniae, S. mastitidis, S. typhimurium, and S. typhosa (Ty2) may be ascribed to the differences in the natural host defense mechanism operative against these pathogens as compared to those for S. aureus and S. flexneri. Moreover, there may be other subtle but important differences in the experimental conditions, animals, molecular weights, cross-linkages, or mode of sterilization which may account for the lack of activity ascribed to neutral dextrans by Bonventre and Black-Schaffer.

The carbon clearance-enhancing effects found with dextran sulfate 500 and 2000 correlated nicely with their effects in increasing the susceptibility of mice to infection. This observation and correlation was in agreement with those findings by Bonventre and Black-Schaffer utilizing the liver perfusion method to determine the effect of dextran sulfate 500 on clearance of S. aureus. However, this correlation of carbon clearance and enhanced susceptibility to infection could not be demonstrated with the neutral dextrans, in that they did not affect carbon clearance rate or phagocytosis of S. typhimurium. This discrepancy in the effects on carbon clearance may underscore the differences in the primary host defense mechanism that may be operative against a specific pathogen, i.e., humoral or cellular factors.

As with endotoxin, in most instances when the dextrans were administered 30 min prior to challenge, mice became more susceptible to infection. The exception in this regard was noted when mice were challenged with S. mastitidis after IV administration of dextran sulfate 500 or 2000 and when dextran sulfate 500 was injected via the IV route and challenged with S. typhimurium. As the time period between the injection of dextrans increased, the animals became less susceptible to bacterial infection.

The results of experiments directed to ascertain the effects of dextrans on protective antibodies indicated that neither the neutral nor acidic dextrans, at doses found to increase the susceptibility of mice to bacterial infections, apparently affected the protective function of antibodies.

We conjectured, as did Bonventre and Black-Schaffer [2], that the increase in susceptibility of mice by dextrans was more an effect on the host than on the infecting bacteria. An experiment was therefore performed to determine if Sephadex G-100 and dextran sulfate 500 might also stimulate the growth of S. typhimurium. The experiment was performed with a diffusion chamber placed in the peritoneal cavity to simulate in vivo conditions without the intervention of phagocytosis which might make it difficult to observe and interpret the effects of dextrans on the growth of S. typhimurium. The results of the experiment indicated that dextrans under the experimental conditions did not affect the growth rate of S. typhimurium.

The potentiation of the lethal action of endotoxin by dextrans, and the reduction of the protective action of endotoxin with Sephadex G-100 and dextran sulfate 500 were found to be comparable with the effects of dextrans on the susceptibility of mice to infection. However, the effect of dextran sulfate 2000 administered via the IP route on the protective effects of endotoxin was not anticipated. Since 1 mg of dextran sulfate 2000 administered via IP route elicited no effect on the susceptibility of mice to S. typhimurium infection (Table XIII), it was surprising to find that dextran sulfate 2000 treatment reduced the amount of endotoxin required to protect mice against S. typhimurium infection.

SUMMARY AND CONCLUSION

1. Neutral dextrans were found to be essentially not toxic for mice when injected via the IP route, but toxic when injected via the IV route.

2. Acidic dextran sulfates were found to be equally toxic for mice when injected by either the IP or IV routes.

3. Neutral, as well as acidic dextrans, generally increased the susceptibility of mice to infection when administered 30 min before infection, but they increased resistance to infection when given 2-4 days before infection.

4. The results of carbon-clearance assays, relating to the function of RES, correlated well only with the effects of acidic dextrans on increasing the susceptibility of mice to infection. Therefore, the basis for the action of neutral dextrans on susceptibility appears to be due to the suppression of host defense factors other than the RES.

5. Neutral and acidic dextrans did not appear to interfere with protective antibodies or affect the growth rate of bacterial pathogens.

6. Dextrans increased the susceptibility of mice to the lethal action of endotoxin and increased the amounts of endotoxin required to protect mice against infection. The only exception noted was that dextran sulfate 2000 appeared to potentiate the protective action of endotoxin against infection with Salmonella typhimurium.

REFERENCES

1. G. Biozzi, B. Benacerraf, and B.N. Halpern, Brit.J.Exptl.Pathol., 36:226, 1955.
2. P.F. Bonventre and B. Black-Schaffer, J.Infect.Diseases, 115:413, 1965.
3. G.M. Fukui, Bacterial Endotoxins. Rahway, New Jersey, Quinn and Boden Co., 1964, p. 373.

4. J.T. Litchfield, Jr. and F. Wilcoxon, J.Pharmacol.Exptl.Therap., 96:99, 1949.
5. L.J. Reed and H. Muench, Am.J.Hyg., 27:493, 1938.
6. M. Shilo, Ann.Rev.Microbiol., 13:255, 1959.
7. M. Shilo, Bacterial Endotoxins, Rahway, New Jersey, Quinn and Boden Co., 1964, p. 382.

Prevention and Treatment of Friend Leukemia Virus (FLV) Infection by Interferon-Inducing Synthetic Polyanions*

W. Regelson †

Department of Medicine A
Roswell Park Memorial Institute
Buffalo, New York

ABSTRACT. Divinyl ether maleic anhydride (MA) copolymers (pyran copolymer, NSC 46015) inhibits Friend leukemia virus (FLV) splenomegaly. Pyran copolymer induces interferon in normal mice and the decreases in splenic FLV titers seen following pretreatment with these polyanions might be explained by the appearance of interferon. In vivo inhibition of FLV splenomegaly has also been obtained by statolon, an anionic polysaccharide, and the plant lectin, phytohemagglutinin, both of which have been reported to induce interferon. Similar inhibition of FLV splenomegaly has also been seen for methyl vinyl ether/MA and styrene/MA copolymers. Pyran copolymer is currently undergoing clinical trial in man. Its animal and human pharmacology indicates uptake in the nucleated formed elements of the blood, and stimulation of reticuloendothelial activity in liver, spleen, and bone marrow.

Some polyanions possess antitumor [1-5] and antiviral activity [6, 7], and Kleinschmidt et al. [8, 9] have shown induction of interferon by statolon, an anionic polysaccharide that inhibits FLV [10]. In this study, polyanionic divinyl ether maleic anhydride (MA) copolymers, which are polycarboxylic

* This work was accomplished with the support of USPHS grants CY-3887, C-5834, and C-2821, and the technical assistance of O. Foltyn in our laboratory. We wish to thank W. J. Kleinschmidt, Lilly Research Laboratories, for interferon assays. Statistical evaluation of data was done with the help of Roger L. Priore, Sc.D., of the Department of Biostatistics, Roswell Park Memorial Institute, Buffalo, New York.

† Currently, Professor, Chief Division of Medical Oncology, Medical College of Virginia, Richmond, Virginia 23219.

Table I

Expt. No.	Drug	Av. MW of Polymer	Mg/kg inj	Treatment Sequence (days) Pre	Post	Mice, Rx/Control	Dead, Rx/Control	Mouse wt. Change, Rx/Control	Spleen wt., mg	± Standard Error, mg Rx/Control	% Inhibition
505	NSC 46015-c (clinical)	17,000	250		6	10/20	2/1	3.8/8.9	430/1192	41/108	64
540	NSC 68988	450,000	250		6	10/10	0/2	6.7/6.5	763/1650	132/71	54
507	NSC 46015-c (clinical)	17,000	250	6		15/15	5/0	6.0/13.2	387/1428	66/164	72
514	NSC 46015 (laboratory)	36,000	62.5	6		20/20	1/3	15.6/16.8	379/1286	24/127	70
			125	6		20/20	3/3	12.8/16.8	378/1286	17/127	71
			250	6		20/20	5/3	10.3/16.8	432/1286	26/127	66
528	NSC 46015 (laboratory)	36,000	15.6	6		10/20	3/3	13.2/13.6	274/1741	43/144	84
			31.25	6		10/20	0/3	13.4/13.6	556/1741	196/144	68
			62.5	6		10/20	3/3	11.8/13.6	548/1741	54/144	68
536	NSC 46015 (laboratory)	36,000	125	1		10/10	1/0	13.6/10.2	378/1640	88/216	72
529	NSC 46015 (laboratory)	36,000	125	1		10/10	0/0	14.1/13.1	441/1669	62/207	74

copolymers in similar fashion to statolon, increased host resistance to FLV splenomegaly, and were shown to induce serum interferon in normal mice. Decreases in splenic FLV titers following pretreatment with these synthetic polyanions might be explained by the appearance of interferon.

One of these divinyl ether maleic anhydride copolymers of molecular weight 17,000, pyran 3,4-dicarboxylic anhydride (Pyran copolymer, NSC 46015-c), is undergoing clinical trial against advanced cancer in man. Its animal and clinical pharmacology indicates uptake in the nucleated formed elements of the blood and stimulation of reticuloendothelial (RE) activity in liver, spleen, and bone marrow.

The action of these polyanions may be similar to that of kidney bean phytohemagglutinin (PHA) which similarly inhibits Friend Virus splenomegaly [10], and which has been shown by Wheelock to induce interferon-like activity in vitro [11].

MATERIALS AND METHODS

Friend Leukemia Virus is obtained from the spleens of male Ha/ICR Swiss mice four weeks after infection. Donor mice are four weeks old at the time of FLV infection and virus is obtained immediately after sacrifice by filtering a 10% homogenate of pooled spleens in cold Locke–Ringer solution through a 0.45-μ Millipore filter. Unless otherwise indicated, 0.2 ml of this virus suspension is given intraperitoneally to male Ha/ICR recipient mice which are uniform in age and weight, randomized, kept ten per cage, and fed Derwood–Morris pellets. Wherever possible, an attempt was made to use mice between 15 and 20 g. For studies of viral titers in treated animals, 0.2 ml virus suspension was given as described above after dilution in Locke–Ringer solution to 10^{-1}-10^{-6}.

Mice were usually sacrificed eight days after virus inoculation, or at intervals as indicated, and their spleens were weighed. The time of drug injection and evaluation of splenic weights are indicated for each experiment reported. All compounds used were dissolved in saline and given in a volume of 0.5 ml intraperitoneally and compared to saline-injected controls.

The "t" test was used to determine the significance of differences in average splenic weights between the treated and control. In all cases the difference was significant at the 5% level.

Periodic checks of splenic morphology showed no departure from the pathology originally described by Friend and others.

Interferon induction assays using inhibition of plaque formation induced by MCN mouse cell vesicular stomatitis virus (VSV) on mouse embryo cells

Table II. Pretreatment for 6 Days. Experiment No. 528

Drug	Dose, mg/kg	No. of Mice, Start/End	Wt. Gain of mice, g	Spleen,* mg	% Inhibition
Saline	0.5 cc	20/17	13.6	1741	
Phytohemagglutinin	83	10/10	13.6	622	64
	41.5	10/10	13.9	617	64
Pyran polymer† (NSC 46015)	62.5	10/7	11.8	548	68
	31.25	10/10	13.4	556	68
	15.6	10/7	13.2	274	84
Statolon	250	10/8	13.2	369	79
	125	10/10	14.4	310	82
	62.5	10/9	12.1	583	67
	31.25	10/9	16.6	912	48
Saline	0.5 cc	10/10	12.3	153‡	
Phytohemagglutinin	83	10/10	12.6	149‡	
Pyran polymer	125	10/9	11.9	482‡	
Statolon	250	10/9	13.2	200‡	

*Spleens were evaluated eight days after FLV inoculation.
†All studies on laboratory fraction MW 36,000.
‡Normal spleens.

[7] were done through the courtesy of W.J. Kleinschmidt.* Interferon activity was determined from pooled serum samples obtained at intervals following intraperitoneal pyran copolymer injection into uniform groups of normal Ha/ICR mice.

RESULTS

Table I summarizes 11 typical consecutive experiments where divinyl ether/MA copolymers† were given at daily intervals 24 hr past FLV inoculation, as pretreatment for six days or by single injection up to 24 hr prior to FLV inoculation and compared to saline-injected controls. Out of 17 consecutive experiments performed, inhibition ranged from 54-84% for a median of 71%. In each experiment, the inhibition was statistically significant at the 5% level, as measured by the difference between the mean of each treatment group and its saline-injected control. In no experiment was weight loss found, although at higher repetitive doses treated mice gained

*Eli Lilly Laboratories, Indianapolis, Indiana.
† Courtesy of Dr. H. Wood, Jr., 7550 Wisconsin Avenue, Bethesda, Maryland and H. Espy, Hercules Powder Company, Wilmington, Delaware.

less rapidly. Nowhere did deaths exceed one-third of the animals present at the outset.

Treatment following FLV infection with pyran copolymers was successful only during the first week. Treatment of established splenomegaly (one week after FLV injection) did not produce significant regression of splenic weight.

In Table II (Expt. 528), note that pyran copolymer behaves similarly to phytohemagglutinin (PHA) and statolon* in inhibiting FLV splenomegaly when given for 6 days prior to FLV inoculation. However, unlike statolon and PHA, pyran copolymer produces splenomegaly on treatment of normal mice. Similar effects have been obtained with a pyran copolymer of average MW 17,000 (NSC 46015-c), which is currently under clinical trial.

Single injections of pyran copolymer, statolon, or PHA produced similar degrees of inhibition of FLV splenomegaly. However, distinct differences were seen between the synthetic pyran copolymer, PHA, and statolon, depending on the time of drug injection in relation to viral inoculation. Statolon was effective as a single injection after viral infection, whereas pyran copolymer and PHA were not (Fig. 1), but the reverse was true on treatment prior to FLV infection. In other experiments, statolon was unlike pyran copolymer in that it produced consistent significant regression of established FLV splenomegaly. Thus, the character of the polyanion used seems to affect the results seen, For example, in contrast to pyran copolymer and statolon (Fig. 2), native heparin given 24 hr prior to virus inoculation decreased host resistance, as evidenced by increased splenic growth. In contrast, phytohemagglutinin on pretreatment 24 hr before FLV inoculation behaves similarly to pyran copolymer and statolon in inhibiting eight-day-old FLV splenomegaly (Fig. 2).

In similar fashion to heparin, methyl vinyl ether maleic anhydride copolymers† (Expt. 562, Table III) of MW 1,250,000 and 500,000 appeared to increase FLV splenomegaly. These results may reflect interference with normal host defenses which may be dependent on the dose and timing of the polyanion administered (Expt. 551, Table III). However, regardless of whether FLV splenic growth is stimulated or not, the dicarboxylic copolymers of methyl vinyl ether maleic anhydride and their amide-acid derivatives of MW 250,000 or 1,250,000 can both show inhibitory activity (Table III). These results confirm those of previous in vivo studies of inhibition of transplanted tumors with ethylene maleic anhydride copolymers [4].

Styrene maleic anhydride copolymers of MW 1.4-70,000 also inhibit FLV splenomegaly on pretreatment‡ (Table III).

---

* Eli Lilly Laboratories, Indianapolis, Indiana.

† Courtesy of L. McCory, General Aniline & Film Co., New York, New York.

‡ Courtesy of J. Johnson, Monsanto Co., St. Louis, Missouri.

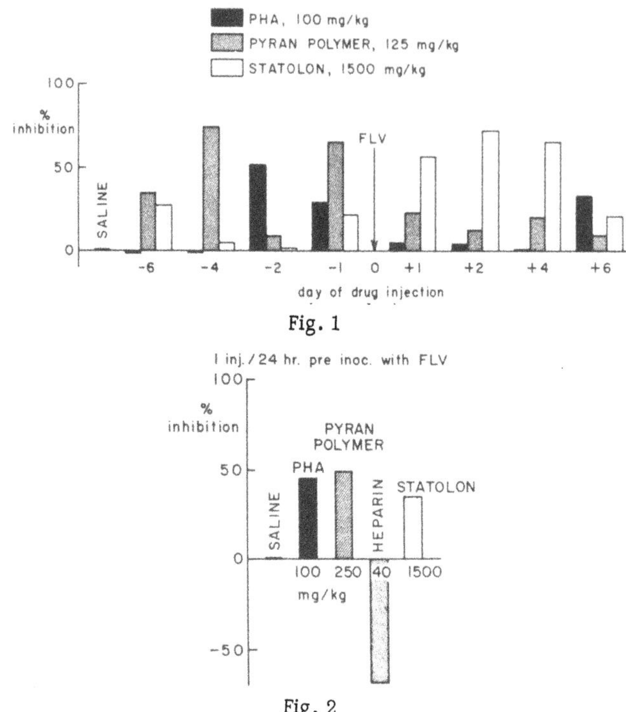

Fig. 1

Fig. 2

Figs. 1 and 2. Percent inhibition of FLV spleen weights following single injection on days indicated. Splenomegaly is evaluated eight days after FLV infection.

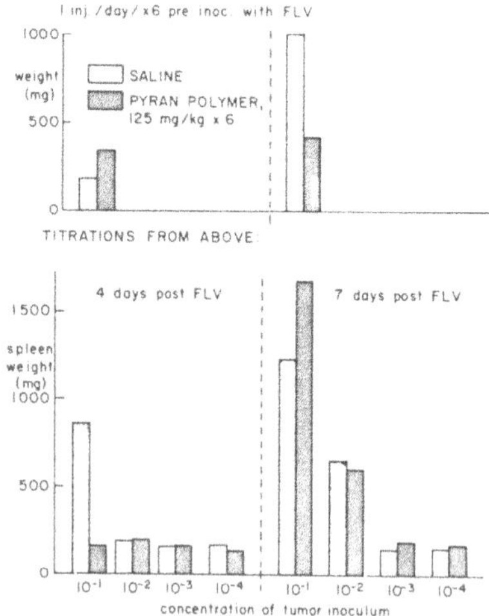

Fig. 3. The effect of FLV titration from infected spleens inhibited by pretreatment for six days 24 hr prior to FLV infection.

Table III. The Effect of Methyl Vinyl Ether/Maleic Anhydride and Styrene Maleic Anhydride Copolymers of Differing Molecular Weights (MW) Given 24 hr Prior to Friend Viral Inoculation

Drug		Average MW	Dose, mg/kg	No. of Mice, Start/End	Wt. Gain of Mice, g	Spleen,* mg	% Inhibition
Experiment 562:							
Saline			0.5 cc	20/20	11.7	1081	
	Methyl Vinyl Ether/MA						
ELMW		<250,000	1500	10/6	8.2	481	55
AN-109	Dicarboxylic	250,000	1000	10/9	9.2	461	57
AN-119	Dicarboxylic	>250,000	1000	10/9	10.2	956	11
AN-4151	Half amide	250,000	500	10/10	6.7	489	55
AN-169	Dicarboxylic	1,250,000	500	10/9	8.4	1616	−49
AN-4651	Half amide	1,250,000	500	10/10	7.2	556	49
AN-3391	Half methyl ester	500,000	150	10/6	9.6	1416	−31
Experiment 551:							
Saline			0.5 cc	20/19	7.8	1640	
	Methyl Vinyl Ether/MA						
AN-169	Dicarboxylic	1,250,000	200	20/19	8.8	1160	29
AN-4651	Half amide	1,250,000	1000	20/19	8.1	600	63
	Styrene/MA						
S-810	Dicarboxylic	1,400	25	20/18	5.8	227	86
S-811	Dicarboxylic	10,000	25	20/12	7.6	353	78
S-812	Dicarboxylic	70,000	25	20/20	9.3	331	80

*Spleens were evaluated eight days after FLV inoculation.

Table IV

Treatment	Dose of Drug, mg/kg of Mouse	Concn. of FLV, %	Wt. Gain of Mice, g	Spleen wt., mg
FLV		10	11.6	1108
		1	12.2	366
		.1	12.4	248
		.01	12.4	146
		.001	11.8	165
Pyran polymer + FLV	100	10	13.0	255
($1.6 \cdot 10^{-5}$ M)	100	1	11.0	264
	100	.1	10.0	304
	100	.01	11.4	286
	100	.001	7.2	256
Pyran polymer + FLV	100	10	11.4	547
	10	10	10.0	1418
	1	10	10.4	1176
	.1	10	10.8	814
	.01	10	10.6	1601

Virus suspension (0.2 cc) and pyran copolymer (NSC 46015, 0.64 mg, MW 36,000 in 0.2 cc) incubated together at room temperature for 30 min before inoculation. Five mice/group studied. Splenomegaly was evaluated eight days after FLV-copolymer inoculation.

Table V

Drug	Dose	No. of Inj.	No. of Mice, Start/End	Wt. Gain of Mice, g	Spleen wt.,mg	% Inhibition
Saline	0.5 cc	6	10/10	13.1	1669	
Saline + pyran *	0.5 + 125	6 + 1	10/10	14.1	441	74
Pertussis vaccine †	0.1 cc	6	10/8	11.5	1021	39
Pertussis vaccine + pyran	0.1 cc + 125	6 + 1	10/6	12.4	1043	37
Pyran polymer	125	6	10/6	11.8	446	73

*Pyran copolymer, 125 mg/kg, was given to the mice 1 hr after the sixth daily injection of saline or pertussis vaccine. FLV was inoculated 24 hr later.

† Pertussis vaccine was obtained through the courtesy of Wyeth Laboratories, Philadelphia, Pennsylvania.

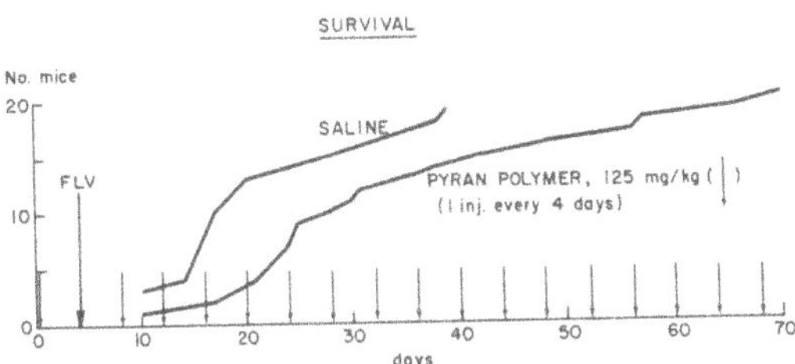

Fig. 4. Number of deaths/day following FLV inoculation. Pyran copolymer treated compared to saline control.

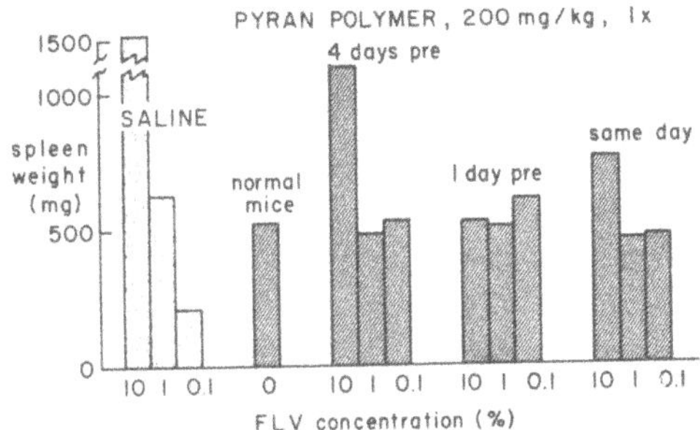

Fig. 5. Spleen weights after intravenous infection with FLV after single intraperitoneal drug injection 4 days, 1 day, and 1 hr before FLV inoculation.

Attempts were made to determine the mechanism of inhibition of FLV splenomegaly (Fig. 3). Virus titers were obtained four and seven days after FLV inoculation from pyran copolymer-inhibited spleens. It can be seen from the subsequent growth of spleens obtained that, at day 4 post-FLV injection following six daily doses of pyran copolymer at 125 mgm/kg, given up to 24 hr prior to virus inoculation, there was significant decrease in virus titer. But this was not true for seven-day-old treated spleens despite the significant reduction (57%) of splenic size. Similar results have been obtained with phytohemagglutinin.

On single injection of pyran copolymer 24 hr prior to virus inoculation, the inhibitory effect was manifested only during the first week. Therefore, it was not surprising to find that a single injection prior to FLV inoculation showed no major effect on survival although injection beginning every fourth day prior to and following virus injection significantly prolonged survival (Fig. 4).

Pyran copolymer showed in vitro viral neutralizing activity when incubated at room temperature for 30 min prior to inoculation into host mice (Table IV). At an in vitro molar concentration of $1.6 \cdot 10^{-5}$, which was equal to an in vivo concentration of 100 mgm/kg of pyran copolymer per mouse, there was little or no active virus present, even with 10% viral suspensions. However, with dilution of pyran copolymer to a level below 10^{-5} molar, the antiviral effect was lost. In another experiment of in vitro neutralization, the inhibitory effect was still present up to four weeks after virus copolymer inoculation with in vitro molar concentrations of pyran copolymer of $2 \cdot 10^{-5}$.

In the mouse the effect may be mediated by other than direct neutralization. In vivo antivirus effect was present when pyran copolymers were given intraperitoneally to intravenous Friend Virus. In this case, pretreatment four days prior to virus inoculation was not effective at the 10% concentration of FLV, but was effective 24 hr before or simultaneously with intravenous virus injection (Fig. 5). Again, it can be seen that pyran copolymer induces splenomegaly in normal mice.

In attempts to determine the role of the reticuloendothelial system (RES) in the antiviral antitumor effects seen, it was found that pretreatment of mice for six days with pertussis vaccine blocked the inhibitory action of pyran copolymer when the polyanion was given 24 hr prior to FLV inoculation (Table V).

Table VI. Interferon Induction

Sample Injected	Dose / 0.5 cc	Interferon Units					
		0 hr	12 hr	24 hr	48 hr	72 hr	144 hr
Experiment A:							
Saline control		<20	<20	<20	<20	<20	<20
Pyran copolymer / NSC 46015 (laboratory)	125 mgm/kg / MW-36,000	<20	90	159	25	<20	<20
Experiment B:							
Saline control		–	–	60	–	–	–
Noninjected control		–	–	53	–	–	–
Pyran copolymers / NSC 46015-c (clinical)	125 mgm/kg / MW-17,000	–	–	187	–	–	–
X13083-57-H6	40,000	–	–	219	–	–	–
NSC 68987	110,000	–	–	246	–	–	–
NSC 68988	450,000	–	–	205	–	–	–

Five normal mice pooled/sample. In experiment B, assays were done 24 hr following drug injection.

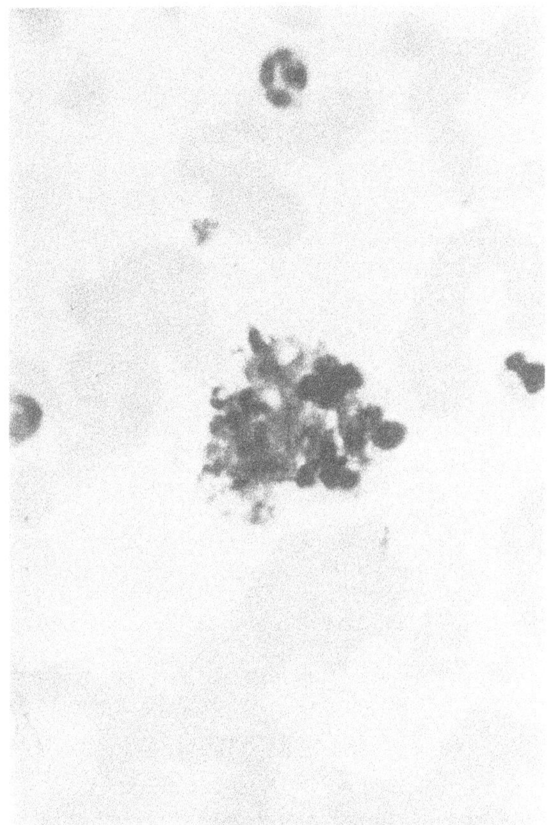

Fig. 6. Bone marrow histiocyte of patient who received intravenous pyran copolymer (NSC 46015, MW 17,000) for two weeks at 8 mg/kg (Wright and Giemsa stain).

Following these observations, interferon assays were made on the serum of normal mice following a single injection of vinyl ether maleic anhydride (pyran) copolymers. It can be seen from Table VI that serum interferon is induced as measured by VSV plaque inhibition. Molecular weight ranges of synthetic pyran copolymers between 17-450,000 did not differ significantly in their ability to induce interferon.

As was suggested by the increases in splenic weight observed in normal mice (Table II, Fig. 5), pyran copolymers histologically stimulate splenic RES activity.

In human pharmacologic study, intravenously administered pyran copolymer (NSC 46015-c; MW 17,000) produces thrombocytopenia, increased histiocytic activity of the liver, spleen, and bone marrow with the appearance of cytoplasmic inclusions in nucleated formed elements of the blood.

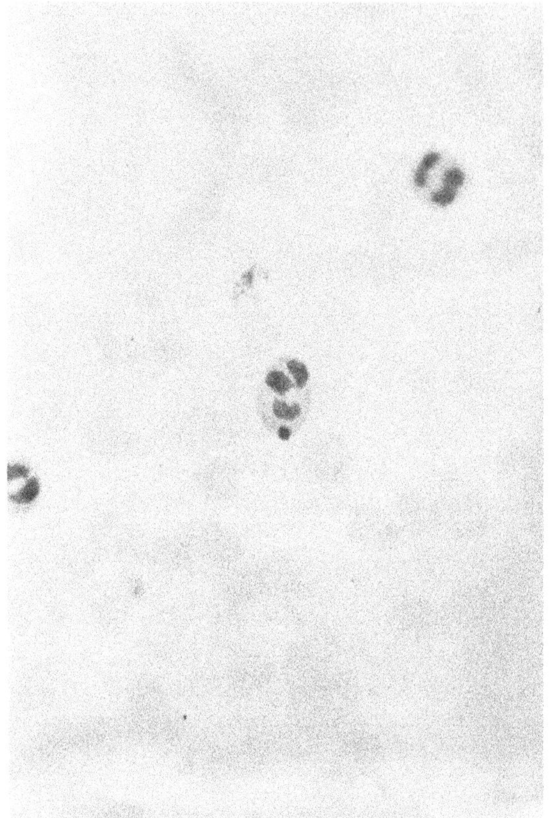

Fig. 7. A neutrophil of same patient as in Fig. 6 showing a basophilic inclusion (Wright–Giemsa stain).

Figures 6-8 show the bone marrow and peripheral blood of a patient who received pyran copolymer (NSC 46015-c) at 8 mg/kg for two weeks as a single rapid daily intravenous injection. Note the basophilic inclusions in a histiocyte of the bone marrow (Fig. 6). Similar inclusions were seen in circulating granulocytes (Fig. 7) and monocytes (Fig. 8) of the peripheral blood, as well as in the histiocytes of liver and spleen at autopsy. These inclusions stain metachromatically and probably represent pyran copolymer deposited within the cell.

DISCUSSION

The foregoing experiments compare the inhibitory effect of synthetic polyanions with statolon, a naturally occurring anionic polysaccharide, and phytohemagglutinin, a plant lectin, on FLV infection. Although past studies have shown that synthetic polyanions show significant inhibitory activity against established transplanted rodent tumors [1-5], the effect against FLV splenomegaly is significant only during the proliferative phase.

Attempts were made to determine the mechanism of the inhibition obtained, and it was found that following Friend Leukemia Virus infection and effective drug-induced inhibition, that there was a decrease of in vivo virus titers in the spleen four days after virus inoculation, but this effect was lost at seven days and beyond. This observation relates to two phenomena. One is suggested by the observed direct in vitro neutralization of the virus which would imply a direct polymer neutralization effect for antiviral activity seen (Table IV). Direct in vitro virus neutralization effects have been seen for phytohemagglutinin with FLV [10] and for polyanions with other viruses [6, 7]. However, it is difficult to accept this as the sole explanation for the in vivo antiviral and antitumor effect, since inhibition of FLV splenomegaly occurs following a single intraperitoneal injection prior to intraperitoneal virus inoculation as long as four days before the introduction of

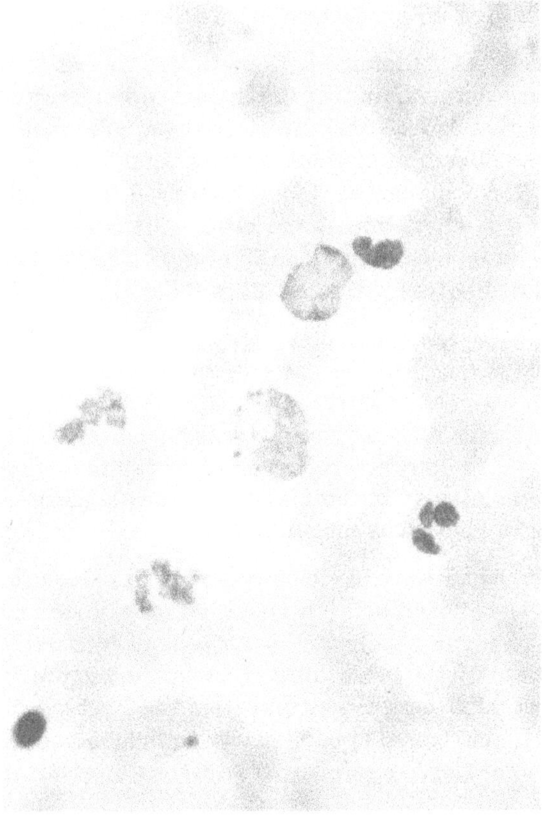

Fig. 8. A circulating monocyte with basophilic cytoplasmic inclusions seen in same patient as in Figs. 6 and 7 (Wright–Giemsa stain).

FLV infection (Fig. 1). Similarly, inhibition was also seen on injection of statolon within the first week, 24-72 hr after virus inoculation (Fig. 1). In addition, inhibition of FLV splenomegaly was obtained despite intravenous virus inoculation following intraperitoneal pyran copolymer injection (Fig.5).

The fact that pretreatment prior to virus inoculation could modify host response to virus-induced splenomegaly growth suggested that the anti-FLV effects of the synthetic polyanions might be mediated through factors altering host resistance. In this regard, the similarity between statolon effects on inhibiting FLV splenic proliferation with that occurring following the administration of synthetic polyanions suggested that both might act in similar fashion.

Statolon is a complex anionic polysaccharide macromolecule containing galacturonic acid, derived from fermentation of Penicillium stoloniferum [13]. It prophylactically inhibits virus infection in animals and tissue culture. Inhibition has been seen against multiple viruses [14-19], including Rous sarcoma [16] as well as Friend leukemia [10]. More recently, statolon has been shown to exert its antiviral action by stimulating the in vitro [8] and in vivo [9] production of interferon [20].

Statolon possesses a biologic action similar to that of lipopolysaccharides derived from bacteria, in that it can on prior injection nonspecifically protect mice and rats from lethal infection from Salmonella and pneumococci [19]. These effects of statolon on host resistance may be similar to what Elliott and Higgenbotham [21] have observed for the effect of sulfated carrageenin which protects mice from encephalomyocarditis (EMC) virus. This was thought to be mediated via RES stimulation secondary to accumulation of the sulfated polysaccharide within the cell.

In this regard, pyran copolymer appears to be phagocytosed by histiocytes (Fig. 6) and these observations may be pertinent to our finding that 24 hr after pyran copolymer injection significant levels of interferon are induced in mice (Table VI). Although the serum levels of interferon obtained for statolon are 10 times those achieved for divinyl ether maleic anhydride copolymers, levels of interferon of 159-426 units may still be capable of inhibiting in vivo virus multiplication.

Phytohemagglutinin has also been reported to induce interferon [11] and, despite the fact that interferon induction may be common to all these compounds, unlike pyran copolymer or phytohemagglutinin, statolon may exert a direct effect on the established FLV splenic growth. Statolon produced significant inhibition when given within the first week after virus inoculation (Fig. 1), and has also been shown to induce regression of established FLV splenomegaly, even one to two weeks after viral inoculation.

It is not surprising that both stimulation and inhibition of FLV splenomegaly can occur dependent on the polyanion used and the timing of its administration (Fig. 2, Table III). Similar effects have been observed on polio virus plaque formation depending on the molecular weight of the dextran sulfate fractions used [22, 23]. This may be pertinent to the observations that large quantities of interferon added exogenously to tissue culture cells block interferon production on subsequent virus infection while small quantities enhance interferon production [24, 25].

We have not yet studied the levels of interferon produced on repeated polyanion administration or subsequent virus infection, but it should be noted that administration of pyran copolymer, every fourth day, enhanced the survival of mice infected with FLV (Fig. 5).

Merigan and Kleinschmidt [26] have shown that splenic interferon is a different species from that found in the serum. The splenic enlargement and RES stimulation produced in normal mouse spleens by pyran copolymer may reflect local increases in interferon production that may interfere with local FLV replication regardless of the serum levels. This is supported by recent work of Fruitstone et al. [27], who found that splenectomy decreases interferon production and enhances viral susceptibility in mice.

On pretreatment of mice with pertussis vaccine for six days, reversal of the inhibiting action of pyran copolymer given 24 hr prior to virus inoculation on FLV splenomegaly was seen (Table V). Pertussis vaccine has been observed to block interferon activity [28]. This also suggests that the mechanism of action of the synthetic polyanions may be mediated via the RES for it is well known that bacterial endotoxins stimulate the release instead of the production of interferon [29]. In this regard, it remains to be seen how the synthetic polyanions produce their effect, inasmuch as statolon and phytohemagglutinin appear to be true inducers of interferon production [8, 9, 11, 26, 30]. However, the induction of interferon need not be a primary effect, as destruction of vulnerable cells by synthetic polyanions could release native nucleic acid polymers which in turn could be the true inducers of the interferon obtained.

Whatever the mechanism, cellular uptake of synthetic polyanions may be necessary for interferon induction or the antiviral effect seen. Leucocytes and the RES have been found to be prime producers of interferon following infection [11, 26, 31, 32] and splenomegaly and cytoplasmic inclusions were seen in hepatic, splenic, and bone marrow histiocytes (Fig. 6) of patients who received pyran copolymer. Inclusions were also found in circulating nucleated formed elements of the blood (Figs. 7 and 8).

Thrombocytopenia that has been observed clinically in eight of 34 patients receiving pyran copolymer suggests that platelet or megakaryocyte uptake may also occur.

Inclusions that were seen in vivo may be similar to what has been seen by Takemoto and Spicer [33] for dextran sulfate in HeLa cells in vitro. Their work with dextran sulfate and previous work we have done in vitro with ethylene maleic anhydride copolymers [6], suggest that the higher molecular weight polymers appeared to be the most active viral inhibitors. We cannot say this for the in vivo data of this study as the evidence supports good inhibition of FLV splenomegaly for a wide range of molecular weights (1400-450,000) and equal interferon-inducing capacity was found for all molecular weight ranges of pyran copolymer studied (Table VI).

In an extensive study, Vaheri [7] tested heparin and a variety of polyanionic polymers of natural and synthetic origin. The degree of viral inhibition produced by these polyanions seemed to correlate with their in vitro ability to agglutinate chicken red cells and with their toxicity to HeLa cells in culture. Also, all these active inhibitors showed potent heparin-like antithrombin action, metachromatic activity, and the ability to alter the growth behavior of HeLa cells on glass [7]. In this regard, both synthetic polyanions [34] and phytohemagglutin [34a] induce cell aggregation of ascites tumor cells in vivo and in vitro, which has been associated with decreases in cellular RNA and protein content [33, 34].

Apart from the above, the action of polyanions as inhibitors of viral action may be mediated through other pathways. In some cases it is obviously a function of electrostatic binding between the virus and the polyanion macromolecule. Pyran copolymer (NSC 46015) probably inhibits T_4 bacteriophage [35] in this way. In other cases, which may be more pertinent to the biologic antiviral activity of the polyanions, it blocks viral adsorption and can interfere with viral recycling as long as it is present in the medium [6, 7]. The need for cells to be present for the antiviral action to be manifested is consistent with the possibility that interferon production may be involved.

The action of polyanions may also be mediated through inhibition of enzymes important for viral adsorption. However, attempts to correlate antiviral action with inhibition of ribonuclease, hyaluronidase, and antithrombin activity has not been successful [7, 36]. Pertinent is the observation that the polyanion, polyethylene sulfonate, inhibits deoxyribonucleotide transferase [37], which may be necessary for viral synthesis.

Although Nahamias et al. [38] suggested that the antiviral action of polyanions may be similar to polyanion interaction with lipoprotein [39], this was not supported by Vaheri's [7] observations. However, it is still possible to consider that lipase and esterase activation or inhibition by polyanions may be pertinent to their mechanism of action, perhaps related to alteration of lipoproteins in lipid-containing viruses or through effects on lipoproteins at cell surfaces [39]. This is of interest in that polyanions can activate lipases to make available free fatty acids [40]. Furthermore, as lipid fractions can provide stimulation of the RES which can increase resistance to Rous and Friend viruses [41], the action of polyanions could be mediated via changes in RES lipid distribution.

It may be that the major in vivo mechanism for virus inhibition by polyanions is interferon induction, but regardless of how they work, the clinical testing of one such polyanion, pyran copolymer (NSC 46015-c), provides an interesting opportunity for study of the biologic and toxicologic consequences of RES stimulation in man. Whatever the results in man, the availability of well-characterized synthetic polyanions provides an opportunity for study of correlation between the physicochemical properties of these compounds and their effects on host resistance, RES response, interferon induction, antiviral activity, and the proliferation of tumors.

REFERENCES

1. W. Regelson and J.F. Holland, Nature, 181:46, 1958.
2. C. Muehbarcher, J. Straumfjord, Jr., J.P. Hummell, and W. Regelson, Cancer Res., 19:907, 1959.
3. W. Regelson, M. Tunis, and S. Kuhar, Acta Unio Intern. Contra. Cancrum, 16:729, 1960.
4. W. Regelson, S. Kuhar, M. Tunis, J. Fields, J. Johnson, and G. Glusenkamp, Nature, 186:778, 1960.
5. W. Regelson and J.F. Holland, Clin. Pharmacol. Therap., 3:270, 1962.
6. G.T. Feltz and W. Regelson, Nature, 196:642, 1962.
7. A. Vaheri, Acta Pathol. Microbiol. Scand. Suppl. 171, 1964.
8. W. Kleinschmidt, Proc. Nat. Acad. Sci. U.S., 52:741, 1964.
9. W. Kleinschmidt and E. Murphy, In press, 1965.
10. W. Regelson and O. Foltyn, Proc. Am. Assoc. Cancer Res., 7:58, 1966.
11. E.F. Wheelock, Science, 149:310, 1965.
12. M. Tunis, J. Immunol., 92:864, 1964.
13. W.J. Kleinschmidt and G.W. Probst, Antibiot. Chemotherapy, 12:298, 1962.
14. H.M. Powell, D.N. Walcher, and C. Mast, Proc. Soc. Exptl. Biol. Med., 107:55, 1961.
15. R.N. Hull and J.M. Lavelle, Proc. Soc. Exptl. Biol. Med., 83:787, 1953.
16. I.S. Johnson and L.A. Baker, Antibiot. Chemotherapy, 8:113, 1958.
17. E. Furusawa, W. Cutting, and A. Furst, Proc. Soc. Exptl. Biol. Med., 112:617, 1963.
18. K.W. Cochran and F.E. Payne, Proc. Soc. Exptl. Biol. Med., 115:471, 1964.
19. C.W. Probst, Eli Lilly Laboratories, Personal Communication, 1965.
20. Z. Rotem, R.A. Cox, and A. Isaacs, Nature, 197:564, 1963.
21. A.Y. Elliott and R.D. Higgenbotham, Texas Reports Biol. Med., 18:362, 1960.
22. K.K. Takemoto and H. Liebhaber, Virology, 17:499, 1962.
23. J.S. Pagano and D. Vaheri, Federation Proc., 24:319, 1965.

24. R.M. Friedman, Personal Communication, 1965.
25. H. Levy, F. Buckler, and S. Baron, Personal Communication, 1966.
26. T.C. Merigan and W.J. Kleinschmidt, Nature, In press, 1966.
27. M. Fruitstone, B. Michaels, D. Rudloff, and M. Sigel, Personal Communication, 1966.
28. L. Borecky and V. Lackoviv, Personal Communication, 1966.
29. J. Youngner and W. Stinebring, Personal Communication, 1966.
30. T.C. Merigan, Proc.Interferon Conf., NIH, December 16, 17, 1965 (Abstract).
31. H. Strander and K. Cantrell, Ann.Med.Exptl.Fenn., In press, 1966.
32. S.H.S. Lee and R.L. Ozere, Proc.Soc.Exptl.Biol.Med., 118:190, 1965.
33. Takemoto, K. K., and S. S. Spicer, Ann. N. Y. Acad. Sci. 130:365, 1965.
34. M. Tunis and W. Regelson, Exptl. Cell Res., 40:383, 1965
34a. M. Tunis, Proc.Am.Assoc.Cancer Res., 7:72, 1966.
35. W. Regelson, Work in progress, 1966.
36. H. Heymann, Z.R. Gulick, C.J. DeBoer, and G.D. Stevens, Arch. Biochem.Biophys., 73:366, 1958.
37. M.K. Bach, Biochem.Biophys.Acta, 91:619, 1964.
38. A.J. Nahamias, S. Kibrick, and P. Bernfeld, Proc.Soc.Exptl.Biol. Med., 115:993, 1964.
39. M.A. Jesaitis and W.F. Goebel, Cold Spring Harbor Symp.Quant. Biol., 18:205, 1953.
40. P. Bernfeld, J.S. Nisselbaum, B.J. Borkley, and R.W. Hanson, J.Biol.Chem., 235:2852, 1960.
41. J.H. Heller, Proc. IV Symp. on the Reticuloendothelial System, May 29-June 1, 1964, p. 77.

Immunoglobulin Synthesis in the Rat*

Mariano F. La Via,† William S. Hammond,‡
Barbara H. Iglewski,‡ Albert E. Vatter,
Michael Bean, and Patricia V. Northup

Department of Pathology
University of Colorado Medical Center
Denver, Colorado

The synthesis of immunoglobulin consists of a complex series of cellular and molecular reactions beginning soon after the injection of a specific antigen. It is established with some certainty that antigen, following administration, is taken up by macrophages and processed by these cells. A stimulus is then transmitted in a still undetermined manner to immunocompetent, undifferentiated reticular cells. These begin dividing very rapidly and give rise to differentiated lymphoid cells which are the main antibody producers. The serum antibody titer begins to rise around the third day after primary immunization, reaches a peak by the end of the first week, and then declines slowly. A second injection of antigen is followed by a more rapid rise and a slower decline of antibody titer [1-4].

The spleen seems to be the major or sole antibody-producing organ in rats when antigen is given intravenously [5-7]. The pattern of cellular and humoral reactions observed in rat spleens after immunization has been extensively studied and described [1, 8-10].

The macrophage has been described by some as being responsible for the elaboration of a ribonucleic acid (RNA) capable of inducing immune response in vitro and in vivo [11]. This phenomenon may be due to contamination of RNA by small amounts of antigen [12].

---

* This work was supported by grant T 290A of the American Cancer Society and by Army Contract DA-18-035-AMC-390.

† Recipient of Research Cancer Development Award K3-AI-19,421 of the U.S.P.H.S.

‡ Trainee, U.S.P.H.S. Training Grant T01 CA-05164 of the National Cancer Institute.

It has been shown that no appreciable antibody synthesis occurs during the 48 hr following immunization [13]. On the other hand, several purine, pyrimidine, and amino acid analogs will depress maximum antibody production when given during the induction period, indicating the importance of this period of immunogenesis [14].

Examination of polyribosomal patterns of immunoglobulin synthesis has been undertaken in several laboratories in the hope of understanding some of the molecular events leading to antibody specificity [15, 16].

Reported here are the results of three series of experiments designed to clarify the following problems. (1) The possible role of RNA synthesized in macrophages exposed to antigen in eliciting immune responses. It appeared that if macrophagic RNA were responsible for the initiation of antibody production, this RNA should be newly made after antigen stimulation. Previous experiments had shown that RNA from rat peritoneal macrophages exposed to Salmonella typhi vaccine was capable of eliciting low antibody titers in recipient, nonimmunized rats [17]. (2) The mechanism of action of beta-3-dl thienylalanine (β-3-TA) in depressing the immune response. β-3-TA had been shown to depress antibody production preferentially when given during the period immediately preceding and following immunization with sheep erythrocytes [18]. This approach should help to gain a further understanding of the induction period of antibody synthesis by learning which steps are affected by the analog. (3) The polysomal species found during immunoglobulin synthesis in the hope of elucidating the mechanism of assembly of L and H chains in finished molecules of antibody. It was known that polysomes ranging in size from dimers to decamers could be isolated from spleen cells during antibody formation and shown to be associated with labeled nascent polypeptide chains [16]. These experiments were expected to clarify some aspects of the genetic basis of antibody specificity.

MATERIALS AND METHODS

Sprague-Dawley rats were used in all experiments. Antigens used were UV inactivated bacteriophage (R17), S. typhi vaccine (S.t.) and sheep erythrocytes (RBC). These were prepared as described [7, 10, 15]. All antigens when injected in rats were given intravenously in 1.0-ml doses. Methods of antibody titration were described previously [19, 20]. Peritoneal macrophages were obtained by washing the peritoneal cavity of rats with PO_4-buffered Hanks balanced salt solution (BSS). In some experiments the rats had received 10 ml of proteose–peptone broth three days prior to sacrifice, to obtain a higher yield of macrophages. Macrophage preparations contained 70% macrophages. Spleen cells were obtained as already described [16]. The analog β-3-TA was purchased from Nutritional Biochemicals Co.; ^{3}H uridine and reconstituted ^{14}C Chlorella hydrolysate were obtained from Schwarz Bio.Research, Inc. The extraction of RNA was carried out by a hot phenol method modified from Mach and Vassalli [21].

Extracted RNA was analyzed by density gradient centrifugation in a 5-20% sucrose gradient with 0.05% sodium dodecylsulfate (SDS). At the end of a 3.5-hr centrifugation at 115,000 × g (maximum) in an SW39 Spinco rotor, the gradient was scanned at 260 mμ and fractions were collected. An aliquot of each fraction was used for counting. This was done in a Packard liquid scintillation spectrometer. Polyribosomes from spleen cells of S. typhi-immunized rats were studied as previously described [22].

Spleen cells from β-3-TA-treated animals were incubated in the same manner as those used in polysome isolation experiments [22]. They were pulsed with ^{3}H uridine or ^{14}C Chlorella hydrolysate and radioactivity was counted in a liquid scintillation spectrometer in the case of ^{3}H or in a low background gas flow counter in the case of ^{14}C.

Polysome fractions for electron microscopy were prepared and studied by the method outlined in previous publications [16, 23]. Fragments of spleen were fixed in glutaraldehyde and post-fixed in OsO_4 buffered with s-collidine (pH 7.3). They were embedded in Epon, sectioned, and viewed with a Philips 200 electron microscope.

RESULTS

The results of experiments designed to test the immunogenicity of newly synthesized RNA from antigen-treated macrophages showed that this RNA has no detectable immunogenic activity. Figure 1 illustrates the types of RNA synthesized by R17-treated and control rat peritoneal macrophages. It is apparent that the major product of synthesis is 3 to 8S RNA, with some incorporation of radioactive uridine in the higher molecular weight RNA peaks. Since removal of soluble RNA from the 4S region reduced radioactivity only moderately, it is concluded that newly synthesized RNA in this region is compatible with messenger RNA (m-RNA). The newly synthesized higher molecular weight RNA may also be m-RNA; however, there are no experimental data to substantiate this.

The total RNA from some preparations, and the highly labeled fraction from other preparations, were injected into the foot pad of normal rats. This treatment has never induced the formation of R17-inactivating antibody in the recipient as one would expect if this material were immunogenic. In another group of experiments R17 was labeled with ^{125}I and exposed to peritoneal macrophages to see whether antigen or labeled material was carried along during the RNA extraction. In no case could ^{125}I label be detected in the RNA prepared from these cells.

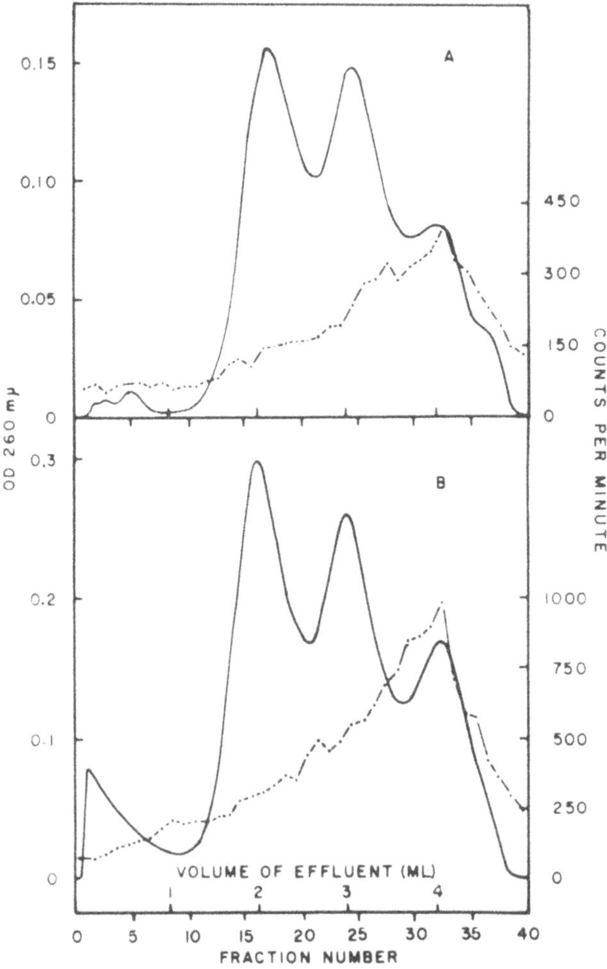

Fig. 1. Optical density scan (solid line) and radioactivity determination (dashed line) of two RNA preparations from normal (A) and R17-treated (B) rat peritoneal macrophages. RNA peaks can be seen at 4S (peak closest to the top of the gradient), 18S (middle peak), and 28S (peak on the left of the graph). Radioactivity is associated with all fractions, but the highest incorporation has occurred in the 3 to 8S area.

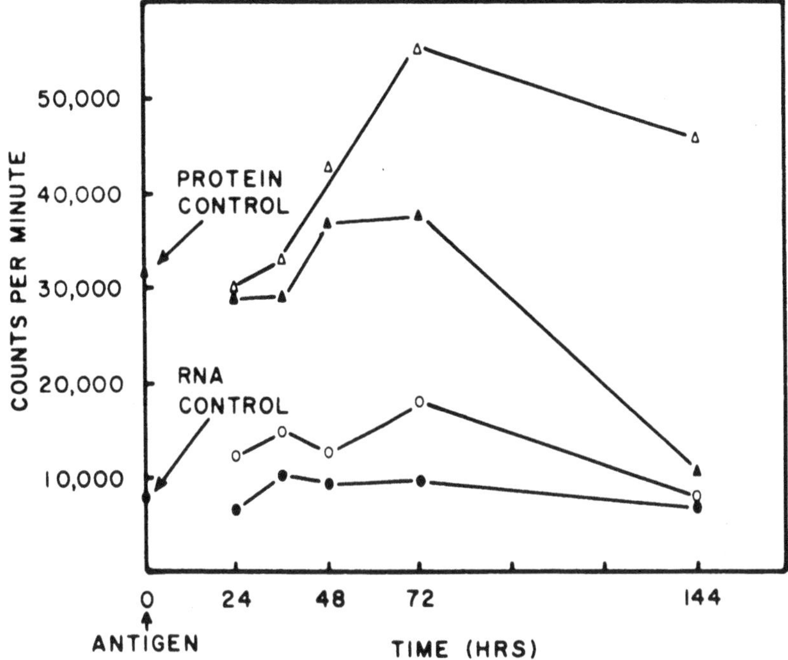

Fig. 2. ^{14}C amino acid incorporation into protein of spleen cells of β-3-TA-treated (▲) and nontreated (△) immunized rats; ^{3}H uridine incorporation into RNA of spleen cells of β-3-TA-treated (●) and nontreated (○) immunized rats. The synthesis of RNA after β-3-TA treatment does not change appreciably from that in normal, nonimmunized rat spleen cells, while spleen cells from antigen-treated rats show a doubling of RNA synthesis by the third day after immunization. As expected, protein synthesis in β-3-TA-treated rats does not rise very much and falls precipitously after the small rise. In immunized rat spleen cells, by comparison, a considerable increase in synthetic activity can be seen.

The phenylalanine analog β-3-TA is known to inhibit antibody synthesis when administered during the induction period. To detect the site of action of this drug, the following experiments were performed. Rats were given 1 ml of RBC on day 0 and 50 mg/day of β-3-TA from day −2 to +4 to obtain maximum depression of antibody synthesis. Spleens were removed at 24, 36, 48, 72, and 144 hr. Cells were incubated and exposed to ^{3}H uridine or ^{14}C amino acids for 15 min to label RNA or protein. Incubation was terminated by addition of excess cold saline. RNA was prepared (see Methods) or protein precipitated with 5% trichloracetic acid onto Millipore HA filters. Radioactivity was counted in the RNA and protein fractions. RNA synthesis proceeds at a high rate in injected rat spleen cells; this process is greatly inhibited in β-3-TA-treated animals. New RNA synthesis never rises much above the value obtained for control, nonimmunized rats. Protein synthesis clearly reflects this phenomenon, since it starts to rise as in immunized animals, but stops and declines to levels much lower than in normal rats (Fig. 2).

The study of polysomes from spleen cells of rats immunized with S. typhi has led to interesting findings. These are compatible with a current hypothesis, based on structural studies of Bence Jones protein, which proposes that L chains may be synthesized as two separate polypeptide chains on separate polysomes [24].

The predominant types of spleen cells which are present at the time the rats are sacrificed for polysome analysis are illustrated in Figs. 3 and 4. One cell type has many free polysomes and very scanty endoplasmic reticulum, while another has abundant endoplasmic reticulum lined with many polysomes. These have the characteristic structure presented in Fig. 5.

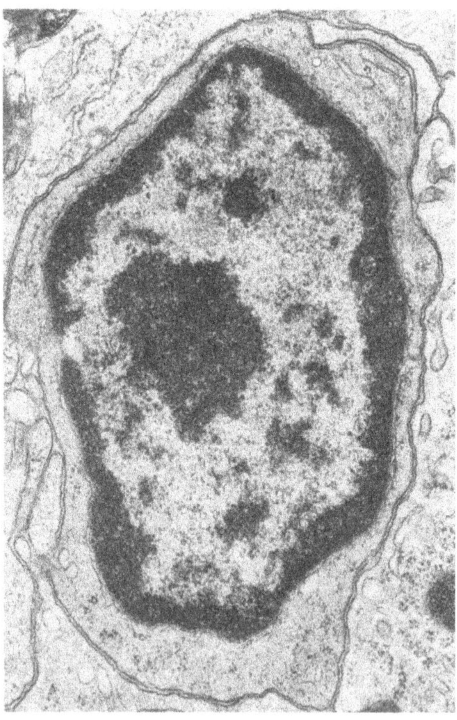

Fig. 3. One of the cell types found to predominate in the red pulp of rat spleens during immune response. This is a lymphoid cell with many non-membrane-bound polysomes and some vesicles of endoplasmic reticulum. It shows a prominent nucleolus in a nucleus with very condensed chromatin. x 25,000. Reduced 40% for reproduction.

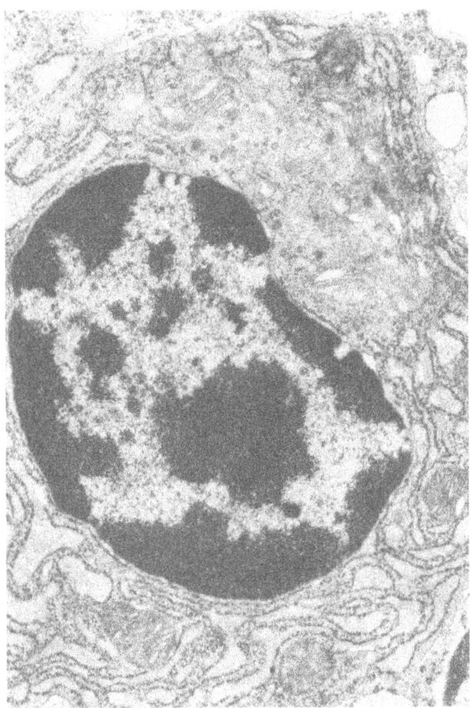

Fig. 4. A cell typical of the six-day response in the red pulp of immunized rats. A very prominent endoplasmic reticulum and Golgi region with typical arrangement of nuclear chromatin identify this as a plasma cell. Note the electron-dense material in dilated cysternae. × 22,000. Reduced 40% for reproduction.

Cells of this type were pulsed with ^{14}C Chlorella hydrolysate to label nascent polypeptide chains. The polysomes were isolated by centrifugation in a 0.3-1.0 M sucrose density gradient. Optical density at 260 mμ was measured to locate peaks of polysomes, and fractions were collected for radioactivity determination and for electron microscopic study. In Fig. 6 are shown the results of a typical experiment. Scanning the preparation at 260 mμ revealed some soluble protein at the very top of the gradient tube, a small peak of single ribosomes, peaks of dimers and trimers and shoulders indicating the position of tetramers, pentamers, and hexamers with larger polysomes toward the bottom of the tube. The nascent polypeptide chains are concentrated in four regions. These correlate with the trimers, with the tetramers, with the pentamers, and with larger polysomes. The size of these polysomes was checked by electron microscopic examination of a drop taken from each fraction. The typical appearance of a sample is shown in Fig. 7. Here, the majority of polysomes are three to five ribosomes in size. Several single ribosomes are also present, as is typical of all fractions examined.

DISCUSSION

From the results of the first series of experiments, two conclusions can be drawn. First, RNA synthesis in control, untreated peritoneal macrophages does not differ appreciably from that seen in antigen-treated macrophages. And, second, in the system studied, RNA from macrophages stimulated with antigen is not immunogenic in the rat. It seems reasonable to assume that if RNA from antigen-stimulated macrophages were capable of transferring antigenic information, this RNA would have to be made after exposure of the cell to antigen. The probability of the existence of an RNA fraction carrying the information necessary for initiation of a specific immune response is very low. It is clear that this new RNA, which may include m-RNA, does not possess the property of transferring immunogenicity. It is of interest to note also that no labeled material is found in this fraction, or in any other RNA fraction, when labeled antigen is used. Although this observation does not prove that antigenic material is not extracted with the RNA, it strongly suggests that no immune response is elicited after injection of RNA from antigen-stimulated macrophages if antigen is not present. Thus, similar observations of other workers appear to be confirmed by these experiments. Whatever the mechanism of induction of immune responses at the level of the immunocompetent cell, it is apparent that it necessitates the transfer of materials other than ribonucleic acid, perhaps in conjunction with RNA. Of interest in this respect are experimental results of Gottlieb [25], who found that the 28S

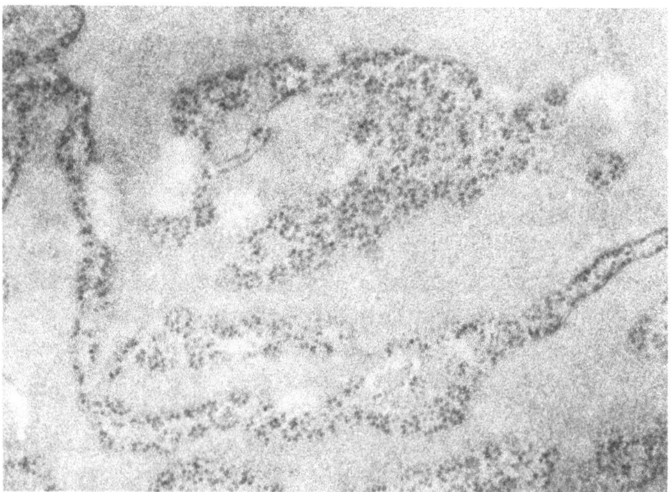

Fig. 5. A tangential section from the endoplasmic reticulum of the cell illustrated in Fig. 4. Polysomes contain numerous ribosomes and are arranged in a spiral fashion.

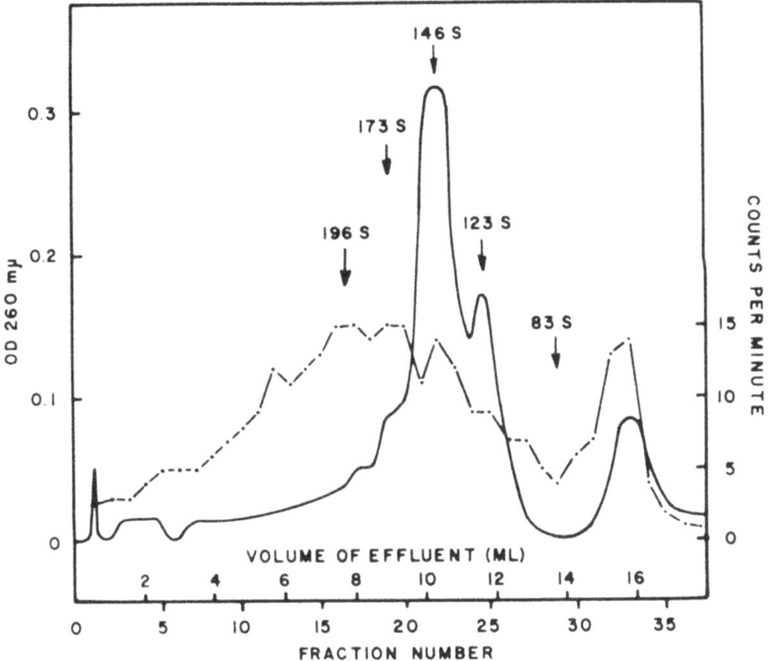

Fig. 6. Optical density scan (solid line) and radioactivity plot (dashed line) of polyribosomes and nascent polypeptide chains from spleen cells of S. typhi-immunized rats. Some soluble labeled protein is present at the top of the gradient. Peaks of dimers and trimers and shoulders of tetramers and pentamers are seen. Radioactive polypeptides peak in the trimer, tetramer, and pentamer regions. Another peak of radioactivity is seen in a region of larger polysomes.

fraction of a preparation similar to that used in these experiments was capable of inducing immune response. The only differences between his procedure and the one used here are the temperature of extraction and the antigen (T2 phage, in Gottlieb's case). It appears that a difference in phenol solubility of T2 phage and R17 at the temperatures used may account for the different results by antigen carryover in the one case and not in the other.

It is surprising that the action of β-3-TA in depressing antibody production is mediated by RNA. One would expect an amino acid analog to act directly on protein synthesis, particularly in the case of an essential amino acid like phenylalanine. The results of the experiments with β-3-TA confirm the well-established fact that protein synthesis is RNA-dependent. These experiments are preliminary, as nothing is yet known about the type of RNA being depressed. They stress the fact that, as expected, the induction period has an active phase of RNA synthesis which is preparatory to the synthesis of antibody. The questions of why β-3-TA acts by depressing

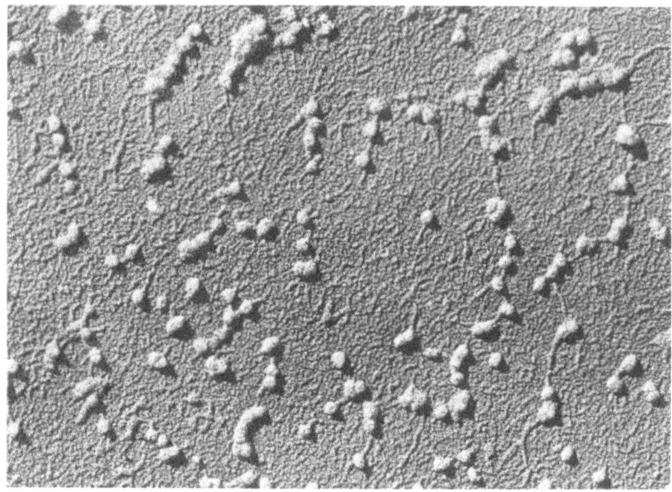

Fig. 7. Typical aspect of polysomes from the 190-200S area of a density gradient. Note the predominance of three-to-five-member polysomes with some single ribosomes scattered throughout.

RNA synthesis and of why the induction period can be several days long are still unanswered. It is of interest to note that in preliminary experiments with ^{3}H labeled β-3-TA, the drug was found to be incorporated into antibody. This antibody was as active as antibody from non-β-3-TA-treated animals.

Nascent polypeptide chains are found to be associated with three or four groups of polysomes from immunized rat spleen cells. Negligible radioactivity can be measured on polysomes from control cells. Because hemoglobin is made in rat spleens by numerous erythropoietic elements, the radioactivity associated with the pentaribosome peak, in all probability, represents hemoglobin chains. By using figures presented by Rich [26] on the basis of studies of reticulocyte polysomes, a polysome which can synthesize L chains of immunoglobulin should consist of seven ribosomes on a strand of m-RNA. The sedimentation coefficient of a seven-member polysome, according to the data of Pfuderer et al. [27], should be approximately 257S. While it is possible that any protein can be made on monomeric polysomes, it is commonly accepted that a direct relationship exists between the size of a protein and that of a polysome, the latter being a function of m-RNA size. In the experiments reported here, the nascent polypeptide chains have been associated with polysomes ranging from two to ten members. They were distributed in such a manner that the peaks of radioactive material were located in the region of trimers, tetramers, pentamers, and larger polysomes with a declining front of radioactive polypeptides covering the rest of the gradient. Pentamers can be considered to be engaged in the synthesis of hemoglobin. No distinct peak exists in the region of seven-member polysomes but two peaks are seen in the trimer and tetramer area. This suggests the possibility that synthesis of L chains may occur on two distinct polysomes, each responsible for the manufacture of half a chain. These would be three- to four-member polysomes. While this idea is in keeping with present concepts of L-chain synthesis derived from structural analysis of these molecules, it is not yet proven and it awaits further experimentation.

SUMMARY

The synthesis of antibody does not appear to be stimulated by RNA extracted from antigen-exposed macrophages if all antigenic material is removed from this RNA.

The action of β-3-TA on antibody inductive period seems to be by depressing RNA synthesis and, in turn, protein synthesis. Antibody which has incorporated the analog does not appear less active than "normal" antibody.

Polysomes of immunized rat spleen cells sediment in several classes of from 2 to 10 members. Nascent polypeptide chains are associated with trimers, tetramers, pentamers, and with larger polysomes. These can be responsible for the synthesis of hemoglobin and of subunits of L and H chains.

REFERENCES

1. M.F. LaVia, F.W. Fitch, C.H. Gunderson, and R.W. Wissler, in: J.H. Heller, Ed., Reticuloendothelial Structure and Function. New York, Ronald Press, 1960.
2. J.W. Uhr, Science, 145:157, 1964.
3. G.J. Nossal, Intern.Rev.Exptl.Pathol., 1:1, 1962.
4. G.J. Nossal, G.C. Ada, and C.M. Austin, Australian J.Exptl.Biol. Med.Sci., 42:311, 1964.
5. D.A. Rowley, J.Immunol., 64:289, 1950.
6. J. Winebright and F.W. Fitch, J.Immunol., 89:891, 1962.
7. P.A. Campbell and M.F. LaVia, Proc.Soc.Exptl.Biol.Med., 124:571, 1967.
8. R.W. Wissler, F.W. Fitch, M.F. LaVia, and C.H. Gunderson, J.Cell.Comp.Physiol., 50, Suppl.1:265, 1957.
9. C.H. Gunderson, D. Juras, M.F. LaVia, and R.W. Wissler, J.Am. Med.Assoc., 180:1038, 1962.
10. M.F. LaVia, J.Immunol., .92:252, 1964.
11. M. Fishman, J.J. van Rood, and F.B. Adler, in: J. Sterzl, Ed., Molecular and Cellular Basis of Antibody Formation. New York, Academic Press, 1964.

12. B.A. Askonas and J.M. Rhodes, in: J. Sterzl, Ed., Molecular and Cellular Basis of Antibody Formation. New York, Academic Press, 1964.
13. W.H. Taliaferro and D.W. Talmage, J.Infect.Diseases, 97:88, 1955.
14. R.S. Schwarz, Progr.Allergy, 9:246, 1965.
15. S. Tawde, M.D. Scharff, and J.W. Uhr, J.Immunol., 96:1, 1966.
16. M.F. LaVia, A.E. Vatter, and P.V. Northup, Exptl.Mol.Pathol., Suppl.3:124, 1966.
17. W.S. Hammond, M. Bean, and M.F. LaVia, In preparation.
18. M.F. LaVia, Proc.Soc.Exptl.Biol.Med., 114:133, 1963.
19. P.R. Cannon, W.E. Chase, and R.W. Wissler, J.Immunol., 47:133, 1943.
20. P.R. Cannon, Ann.Surg., 120:514, 1944.
21. B. Mach and P. Vassalli, Proc.Nat.Acad.Sci.U.S., 54:975, 1965.
22. P. V. Northup, W. S. Hammond, and M. F. La Via, Proc. Nat. Acad. Sci. U. S., 57:273, 1967.
23. M.F. LaVia, A.E. Vatter, W.S. Hammond, and P.V. Northup, Proc. Nat. Acad. Sci. U. S., 57:79, 1967.
24. L. Hood, W. Gray, and W. Dreyer, Proc.Nat.Acad.Sci.U.S., 55:826, 1966.
25. A.A. Gottlieb, in: "Differentiation and growth of hemoglobin and immunoglobulin-synthesizing cells," J.Cell Physiol., 67, Suppl.1:164, 1966.
26. A. Rich, J.R. Warner, and H.M. Goodman, Cold Spring Harbor Symp.Quant.Biol., 28:269, 1963.
27. P. Pfuderer, P. Cammarano, D.R. Holladay, and G.D. Novelli, Biochim.Biophys.Acta, 109:595, 1965.

Modifications of Antibody Synthesis by Chloramphenicol*

Melvin D. Schoenberg, Richard D. Moore,
and Austin S. Weisberger

Department of Pathology and Medicine
Western Reserve University
Cleveland, Ohio

When chloramphenicol (CM) is given in sufficient quantity before immunization or early in the inductive phase of antibody synthesis, there is an attenuation of antibody formation. This has been shown in animals and in cultures of lymphoid tissue [1-8]. Despite these studies, there is little information about the cellular aspects of the immune process in the presence of CM.

In this study the effect of CM on the attenuation of antibody synthesis was considered in relation to the sequence of events thought to occur in a primary immunologic response: phagocytosis of antigen, relay of some stimulus to potential antibody producing cells, and then, proliferation, maturation, and functional expression of the recipient cells.

MATERIALS AND METHODS

Albino rabbits maintained on Purina chow and tap water were used. They were separated into two groups. One received 1 ml of complete Freund's adjuvant containing *Mycobacterium butyricum* followed immediately through the same needle by 80 Lf of soluble diphtheria toxoid. The spleens were removed on 3, 6, 7, 9, 11, 13, 15, 17, and 21 days after immunization. The other group was started on 0.6 g of CM/kg body weight by intramuscular injection the day before immunization and continued on the drug to the end of the experiment. The antibiotic was given in divided doses at 12-hr in-

*Supported by grants AM-07161 (MDS and RDM), H3952 and C4944 (ASW) from the United States Public Health Service. This work was performed during the tenure of a Research Career Development Award (MDS) from the United States Public Health Service.

Table I. Circulating Antibody Response to Diphtheria Toxoid and *Mycobacterium butyricum* With and Without Chloramphenicol (CM)

Days after immunization	Circulating Antitoxoid*		Percent Species of Antitoxoid in Control Animals		Circulating Antibody to *Mycobacterium butyricum**		Percent Species of Antibody to *Mycobacterium butyricum* in Control Animals	
	No CM	CM	γM	γG	No CM	CM	γM	γG
3	0	0	0	0	0	0	0	0
6	20	0	I	I	0	0	0	0
7	40	0	100	I	2-4	0	I	I
9	640	0	100	I	12	0	I	I
11	1280	0	100	I	24	0	I	I
13	2560	0	80	20	32	0	100	I
15	2560	0	80	20	64	0	100	I
17	2560	0	70	30	128	0	100	I
21	2560	0	70	30	192	0	100	I

*Reciprocal of titers of circulating antibody.
I = Insufficient antibody titers for determination of species of antibody.

tervals to maintain adequate blood levels. The rabbits were bled at intervals from the marginal ear vein. At the indicated times, four from each group were anesthetized, blood obtained from the heart, and the spleens removed for histologic, immunofluorescent, and electron microscopic examination.

Complete Freund's adjuvant containing *M. butyricum* was used along with diphtheria toxoid in order to place a greater stress on the immune system. The addition of the adjuvant increases the proliferation of the cells associated with antibody production and results in an accelerated, enhanced, and prolonged synthesis of both γM and γG antibody. In addition, there is a temporal separation of the γM and γG responses, so that they can, to some extent, be studied separately [9-12].

RESULTS

The pattern of the immune response in rabbits treated with complete Freund's adjuvant and diphtheria toxoid has been described [9-12]. Circulating antitoxoid and antibody to *M. butyricum* were not found in the sera from rabbits maintained on CM. This is in contrast to the relatively high levels of circulating antibody obtained from those animals that did not receive the antibiotic (Table I).

The cells eventually concerned with the synthesis of γG antibody are limited to the lymphocytic cells of the nonfollicular white pulp. Those associated with γM antibody synthesis are limited to nonphagocytic mono-

Table II. Response of Antibody-Producing Cells to Diphtheria Toxoid and _Mycobacterium Butyricum_ With and Without Chloramphenicol

Days	Maturation of Mononuclear Cells in Red Pulp		Estimated % of Mononuclear Cells with Either Antitoxoid or Antibody to _M. b._				Development of Mature Plasma Cells		Estimated % of Plasma Cells with Either Antitoxoid or Antibody to _M. b._			
	No CM	CM	No CM		CM		No CM	CM	No CM		CM	
			Anti-toxoid	_M.b._	Anti-toxoid	_M.b._			Anti-toxoid	_M.b._	Anti-toxoid	_M.b._
3	Few	0	0	0	0	0	0	0	0	0	0	0
6	+	0	75	25	0	0	0	0	0	0	0	0
7	+	0	75	25	0	0	0	0	0	0	0	0
9	2+	0	75	25	0	0	Few	0	50	50	0	0
11	2+	Few	75	25	0	0	+	Few	50	50	0	0
13	3+	Few	75	25	0	0	2+	+	50	50	0	0
15	3+	+	25	75	0	0	3+	2+	50	50	0	0
17	3+	2+	5	95	5	0	3+	2+	50	50	0	0
21	4+	3+	5	95	5	5	4+	2+	50	50	5	5

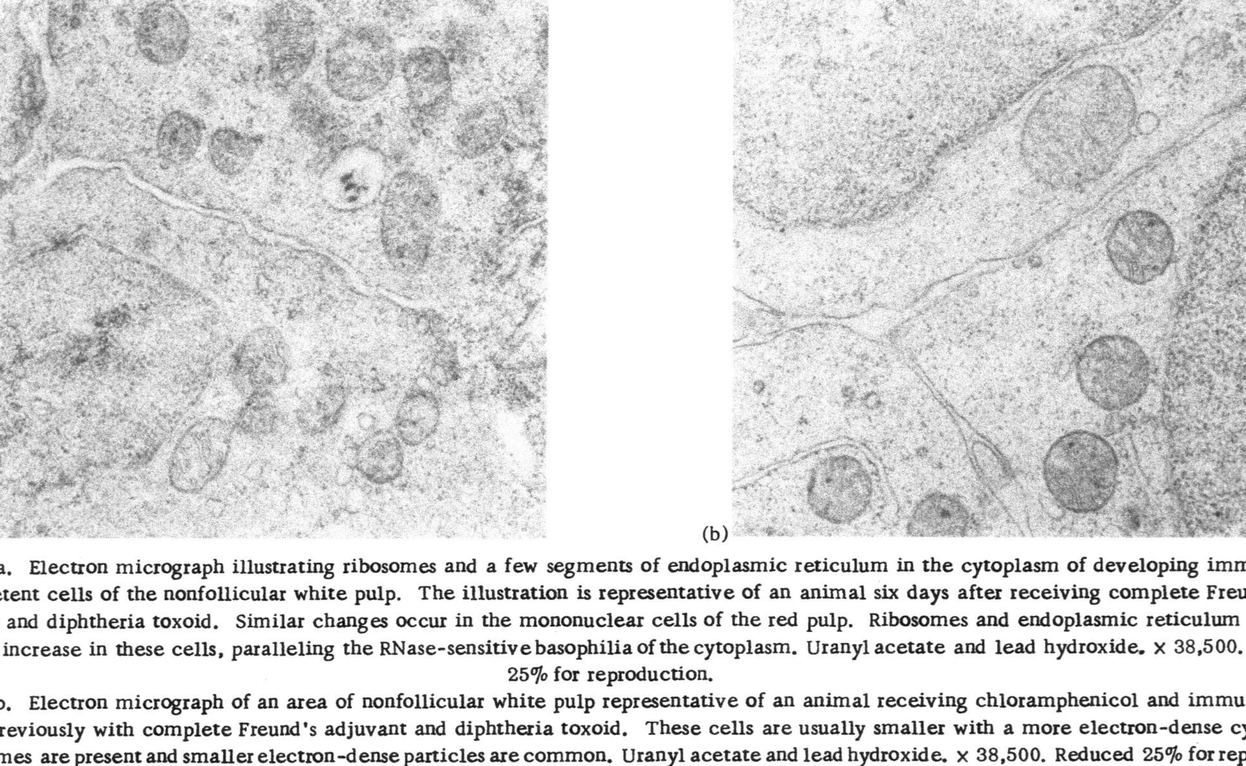

Fig. 1a. Electron micrograph illustrating ribosomes and a few segments of endoplasmic reticulum in the cytoplasm of developing immunologic competent cells of the nonfollicular white pulp. The illustration is representative of an animal six days after receiving complete Freund's adjuvant and diphtheria toxoid. Similar changes occur in the mononuclear cells of the red pulp. Ribosomes and endoplasmic reticulum progressively increase in these cells, paralleling the RNase-sensitive basophilia of the cytoplasm. Uranyl acetate and lead hydroxide. × 38,500. Reduced 25% for reproduction.

Fig. 1b. Electron micrograph of an area of nonfollicular white pulp representative of an animal receiving chloramphenicol and immunized six days previously with complete Freund's adjuvant and diphtheria toxoid. These cells are usually smaller with a more electron-dense cytoplasm; ribosomes are present and smaller electron-dense particles are common. Uranyl acetate and lead hydroxide. × 38,500. Reduced 25% for reproduction.

nuclear cells (large lymphocytic cells) in the walls of the sinusoids of the red pulp. The cells contain specific antibody several days before it is demonstrated in the circulation. It is emphasized that the absence of antibody in the circulation does not necessarily indicate inhibition of antibody synthesis. In studies of this kind it is necessary to consider intracellular antibody synthesis as well as circulating antibody.

By combining electron microscopy with conventional methods, it was possible to trace the sequence of events in the development of immunologic competent cells in the red and white pulp. The response of the antibody-producing cells to the antigens is summarized in Table II.

Mononuclear Cells

Within three days after immunization without CM, certain nonphagocytic, mononuclear cells in the walls of the sinusoids of the red pulp showed an increase in the amount and in the basophilia of the cytoplasm. The latter was sensitive to digestion with RNase. At this time the ribosomal population was substantially increased. The ribosomes were found randomly scattered and arranged in aggregates through the cytoplasm. Associated with this was an increment in mitotic activity that correlated with the larger number of these cells eventually found. A prominent Golgi apparatus and segments of endoplasmic reticulum were seen by seven days. With the development of the endoplasmic reticulum there was attachment of some of the ribosomes to the lamellae (Fig. 1a). It was at this stage that the RNase-sensitive basophilia of the cytoplasm was most intense and γ-globulin and γM antibody were first demonstrated in the cytoplasm of these cells. Once the mononuclear cells attained this level of morphologic development, no further change occurred. At no time did they achieve the ultrastructural details of the plasma cell. The number of cells containing γM antitoxoid steadily increased to 13 days and then sharply declined, so that after this point antitoxoid was rarely found in these cells. In contrast, γM antibody to M. butyricum was found in fewer of these cells during the first 13 days, and then in more throughout the experiment.

In contrast, in those animals given CM there was a delay in the development of these cells. Though the amount of cytoplasm increased, it did so more slowly than in the controls. RNase-sensitive basophilia of the cytoplasm was not appreciated until 11 or 12 days after immunization. On an ultrastructural level there was a corresponding delay in the cytoplasmic maturation of two or three days. During this period of development, the cells differed in several respects from those of the control group. Their cytoplasm did not increase to the same extent. Ribosomal particles were common but aggregation into polyribosomes was not as extensive. In addition, the cytoplasm was packed with small electron-dense particles that may represent incomplete ribosomes (Fig. 1b). The marked accumulation of these particles is not found in the usual sequence of development of these cells in

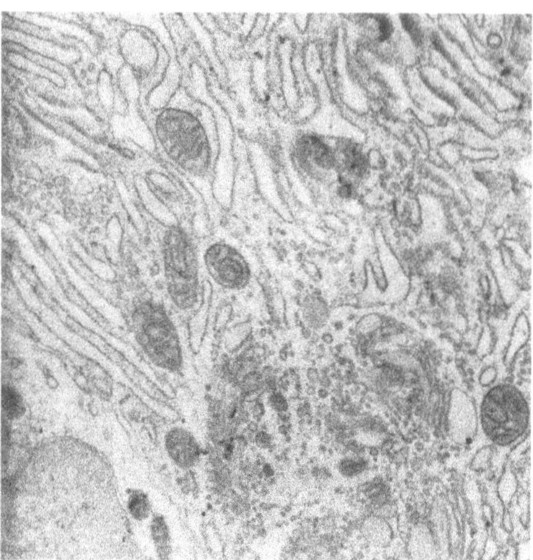

Fig. 2. Electron micrograph illustrating the presence of a "typical" plasma cell 17 days after immunization in a chloramphenicol-treated animal. Note the elaborate Golgi apparatus and endoplasmic reticulum, the numerous RNP particles, and the presence of slightly electron-dense amorphous material in the channels between the lamellae. Though well differentiated, only a few of these cells contained specific antibody and gamma globulin. Uranyl acetate and lead hydroxide. × 13,750. Reduced 25% for reproduction.

animals not receiving the antibiotic. There were fewer profiles of endoplasmic reticulum and a corresponding decrease or delay in the development of the Golgi apparatus. By 17 days, however, these cells were morphologically similar to those of the control group. It was only toward the end of the experiment that antibody was found in a small percentage of these cells. The delay and slower rate of maturation was substantial, indicating a suppressive effect of CM on structural protein synthesis as well as on antibody synthesis. In addition, the surge in mitotic activity experienced after immunization with adjuvant and toxoid was less. Mitotic figures were not as frequent under the influence of CM, but were more numerous than in nonimmunized animals or in those receiving toxoid without adjuvant.

Plasma Cells

Plasma cells containing γG antibody were found in and adjacent to the nonfollicular white pulp and seemed to develop from the small and medium lymphocytes in these areas. By three days some of these cells had acquired some endoplasmic reticulum, a complicated Golgi apparatus, and a large number of ribosomes. The ribosomes were free in the cytoplasm, in aggregates, and attached to the lamellae of the endoplasmic reticulum by six or seven days. By optical microscopy these ultrastructural features were reflected as enlarged lymphocytic cells with abundant RNase-sensitive, basophilic cytoplasm. Thirteen days after immunization the majority of these cells had the currently accepted features of the plasma cell.

After 13 days there was a gradual reduction in cytoplasmic basophilia and a transition toward acidophilia. Gamma globulin, γG antitoxoid, and γG antibody to M. butyricum were found in the plasma cells by nine days, and then in an increasing number of these cells. As the number of plasma cells containing antibody and the intensity of fluorescence increased and the cytoplasmic basophilia decreased, amorphous, moderately electron-dense material accumulated in the cisternae of the endoplasmic reticulum.

The delay in the maturation of the plasma cells was similar to that of the mononuclear cells in the animals that received CM. Ribosomal synthesis, the development of endoplasmic reticulum, and the Golgi apparatus were delayed, but eventually most of the cells that started to mature completed the process at least in a morphologic sense (Fig. 2). However, only a few of these contained gamma globulin and specific antibody. Here, again, mitotic activity was less than in the control group, but not suppressed to the level that might account for the lack of identifiable antibody synthesis.

DISCUSSION

It is clear that CM interfered significantly with the synthesis of specific antibody (i.e., γM and γG antibody) and to a lesser but significant extent with the structural protein synthesis (i.e., proteins necessary for cellular replication and maturation).

The failure of the animals to respond to the antigenic stimulus cannot be attributed to impairment of phagocytosis. There is no significant alteration in antigen uptake by the splenic macrophages in the animals given CM [13].

Though mitotic activity was not quantitatively determined, it was clear that mitoses were delayed and fewer in the group given CM. Despite this reduction in replication, mitotic activity was greater than in nonimmunized animals or in those given toxoid without adjuvant. A sufficient number of cells proliferated, so that significant antibody synthesis should have occurred if the number of immunologic competent cells available were the only consideration.

Further evidence that some stimulus was received by the potential immunologic competent cells in the presence of CM is illustrated by the development of ribosomes, endoplasmic reticulum, an elaborate Golgi complex, and the eventual synthesis of antibody by a few of these cells. The rapid progression of the immune response following cessation of the antibiotic [5] and a characteristic secondary response on reexposure to the antigen is additional support that immunocompetent cells have been prepared [2].

Despite the delay in the maturation of immunocompetent cells, a substantial number of ribosomes similar in size and morphologic appearance to those in animals that did not receive CM were formed. However, early in the course of maturation in the CM group there were many smaller particles (electron-dense) in the cytoplasm of these cells. The incidence of these smaller particles preceded and then paralleled the RNase-sensitive basophilia of the cytoplasm. Some probably represent the synthesis of new ribosomal RNA and/or protein-poor ribosomes. It has been reported that the injection of antigen results initially in a rapid synthesis of RNA mostly of the ribosomal type instead of the DNA-directed m-RNA for specific antibody synthesis, which occurs later and in smaller amounts [14-16]. If both m-RNA and r-RNA synthesis is maintained in the immunologic-competent cells in the presence of CM and the prime effect of CM is on protein synthesis, then the assembly of the synthetic machines for protein synthesis, the ribosomes or polyribosomes, would be impaired (i.e., protein-poor ribosomes) [17-23]. Quantitatively, this would be expressed to a greater extent in antibody synthesis than in structural protein synthesis.

It is fairly well established that CM does not significantly affect protein synthesis by endogenous m-RNA associated with mammalian ribosomes. This has been shown with rat liver ribosomes [24] and microsomes [25] and rabbit reticulocyte ribosomes [26-28]. The synthesis of some of the structural proteins in the immunocompetent cells in the presence of CM may be on a similar basis. Endogenous m-RNA-ribosome (polyribosomes) complexes already formed would not be expected to be materially affected by CM. In this respect a certain amount of mitotic activity, synthesis of endoplasmic reticulum, Golgi apparatus, functional ribosomes, and mitochondrial replication would be anticipated. The delayed and decreased morphologic response could be accounted for by the necessity of manufacturing additional protein-synthesizing systems directed to the reproduction and replication of structural protein elements. CM apparently interferes with these processes.

With respect to antibody synthesis, an entire new message must be transcribed (m-RNA) and then introduced in the translation device (m-RNA—ribosome or polyribosome—s-RNA). The fact that the synthesis of m-RNA for antibody translation is very likely later than r-RNA synthesis would make more difficult the assembly of the ribosome or polyribosome complex necessary for the formation of antibody. In effect, there would be a competition for those normal, preantibiotic ribosomes with the advantage on the side of the endogenous m-RNA directed to structural protein synthesis. This is not an unusual expectation, since the current data do not indicate any ribosomal specificity for any particular m-RNA, but instead competitive access to preformed or intact ribosomes. That some m-RNA directed to antibody synthesis becomes attached to functional ribosomes is shown by the small percent of cells that eventually synthesized antibody even in the presence of large doses of CM.

An analogous situation was found in the effect of CM on total protein synthesis in chick fibroblasts [29]. When these cells were making protein at or near maximal rate, CM was without effect. In cells just initiating protein synthesis, the drug sharply reduced the amount of protein synthesized. Even in this case, while protein synthesis was inhibited, RNA synthesis was unchanged. Withdrawal of CM in this instance, as in that of antibody synthesis, resulted in a prompt restoration of protein synthesis [5, 29].

The critical time at which CM must be administered to be effective supports the concept that the drug interferes with an important stage early in the synthesis of antibody. The administration of CM must precede immunization or be given early in the inductive phase [3, 4], or antibody synthesis is not sufficiently altered to be recognized by the procedures used. If sufficient r-RNA and m-RNA synthesis occurs prior to giving CM, then the drug should have little effect. Presumably, sufficient assembly of normal functional synthetic units has taken place so that expression, antibody synthesis, is seen. The prompt recovery of the immune system after withdrawal of CM indicates that some of the machinery for antibody synthesis has been constructed in the presence of CM.

Another effect of CM that may account for the greater suppression of antibody synthesis compared to structural protein synthesis has been reported. There is apparently a differential sensitivity to CM of the two general classes of ribosomes, those free in the cytoplasm and those bound to the membranes of the endoplasmic reticulum. In an in vitro system the membrane-bound ribosomes are inhibited more completely and at lower concentrations of the drug than the free ribosomes [30]. The synthesis of antibody protein is apparently associated with membrane-bound ribosomes (presumably polyribosomes). If this is the case, a greater effect on antibody synthesis would result from CM treatment. The protein synthesis for cellular replication and development probably occurs on the ribosomes free in the cytoplasm and would not be expected to be as susceptible to the drug.

In this same respect, the delay in the formation of endoplasmic reticulum and the attachment of ribosomes to the lamellae may also influence antibody synthesis. The relationship of the endoplasmic reticulum and the distribution of ribosomes with respect to protein synthesis has been considered in cells from a number of tissues [31, 32]. While ribosomes may occur free in the cytoplasm in rapidly dividing cells and in some so-called resting cells, they are usually attached to membranes in cells that synthesize "proteins for export." Cells of the latter variety treated in such a manner that the endoplasmic reticulum is destroyed or solubilized have a decreased capacity for protein synthesis even though there are a large number of ribosomal particles remaining free in the cytoplasm. The delayed development of the endoplasmic reticulum in the potential immunocompetent cells in these experiments could result in a delay and decrease in antibody synthesis.

REFERENCES

1. A.S. Weisberger and S. Wolfe, "Effect of chloramphenicol on protein synthesis," Federation Proc., 23:976, 1964.
2. A.S. Weisberger, T. Daniel, and A. Hoffman, "Suppression of antibody synthesis and prolongation of homograft survival by chloramphenicol," J. Exptl. Med., 120:183, 1964.
3. W.T. Butler and A.H. Coons, "Studies on antibody production. XII. Inhibition of priming by drugs," J. Exptl. Med., 120:1051, 1964.
4. A. Cruchaud and A.H. Coons, "Studies on antibody production. XIII. The effect of chloramphenicol on priming in mice," J. Exptl. Med., 120:1061, 1964.
5. A.S. Weisberger, R.D. Moore, and M.D. Schoenberg, "Modification of experimental immune nephritis by chloramphenicol," J. Lab. Clin. Med., 67:58, 1966.
6. C.T. Ambrose and A.H. Coons, "Studies on antibody production. VIII. The inhibitory effect of chloramphenicol on the synthesis of antibody in tissue culture," J. Exptl. Med., 117:1075, 1963.
7. S.E. Svehag, "Antibody formation in vitro by separated spleen cells: Inhibition by actinomycin and chloramphenicol," Science, 146:659, 1964.
8. S.E. Svehag, "In vitro secondary 19S and 7S antibody responses to poliovirus in membrane cultures of separated spleen cells," Arch. Ges. Virusforsch., 15:261, 1965.
9. M.D. Schoenberg, A.B. Stavitsky, R.D. Moore, and M.J. Freeman, "Cellular synthesis of rabbit immunoglobulins during primary response to diphtheria toxoid – Freund's adjuvant," J. Exptl. Med., 121:577, 1965.
10. M.D. Schoenberg, J.C. Rupp, and R.D. Moore, "The cellular response of the spleen and its relationship to the circulating 19S and 7S antibody in the rabbit," Brit. J. Exptl. Pathol., 45:111, 1964.
11. A.B. Stavitsky, "Micromethods for the study of proteins and antibodies. I. Procedure and general applications of hemagglutination and hemagglutination–inhibition reactions with tannic acid and protein-treated red blood cells," J. Immunol., 72:360, 1954.
12. R.D. Moore, V.R. Mumaw, and M.D. Schoenberg, "Changes in antibody-producing cells in the spleen during the primary response," J. Exptl. Mol. Pathol., 4:370, 1965.
13. R.D. Moore and M.D. Schoenberg, Unpublished observations.
14. J. Mitchell, "Autoradiographic studies of nucleic acid and protein metabolism in lymphoid cells. I. Differences among members of the plasma cell sequence," Australian J. Exptl. Biol. Med. Sci., 42:347, 1964.

15. J. Mitchell, "Autoradiographic studies of nucleic acid and protein metabolism in lymphoid cells. II. Stability and actinomycin sensitivity of rapidly formed RNA and protein," Australian J. Exptl. Biol. Med. Sci., 42:363, 1964.
16. B. Mach and P. Vassalli, "Biosynthesis of RNA in antibody-producing tissues," Proc. Nat. Acad. Sci. U.S., 54:975, 1965.
17. M. Nomura and J.D. Watson, "Ribonucleoprotein particles within chloromycetin-inhibited E. coli," J. Mol. Biol., 1:204, 1952.
18. A.B. Pardee, K. Paigen, and L.S. Prestidge, "A study of the ribonucleic acid of normal and chloromycetin-inhibited bacteria by zone electrophoresis," Biochim. Biophys. Acta, 23:162, 1957.
19. S. Dagley and J. Sykes, "Effect of drugs upon components of bacterial cytoplasm," Nature, 183:1608, 1959.
20. S. Dagley, A.E. White, and D.G. Wild, "Synthesis of protein and ribosomes by bacteria," Nature, 194:25, 1962.
21. K. Hosokawa and M. Nomura, "Incomplete ribosomes produced in chloramphenicol and puromycin-inhibited E. coli," J. Mol. Biol., 12:225, 1965.
22. D. Vazques, "The binding of chloramphenicol by ribosomes from Bacillus megaterium," Biochem. Biophys. Res. Commun., 15:464, 1964.
23. D.T. Dubin and A.T. Elkert, "Some abnormal properties of chloramphenicol RNA," J. Mol. Biol., 10:508, 1964.
24. R. Rendi and S. Ochoa, "Effect of chloramphenicol on protein synthesis in cell-free preparations of E. coli," J. Biol. Chem., 237:3711, 1962.
25. R. Rendi, "The effect of chloramphenicol on the incorporation of labeled amino acids into proteins by isolated subcellular fractions from rat liver," Exptl. Cell. Res., 18:187, 1959.
26. G. von Ehrenstein and F. Lipmann, "Experiments on hemoglobin biosynthesis," Proc. Nat. Acad. Sci. U.S., 47:941, 1961.
27. E.H. Allen and R.S. Schweet, "Synthesis of hemoglobin in a cell-free system. I. Properties of the complete system," J. Biol. Chem., 237:760, 1962.
28. A.S. Weisberger, S. Wolfe, and S. Armentrout, "Inhibition of protein synthesis in mammalian cell-free systems by chloramphenicol," J. Exptl. Med., 120:161, 1964.
29. H. Amos, "Effect of actinomycin D and chloramphenicol on protein synthesis in chick fibroblasts," Biochim. Biophys. Acta, 80:269, 1964.
30. N. Talal and E.D. Exum, "Two classes of spleen ribosomes with different sensitivities to chloramphenicol," Proc. Nat. Acad. Sci. U.S., 55:1288, 1966.

31. G.E. Palade, "A small particulate component of the cytoplasm," J.Biophys.Biochem.Cytol., 1:59, 1955.
32. M.L. Peterman, The Physical and Chemical Properties of Ribosomes. New York, Elsevier Publishing Co., 1964. (Page 11 contains an extensive list of references on the relationship of endoplasmic reticulum to protein synthesis.)

Arthritis—An Example of Inflammation Based on Particles*

Jeanne M. Riddle, Gilbert B. Bluhm, and Marion I. Barnhart

Departments of Pathology and Medicine, Henry Ford Hospital and Department of Physiology and Pharmacology Wayne State University School of Medicine Detroit, Michigan

ABSTRACT. Exudative leukocytes from synovial fluids of patients with several types of arthritis were examined by light microscopy, immunofluorescence, and electron microscopy. The fine structure of these leukocytes and their associated intracellular particles was examined in rheumatoid arthritis, gout, and pseudogout. Immune complexes and crystals served as examples of disease-related particles. A variety of particulate materials was observed within the neutrophils from patients with rheumatoid arthritis. These were segregated in phagosomes. Intraleukocytic crystals of sodium urate observed only in gouty arthritis were frequently not contained within a membrane-bounded vacuole. In contrast, crystals of calcium pyrophosphate found only in pseudogout were consistently within membrane-limited vacuoles at their intraleukocytic location. Other particles such as fibrin flakes and cytoplasmic buds shed from the exudative leukocytes were not disease related. Neutrophil granules interacted with each of these intracellular particles. A unifying concept of joint inflammation is presented which illustrates interrelationships between the various types of arthritis when particles serve as the common denominator.

INTRODUCTION

Synovial fluid in the diseased joint may contain several cell types and a variety of particles. Emigrated neutrophils and mononuclear leucocytes constitute a large percentage of the cytopopulation, since the various particulate materials exert a positive chemotactic response. Subsequent interactions between the particles and exudative leucocytes contribute to several facets of the inflammatory process observed in the various types of arthritis.

---

*Supported in part by grant HE 09464-02.

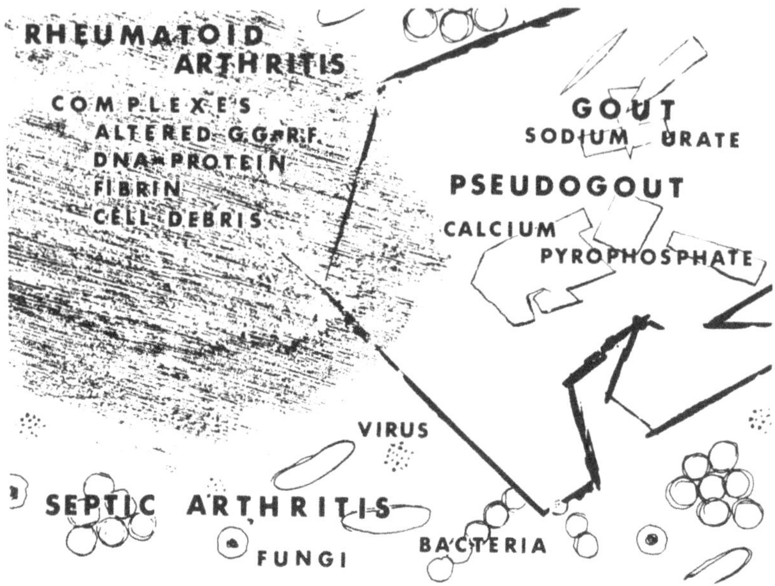

Fig. 1. Various particles are found either extracellularly in the synovial fluid or within the exudative leucocytes in rhematoid arthritis, gout, pseudogout or septic arthritis. Some particles are disease-related while others are common to the various types of arthritis.

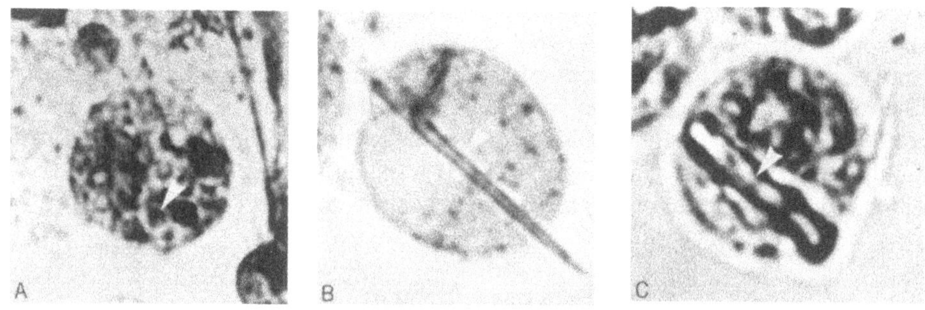

Fig. 2. Exudative neutrophils from synovial fluids of patients with rhematoid arthritis exhibit cytoplasmic inclusions by light microscopy (A). These inclusions (arrows) were larger than neutrophil granules and showed several densities. × 2700. Intraleucocytic crystals of sodium urate (arrow) were observed easily in gouty arthritis (B). × 4400. Likewise in pseudogout, crystals of calcium pyrophosphate were intracellular (C). × 4200. Reduced 30% for reproduction.

The purposes of this presentation were twofold. First, the fine structure of exudative neutrophils and their associated intracellular particles was studied in neutrophil populations from synovial fluids of patients with rheumatoid arthritis, gout and pseudogout. Second, we have illustrated diagrammatically the central role played by particles in initiating or resolving or sustaining the inflammatory reaction accompanying synovitis.

MATERIALS AND METHODS

Samples of synovial fluid were obtained by arthrocentesis and anticoagulated as described previously [1]. A leucocyte count was performed and the total volume aspirated was recorded. Fibrin flakes, if present, were removed by filtering the sample through several layers of gauze. The approximate volume of in vivo formed fibrin was calculated by subtracting the volume of fluid, after the sample was filtered, from the total volume aspirated. Cellular elements were removed from the filtered sample of synovial fluid by centrifugation. Viability studies were performed on one portion of these concentrated leucocytes. Other representative samples of the leucocyte concentrate were processed for electron microscopy and smeared onto glass slides for subsequent staining and study by light microscopy and immunofluorescence [2]. Maraglas was used to embed the samples of concentrated leucocytes processed for ultrathin sections and sections were double-stained with uranyl acetate [3] and potassium permanganate [4]. A modified RCA EMU-2 and an RCA EMU-3H electron microscope were used to examine and photograph our material.

RESULTS

The inflammatory reaction which characterized the disease states of rheumatoid arthritis, gout and pseudogout exhibited several common features. Leucocyte counts per mm^3 varied over a wide range. However, neutrophils constituted the predominant leucocyte in the differential counts from all patients with the various types of arthritis included in our study. From 90-100% of the leucocytes present in the synovial fluids studied were viable.

Certain of the particles present in the samples of synovial fluid from our patient group were disease-related. For instance, complexes with antigenic determinants of 7S gamma globulin and 19S macroglobulin [5] as well as DNA-protein complexes [6] were found in leucocytes from the synovial fluids of patients with rheumatoid arthritis. Likewise, crystals of sodium urate and calcium pyrophosphate were demonstrated only in synovial fluids from patients with gout and pseudogout, respectively [7]. In septic arthritis the synovial fluid may contain bacteria, fungi, or viruses as particulate material (Fig. 1).

In contrast to particles which were present in only specific forms of arthritis, we noted that flakes of fibrin or altered fibrin were found in the synovial fluids from certain patients with rheumatoid arthritis, gout and septic arthritis. The exclusion of fibrin flakes from the synovial fluids of patients with pseudogout probably was a reflection of the small number of samples available for study. These free-floating, in vivo formed particles were identified as fibrin or altered fibrin after the application of a fluorescent-tagged antisera specific for human fibrinogen, fibrin, or related molecules. The number of synovial fluids which contained in vivo formed fibrin flakes varied in each type of arthritis studied. Likewise, the quantity of fibrin flakes present in the samples of synovial fluid was different from one patient to another in a single type of arthritis. In 30 of 42 patients (71%) with rheumatoid arthritis, fibrin flakes constituted as much as 38% of the total volume aspirated from the knee. Fibrin flakes were observed in synovial fluids from 5 of 16 patients (31%) with gout, but they accounted at maximum for only 0.8% of the volume aspirated. Only 1 of 4 patients (25%) with septic arthritis had fibrin flakes in the synovial fluid. These flakes constituted only 1% of the total volume aspirated.

Another particle common to the synovial fluids from the various types of arthritis was shed cytoplasmic buds of leucocytes, especially exudative neutrophils. These available particles either floated freely in the synovial fluid, adhered to the outer surface of the leucocyte membrane, or were contained within phagosomes. In gout, pseudogout, and septic arthritis, the shed buds were phagocytized mainly by macrophages. However, in rheumatoid arthritis it was not unusual to observe cytoplasmic buds of the neutrophils adjacent to the plasma membrane and inside membrane-bound structures of other neutrophils. A few buds were also phagocytized by macrophages present in the synovial fluids from patients with rheumatoid arthritis.

Rheumatoid Arthritis

Neutrophils and mononuclear leucocytes which emigrate into the synovial fluid of patients with rheumatoid arthritis are confronted with a variety of molecular aggregates (Fig. 1). It was demonstrated by the examination of ultrathin sections that the available extracellular particles were phagocytized by the leucocytes and segregated into phagosomes [2, 8]. These membrane-bound structures were observed previously by examining fresh preparations of leucocytes from the synovial fluids of nearly all patients with rheumatoid arthritis by light or phase microscopy. Using these methods of observation, the phagosomes were described as dense, black granules (Fig. 2A) measuring about 0.5 to 1.5 μ in diameter [9]. The chemical heterogeneity of the contents of the phagosomes was expressed morphologically by a diversification of their substructure [2]. Some phagosomes were filled with a homogeneous material of varying electron density. In others, smaller particles with increased density were intermixed with the homogeneous material (Fig. 3). Still other phagosomes contained obvious cellular organelles or a material reminiscent of altered fibrin. The con-

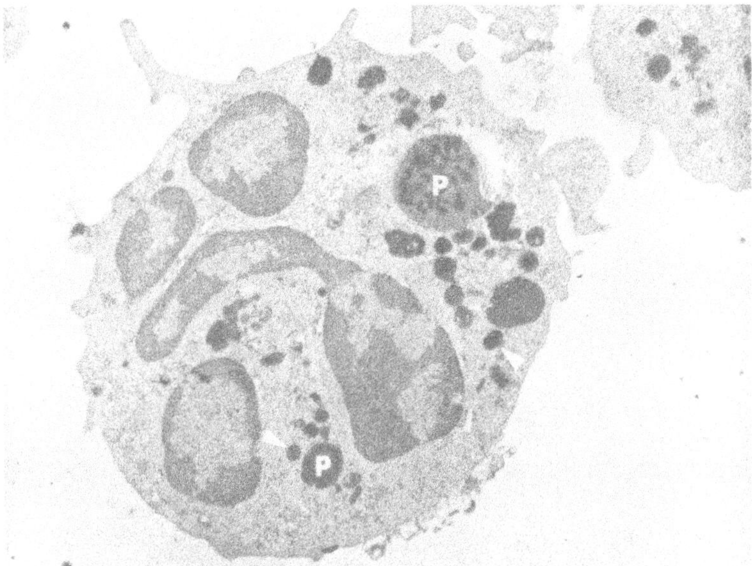

Fig. 3. Using ultrathin sections, numerous phagosomes (P) were observed in the cytoplasm of exudative neutrophils from rheumatoid arthritis patients. These membrane-bounded structures were larger than neutrophil granules (arrows) and their contents exhibited a diversified substructure. × 13,125. Reduced 35% for reproduction.

tents of these phagosomes were not separated from the limiting membrane by a large vacuole. The number of neutrophil granules was decreased in the majority of the exudative neutrophils and evidence for their utilization was obvious, since they were adjacent to the membranes of phagosomes or released into the phagosome interior. Some specific granules in the cytoplasm of neutrophils appeared to coalesce with other neutrophil granules forming a single large granule presumably with an increase enzyme potential.

Crystal Deposition Diseases

The clinical expression of crystal deposition in a joint is identical in both gout and pseudogout. Like rheumatoid arthritis, exudative neutrophils are the leucocytes which predominate most frequently in the synovial fluid. In ultrathin sections crystals were either extracellular, contained within the cytoplasm of intact neutrophils and mononuclear leucocytes or were present in buds shed from the cytoplasm of leucocytes.

Gout

The crystals of sodium urate found in the synovial fluids from patients with gout were identified by their digestion with uricase and their optical properties in a polarizing microscope as described previously [10]. Al-

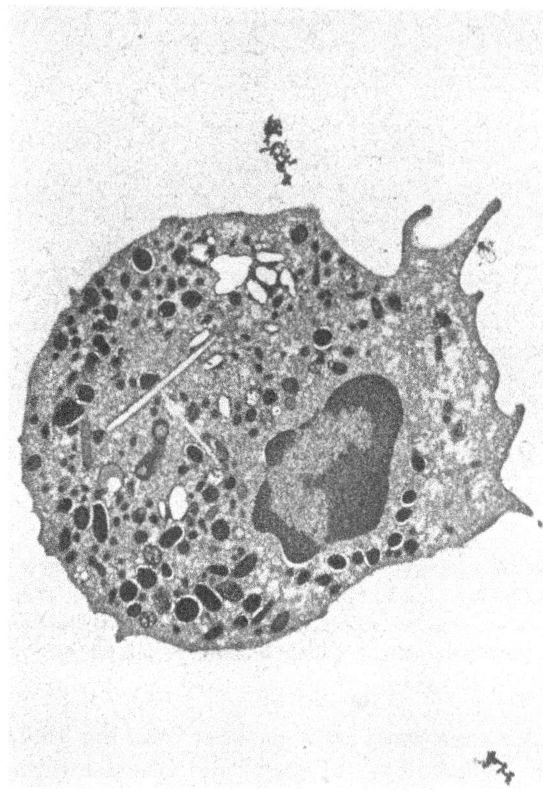

Fig. 4. The majority of sodium urate crystals (arrow) inside exudative neutrophils in gouty arthritis were not contained within a membrane-bounded structure, but seemed to be in direct contact with the cytoplasmic matrix. × 13,230. Reduced 35% for reproduction.

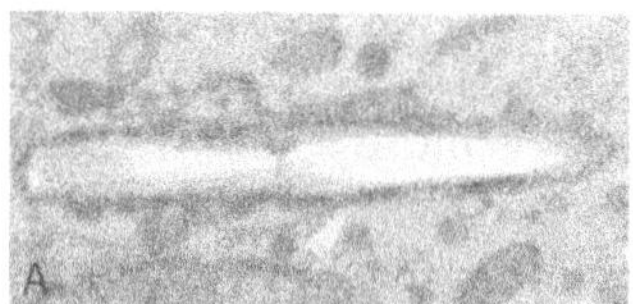

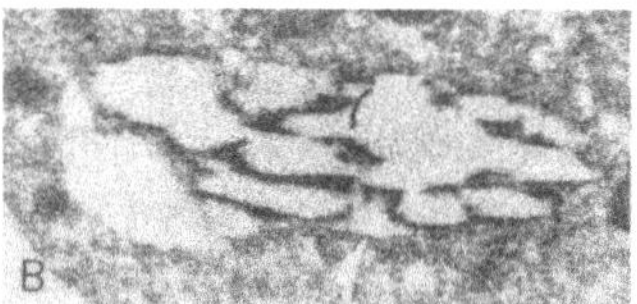

Fig. 5. A few intraleucocytic crystals of sodium urate (arrow) were contained within a typical phagosome. The contents of neutrophil granules frequently aligned the edges of the engulfed crystal (A). × 21,390. Other crystal-like profiles observed within exudative neutrophils from gouty arthritis appeared to be composed of subunits (arrow). These profiles may reflect morphological evidence of intraleucocytic uricolysis or they may indicate that large sodium urate crystals are formed within the cytoplasm of these exudative leucocytes (B). × 31,120. Reduced 30% for reproduction.

though we could ascertain that sodium urate crystals were intraleucocytic, it was not possible by light or polarizing microscopy to discern whether or not these crystals were membrane-bound (Fig. 2B). By examining serial, ultrathin sections of single crystal-containing neutrophils we observed that many of the intracellular crystals of sodium urate were not surrounded by a typical plasma membrane. In fact, some sodium urate crystals appeared to lie in direct contact with the cytoplasmic matrix of the exudative neutrophil (Fig. 4). The edges of other crystals inside the neutrophil were covered by a thin, dense line which was either continuous or interrupted at intervals and gave the surface of the crystal a beaded appearance. Only occasionally was a crystal of sodium urate found within a membrane-limited structure. Rarely was the crystal surrounded by a vacuole which separated the surface of the crystal from the limiting membrane (Fig. 5A).

Profiles of some structures which had a crystal-like appearance were demarcated into numerous smaller subunits by areas of electron-dense material (Fig. 5B). This finding can be interpreted in two ways. First, we considered that larger crystals of sodium urate were in the process of being degraded into smaller subunits. However, the opposite possibility that the

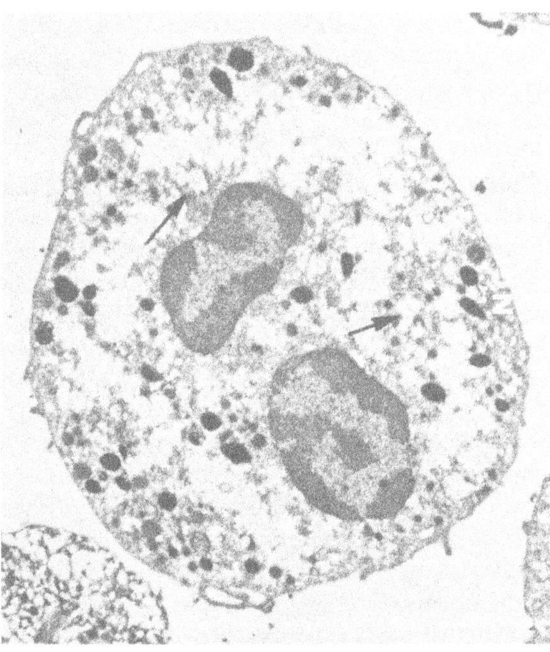

Fig. 6. The cytoplasm of certain exudative neutrophils from gouty arthritis exhibited a striking "honeycomb" appearance. Numerous electron-lucent "spaces" (arrows) were demarcated from the more dense cytoplasmic matrix. The "spaces" contained a finely granular material and neutrophil granules (NG) frequently rimmed their outer limits. x 19,490. Reduced 35% for reproduction.

smaller crystals of sodium urate were being assembled intracellularly to form the typical large crystal was not unreasonable. Our data at present do not permit a selection between these two points of view. However, in vitro experiments in progress may ultimately provide a definitive answer.

Neutrophil granules were associated with the intracellular crystals. Intact granules lay adjacent to the edge of the crystals or were released into the interior of a crystal-containing phagosome. In some micrographs it appeared that the contents of neutrophil granules were distributed along the surface of the crystal lying free within the neutrophil cytoplasm.

In addition to our observations on the orientations between intracellular crystals of sodium urate and structural components of the exudative neutrophil, the cytoplasm of other neutrophils from gouty arthritis revealed a striking "honeycomb" apparence. These "spaces" were prominent also when certain of these exudative neutrophils were examined by phase-fluorescence microscopy. In ultrathin section the more dense cytoplasmic matrix of the neutrophil was separated by numerous electron-lucent "spaces." These varied in size and shape and were devoid of a limiting membrane. The content of these "spaces" was dispersed widely and consisted of granules with a low electron-density. Neutrophil granules were poised frequently on the outer limits of these "spaces" (Fig. 6).

Phagocytic macrophages contained intracellular crystals of sodium urate, pyknotic and nonviable neutrophils, as well as cytoplasmic buds of neutrophils which frequently contained smaller crystals.

Pseudogout

Calcium pyrophosphate crystals were also observed easily in their intraleucocytic location by light and phase microscopic examination (Fig. 2C). The problem of whether or not these crystals were contained within a membrane-bound structure was similar to that encountered in gout. Again our examination of numerous ultrathin sections of neutrophils containing crystals of calcium pyrophosphate resolved this difficulty. Calcium pyrophosphate crystals varied greatly in size and most frequently showed a rectangular shape. These crystals were almost uniformly contained within a membrane-limited structure (Fig. 7). This observation was in sharp contrast to our finding that the majority of the intracellular crystals of sodium urate were not restricted to membrane-limited structures. These membrane-bounded structures which contained crystals of calcium pyrophosphate were often large. Frequently, one or more sides of the crystal were separated from the limiting membrane by a huge vacuole. Other large membrane-limited vacuoles devoid of crystals contained intact neutrophil granules or disintegrating granules. The outer surface of the crystals of calcium pyrophosphate was not generally outlined with the thin, dense line observed to surround the surface of sodium urate crystals. Neutrophil granules were also adjacent to the surfaces of the crystals of calcium pyrophosphate.

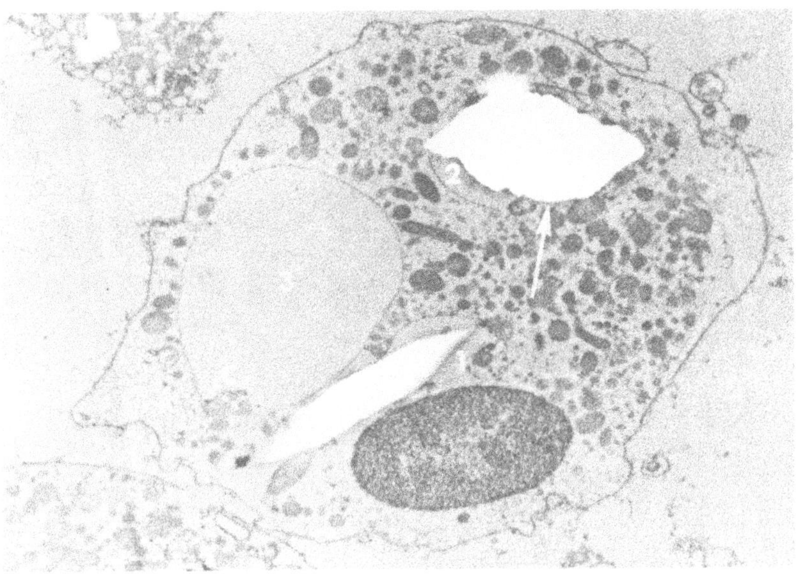

Fig. 7. Exudative neutrophils from pseudogout patients contained intracellular crystals of calcium pyrophosphate (arrow). Large membrane-bounded vacuoles either containing the crystals (1 and 2) or devoid of crystals (3) were present within these neutrophils. Neutrophil granules released their contents (C) into the interior of these vacuoles. x 14,780. Reduced 35% for reproduction.

These granules appeared to disintegrate into small subunits which were vesicular in nature and were surrounded by a finely granular, electron-dense material (Fig. 7). Morphological evidence suggested that some large crystals of calcium pyrophosphate were also composed of smaller subunits which were either being assembled or degraded at their intracellular location.

Again, phagocytic macrophages contained crystals of calcium pyrophosphate, disintegrating neutrophils and shed cytoplasmic buds of other exudative neutrophils.

DISCUSSION

Several schemes representing a series of sequential events which explain the chronic synovitis associated with rheumatoid arthritis and gout have been introduced into the literature. Some of these diagrams stress the importance of a single particle such as immune complexes [9], or crystals of sodium urate [7] in the pathogenesis of joint inflammation. Our study using light, fluorescent and electron microscopy shows that other particles such as fibrin flakes and organized cellular debris were also present in the synovial fluids of patients with rheumatoid arthritis [2]. These particles plus the immune complexes elicited a similar sequence of neutro-

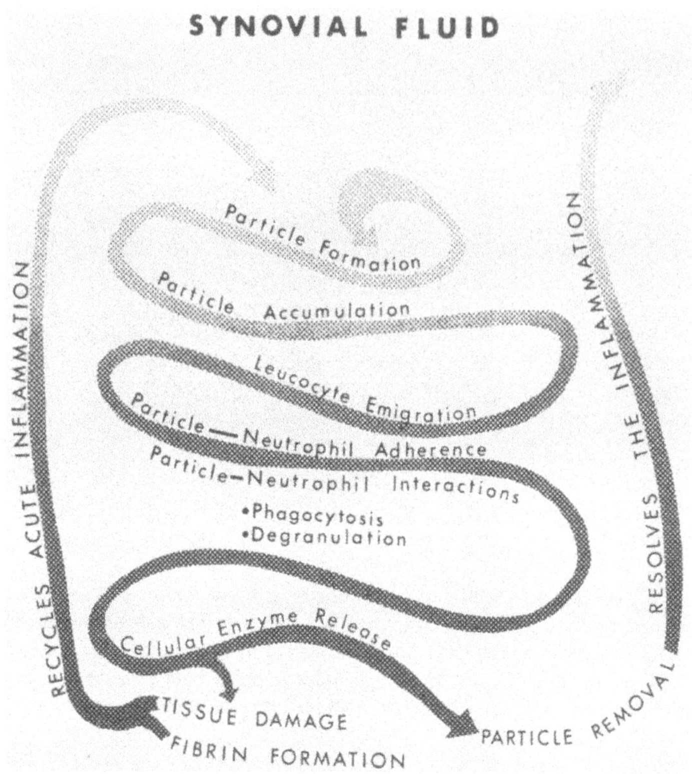

Fig. 8. A unifying concept of joint inflammation based on particle–leucocyte interactions.

phil emigration, particle phagocytosis, interaction of neutrophil granules with phagosomes and subsequent enzyme release. Fibrin formed at an inflammatory site may assume a dual importance. We have shown previously that when a fibrin network is introduced into an experimental lesion neutrophils, and at key hours eosinophils, are attracted selectively [11]. It is known also that fibrin forms and occludes small blood vessels and lymphatics during the dynamic course of inflammation. Fluid is thereby retained and other macromolecular substances might accumulate in an area such as the joint. Resolution of the inflammatory process would then depend in part on the removal of the obstructing fibrin by either chemical or cellular mechanisms.

Our ultrastructural survey of the morphology of exudative leucocytes and associated particles from patients with gout and pseudogout has revealed certain differences in the neutrophil–particle interaction. For example, the majority of sodium urate crystals are not surrounded by a typical continuous limiting membrane. It may be that the sharp needlelike crystals of sodium urate gained entrance into the neutrophil by piercing the cell membrane. Or, crystalline sodium urate may in some unknown way damage or destroy the phagosomal membrane. Finally, we must consider that the sodium urate crystals may be assembled within the cytoplasm of the exudative neutrophil. In contrast, nearly all of the crystals of calcium pyrophosphate were contained within large, membrane-bounded vacuoles.

Regardless of the way in which these various particles are segregated inside the cytoplasm of the neutrophil, our fine structural data show that neutrophil granules interact with all of these intracellular particles regardless of their chemical composition. Proteolytic enzymes such as cathepsin are increased in the synovial fluid during the course of joint inflammation [12]. These findings suggest that neutrophil granules rupture and release their enzymes which possibly mediate tissue damage. From our studies and the work of others [2, 7, 9, 13], particles appear to be one common denominator of the inflammatory reaction in rheumatoid arthritis, gout, pseudogout and septic arthritis. However, we have noted also that some parameters of the inflammatory reaction differ in the various types of arthritis. These distinctive findings may relate directly to characteristic features of the particles. We have represented diagrammatically a unifying concept of joint inflammation which interrelates the various types of arthritis and highlights the role of particles (Fig. 8). Our scheme demonstrates that the inflammatory reaction in a joint may be initiated when particles are formed within the synovial fluid and synovial membrane, resolved when these particles are removed or recycled when the particles accumulate.

ACKNOWLEDGMENTS

The authors wish to express their appreciation to Mr. Wayne Pitchford and Miss Linda Forrest for their technical assistance.

REFERENCES

1. G.B. Bluhm, J.M. Riddle, and M.I. Barnhart, Henry Ford Hosp. Med.Bull., 14:119, 1966.
2. J.M. Riddle, G.B. Bluhm, and M.I. Barnhart, J.Reticuloendothelial Soc., 2:420, 1965.
3. M.L. Watson, J.Biophys.Biochem.Cytol., 4:475, 1958.
4. D.C. Pease, Histological Techniques for Electron Microscopy. New York, Academic Press, 1964, p. 239.
5. A.J. Rawson, N.M. Abelson, and J.L. Hollander, Ann.Internal. Med., 62:281, 1965.
6. T.J. Pekin, Jr., H. Bauer, and N.J. Zvaifler, Arthritis Rheumat., 8:461, 1965.
7. D.J. McCarty, Jr., R.A. Gatter, and J.M. Brill, GP, 31:96, 1965.
8. D. Zucker-Franklin, Arthritis Rheumat., 9:24, 1966.
9. J.L. Hollander, D.J. McCarty, Jr., G. Astorga, and E. Castro-Murillo, Ann.Internal. Med., 62:271, 1965.

10. D.J. McCarty, Jr. and J.L. Hollander, Ann. Internal. Med., 54:452, 1961.
11. J.M. Riddle and M.I. Barnhart, Am.J. Pathol., 45:805, 1964.
12. M.I. Barnhart, C. Quintana, J.M. Riddle, and G.B. Bluhm, Ann. N.Y.Acad.Sci. In press.
13. D. Hamerman, Am.J.Med., 40:1, 1966.

A Major Fault in Diabetic Inflammation: Failure of Leucocytic Glycogen Transfer to Histiocytes

J. W. Rebuck, F. W. Whitehouse, and S. M. Noonan

The Henry Ford Hospital
Detroit, Michigan

INTRODUCTION

The diabetic is allegedly more susceptible to infection than the non-diabetic. Particularly, there has been noted a frequent association of extensive local or systemic infection with the presence of diabetic acidosis. Perillie, Nolan, and Finch [18] have reviewed the humoral immunologic studies in this area and concluded that if lowered resistance to infection is present in patients with diabetes, immunologic factors did not play the essential role in impaired resistance. In contrast, these workers showed that the early neutrophilic phase of the local inflammatory response was significantly delayed and diminished in diabetic patients with acidosis in comparison with normals or nonacidotic patients. The advent of the human skin window technique [20] presents the inflammatory leucocytes with the same clarity of cytologic detail previously available only in the classic hematologic preparations of peripheral blood or marrow aspirates. With this, a new neutrophilic function of cytoplasmic shedding into the exudative fluids was apparent. Before death of the granulocyte in the later stages of inflammation, it could be demonstrated that the neutrophilic cytoplasm peripheral to its nuclear lobes was fragmented in granular or particulate form and shed into the exudative fluids.

The lymphocytes, monocytes, and histiocytes of the inflammatory exudate avidly ingested such neutrophilic cytoplasmic fragments, suggesting their ultimate use in further mononuclear function, especially in mononuclear energization. Following this finding, Page and Good [17] demonstrated that the condition of agranulocytosis produced not only absence of granulocytic migration at the local inflammatory site, but failure of subsequent mononuclear migrations as well. However, when these workers applied viable granulocytes to agranulocytic test lesions, normal mononuclear migrations and functions were restored in the local inflammatory site. This concept has been recently fortified by the observation that growth of homologous and autochthonous tumor cells in inflammatory sites in patients suffering from far-advanced malignancy was accompanied by their ingestion of shed neutrophilic material and usurpation of such normal leucocytic trophocytic transfer to mononuclears [19].

Because of the paucity of reports on actual leucocytic abnormalities in the diabetic patient, it became the purpose of this study to evaluate possible faults in leucocytic–mononuclear transfer and interaction. For obvious reasons our attention was primarily attracted to the glycogen interactions of the various inflammatory cell types. Ackerman [1] has demonstrated that glycogen appears usually during the late neutrophilic myelocytic phase of development and increases rapidly during the metamyelocyte and band-form stages of development. Furthermore, the metabolism of carbohydrates, and especially the pathways of glycogen formation, have been the object of intensive study in the leucocytes [25]. This is of special interest in view of Karnovsky's [12] demonstration that phagocytosis by polymorphonuclear leucocytes requires glycolysis.

MATERIALS AND METHODS

Inflammatory Excitants

Local inflammatory stimuli applied to the test lesions in 0.05 ml amounts included crystalline zinc insulin of u 40 strength (2 units) in 24 lesions, a suspension of killed Escherichia coli (16 lesions), diphtheria toxoid (Parke-Davis and Co.) in 34 lesions, and butter in 2 lesions in diabetic patients.

Method for Human Skin Windows

The method for obtaining timed samples of inflammatory cells from individual test lesions in man has been described in detail previously [20]. Essentially, the technique consists in scraping the epidermis from a 4-mm diameter circular area on the volar surface of the forearm. One of the inflammatory excitants listed above (0.05 ml) was placed on the abraded surface and the entire lesion was next covered with a small, sterile coverslip under a large square of surgical adhesive tape. The exudative cells responding to the stimulus migrate to the undersurface of the coverslip in 30 min to an hour. At 2- to 3-hr intervals, the coverslip was removed and another immediately put in its place. In this way permanent mounts of consecutive samples of the exudative cells from individual investigative lesions were obtained for the special studies listed below.

Listing of Windows

Crystalline zinc insulin, as above, was placed in the paired windows of 12 diabetic patients and 2 normal controls. Killed E. coli suspension was placed in the lesions, again paired, of 8 diabetic patients and 1 normal control. Diphtheria toxoid was placed in the lesions of 17 diabetics and 3 normal controls. And butter was placed in the lesions of one diabetic and two normal controls. In this fashion the exudative responses were studied in a total of 76 lesions in diabetic patients and 16 lesions in normal controls.

Staining Procedures

Leishman's blood-staining procedure was utilized in the study of all insulin-stimulated lesions and in all but 48 of the responses elicited by the bacterial products. The coverslip preparations obtained from the latter 48 lesions in 21 diabetics and 3 normal controls were stained with the Hotchkiss-Lillie alcoholic PAS method [14, 21, 26] with and without diastase digestion for the demonstration of neutrophilic and mononuclear glycogen. Figures 1-4 are illustrations of the undigested PAS reaction, and Fig. 5 shows the same reaction after diastase digestion. Prefixation was accomplished for the Hotchkiss–Lillie method by immersion in 1% HgCl in absolute alcohol for 30 min followed by direct transfer to the first step 70% alcohol of the above-mentioned method. The preparations were counterstained in hematoxylin. Preliminary studies of the reaction to butter utilized the Sudan Black B method of Baillif and Kimbrough [2].

Tests for Phagocytic Ability

When the phagocytic ability of a particular timed stage of leucocytic exudation was to be tested, India ink was applied with a platinum loop to the surface of the lesion at the time of one prior coverslip change.

The number of phagocytic neutrophils per 1000 neutrophils counted was noted at the time of the next coverslip removal. Four lesions in diabetics and two in controls were studied for their phagocytic characteristics.

RESULTS

Quantitatively, the cellular response in the diabetic did not differ significantly from the controls except in the immediate postacidotic state and in insulin resistance.

Response to Insulin

The response to insulin was modest and less marked than that elicited by bacterial antigenic stimuli in 11 of the 12 patients on long-term insulin therapy so studied. A sparse early neutrophilic migration was joined by a few monocytes and moderate numbers of lymphocytes at 9-12 hr. Hypertrophy of both lymphocytes and monocytes resulted in their transformation into histiocytes at 20-24 hr. In the two windows from the remaining patient in this group, who presented with chronic insulin resistance requiring 1000 to 1500 units of insulin per day, there was a massive leucocytic outpouring at the first hour of inflammation. This was marked by superimposition of large numbers of eosinophilic granulocytes and occasional basophilic leucocytes on the customary initial neutrophilic migrations. At 3 hr inflamma-

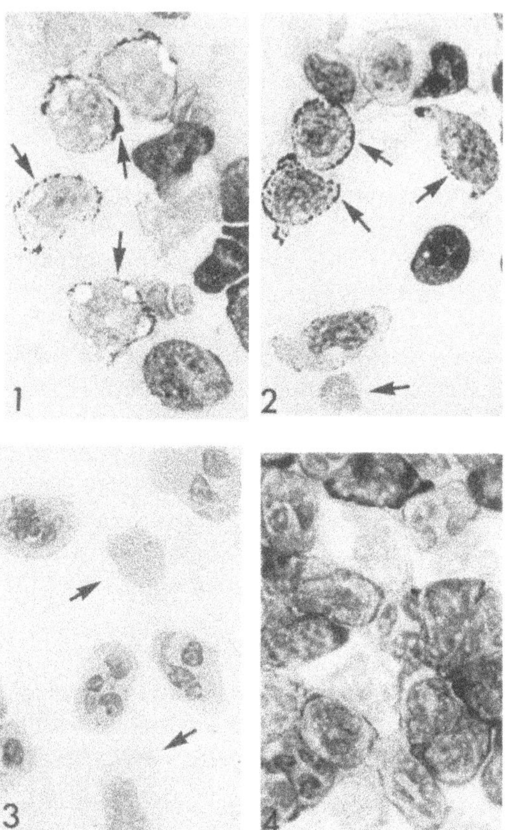

Fig. 1. 6 hr inflammation in nondiabetic control. Arrows point to membranous and submembranous glycogen of lymphocytes, monocytes, and small histiocytes. PAS. × 1100. Reduced 40% for reproduction.

Fig. 2. 12 hr inflammation in nondiabetic control. Arrows point to submembranous glycogen aggregates of lymphocytes and small histiocytes. Bottom arrow designates neutrophilic cytoplasmic fragment. PAS. × 1100. Reduced 40% for reproduction.

Fig. 3. 6 hr inflammation in convalescent phase of diabetic acidosis. Arrows point to absence of membranous or submembranous glycogen. PAS. × 1100. Reduced 40% for reproduction.

Fig. 4. 12 hr inflammation in immediate recovery phase of diabetic acidosis. PAS. × 1100. Reduced 40% for reproduction.

tion (Fig. 6) the eosinophils were found within and about numerous fibrin strands to which they had been attracted. Individual eosinophilic granules had been discharged in large quantities into the fibrin strands and surrounding exudate. This abnormal influx of eosinophilic leucocytes with a few basophilic companions persisted through the 7-, 9-, 12-, 14-, 24-, and 30-hr stages of inflammation in addition to the more normal lymphocyte–histiocyte representations. Many distinct, thin fibrin strands were observed as late as 24 hr with adherent eosinophil granules in view.

Response to Bacterial Antigens

A. Leishman's Stain

As studied with the customary Romanowsky hematologic staining procedures, there was little appreciable difference in the leucocytic exudates responding to the killed E. coli suspensions or diphtheria toxoid stimulation in diabetic patients, when similar responses were elicited in controls. In all but the five postacidotic patients the migrations consisted of an early neutrophilic phase with concurrent lymphocytic appearance at 8-12 hr followed by steady diminution of neutrophilic numbers with gradual small mononuclear transformation to histiocytes by the 24-hr stage. However, responses to the E. coli suspensions in both patients and controls differed from the responses to diphtheria toxoid in that the first-mentioned pyogenic organisms elicited an absolute and relative increase in neutrophilic leucocytes throughout the entire first 14 hr of inflammation. In the five patients studied in the postacidotic state, there was a decrease noted in neutrophilic numbers responding at the third hour of inflammation.

B. PAS Reaction

Of the six lesions in the three normal human volunteers, five were studied without prior diastase digestion and one with prior digestion. In the five without prior digestion at 3 hr of inflammation, the predominant neutrophilic leucocytes showed PAS positive material in abundance as a peripheral cytoplasmic rim of aggregates and in their cytoplasmic frag-

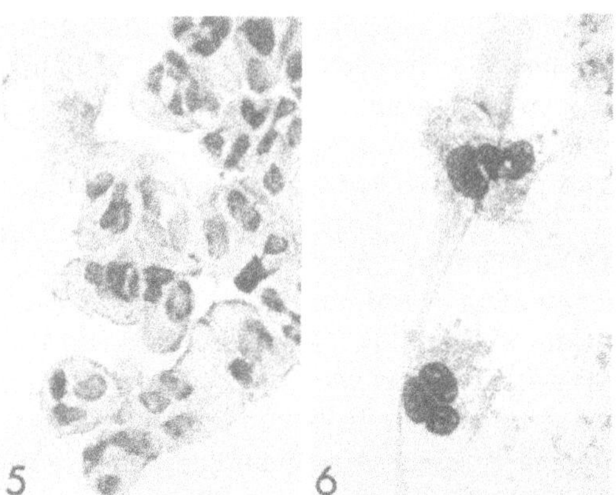

Fig. 5. 6 hr inflammation in immediate recovery phase of diabetic acidosis. Diastase digestion followed by PAS. Note absence of PAS positive material in histiocytes and neutrophils. × 1100. Reduced 40% for reproduction.

Fig. 6. 3 hr inflammation in patient with chronic insulin resistance. Insulin as antigen. Note eosinophils and free eosinophil granulations enmeshed in fibrin strands. Leishman stain. × 1100. Reduced 40% for reproduction.

ments or buds extruded in varying sizes into the surrounding exudative fluids.

At 6 hr inflammation in the control lesions, PAS positivity continued in cytoplasm both intact and extruded pertaining to neutrophilic leucocytes. As the lymphocytes and occasional blood monocytes made their appearance in the field of inflammation (Fig. 1) there was a marked change in their PAS reactivity. Lymphocytes of the blood normally show a sparse, finely granular glycogen content, while monocytes are usually devoid of this material [26]. After a brief sojourn in the field of inflammation, both lymphocytes (top arrow, Fig. 1) and monocytes (bottom arrow, Fig. 1) showed definite massed membranous aggregation of PAS positive material. Inasmuch as the diastase-digested controls showed almost complete elimination of this reactivity in neutrophils, lymphocytes, monocytes, and histiocytes in the field of inflammation in the present study (Fig. 5) and in prior reports [26], the PAS positive aggregates will henceforth be referred to as glycogen. In any instances, there was close apposition of mononuclear to neutrophil. At the top of Fig. 1 a lymphocyte with peripheral glycogen aggregates is found adherent to a neutrophil which has shed its cytoplasm and lost its glycogen. At the bottom of Fig. 1, the aforementioned monocyte with peripheral glycogen aggregates is closely bound to a second neutrophil which has lost much of its cytoplasm as well as most of its glycogen. In the lymphocyte at the right center of Fig. 1, the apposed neutrophil above has its normal glycogen content, while the partially overlying lymphocytic cytoplasm presents only the modest finely granular glycogen of a recently migrated blood lymphocyte.

At 9.5 hr of inflammation in controls the perimembranous massing of glycogen aggregates about the increasing numbers of lymphocytes was itself increased. Pinocytotic activity became apparent just beneath the lymphocytic cytoplasmic membrane with gradual movement of the perimembranous glycogen masses to underlying submembranous, individualized glycogen-containing vacuoles. A beginning of this submembranous localization was apparent at 6 hr (left arrow, Fig. 1). At times a histiocytic foot process rich in glycogen was found attached to a glycogen-depeleted neutrophil. At 12 hr of inflammation (Fig. 2) control migrations were marked by a steady loss of neutrophilic cytoplasm and neutrophilic glycogen content, while a steady increase took place in perimembranous and submembranous glycogen in the numerically increasing lymphocytes and the smaller histiocytes into which they were rapidly transforming.

Direct mononuclear ingestion of shed neutrophilic cytoplasmic fragments was also observed. At 14 hr inflammation there were still some perimembranous and submembranous accumulations of mononuclear glycogen, but as hypertrophy toward the histiocytic state continued, there was at first dispersion of the glycogen aggregates throughout the cytoplasm (lower cell, Fig. 2) followed by a gradual decrease in glycogen content in the histiocytes at 24 hr.

Of the 42 lesions in the 21 diabetic patients, 37 were studied without prior diastase digestion and 5 with prior digestion. In the latter five groups of coverslip exudative samplings, almost complete absence of PAS reacting material in the responding leucocytes, again attested to its glycogen nature. Since at least one series from each patient was studied without prior diastase digestion, the gradual diminution of neutrophilic cytoplasm and glycogen, together with perimembranous, membranous, and submembranous glycogen aggregation about lymphocytes, monocytes, and small histiocytes, proceeded as described above for the controls in 10 of the diabetic patients. In the remaining 11 diabetic patients their lesions showed a marked deviation from the findings with regard to PAS reactivity in both the controls and the aforementioned diabetic patients. All five postacidotic diabetics fell into the affected group depicted in Figs. 3 and 4. In these remaining 11 diabetic patients, PAS reactivity, at first slow to develop in the neutrophils at the 3- to 6-hr stage, actually increased in intensity in the intermediate stages. Large aggregations of glycogen filled the cytoplasm or were massed at the peripheries of these intact neutrophils as late as 14 hr of inflammation. Neutrophilic cytoplasmic shedding and fragmentation were decreased. The most remarkable abnormality was the almost complete failure of membranous or submembranous accumulation of glycogen aggregates in the histiocytes (arrows, Fig. 3) at 6 hr or in the mononuclears of hematogenous origin depicted at 12 hr of inflammation in Fig. 4. In one instance, mononuclear glycogen reactivity began to appear at 14 hr, in another it began at 24 hr, and as late as 30 hr of the inflammatory response. Analysis of the clinical features of these 11 diabetics with delay or absence of mononuclear glycogen activity revealed a parallel severity in their clinical state, there occurring combinations of the following: postacidotic (5), acutely infected (5), severely affected vasculature (4), incapable of control (3), afflicted with advanced diabetic nephropathy (2), insulin-resistant (1), and newly discovered diabetic (1).

Tests for Phagocytic Ability

The number of neutrophils phagocytic for India ink at 12 hr of inflammation was noted in four lesions in diabetics and two in controls, as listed in Table I. It will be seen that phagocytic ability of the neutrophils was significantly decreased in diabetic patients D, E, and F when compared with that of control leucocytes. The phagocytic ability of patient C's leucocytes fell within the normal range. Clinical study of patient C revealed that he was well controlled without noteworthy clinical findings. Diabetic patients

Table I. Number of Neutrophils Phagocytic for India Ink at 12 hr per 1000 Neutrophils Responding

Controls	Diabetics
A 294	C 399
B 429	D 101
	E 115
	F 79

D, E, and F were members of the severely affected group described above as lacking in mononuclear glycogen assimilation.

The exudative samplings from two diabetic patients were studied simultaneously for phagocytic ability and PAS reactivity. These leucocytes were characterized by at least two abnormalities: (1) significantly inhibited phagocytic ability, especially on the part of those neutrophils stuffed with glycogen; and, (2) absence of mononuclear membranous or submembranous glycogen aggregation.

Response to Butter

In the preliminary studies in this group, Sudan Black B-stainable material was depleted in the mononuclears of the diabetic lesions, but the preparations were deemed insufficient for interpretation.

DISCUSSION

The interaction between cells in the living organism has been known for a century. The practical importance of such cellular interrelationships has been appreciated by the embryologist for almost as long. Realization that such cellular interactions persist throughout the life of the organism, as a prequisite of normal function, and that breakdown of cellular interfunctions can lead to the disruptions of disease, has more recently attained importance in biologic thought. The leucocytic sequences initiated in inflammation as outlined by Metschnikoff have been one of the most fertile fields for such exploration. The improved cellular detail afforded by the skin window technique revealed the transfer of granular, particulate, and fragmented portions of neutrophilic cytoplasm from the granulocyte to the mononuclears in the field of inflammation [20]. Direct in vitro observations [21] revealed that such transfer was effected in two ways: (1) by shedding of neutrophilic cytoplasmic material into the exudative fluids from which the mononuclears ingested it; and, (2) by direct apposition of neutrophil to mononuclear. Direct intercellular transfer between lymphocyte and mononuclear has been demonstrated in numerous recent studies [10]. Especially pertinent are those of McFarland and Heilman [15] and Berman [5]. Nor have such observations been confined to interleucocytic transferrals, since

McKhan [16], in this connection, found that tritiated thymidine-labeled lymphocytes injected into tumor-bearing mice soon yielded their label to the tumor cells themselves. Our own observations [19] revealed similar transfer of neutrophilic cytoplasmic materials to growing implanted tumor cells.

The present finding indicates that neutrophils in the field of inflammation in controls yield their glycogen to the lymphocytes, monocytes, and histiocytes in such a fashion that these cells present distinct structural manifestations of the process. This is characterized by perimembranous aggregation of glycogen, membranous, submembranous vacuolar dispositions, and finally intracytoplasmic mononuclear dispersion and glycogenolysis. In the severely insulin-deficient diabetic patient, especially in the immediate postacidotic state, there is retention of glycogen within the neutrophil and partial or more often complete absence of the membrane-related glycogen in the mononuclears. Such a failure of glycogen transfer, and especially interference, with the observed manner of transfer in insulin deprivation is in keeping with current studies on insulin-cellular interactions. Barnhart and Ball [4] found foremost among the ultrastructural changes induced by insulin in rat adipose cells in vitro, a propensity for insulin to initiate pinocytosis by invagination of plasma membranes to form numerous membrane-bounded vesicles. A similar process was observed in our control mononuclears at the time when minute submembranous aggregates of glycogen within vacuoles shifted from their membranous location. Recently, Levine [13], in discussing the action of insulin at the cell membrane, suggested that the glucose transport system is a system of patches on the cell membrane attached structurally to the glycogen-storage apparatus, and noted that the faster rate of glucose entry caused by insulin favored the glycogen storage pathway. Indeed, Bessman [6] emphasizes that insulin stimulated small permeable fragments of diaphragm tissue to synthesize glycogen as measured by a net increase in glycogen. He stated further that insulin provides a mechanical connection between hexokinase and the mitochondrion, so as to facilitate operation of an acceptor effect. Zierler [27] has brought forth evidence that insulin increases resting membrane potential. After the extrusion of glycogen from the neutrophil, the exact manner of its transmission to the mononuclear perimembranous site is not clear. Direct ingestion of neutrophilic glycogen-containing cytoplasmic fragments by the lymphocytes, monocytes, and histiocytes was observed. The structural manifestations of this type of transfer were of a phagocytic nature lodged within the cytoplasm unlike the more characteristic membranous location. Cellular apposition of neutrophil to mononuclear was exceedingly frequent and, as stated above, in prior experiments we have watched direct transfer of neutrophilic neutral red vacuoles and ingested antigen from neutrophilic cytoplasmic buds to lymphocytes [21]. There are so many instances, in our timed preparations, of neutrophilic cytoplasm adherent to adjacent mononuclear cell bodies, that direct cellular transfer of glycogen appears to be the most common manner of such access. Neutrophilic glycogen particulate extrusion into the fluids as microscopic or submicroscopic particulates, with transmission to the mononuclear perimembranous location, is another possibility. In such a pathway, the glycogen could remain intact or glycogenolysis could be followed by glycogen resynthesis at or near the mononuclear membrane.

Shohl and Field [24] felt that most of the insulin binding among the white blood cells was done by the granular leucocytes. Clinical difference in the types of diabetes did not seem to be related to the ability of the white blood cell to bind insulin. However, Cruickshank and Payne [9] found that leucocytes from rabbits with alloxan diabetes and acidosis had reduced destructive power for the ingested pneumococci. Later, Cruickshank [8] observed impairment of the inflammatory reaction in staphylococcal skin lesions of rabbits with acute alloxan diabetes and ketosis. Sheldon and Bauer [23] extended our knowledge of inflammatory events in cutaneous mycormycosis infection in the alloxan diabetic and acidotic rat. He noted first complete failure of tissue mast cells to discharge their granules, then delay of granulocyte clustering, decreased participation of large mononuclears, and, finally, facilitation of massive fungus invasion. Gabrielli and his associates [11] reported significantly depressed leucocytic motility in tubes filled with leucocytes from severely affected diabetic patients. As mentioned before, Perillie, Nolan, and Finch [18] had noted delayed neutrophilic migrations in the local cellular response to inflammation in patients with poorly controlled diabetes, with acidosis, and ketosis. Re-examination of the poorly controlled diabetic group, after acidosis and ketosis had cleared, resulted in restoration of normal leucocytic response at the local inflammatory site. In addition, they were able to demonstrate ketone bodies at the site of inflammation during the acidotic phase. In this connection, it should be recalled that Chernew and Braude [7] have shown that phagocytosis in vitro is inhibited by glucose in concentrations above 2.0%. Our finding of impaired phagocytosis in those inflammatory neutrophils with increased glycogen content suggests that a membrane fault interfering with carbon particle ingestion was on the same basis as inhibition of neutrophilic cytoplasmic glycogen extrusion.

The unusual finding of marked eosinophilic leucocytic responses to local insulin as a stimulus at the early first and third hours of inflammation in the patient resistant to insulin therapy, was accompanied by excess fibrin deposition in the lesion. Although the reason for excessive fibrin deposition is not clear, the abnormal influx of eosinophils agrees with the finding of Barnhart and Riddle [3] that profibrinolysin localization is within the specific granules of the eosinophilic leucocytes and that their presence in inflammation is a prerequisite for neutrophilic dissolution of the fibrin meshwork [22].

SUMMARY

The severely affected diabetic is more susceptible to infection than the nondiabetic. We have studied the local leucocytic reactions to inflammatory stimuli in the diabetic in an attempt to elucidate this problem.

Using our skin window technique to study the cellular reaction to inflammatory excitants, 76 test lesions were performed in 37 diabetic patients. Local stimuli included insulin (24 lesions), a suspension of killed _E. coli_ (16 lesions), and diphtheria toxoid (34 lesions). Appropriate controls were included in the study. The cellular exudate was stained by the Leishman and Periodic Acid Schiff (PAS) techniques.

The response to insulin was less marked than that elicited by bacterial antigens in 11 of the 12 patients so studied. Early and excessive fibrin deposition accompanied by massed eosinophilic granulocytic migrations marked one patient with chronic insulin resistance.

Study of PAS reactivity in the inflammatory responses to bacterial antigens in severely affected diabetic patients, particularly in the postacidotic state, revealed failure of transfer of neutrophilic cytoplasmic glycogen to lymphocytes, monocytes, and histiocytes at the 6- to 14-hr stages. This was in contrast to controls and well-controlled diabetic patients in which glycogen from neutrophils was shed into the exudative fluids in fragments and particulate form to gain access to mononuclears. More commonly, transfer was effected by neutrophilic–mononuclear apposition. In successful transfer, the glycogen first surrounded the mononuclear cell membrane, became incorporated into the membrane, next appeared in vacuolar aggregates immediately beneath the membrane, and, finally, was dispersed throughout the cytoplasm to disappear in glycolysis. In the severely diabetic patients such membranous-glycogen relationships were absent or greatly delayed in their mononuclear responses. Furthermore, in the same patients the neutrophils showed abnormally increased glycogen concentrations accompanied by decreased neutrophilic phagocytic function, and in the postacidotic state neutrophilic migration itself was delayed.

REFERENCES

1. G.A. Ackerman, "Histochemical differentiation during neutrophil development and maturation," Ann. N. Y. Acad. Sci., 113 : 537-565, 1964.
2. R.N. Baillif and C. Kimbrough, "Studies on leucocyte granules after staining with Sudan Black B and May–Grünwald–Giemsa," J. Lab. Clin. Med., 32 : 155-166, 1947.
3. M.I. Barnhart and J.M. Riddle, "Cellular localization of profibrinolysin (plasminogen)," Blood, 21: 306-321, 1963.

4. R.J. Barnhart and E.G. Ball, "Metabolic and ultrastructural changes induced in adipose tissue by insulin," J. Biophysic. Biochem. Cytol., 8: 83-101, 1960.
5. L. Berman, "Lymphocytes and macrophages in vitro, their activities in relation to functions of small lymphocytes," Lab. Invest., 15: 1084-1099, 1966.
6. S.P. Bessman, "A molecular basis for the mechanism of insulin action," Am. J. Med., 40: 740-749, 1966.
7. I. Chernew and A.I. Braude, "Depression of phagocytosis by solutes in concentrations found in the kidney and urine," J. Clin. Invest., 41: 1945-1953, 1962.
8. A.H. Cruickshank, "Resistance to infection in the alloxan diabetic rabbit," J. Pathol. Bacteriol., 67: 232, 1959.
9. A.H. Cruickshank and T.P.B. Payne, "Anti-pneumococcal powers of the blood in alloxan diabetes in the rabbit," Bull. Johns Hopkins Hosp., 84: 334, 1948.
10. M. Fishman, R.A. Hammerstrom, and V.P. Bond, "In vitro transfer of macrophage RNA to lymph node cells," Nature, 198: 549, 1963.
11. E.R. Gabrielli, T. Pyzikiewicz, and P.A. Seamans, "Reticuloendothelial activity and leucocyte motility in diabetes mellitus," Federation Proc., 22: 433, 1963.
12. M.L. Karnovsky, in G.E.W. Wolstenholme and M. O'Connor, Eds., Biological Activity of the Leucocyte. London, Churchill, 1961, pp. 60-78.
13. R. Levine, "The action of insulin at the cell membrane," Am. J. Med., 40: 691-694, 1966.
14. R.D. Lillie, Histopathologic Technic and Practical Histochemistry, 3rd ed. New York, McGraw-Hill, 1965.
15. W. McFarland and D.H. Heilman, "Lymphocyte foot appendage: Its role in lymphocyte function and in immunological reactions," Nature, 205: 887, 1965.
16. C.F. McKhan, "In vivo destruction of immune lymphoid cells in transplantation immunity," Federation Proc., 22: 275, 1963.
17. A.R. Page and R.A. Good, "A clinical and experimental study of the function of neutrophils in the inflammatory response," Am. J. Pathol., 34: 645-670, 1958.
18. P.E. Perillie, J.P. Nolan, and S.C. Finch, "Studies of the resistance to infection in diabetes mellitus: Local exudate cellular response," J. Lab. Clin. Med., 59: 1008-1015, 1962.
19. J.W. Rebuck, M.J. Brennan, J.A. Hall, and C.L. Barth, "Leucocytic trophism for inflammation and autochthonous and homologous tumor cells," J. Reticuloendothelial Soc., 1: 450-463, 1964.
20. J.W. Rebuck and J.H. Crowley, "A method of studying leucocytic functions in vivo," Ann. N.Y. Acad. Sci., 59: 757-805, 1955.

21. J.W. Rebuck, R.A. Monto, E.A. Monaghan, and J.M. Riddle, "Potentialities of the lymphocyte with an additional reference to its dysfunction in Hodgkin's disease," Ann.N.Y.Acad.Sci., 73 : 8-39, 1958.
22. J.M. Riddle and M.I. Barnhart, "Ultrastructural study of fibrin dissolution via emigrated polymorphonuclear neutrophils," Am.J.Pathol., 45 : 805-823, 1964.
23. W.H. Sheldon and H. Bauer, "Tissue mast cells and acute inflammation in experimental cutaneous mucormycosis of normal, 48/80 treated and diabetic rats," J.Exptl.Med., 112 : 1069, 1960.
24. J. Shohl and J.B. Field, "Insulin binding in vitro by leucocytes from normal and diabetic subjects," J.Lab.Clin.Med., 51 : 288-292, 1958.
25. R.L. Stjernholm and E.P. Noble, "Carbohydrate metabolism in leucocytes," J.Biol.Chem., 236 : 3093-3096, 1961.
26. H.R. Wulff, "Histochemical studies of leucocytes from an inflammatory exudate. Glycogen and phosphorylase," Acta.Hematol., 28 : 86-94, 1962.
27. K.L. Zierler, "Possible mechanisms of insulin action on membrane potential and ion fluxes," Am.J.Med., 40 : 735-739, 1966.

Participation of Hepatic Parenchymal and Kupffer Cells in Chylomicron and Cholesterol Metabolism*

N. R. Di Luzio and S. J. Riggi†

Department of Physiology and Biophysics
University of Tennessee Medical Units
Memphis, Tennessee

ABSTRACT. The administration of reticuloendothelial (RE) stimulants produced an increased growth and functional activity of RE cells. Parenchymal cell number, structure, and function, as indicated by BSP removal, and histological and electron-microscopic observations were unaltered in RE-stimulated rats. The RE hyperactive group manifested an increased intravascular removal of colloidal carbon which was associated with enhanced accumulation of carbon in Kupffer cells.

The technique of selectively and exclusively producing an RE hyperfunctional state was employed to evaluate the metabolic behavior of labeled chyle, chylomicrons, and an artificial lipid emulsion, designated as "RE test lipid emulsion." The intravascular removal of chyle and chylomicrons was not enhanced in RE-stimulated rats. The predominant uptake of injected chyle and chylomicrons was hepatic in nature with lung and spleen manifesting 1-3% removal. Cholesterol-containing chylomicrons demonstrated a behavior similar to that of triglyceride-containing chylomicrons and unlike colloidal carbon and the RE test lipid emulsion. Significant differences existed, however, between the organ uptake of cholesterol and triglyceride-labeled chylomicrons.

An artificial lipid emulsion was developed that possessed an intravascular behavior and an organ distribution which was comparable to colloidal and particulate materials which are removed by phagocytosis. This RE test lipid emulsion has been employed in the evaluation of RE function in experimental and clinical subjects.

* These studies were supported in part by the USPHS (HE-05367) and the Atomic Energy Commission.

† These studies were conducted during the tenure of a USPHS Predoctoral Fellowship. Present address: Lederle Laboratories, Pearl River, New York.

Normal chylomicrons containing cholesterol or triglyceride are relatively immune to RE cell uptake and the hepatic mechanism of chylomicron removal involves essentially their removal by the parenchymal cell.

INTRODUCTION

The term "chylomicron," to designate the lipid particle which appeared in blood after fat feeding, was first employed by Gage in 1920 [1] to replace Gulliver's phrase "molecular base of the chyle" [2, 3]. Gage and Fish, in 1924, investigated the problems of fat digestion, absorption, and assimilation in man and experimental animals [3] and in an excellent and classical paper contributed greatly to the early comprehension of various problems of lipid metabolism by defining the nature, source, size, and distribution of chylomicrons. It is of interest that among the unsolved problems of fat metabolism, as proposed by Gage and Fish [3], was "How, and in what form, does the fat leave the blood stream and become incorporated into the substance of adipose cell or the protoplasm of the active cells of the body?"

This report is limited to the consideration of the possible role of the liver parenchymal and Kupffer cells in the metabolism of triglyceride and cholesterol-containing chylomicrons and artificial lipid emulsions. Extensive and excellent reviews of the metabolism of chylomicrons have been published by Dole and Hamlin [4], Olivecrona et al. [5], and Olson and Vester [6].

Chylomicrons are essentially composed of a central core of triglyceride [4-6] associated with phospholipid and free and ester cholesterol [7, 8], the former serving as a surfactant material. Free fatty acids as well as mono- and diglycerides have also been identified as constituents [4, 6, 8]. The protein absorbed on the surface of the lipid particle contributes to the negative charge which the particle possesses [9]. The triglyceride, which constitutes 85-90% of the lipid, is synthesized in the intestinal mucosa from dietary fatty acids possessing a chain length of twelve carbons or more [10]. The term "chylomicron" therefore denotes a particulate transport form of exogenous fat from the alimentary tract.

Previous studies have demonstrated that labeled chylomicrons rapidly disappear from the circulation at an exponential rate [11-19]. The composite nature of the disappearance curve revealed the presence of a fast and a slow component [11]. The disappearance rate of chylomicrons decreased with increasing fat loads and a previous injection of chylomicrons delayed the removal of subsequently injected lipid particles [11].

Among various factors which influence chylomicron removal, heparin has been shown to cause a significant increase in the rate of intravascular disappearance, while Triton, a lipemic agent, significantly inhibited the removal mechanism [11].

The importance of the liver in the removal of both plasma free fatty acids (FFA) as well as chylomicron cholesterol and triglyceride has been amply demonstrated [14-20]. It appears that approximately 50% of the injected chylomicrons disappear from the vascular system due to an as yet undefined hepatic removal mechanism [19]. Goodman [20] has reported that more than 90% of chylomicron cholesterol ester is removed by the liver within 60 min following the intravenous injection of labeled chylomicrons.

The liver has been demonstrated by Doaust to be composed of five different types of cells, of which parenchymal and Kupffer cells are present in greatest numbers [21]. The cellular composition of liver is approximately 61% parenchymal and 33% littoral or endothelial cells. The relative roles of parenchymal and Kupffer cells in the removal of triglyceride or cholesterol-containing chylomicrons remains to be established.

Jaffe [22] stressed the importance of the Kupffer cell in the removal of chylomicrons. He also reviewed the earlier literature on RE involvement in lipid metabolism [23]. These studies, based principally upon the presence of lipid droplets in hepatic cells, resulted in the concept that Kupffer cells, in contact with the vascular compartment, phagocytized chylomicrons. Jaffe felt that the lipid material would then be transferred to the parenchymal cell for subsequent alteration and metabolism [23]. A physiological role of the Kupffer cell in removal of chylomicrons was therefore proposed, as well as the hypothesis that the liver cell extracted lipid from the Kupffer cell after the latter removed it from blood.

Based on the cellular localization of cholesterol 6 hr after feeding cholesterol and oil, as well as the fact that the injection of India ink, chromium phosphate, or saccharated iron resulted in a reduction in the liver deposition of cholesterol and in the development of chylomicronemia, Byers et al. reported that the RES was essential for the normal disposition of cholesterol-containing chylomicrons [24,25]. Neveu et al. [26] also concluded that reticuloendothelial (RE) cells removed cholesterol-containing lipoproteins and chylomicrons. However, this study involved the use of heterologous (rabbit) lipoproteins and chylomicrons which were injected into rats. The significance of these observations, as related to isologous chylomicron behavior, is as yet unanswered.

The accumulation of lipid in the reticuloendothelial system (RES) in reticuloendotheliosis seems to support the concept of RE involvement in lipid metabolism [27]. The particulate nature of the chylomicron, its negative charge, and the exponential removal rate, as well as an inverse relationship between the rate of removal and chylomicron load were taken as further evidence of RE involvement. Variant concepts of hepatic removal of chylomicrons are presented in Fig. 1.

The involvement of the RES in certain areas of cholesterol metabolism was also suggested by studies which demonstrated the inhibition of dietary-

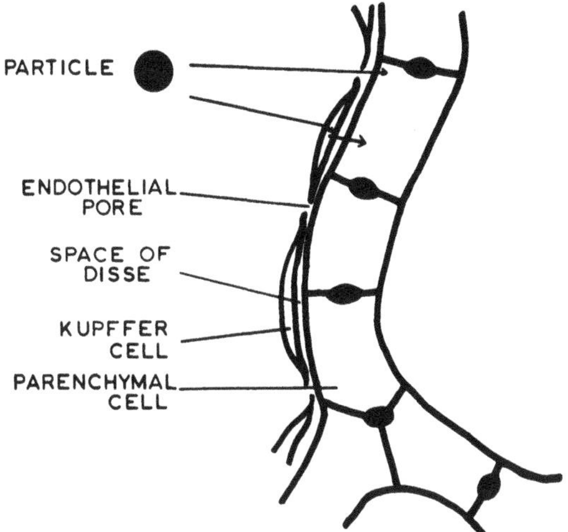

Fig. 1. Potential mechanisms of the removal of the chylomicron triglyceride or cholesterol involving: (a) phagocytosis by the Kupffer cell, or (b) removal by the parenchymal cell.

induced hypercholesterolemia and hepatic cholesterosis in RE hyperfunctional rats [28-32].

The liver has been demonstrated to be the principal site of removal of artificial fat emulsions [33-35]. In evaluating whether the RES played a role in the removal of emulsified fat from blood, Waddell et al. [33] reported that the prior injection of either lithium carmine, carbon black, or trypan blue (agents which localized in Kupffer cells), did not alter the removal rate of injected lipid emulsion. Histological studies showed fat droplets in the parenchymal cells whether or not the RE cells were capable of uptake. In a study in which corn oil, coconut oil, and mineral oil emulsions were employed with essentially similar results, Waddell et al. [33] concluded that free permeation of fat particles from the sinusoids into the hepatic cell was the mechanism of lipid uptake. Murray and Freeman [34] concluded that while certain synthetic fat emulsions may be of the same size as chylomicrons, they are not handled in a comparable fashion, but like foreign particulate material are removed by a phagocytic process.

Fine structural studies of Ashworth et al. [34, 37] demonstrated that hepatic parenchymal cells were more actively engaged in the removal of chylomicrons than were Kupffer cells.

Since the relative participation of various types of hepatic cells in lipid metabolism has not been fully delineated, the following series of experiments detail our studies to evaluate the role of hepatic, parenchymal, and Kupffer cells in the intravascular removal of triglyceride and cholesterol-containing chylomicrons. The Kupffer cell constitutes the major functional element of the RES.

Comprehensive understanding of the initial phase of triglycerides and cholesterol metabolism should not only contribute to a basic understanding of lipid metabolism, but also aid the development of a physiological lipid emulsion for intravenous alimentation.

EXPERIMENTAL PROCEDURE AND RESULTS

Our initial study to define the role of the RES in the vascular clearance of chylomicrons made use of the Halpern effect, i.e., the rate of clearance of intravenously injected colloidal or particulate material is inversely proportional to the initial mass of the administered material [38]. This effect is readily demonstrated when increased carbon loads are injected (Table I). If chylomicrons were handled in a manner similar to colloidal gold or carbon, materials known to be removed by phagocytosis, it would be antici-

Table I. Phagocytic Function and Sulfobromophthalein Concentration in Normal and RE Hyperfunctional Rats*

Group	Colloidal carbon t/2 (min)		Plasma BSP*
	8 mg/100 g	25 mg/100 g	mg/cc
Saline	7.4	27.7	0.32
Glucan	0.7	1.7	0.30

*Means are derived from 6-9 rats/group. Sulfobromophthalein (BSP) was injected in the amount of 50 mg/kg and plasma concentrations determined 10 min after injection.

Table II. Phagocytic Activity in Normal and Hyperlipemic Dogs

Group	Intravascular Removal Rate		Organ Distribution* Colloidal ^{198}Au		
	Carbon (min)	Gold (sec)	Liver	Lung	Spleen
Normal	12.2	123	90.5	0.38	1.34
Lipemic: olive-oil fed	–	99	86.5	0.19	1.38
Lipemic: lard-fed	9.5	87	86.8	0.17	1.02

*Values expressed as percent of the injected dose per organ. Means are derived from 7-10 dogs/group.

pated that during alimentary lipemia, when myriads of chylomicrons were present, a decrease in the removal rate of the test colloid would occur. Alimentary lipemia was induced in dogs by feeding 4.5 g/kg of either lard or olive oil. Phagocytic activity of the RES was determined during the peak of the lipemia [39]. The results indicated that the presence of chylomicrons did not depress the disappearance rate of colloidal carbon (200 mg/kg) or colloidal radio-gold (Table II). In fact, an enhancement in removal rate of the test colloid was observed. The tissue distribution of the colloidal gold was unaltered in lipemic dogs (Table II).

Failure to induce an effective RE blockade [40, 41] led to attempts to evaluate the role of the RES in triglyceride and cholesterol metabolism by the technique of selective RE stimulation.

The cell wall preparation from Saccharomyces cerevisiae, designated as zymosan, has the ability to induce an increase in the functional activity of the RES [42-46]. Phagocytic efficiency in these RE-stimulated animals as measured by the removal rate of colloidal carbon is approximately 100%, i.e., complete extraction of the colloidal carbon in one pass through the liver. This hyperphagocytic state was associated with pronounced hypertrophy and hyperplasia of organs such as liver, lung, and spleen, which contain large populations of RE cells [37, 44-46].

Subsequent studies indicated that glucan, a polysaccharide which constitutes a portion of the yeast cell wall, is an active RES stimulating agent or RES growth factor [44]. Glucan is characterized by a chain of glucopyranose units united by a 1-3 β-glucosidic linkage. Studies conducted in our laboratory have demonstrated the importance of the 1-3 β-type linkage in RES activation. Because of the reduced toxicity and known purity of the glucan fraction, the studies reported involve the use of intravenously administered glucan to selectively stimulate the RES.

The measurement of sulfobromophthalein (BSP) removal in normal and RE-stimulated rats demonstrated that during intense hyperphagocytosis and hyperplasia of the RES, the removal of BSP was unaltered (Table I). These studies indicate that parenchymal cell activity is unchanged in RE-stimulated animals [45].

The specificity of the hepatic response to RES stimulants indicates that these agents offer a unique method by which a controlled and selective growth and hyperfunction of RE cells can be induced. Histological observations of our RE-stimulated and control rats indicate approximately one endothelial or Kupffer cell for every 2.5 parenchymal cells in control animals to one Kupffer cell for every parenchymal cell in the glucan-treated group. The size of the Kupffer cell was also profoundly increased in glucan-treated rats.

Since studies indicated that the morphology, number, and functional activity of parenchymal cells were unaltered in RE hyperactive mice and rats, this RE activation technique lends itself to the elucidation of the contribution of hepatic and parenchymal cells in the intravascular removal of triglyceride and cholesterol-containing chylomicrons and artificial lipid emulsions.

Radioactive chyle was obtained following the administration of either ^{131}I-labeled triolein, glyceryl tripalmitate-1-^{14}C, or 4-^{14}C-cholesterol in corn oil to rats with thoracic dust fistulas [47]. The chyle was collected in an iced sealed container, filtered, and injected intravenously either into saline-injected control rats or into glucan-injected rats. The analysis of ^{14}C-tripalmitin-labeled chyle by thin-layer chromatography and subsequent liquid scintillation counting indicated that 92% of the total radioactivity was

Table III. Intravascular Clearance and Tissue Distribution of ^{131}I Triolein-Labeled Chyle in Normal and RE-Stimulated Rats*

Group	t/2 (min)	Blood %ID/ml	Liver %ID/TO†	Spleen %ID/TO	Lung %ID/TO
Saline	10.4 ±1.3	2.86 ±0.32	12.60 ±0.90	2.02 ±0.14	0.96 ±0.13
Glucan	8.4 ±0.5	2.35 ±0.17	11.36 ±0.71	2.58 ±0.36	1.89 ±0.29

*Male rats weighing approximately 270 g were injected with either 0.5 mg glucan per 100 g for 5 days or saline. The rats were killed 10 min after injection of labeled chyle in the amount of 4 mg triglyceride/100 g.
†%ID/TO = percent of administered dose per organ.
Values are expressed as mean ± standard error and are derived from 9 rats per group.

Table IV. Tissue Distribution of Tripalmitin-^{14}C-Labeled Lymph Chylomicrons in Normal and RE Hyperfunctional Rats*

Group	Body Weight (g)	Liver %ID/TO†	Spleen %ID/TO	Lung %ID/TO
Saline	198 ±4	25.7 ±0.8	1.3 ±0.2	1.4 ±0.1
Glucan	195 ±2	27.7 ±1.1	3.3 ±0.2	2.4 ±0.2

*Female rats were injected with either saline or glucan daily for 6 days. Animals were killed 10 min after intravenous injection of labeled chyle in a dose of 4 mg triglyceride/100 g.
†%ID/TO = percentage of injected labeled triglyceride per total organ (TO). Values are mean ± standard error of 5 saline- and 6 glucan-treated rats.

in the triglyceride fraction. Approximately 3% was recovered in the phospholipid fraction and 8% in the mono- and diglycerides and free fatty acid (FFA) fractions. These results are similar to the values obtained by Olivecrona and others [8, 11-16]. Chylomicrons were isolated by centrifuging chyle at a density of 1.006 for 4 hr at 21,600 × g. Approximately 85% of the total activity of chyle was in the supernatant or chylomicron fraction with 92% of the recovered radioactivity localized in the triglyceride fraction.

The intravascular removal rate was determined by plotting, semilogarithmically, the blood radioactivity levels against time. The injected dose

Table V. Intravascular Clearance and Tissue Distribution of Isolated Chylomicrons Labeled with Glyceryl Tripalmitate-1-^{14}C in Control and RE-Stimulated Rats*

Group	Body weight (g)	t/2 (min)	Liver %ID/TO†	Spleen %ID/TO	Lung %ID/TO
Saline	220 ± 4	8.4 ±2.0	21.3 ±0.6	2.3 ±0.2	4.5 ±0.4
Glucan	223 ± 2	9.0 ±0.9	27.3 ± 0.6	4.7 ±0.4	4.9 ±0.5

*Female rats received intravenous injections of either glucan or saline for 5 days and were then injected with 23 mg triglyceride/100 g. All rats were killed 10 min after injection. Values are mean ± standard error of 5 saline- and 6 glucan-treated rats.
†%ID/TO = percentage of injected ^{14}C lipid activity per total organ.

Table VI. Tissue Distribution of Triolein ^{131}I-Labeled Triglyceride 24 Hr after Injection of Lymph Chylomicrons in Saline- and Glucan-Treated Rats*

Group	Liver %ID/TO†	Lung %ID/TO	Urine ^{131}I %ID
Saline	0.57 ± 0.05	0.51 ± 0.09	31.5 ± 6.4
Glucan	0.58 ± 0.06	0.45 ± 0.09	38.0 ± 2.5

*Male rats weighing approximately 240 g were treated with saline or glucan for 5 days and were injected with 4 mg triglyceride/100 g as chyle. All animals were killed 24 hr after injection, and the organ distribution of lipid-bound ^{131}I and urinary excretion of inorganic ^{131}I were determined. Values are mean ± standard error of 7 rats per group.
†%ID/TO = percentage of injected lipid ^{131}I activity per organ.

of ^{131}I triolein-labeled whole chyle was 4 mg of triglyceride/ 100 g body weight. The intravascular removal rate (t/ 2) of labeled chyle was 10.4 and 8.4 min, respectively, in the control and RE hyperfunctional groups (Table III). These values are not significantly different. The radioactivity of blood at 10 min was similar in both groups. Approximately 12% of the injected dose was recovered in liver, whereas 2% was found in the spleen. A significant increase in the activity of lung occurred on an organ basis in the RE-stimulated group, which reflects the increased weight of the lung.

The tissue distribution of ^{14}C-tripalmitin-labeled chyle 10 min after injection was similar to that of the ^{131}I triolein chyle. The injected dose of ^{14}C tripalmitin was also 4 mg triglyceride/ 100 g. No difference existed insofar as the degree of hepatic uptake between the RE hyperfunctional and normal animals (Table IV). However, when compared to the percent uptake of ^{131}I triolein chyle, a significantly larger fraction of ^{14}C tripalmitin chyle was localized in liver. Spleen and lung of the RE-stimulated animals showed increased accumulation of the labeled chyle on a total organ basis, reflecting their increased size.

The intravascular clearance and early tissue distribution of isolated washed rat chylomicrons labeled with ^{14}C tripalmitin was also determined to evaluate whether the washing procedure altered the physiological behavior of isologous chylomicrons. Microscopic examination revealed a significant increase in particle size with a large number of particles ranging 3-4 μ. The injected dose of washed chylomicrons was 23 mg triglyceride per 100 g.

The intravascular removal rate of the washed chylomicron preparation was 8.4 and 9.0 min in the normal and RE-hyperfunctional animals, respectively (Table V). Liver uptake at 10 min was 21 and 27% in the two groups, respectively, which was in agreement with the distribution of whole chyle similarly labeled. However, a significant difference of about 27% was noted between the hepatic content of the normal and hyperfunctional groups. This increased localization difference may be a reflection of the phagocytosis of the larger washed chylomicron particle. Spleen uptake was significantly greater in the RE-hyperfunctional group, whereas lung content was not altered.

These findings demonstrate that, in contrast to the behavior of colloidal carbon, no increase in the removal rate of isologous chyle triglyceride occurred in the RE-hyperfunctional group. These data also indicate that the intravascular removal and initial tissue distribution of normal isologous chylomicrons are not a function of the phagocytic activity of RE cells. In an effort to determine whether the late tissue distribution or overall metabolism of chylomicron triglyceride was altered in the presence of an RE-hyperfunctional state, the tissue distribution of lipid-bound ^{131}I and the urinary ex-

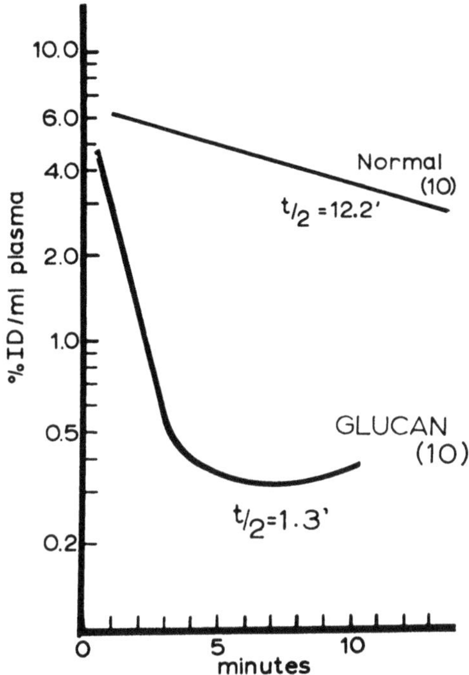

Fig. 2. Mean intravascular removal rate of triolein-^{131}I-labeled lipid emulsion of 10 normal saline-injected and 10 glucan-injected rats. The increased lipid radioactivity of blood after 5 min was observed in all rats in the RE hyperfunctional group.

cretion of inorganic ^{131}I were determined 24 hr following the injection of ^{131}I triolein-labeled chyle (Table VI). No significant difference was observed in the glucan group.

These observations demonstrated that the normal metabolism of chylomicrons is not modified initially or at 24 hr by the presence of a hyperactive and hyperplastic RES. The disposition of normal triglyceride-containing chylomicrons is therefore not dependent upon the functional state of the phagocytic system [48].

Various artificial lipid emulsions were tested relative to their intravascular behavior in normal and RE-hyperfunctional rats [49, 50]. One of these emulsions was prepared as an anhydrous base with corn oil, glycerol, and phospholipid in the ratio of 10 : 10 : 1, respectively. This emulsion was labeled with ^{131}I triolein and injected intravenously into normal and RE-hyperfunctional rats in the amount of 25 mg/ 100 g. In contrast to the unaltered removal of ^{131}I triolein-labeled chyle, the intravascular removal of this emulsion was increased 90% in the hyperfunctional group (Table VII). The 10-min blood radioactivity was, as expected, reduced correspondingly in the stimulated rats.

A study of the organ distribution of lipid bound ^{131}I triolein 10 min following its injection revealed that liver uptake of this emulsion was 32% in the normal group and 72% in the RE-hyperactive group. It is of interest that with an identical intravascular half-time being manifested in the chyle-injected and triglyceride emulsion-injected normal rats, the liver uptake was increased approximately 150% in the emulsion-injected group. Hepatic uptake of the emulsion would account for over 80% of the injected dose.

Table VII. Intravascular Clearance and Initial Tissue Distribution of Artificial Lipid Emulsion in RE-Hyperfunctional Rats*

Group	t/2 (min)	Blood %ID/ml	Liver %ID/TO	Spleen %ID/TO	Lung %ID/TO
Saline	12.3 ±1.20	3.3 ±0.19	31.84 ±1.86	4.6 ±0.28	0.8 ±0.06
Glucan	1.3 ±0.12	0.3 ±0.02	71.7 ±1.6	1.0 ±0.03	0.5 ±0.05

*Female rats, weighing approximately 220 g, were injected with either saline or glucan (0.5 mg/100 g for 5 days). On the 6th day, the rats were killed 10 min after the injection of the RE test lipid emulsion in the amount of 25 mg/100 g. Values are expressed as the percent of the injected dose (%ID) recovered as lipid-bound ^{131}I per total organ (TO). Means and standard errors are derived from 10 rats/group.

Table VIII. Vascular Removal and Tissue Distribution of Tripalmitin-^{14}C-Labeled Artificial Lipid Emulsion in Glucan-Treated Rats*

Group	t/2 (min)	Liver %ID/TO†	Spleen %ID/TO	Lung %ID/TO
Saline	30.4 ± 6.0	30.7 ± 3.2	4.1 ± 0.09	1.5 ± 0.13
Glucan	3.5 ± 0.2	67.9 ± 4.7	1.6 ± 0.08	1.1 ± 0.06

*Male rats weighing approximately 200 g were injected with either saline or glucan for 5 days. On the 6th day, the rats were killed 10 min after administration of the RE test lipid emulsion in the amount of 61 mg of triglyceride/100 g of body weight. Mean and standard error values are derived from 8 saline- and 6 glucan-treated rats.

†%ID/TO = percent of the injected tripalmitin-^{14}C-recovered per total organ.

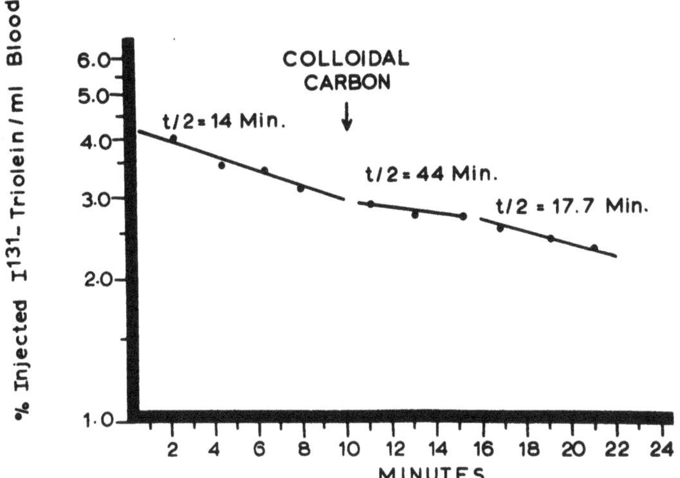

Fig. 3. The inhibitory effect of colloidal carbon on the intravascular removal rate of ^{131}I-triolein-labeled RE test emulsion. The above figure, derived from a single animal, is representative of the response seen in the group of 8 rats.

Spleen and lung collectively removed approximately 5% of the injected lipid in the control group. The uptake by spleen and lung of the triglyceride emulsion was significantly reduced in the RE-hyperfunctional group, possibly due to the predominant liver uptake and a resulting reduced availability of the lipid particle to the macrophages of spleen and lung.

The increased vascular removal was not associated with an elevation in plasma free fatty acids and the neutral polysaccharide, glucan, possessed no clearing activity in lipemic animals. The increasing plasma lipid radioactivity which occurred in the glucan group is suggestive of re-entry of the labeled lipid in an as yet unidentified lipoprotein fraction (Fig. 2).

In an effort to demonstrate that ^{14}C-labeled triglycerides would behave in a manner similar to the ^{131}I-labeled emulsion, the anhydrous emulsions were prepared with glyceryl tripalmitate-1-^{14}C (Table VIII). The rats received 61 mg triglyceride per 100 g body weight. In agreement with previous results with the ^{131}I triolein-labeled emulsion, an increased removal of the ^{14}C tripalmitin emulsion was manifested in the hyperactive group. The enhanced clearing was associated with an increased liver uptake and a reduction in the localization in spleen. Lung content on a gram basis was reduced 50%, whereas total organ uptake was unaltered.

Based upon these observations, it became apparent that this artificial lipid emulsion might be advantageously employed in the measurement of RE

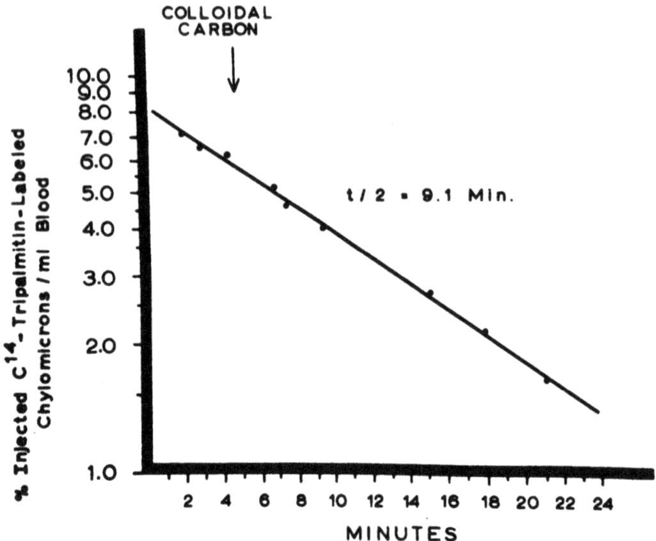

Fig. 4. The mean intravascular removal of ^{14}C-tripalmitin-labeled chylomicrons in 5 normal rats. Colloidal carbon (8 mg/100 g) which was administered 5 min following the chylomicron injection did not alter the vascular clearance of chylomicrons. This is in marked contrast to the inhibitory effect observed with the RE test emulsion (Fig. 3).

function. In an effort to further substantiate the validity of employing this anhydrous emulsion as a functional test for RE activity, the influence of colloidal carbon on the intravascular removal of the artificial lipid emulsion was determined. If this lipid emulsion is handled by the process of phagocytosis, then a significant impairment in removal rate due to competitive inhibition should be manifested in the presence of colloidal carbon.

Eight rats were injected intravenously with the ^{131}I-triolein labeled artificial emulsion in the amount of 20 mg/100 g as triglyceride and tail blood samples were taken at 2, 4, 6, and 8 min. After the fourth sample, colloidal carbon (8 mg/100 g) was administered intravenously and six additional samples were obtained at intervals of 2 min. The radioactivity of the blood samples was plotted semilogarithmically and half-times determined (Fig. 3). In agreement with our previous observations, the initial t/2 of the labeled emulsion was 13.8 min (Table IX). Immediately after the injection of carbon, the t/2 increased to a mean of 34.3 min in six rats, with two rats manifesting no measurable removal of labeled lipid. The impaired removal of the RE test lipid emulsion persisted for a duration of 6-7 min after which a t/2 comparable to the initial value was observed.

The impaired removal of RE test emulsion following the administration of colloidal carbon demonstrates that similar removal, i.e., phagocytic mechanisms, are involved. In contrast to the behavior of the RE test emulsion, the vascular clearance of ^{14}C tripalmitin-labeled chylomicrons was not modified after the injection of colloidal carbon (Fig. 4), demonstrating again that RE test lipid emulsion particles do not behave like native lipid particles which are removed by parenchymal cell activity.

To further support the conclusion that this artificial lipid emulsion was removed by phagocytosis, additional histological, as well as electron-microscopic studies were conducted [37]. The results of these studies fully supported the concept of an exclusive removal of this emulsion by RE cells, particularly the Kupffer cell [37]. This emulsion has been designated as an RE test lipid emulsion [49-51].

Since cholesterol-containing chylomicrons may have a different removal mechanism than triglyceride-labeled chylomicrons, the influence of RE hyperfunction on the intravascular removal and initial tissue distribution of

Table IX. Effect of Colloidal Carbon Administration on the Intravascular Removal of Artificial Lipid Emulsion*

Initial t/2 (min)	After carbon t/2 (min)	Final t/2 (min)
13.8 ± 0.1	34.3† ± 7.0	13.1 ± 0.7

*Male rats weighing approximately 325 g were injected with the triolein-^{131}I-labeled emulsion in the amount of 20 mg triglyceride per 100 g. Colloidal carbon (8 mg/100 g) was injected after 10 min. Values are means and standard errors of 8 rats.
†Two animals showed no clearance of the lipid emulsion during this phase. These values were not computed in the determination of the mean.

Table X. Vascular Clearance and Tissue Distribution of Cholesterol-4-^{14}C-Labeled Chyle in Control and RE-Hyperfunctional Rats*

Group	Liver %ID†/TO	Lung %ID/TO‡	Spleen %ID/TO	Plasma %ID/ml	t/2 (min)
Saline	28.3 ± 3.4	1.1 ± 0.1	1.1 ± 0.3	6.2 ± 0.3	12.2 ± 1.0
Glucan	25.4 ± 3.0	1.5 ± 0.2	1.9 ± 0.3	5.8 ± 0.4	14.0 ± 0.8

*Male rats received saline or 0.5 mg glucan per 100 g for 5 days. The cholesterol load injected was 0.48 mg of cholesterol ester per 100 g body weight. The tissue data, expressed as mean ± standard error were derived from 4 rats/group, while the intravascular removal rate was compiled from 8 rats/group. All rats were killed 10 min after injection.
†%ID = percent of the injected dose.
‡%ID/TO = percent of the injected dose per organ.

cholesterol-4-^{14}C labeled chyle was also studied (Table X). The t/2 of cholesterol-containing chyle was approximately 12 min in the saline control group and 14 min in the RE-hyperfunctional group. The 10-min tissue distribution was not significantly changed in the glucan group. The predominant uptake was by liver, with lung and spleen showing a small and comparable removal.

Preliminary studies of the influence of RE hyperfunction on the removal of albumin-bound palmitic acid-^{14}C have been undertaken. The clearance of albumin-bound palmitic acid was studied in five control and six RE-hyperfunctional rats. The t/2 of intravenously administered albumin-bound palmitate was 1.19 ± 0.08 min in the saline group and 0.85 ± 0.08 min in the glucan group. In contrast to the behavior of triglyceride or cholesterol-containing chyle, a significant increase in the removal of albumin-bound FFA occurred in the RE-stimulated group. These findings are suggestive that plasma FFA are removed to some extent by Kupffer cells.

DISCUSSION

The present studies on the rapid intravascular removal of injected chyle and chylomicrons are in agreement with previous results [11-16]. The t/2 of approximately 8-10 min is similar to the values reported by French and Morris [11], who injected 47.5 mg total fatty acids. The determination of the location of the label in French and Morris' study indicated that 2-3% was in the phospholipid fraction with the remainder in the triglycerides. Our results are comparable.

In the present study, we initially selected chyle in order to study the metabolism of triglyceride-labeled chylomicrons in their physiological environment. Other factors initially considered in selecting chyle, rather than isolated chylomicrons, were the possible heterogeneity of the isolated particulate fraction, the possibility of removing the surface coat, and an attempt to avoid exceeding the load of triglyceride which enters the vascular system during fat feeding, which in the rat approximates 60-80 mg/hr [52].

Electron microscopic studies of a Hungarian commercial preparation of India ink demonstrated that these India ink particles in the hepatic sinusoids are covered by a coat of medium-density material which was presumably formed by blood proteins upon injection [53]. The importance of the surface coat and charge to the phagocytic mechanism was stressed by the observations of Kojima and Imai [54], which indicated that removal of the protein coat of the carbon particle renders it less susceptible to phagocytosis. These observations, which demonstrate the importance of the particle surface to phagocytosis, indicate that extreme care should be employed in the preparation of chylomicrons as well as artificial lipid emulsions.

It is apparent from the studies conducted to date that the liver is the most important single organ relative to the mechanism of removal of exogenously derived triglyceride and cholesterol. Olivecrona [16] reported that maximum liver uptake is reached in 15-30 min following the injection of chylomicrons and approximates a minimum of 40% of the injected dose. Similarly, our results indicate that the greatest uptake of triglyceride or cholesterol-containing chylomicrons occurs in liver. Our studies indicate that approximately 30% of the injected triglyceride or cholesterol-containing chylomicrons would be localized in liver in the normal animals 10 min following their injection. These figures on hepatic uptake of cholesterol-labeled chyle are in agreement with previous results [20, 55].

The uptake of ^{131}I labeled triglyceride or ^{14}C cholesterol-containing chylomicrons by lung and spleen was relatively minor, being of the order of 1-3% of the injected dose at the 10-min interval. These studies are in basic agreement with previous observations, and clearly indicate that lung and spleen play relatively unimportant roles in the vascular clearance of various chylomicrons.

Friedman et al. found no localization of cholesterol in spleen and lung after the feeding of cholesterol and oil to rats [24, 25]. Markowitz and Mann [56] evaluated the role of the lung in the metabolism of fat and observed that intravenous administration of a lipid emulsion resulted in increased lipid content of lung. The intravenous injection of citrated chyle, however, produced no increase in lung content of lipid. Stein and Shapiro [57] observed that when artificial emulsions were employed, considerable localization occurred in lung. They indicated that deposition in the liver is the rule when physiological emulsions were employed. These findings, and those of Goodman [20], however, are in contrast to the observations of Berliner and Dougherty [58, 59] on the importance of lung in the metabolism of cholesterol. The latter investigators employed, however, an artificial cholesterol 4-^{14}C emulsion prepared in propylene glycol or horse serum instead of physiological chyle or chylomicrons. Thus, these findings are not apparently relevant to the behavior of normal cholesterol-containing chylomicrons.

The compiled data of the obvious differences in intravascular removal rates between chylomicrons and colloidal carbon, of the "RE test lipid emulsion," in RE-stimulated rats, demonstrate marked metabolic differences between chylomicrons and these foreign particulate lipids. These data demonstrate that the particulate chylomicrons are not handled by a phagocytic mechanism. The liver cell isolation studies [39], as well as the electron microscopic observations [37], demonstrate that chylomicrons are localized primarily in hepatic parenchymal cells.

Although evidence has been obtained that demonstrate RE cells are relatively unimportant in the vascular clearance of triglyceride and cholesterol-containing chylomicrons, this does not exclude their possible participation in vascular clearance under various nonphysiological conditions.

Jones et al. [60] studied the size of chylomicrons in rats fed either butter or corn oil. In the butter-fed rats three different types of osmiophilic materials were identified. The chylomicrons observed in butter-fed rats ranged from 50 mμ to 20 μ. The chylomicrons over 15 μ were classified as "giant chylomicrons." In contrast, no "giant chylomicrons" were seen in the chyle of corn oil-fed rats. The chylomicrons derived from butter-fed rats not only were larger, but also had scalloped borders, in contrast to the smooth surface of the chylomicrons from corn oil-fed rats. Although it has not as yet been determined, it is entirely possible that these "giant chylomicrons" might be removed by a phagocytic mechanism. Indeed, French and Morris noted that the removal rate for larger particles of chylomicron fat was at a faster rate than that of the smaller particles [11]. Nestel and Scow [61] reported that chylomicrons from cream-fed animals were removed more rapidly from the circulation than chylomicrons obtained from corn oil-fed animals, suggesting that the fatty acid composition of the chylomicron may also influence its removal rate.

Bierman et al. [62] isolated and characterized two distinct lipid particles which were designated as primary and secondary particles. The primary particles migrated in the region of the α 2-globulin fraction, while the secondary particles migrated in the region of the β-globulin fraction. The primary particles were larger in size, appeared early during fat absorption, contained a greater portion of dietary fatty acid, and originated in the intestine. The removal rate and organ distribution of a particulate ^{14}C-labeled triglyceride complex, which has the physical characteristics of the primary particle derived from lymph, was not influenced by RE hyperfunction, suggesting that this particulate lipid behaves more like native lipid particles than like foreign emulsified material [63].

The possible mechanisms of removal of chylomicrons from the vascular compartment involve the processes of: (1) intravascular hydrolysis, (2) removal as an intact particle, or (3) hydrolysis at the cell surface. Presently all three have been proposed as the mechanism of removal of triglyceride-containing chylomicrons, with the greatest evidence favoring the second hypothesis.

Bragdon and Gordon [17] compared the tissue distribution of ^{14}C-labeled chylomicrons and ^{14}C-labeled free fatty acids. The rats received 18 or 44 mg of chylomicron lipid and were killed from 10-200 min after injection. Chylomicron radioactivity was found primarily in the liver in the fasted state and in adipose tissue in the carbohydrate-fed rats. Since the tissue distribution of the injected labeled chylomicrons differed from that of injected FFA, which were found primarily in liver and muscle, it was concluded that the major fraction of the triglyceride does not undergo intravascular hydrolysis. The observation that the isolated perfused liver can remove chylomicrons from the perfusing medium, coupled with the observation that lipoprotein lipase is absent in the liver, supports the hypothesis that the liver can remove chylomicrons intact [64]. The histology of the liver after perfusion with ^{14}C tripalmitin-labeled chylomicrons revealed that most of the fat was located in the parenchymal cells with some fat droplets found in Kupffer cells.

Additional possible support for the concept of direct hepatic removal of particulate lipid was obtained by Edgren and Ivemark [65]. They reported that particulate lipid of artificial lipid emulsion is removed by a nonhydrolytic mechanism, since paraffin emulsions, which cannot be hydrolyzed, were effectively cleared from blood. Belfrage et al. [66] indicated that particles of a different type of fat emulsion were also removed from the vascular compartment without extensive intravascular lipolysis, and localized preferentially in liver and spleen, a tissue distribution unlike that of labeled chylomicrons [19].

Direct evidence that some of the chylomicrons can leave the vascular system as intact particles was reported by French and Morris [11] and Morris and Courtice [67], in which labeled chylomicrons obtained from a donor animal were found to be present in the lymph collected from various portions of the body following the intravenous injection of chyle into a recipient animal.

Experiments with doubly labeled lipids have been most productive in delineating the hepatic removal mechanism. Reiser et al. [68], employing glycerol and palmitic acid-labeled tripalmitin, compared the tissue distribution as well as the glycerol-fatty acid ratios at 3-72 hr after feeding. They concluded that plasma triglycerides are removed by the liver without hydrolysis.

Similar conclusions were reached by Olivecrona [15] who studied removal rates and tissue distributions of chylomicrons labeled with ^{14}C glycerol and ^{3}H palmitic acid 5-160 min after injection. Olivecrona concluded that the major part of the chylomicron glyceride leaves the circulating blood without hydrolysis. This conclusion was based upon: (1) a hepatic $^{14}C:{}^{3}H$ ratio of 1 during the early phase of removal, (2) absence of any appreciable amount of radioactivity in the mono- or diglycerides, and (3) low FFA specific activity. These observations were similar to the findings of Borgstrom and Jordan [69], who injected chylomicrons labeled in the glycerol and fatty acid positions and observed a parallel uptake of glycerol and fatty acids by the liver. Fredrickson et al. [70] also reported that retransport as plasma FFA is not obligatory in the utilization of chylomicron triglyceride fatty acids, and demonstrated that chylomicrons can be removed as such from blood. Havel and Fredrickson [12] demonstrated that the triglyceride and phospholipids of chylomicrons disappear from the vascular compartment at the same rate, indicating removal of the particle as an intact unit.

Stein and Shapiro [57] demonstrated also that chylomicron triglyceride penetrate the liver cell as such and are absorbed on the mitochondria and microsome fractions without prior hydrolysis. Stein and Shapiro observed that 15 min after palmitate administration, most of the radioactivity was found in the mitochondria and microsome fractions, designated as "active metabolizing sites" and very little activity was located in the floating fat fraction. At later intervals, the specific activity of the various liver cell fractions became similar, indicating complete mixing. The observations of Stein and Shapiro [57] and Shapiro [71] also contribute to the concept that intravascular hydrolysis is relatively unimportant in the removal of chylomicron triglyceride. When approximately 60% of the palmitic acid-1-^{14}C labeled chylomicrons were removed, no labeled FFA was found in blood.

There appears to be rather general agreement that the liver can remove particulate lipid intact. The mechanism of direct particulate uptake by the liver (Fig. 1) in which the Kupffer cell is bypassed, is possibly by way of the sinusoidal pore [37, 72-73]. The discontinuity of the sinusoidal surface, in which pore sizes up to 2 μ in diameter are found, would allow the direct passage of chylomicrons into the space of Disse, which exists between the endothelial cell and the hepatic parenchymal cell. This perisinusoidal space of Disse now assumes great importance in the exchange of material between the parenchymal cell and plasma. Holle [74] considers this space as the reaction chamber through which all traffic between liver cells and blood must pass. The existence of microvilli of the parenchymal cell, whereby the surface area is markedly increased, enhances the effective transfer of materials.

Felts and Mayes reported that there is little net uptake or catabolism of chylomicron triglyceride by the isolated perfused liver in the absence of triglyceride hydrolysis by lipoprotein lipase. These investigators, therefore, questioned the concept that chylomicron triglyceride has direct access to hepatic parenchymal cells and proposed that lipolysis of triglyceride had to occur before uptake by the liver [75, 76]. In marked contrast to these conclusions, Higgins and Green [77], employing isolated hepatic parenchymal cells, observed that different chylomicron components such as unesterified cholesterol, cholesterol ester, and triglyceride were taken up at the same rate, indicating that the whole chylomicron is bound to the hepatic cell. Higgins and Green proposed that the site of hydrolysis of chylomicron triglyceride was the plasma membrane [76, 77].

The removal of an artificial RE test lipid emulsion, in contrast to that of chylomicrons, was greatly dependent upon the functional status of the RES. This particular emulsion, which differed somewhat from certain other commercial emulsions tested in this laboratory, manifested a behavior which was identical to colloidal and particulate materials which are known to be phagocytized by the RE cells. The rate of clearance of the anhydrous lipid emulsion was significantly altered when colloidal carbon was injected, which demonstrated a competitive effect on the phagocytic mechanisms. This anhydrous lipid emulsion, which undergoes rapid hydrolysis and oxidation, offered a unique method to evaluate the functional activity of the RES in both experimental and clinical subjects [49, 50, 51, 78].

Since synthetic emulsions differ in respect to particle size, stabilizing agents, lipid content, and composition, no generalization about their physiological behavior can be made. It is obvious that artificial emulsions must be employed with great caution when used in the investigation of normal chylomicron metabolism.

While demonstrating no significant RE involvement in the metabolism of normal chylomicrons, our data in no way imply that RE cells cannot, or do not, remove particulate lipid either during pronounced lipemias or in the presence of abnormal lipid complexes, or in situations of poor chylomicron stability and resulting particle aggregation.

REFERENCES

1. S. H. Gage, Cornell Vet., 10:154, 1920.
2. G. Gulliver, Gerber's General Anatomy, 1847, p. 88.
3. S.H. Gage and P.A. Fish, Am.J.Anat., 34:1, 1924.
4. V.P. Dole and J.T. Hamlin, III, Physiol. Rev., 42:674, 1962.
5. T. Olivecrona, E.P. George, and B. Borgstrom, Federation Proc., 20:928, 1961.
6. R.E. Olson and J.W. Vester, Physiol. Rev., 40:677, 1960.
7. B. Borgstrom and N. Tryding, Acta Physiol. Scand., 37:127, 1956.
8. R.J. Havel, Am.J.Clin.Nutr., 6:662, 1958.
9. C.B. Laurell, Scand.J.Clin.Lab.Invest., 6:22, 1954.
10. B. Borgstrom, in: K. Bloch, Ed., Lipide Metabolism. New York, John Wiley & Sons, 1960, p. 128.
11. J.E. French and B. Morris, J.Physiol., 138:326, 1957.
12. R.J. Havel and D.S. Fredrickson, J.Clin.Invest., 35:1025, 1956.
13. J.E. French and B. Morris, J.Physiol., 140:262, 1958.
14. B. Borgstrom, P. Wlodawer, and C. Naito, Digestion, Absorption Intestinale et Transport des Glycerides Chez Les Animaux Superieurs. Paris, Centre National de la Recherche Scientifique, 1961, p. 125.
15. T. Olivecrona, J.Lipid Res., 3:439, 1962.
16. T. Olivecrona, Acta Physiol. Scand., 55:170, 1962.
17. J.H. Bragdon and R.S. Gordon, J.Clin.Invest., 37:574, 1958.
18. R.J. Havel and A. Golfien, J.Lipid Res., 2:389, 1961.
19. P. Belfrage, B. Borgstrom, and T. Olivecrona, Acta Physiol. Scand., 58:111, 1963.
20. D.S. Goodman, J.Clin.Invest., 41:1886, 1962.
21. R. Daoust, In: R.W. Brauer, Ed., Liver Function. Washington, D.C., Am.Inst.Biol.Sciences, 1958, p. 3.
22. R.H. Jaffe and S.L. Berman, Arch.Pathol.Lab.Med., 5:1020, 1928.
23. R.H. Jaffe, in: H. Downey, Ed., Handbook of Hematology. New York, P.B. Hoeber, 1938, p. 977.

24. M. Friedman, S.O. Byers, and S.St.George, Am.J.Physiol., 184:141, 1956.
25. S.O. Byers, S.St.George, and M. Friedman, in: B.N. Halpern, Ed., Physiopathology of the Reticuloendothelial System. Springfield, Illinois, Charles C. Thomas, 1957, p. 128.
26. T. Neveu, G. Biozzi, B. Benacerraf, C. Stiffel, and B.N. Halpern, Am.J.Physiol., 187:269, 1956.
27. S.J. Thannhauser, Lipidoses. New York, Oxford University Press, 1950.
28. N.R. DiLuzio, Ann.N.Y.Acad.Sci., 88:244, 1960.
29. N.R. DiLuzio, Nature, 185:616, 1960.
30. N.R. DiLuzio, J. Houston, and E.E. Elko, in: S. Garattini and R. Paoletti, Eds., Drugs Affecting Lipid Metabolism. Amsterdam, Elsevier Publishing Co., 1961, p. 228.
31. S.J. Riggi and N.R. DiLuzio, J.Lipid Res., 3:339, 1962.
32. N.R. DiLuzio and S.J. Riggi, J. Reticuloendothelial Soc., 3:135, 1966.
33. W.R. Waddell, B.P. Geyer, E. Clarke, and F.J. Stare, Am.J. Physiol., 177:90, 1954.
34. R.G. Murray and S. Freeman, J.Lab.Clin.Med., 38:56, 1951.
35. J. Van Den Bosch, E. Evrard, A. Billiau, J.V. Joossens, and P. DeSomer, J.Exptl.Med., 114:1035, 1961.
36. C.T. Ashworth, V.A. Stembridge, and E. Sanders, Am.J.Physiol., 198:1326, 1960.
37. C.T. Ashworth, N.R. DiLuzio, and S.J. Riggi, Exptl.Mol.Pathol. Suppl., 1:83, 1963.
38. G. Biozzi, B. Bencerraf, and B.N. Halpern, Brit.J.Exptl.Pathol., 34:441, 1953.
39. N.R. DiLuzio, J.Am.Oil Chemists' Soc., 37:163, 1960.
40. N.R. DiLuzio, K.A. Simon, and A.C. Upton, Arch. Pathol., 64:649, 1957.
41. D.A. Blickens and N.R. DiLuzio, J. Reticuloendothelial Soc., 1:68, 1964.
42. B. Benacerraf and M.M. Sebestyen, Federation Proc., 16:860, 1957.
43. L.S. Kelly, E.L. Dobson, C.R. Finney, and J.D. Hirsch, Am.J. Physiol., 198:1134, 1960.
44. S.J. Riggi and N.R. DiLuzio, Am.J.Physiol., 200:297, 1961.
45. S.J. Riggi and N.R. DiLuzio, Nature, 193:1292, 1962.
46. W.R. Wooles and N.R. DiLuzio, J. Reticuloendothelial Soc., 1:160, 1964.
47. J.L. Bollman, J.C. Cain, and J.H. Grindlay, J.Lab.Clin.Med., 33:1349, 1948.
48. N.R. DiLuzio and S.J. Riggi, J.Reticuloendothelial Soc., 1:248, 1964.
49. N.K. Salky, N.R. DiLuzio, D.P. P'Pool, and A.J. Sutherland, J.Am. Med.Ass., 187:744, 1964.
50. N.R. DiLuzio, N.K. Salky, S.J. Riggi, and A.J. Ladman, in: The Reticuloendothelial System, Morphology, Immunology and Regulation. Kyoto, Japan, "Nissha" Printing Co., 1965, p. 389.

51. N.R. DiLuzio and S.J. Riggi, J.Reticuloendothelial Soc., 1:136, 1964.
52. V. Aberdeen, P.A. Shepherd, and W.J. Simmonds, Quart.J.Exptl. Physiol., 45:265, 1960.
53. I. Toro, P. Ruzsa, and P. Rohlich, Exptl.Cell Res., 26:601, 1962.
54. M. Kojima and Y. Imai, Proc.Japan Soc. Reticuloendothelial System, 1:61, 1961.
55. W.J. Lossow, N. Brot, and I.L. Chaikoff, J. Lipid Res., 3:207, 1962.
56. C. Markowitz and F.C. Mann, Am.J.Physiol., 93:521, 1930.
57. Y. Stein and B. Shapiro, J. Lipid Res., 1:326, 1960.
58. D.L. Berliner and T.F. Dougherty, in: J.H. Heller, Ed., Reticuloendothelial Structure and Function. New York, Ronald Press Co., 1960, p. 403.
59. T.F. Dougherty and D.L. Berliner, in: G. Pincus, Ed., Conference on Hormones and Atherosclerosis. New York, Academic Press, Inc., 1959, p. 103.
60. R. Jones, W.A. Thomas, and R.F. Scott, J.Exptl. and Mol.Pathol., 1:65, 1962.
61. P.J. Nestel and R.O. Scow, J. Lipid Res., 5:46, 1964.
62. E.L. Bierman, E. Gordis, and J.T. Hamlin,III, J.Clin.Invest., 41:2254, 1962.
63. N.R. DiLuzio and E.L. Bierman, Proc.Soc.Exptl.Biol.and Med., 116:1045, 1964.
64. B. Morris and J.E. French, Quart.J.Exptl.Physiol., 43:180, 1958.
65. B. Edgren and B. Ivemark, Acta Physiol.Scand., 48:402, 1960.
66. P. Belfrage, B. Edgren, and T. Olivecrona, Acta Physiol.Scand., 62:344, 1964.
67. B. Morris and F.C. Courtice, Quart.J.Exptl.Physiol., 41:341, 1956.
68. R. Reiser, M.C. Williams, and M.F. Sorrels, J.Lipid Res., 1:241, 1960.
69. B. Borgstrom and P. Jordan, Acta Soc.Med. Upsalien., 64:185, 1959.
70. D.S. Fredrickson, D.L. McCollester, and K. Ono, J.Clin.Invest., 37:1333, 1958.
71. B. Shapiro, Digestion, Absorption Intestinale et Transport des Glycerides Chez Les Animaux Superieurs. Paris, Centre National de la Recherche Scientifique, 1961, p. 165.
72. D.W. Fawcett, J.Nat.Cancer Inst., 15:1475, 1955.
73. J.C. Hampton, Texas Rep.Biol. and Med., 18:602, 1960.
74. G. Holle, German Med.Monthly, 7:91, 1962.
75. J.M. Felts and P.A. Mayes, Nature, 206:195, 1965.
76. J.M. Felts, Ann.N.Y.Acad.Sci., 131:24, 1965.
77. J.A. Higgins and C. Green, Biochem.J., 99:631, 1966.
78. N.K. Salky, D. Mills, and N.R. DiLuzio, J.Lab. and Clin.Med., 66:952, 1965.

Importance of Aging in the Relationships Between the Reticuloendothelial System and Cholesterol Transport

F. M. Antonini

Department of Gerontology
University of Florence
Florence, Italy

The cells of the reticuloendothelial system, whatever their anatomic position, have, as a common physiologic property, a potent phagocytic activity.

An important group of the cells of the reticuloendothelial system is located in the sinusoid wall. Owing to this position, such cells exert their phagocytic activity on the substance contained in the blood.

Some colloidal particles, provided they have determinate requisites [1], can be employed for quantitative sounding of the phagocytic status of the RES. In fact, it is possible to obtain measurements of this activity from the clearance rate from the blood of intravenously injected colloidal carbon [2], colloidal gold [3], albumin aggregates [4], etc., in quantities exceeding the critical dose, according to the well-known relation

$$K = \frac{0.693}{T_{1/2}}$$

where K is the characteristic constant of the phenomenon, which measures the phagocytic activity of the RES.

Through such techniques, several authors [5] have measured the phagocytic activity of the RES in men and animals under various experimental conditions.

Stiffel, Biozzi, and Benacerraf [6] examined first the modifications of the phagocytic activity of the reticuloendothelial system in rats and rabbits in connection with age. They observed a sensible reduction of this function in old animals, but they did not know whether to interpret such variation as a consequence of the altered weight of organs and tissues or as a phenomenon connected with age.

Some years ago we studied the phagocytic function of the RES by means of radioactive colloidal gold ^{198}Au [7]. Such studies were performed in 26 healthy subjects ranging in age from 20 to 84 years. Doses of ^{198}Au equivalent to 10 μg/kg body weight were intravenously injected into the left arm.

This dose was larger than the critical one (Fig. 1) and therefore suitable to explore the phagocytic function of the RES.

The radioactivity was measured by means of a scintillation detector connected with an integrator, in its turn connected with a writing canal provided with logarithmic preamplifier. The detector was shielded with a lead collimator with rectangular opening 10 by 15 cm, which was put into contact with the sural region of a leg of the examined subject and fastened to it with elastic bandages.

In this way, a curve was obtained which, after a first stage of sharp increase, presented a short period of equilibrium and then a descending stage in which two components with exponential course are easily recognizable (Fig. 2). The second exponential of minor gradient is due to the smaller colloidal particles which are more slowly taken up by the cells of the RES [8].

The method we used seems to be suitable for measurements of the activity of the RES. In fact, the particular type of collimation allows the patient a comfortable position during the entire test, which is confirmed by the reproducibility of the curves.

Moreover, the area chosen for the record is far enough from the liver, where remarkable quantities of tracer gather during the test, as well as from the injection point. In this way all interference not related to the phenomenon represented by the curve is excluded from the curve itself.

On the contrary, one could think that the modification of the slope of the curve is due to the dose of colloidal gold taken up by the bone marrow following a course opposite that of the clearance rate of tracer from the blood. But, consider that the share taken up by the bone marrow represents only 1% of the whole injected dose [9] and that the portion of bone marrow seen through the detector is a very small part of the whole quantity contained in the human body. One can understand that the error made is less serious than the experimental one and therefore negligible.

Such a method has the advantage over that of the multiple hematic drawings of being practical particularly when, as in our case, studies are carried out in old subjects.

To calculate $T_{1/2}$, the second curve, b, was deducted from the first curve, a (Fig. 2). The result was a third line, c, half-time of which was measured.

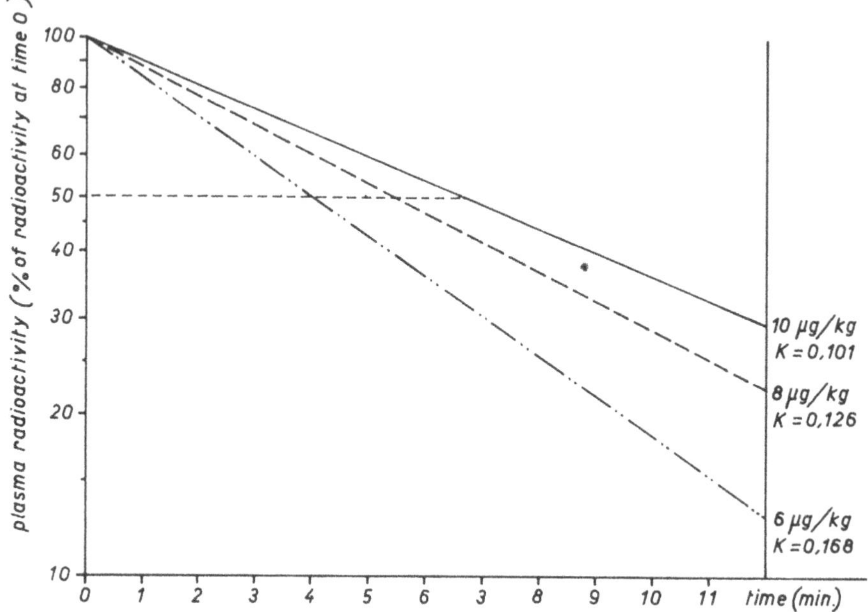

Fig. 1. The relationship between dose and plasma decrease of ^{198}Au : K × dose = const.

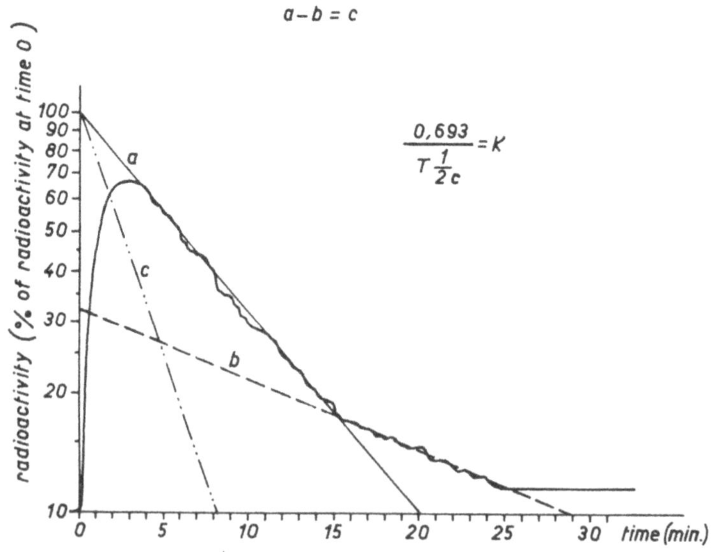

Fig. 2. The calculation of decrease rate of plasma ^{198}Au. The exponential curve c was obtained with graphic subtraction of exponential curve b from exponential curve a.

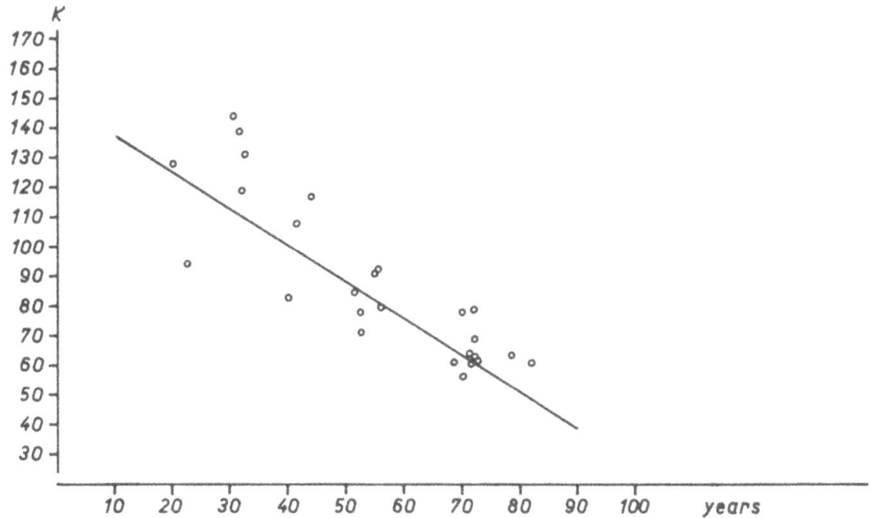

Fig. 3. The relationship between the rate of ^{198}Au clearance and age. The regression equation is $y = 0.15 - 0.001232x$. Correlation coefficient (r) = 0.845 ($P < 0.01$).

The constant characteristic of the phenomenon was calculated on the basis of the well-known formula

$$K = \frac{\ln^2}{T_{1/2}}$$

The coefficient of correlation r between phagocytic function of the RES (represented by K) and age, as well as the relative regression equation were calculated according to the covariance method.

As shown in Fig. 3, phagocytic activity of the RES grows less with age ($P < 0.01$).

Still to be established is how much these variations do actually depend upon a modification of the phagocytic function of the RES induced by aging.

Actually, the gradient of the curve showing the clearance of colloid from the blood depends upon several elements [10]: (1) the administered dose of colloid; (2) the sizes of colloidal micelles; (3) eventual intrahepatic arteriovenous or venovenous shunts; (4) the weight of the liver (in fact, the number of Kupffer cells which come into contact with the blood increases with increase of the liver weight); (5) the hepatic blood flow; and, (6) the variation of hepatic phagocytic activity.

As to point (1) the possibility of error has to be exluded. In fact, the same dose for its weight in gold was administered to every subject (10 μg/kg body weight).

As to point (2), the diameter of particles to the variability of which the two-phase curve is due (in fact, the smallest micelles, as said above, are removed more slowly from the circle) was always 30 mμ on the average.

Also, the possibility mentioned in point (3), particularly important in some pathologic conditions [11], can be excluded from our experiments, since we chose subjects free from any hepatic disease.

On the contrary, we cannot exclude that aging, together with a reduction in the liver weight, also causes a numerical decrease of the Kupffer cells [12]. In any case, such an event would be part of the phenomenon we intended to study (modifications of the functions of the RES). Moreover, we chose for our experiments subjects of normal weight ranging from 62 to 71 kg.

But the possibility still exists that the increase of $T_{1/2}$ that we observed in connection with aging can be due to a reduction in hepatic blood flow [point (5)], and not merely to a reduction in the phagocytic function.

By the doses we employed (larger than the critical one) the clearance rate of colloidal particles from the blood measures in fact the phagocytic function of the RES, the hepatic blood flow being equal. But as is well known [13], hepatic blood flow is reduced in old people.

One should therefore be able to distinguish the two phenomena, i.e., phagocytic power of the RES, and hepatic blood flow.

Therefore, we repeatedly tried to measure the extraction ratio of intravenously injected colloidal substances in doses larger than the critical one by catheterizing the overhepatic veins. In these conditions the extraction ratio gives the percent of the colloid taken up by Kupffer cells from the blood and therefore it is independent of the hepatic blood flow. In case clearance rates in old people could be found lower than in young people, it would have unquestionably proved that the function of the RES in senescence is reduced. However, during catheterizing, auricle fibrillation was observed in most old subjects. We were therefore obliged to interrupt our research.

Our first observation, however, seemed to reveal the existence of a progressive reduction in the phagocytic functions of the RES induced by aging.

More recently, Wagner, Migita, and Solomon [14], employing albumin aggregates and colloidal radioactive gold in man, confirmed our first results proving there, too, a reduction in the phagocytic function of the RES during senescence. In this case, too, the same reservations made about our first experiments are to be kept in mind.

Some years ago it was observed that cholesterol is phagocytosed by the cells of the RES [15]. We observed it ourselves during studies we performed in cooperation with Weber and Zampi [16] on experimental atherosclerosis of rabbits. Cholesterol, if administered to the animals together with Tween 80, instead of storing on the arterial walls, was phagocytized by the cells of the RES, particularly by the Kupffer cells of the liver, and by the spleen reticulum cells. After some months, if administration of Tween 80 was suspended, cholesterol disappeared from the reticuloendothelial cells and was stored in the arterial walls.

Such observations proved that the RES was involved in the transport of cholesterol and that this phenomenon was provided with a dynamics of its own, since it was demonstrated to be reversible.

More recently, DiLuzio and others [17] demonstrated that some lipid emulsions containing triglycerides were phagocytized by the RES, in greater quantities by the Kupffer cells of the liver, and in smaller quantities by the spleen and lung cells.

The same authors demonstrated that these lipid emulsions are suitable to measure the phagocytic function of the RES because they behave similarly to colloidal substances. More precisely, their clearance rate from the blood is proportional to the phagocytic activity of the RES and inversely proportional to the dose.

This way it was possible to study the phagocytic function of the RES in animals [18] and men [19] under various pathologic and experimental conditions.

Therefore, an inversely proportional relationship between phagocytic activity of the RES and levels of serum cholesterol in men was observed [20]. More precisely, the portion which seemed to be most connected with phagocytic activity of the RES was larger than cholesterol.

Through employment of colloidal carbon a reduced phagocytic activity was observed in hypothyroid animals [21] which normally present high levels of serum cholesterol. Following administration of thyroid hormones both the phagocytic activity and the serum cholesterol rates become normal again.

Also, in leukemic subjects, who generally present a hyperfunction of the RES, very low levels of cholesterol are often observed [23].

Finally, it was proved that drugs which are able to stimulate the phagocytic activity of the RES reduce hypercholesterolemia and prevent hepatic cholesterosis in animals kept on a diet rich in cholesterol [24].

By all these observations, evidence is given to the important relationships existing between the RES and cholesterol transport and metabolism. Actually, serum cholesterol levels appear to be reduced in situations in which the phagocytic activity of the RES results increased in comparison with the normal activity, and vice versa. Moreover, stimulation of the RES is also able to prevent metabolic losses induced by diets rich in cholesterol.

Not yet completely known are the processes through which cholesterol is taken up by the cells of the RES [24]. It was proved that cholesterol is taken up by the cells of the RES slower than triglycerides are, and that some cholesterol esters remain in these cells as long as 18 months, whereas triglycerides disappear in a few days [26].

Nevertheless, it is evident that the uptake of cholesterol by the cells of the RES is generally connected with some metabolic process. In fact, owing to the uptake of cholesterol, phospholipids, as well, are stored in the cells of the RES [28]. Moreover, it was proved that the uptake of cholesterol in the macrophages of the rabbits is associated with an accelerated synthesis of phospholipids [29] and that cholesterol, phagocytosed in particulate form by the macrophages in vitro is quickly incorporated by lipoproteins afterward [30]. It is well known that phosholipids are necessary for the formation of lipoproteic complexes. Therefore, it is logical to think that phospholipids play an important part in facilitating the formation of lipoproteins in macrophages, thus causing the solubility of cholesterol.

Some authors [32] having observed that cholesterol is esterified at the surface of macrophages, concluded that the esterification process played an important role in the incorporation of said sterol into lipoprotein. But it has been proved that not only cholesterol esters, but also free cholesterol, are present in an increased amount in lipoproteins of the medium after incubation of the macrophages [33].

Moreover, esterification follows incorporation of cholesterol into lipoproteins [34]. Inside the macrophages, also, active hydrolysis processes, activated by addition of lecithin, take place at the same time [35].

Therefore, it is reasonable to think that macrophages take up cholesterol only in the form of micellar suspension or when cholesterol is bound to lipoproteins [36]. Inside the macrophages, cholesterol would be quickly esterified, hydrolized, incorporated into lipoproteins, and subsequently mobilized [37].

In conclusion, the RES would have in the metabolism of cholesterol the function of mobilizing and clearing. Owing to these functions, the catabolism of cholesterol would be accelerated during hyperactive states of the RES and therefore the levels of such sterol in the blood would be reduced.

It is then reasonable to think that the reduction of the metabolic rate of cholesterol in senescence [38] is in part connected with the reduction of the phagocytic function of the RES.

Therefore, stimulation of the phagocytic activity of the RES could favorably affect, by means of suitable drugs, e.g., Zymosan [39], some metabolic process during aging.

REFERENCES

1. B. Benacerraf, G. Biozzi, B.N. Halpern, and C. Stiffel, Physiopathology of Reticuloendothelial Systems. Oxford, Blackwell Scientific Publications, 1957, pp. 52.
2. W.O. Fenn, J.Gen.Physiol., 3 : 575, 1821.
3. H. Vetter, R. Falkner, and A. Neumayr, J.Clin.Invest., 3 : 1594, 1954.
4. B.N. Halpern, G. Biozzi, G. Pequignot, B. Delaloye, and D. Mouton, J.Pathol.Biol., 7 : 1637, 1959.
5a. E.L. Dobson, G.F. Warner, C.R. Finney, and M.E. Johnston, Circulation, 7 : 690, 1953.
5b. R. Fauvert and J.P. Benhanon, Bull.Soc.Hop., 73 : 79, 1953.
5c. B. Benacerraf, G. Biozzi, B.N. Halpern, C. Stiffel, and D. Mouton, Brit.J.Exptl.Pathol., 38 : 35, 1957.
5d. G. Biozzi, C. Stiffel, B.N. Halpern, and D. Mouton, Rev.Franc. Etudes Clin.Biol., 9: 876, 1960.
5e. A. Ruol and D. Ziliotto, Min.Nucl., 6 : 140, 1962.
6. C. Stiffel, G. Biozzi, B. Benacerraf, and B.N. Halpern, Compt. Rend.Soc.Biol., 150: 1075, 1956.
7. F.M. Antonini, G. Cappelli, S. Citi, and M. Serio, Giorn.Gerontol., 12 : 741, 1964.
8a. C.W. Sheppard, G. Jordan, and P.F. Hahn, Ann.J.Physiol., 164 : 345, 1951.
8b. D.B. Zilversmit, G.A. Boyd, and M. Brucer, J.Lab.Clin.Med., 40 : 255, 1952.
9. A. Billiteri, S. Ramo, and G. Gasso, Min.Nucl., 7: 536, 1963.
10. B.N. Halpern, B. Benacerraf, G. Biozzi, and C. Stiffel, Rev.Hematol., 9 : 619, 1954.
11. B.N. Halpern, G. Biozzi, G. Pequignot, B. Delaloye, C. Stiffel, and D. Mouton, Pathol.Biol., 7: 1637, 1959.
12. Y.T. Culbertson, Arch.Pathol., 27: 212, 1939.
13. S.E. Bradley, F. Ingelfinger, G.P. Bradley, and J.J. Curry, J.Clin.Invest., 24 : 899, 1945.
14. H.N. Wagner,Jr., T. Migita, and E. Solomon, J.Gerontol., 21 : 57, 1966.
15a. M. Friedman and S.O. Byers, Circulation, 10 : 491, 1954.
15b. M. Friedman, S.O. Byers, R.H.Rosenman, Am.J.Physiol., 177: 77, 1954.
15c. M. Friedman, S.O. Byers, and S.O. George, Am.J.Physiol., 184 : 141, 1956.
16. F.M. Antonini, G. Weber, and G. Zampi, in: J.H. Heller, Ed., Reticuloendothelial Structure and Function. New York, Ronald Press, 1958, p. 431.

17a. N.R. DiLuzio and E.L. Bierman, Proc.Soc.Exptl.Biol.Med., 116:1045, 1964.
17b. N.R. DiLuzio and S.J. Riggi, J.Reticuloendothelial Soc., 1:248, 1964.
18. G.T. Ashworth, N.R. DiLuzio, and S.J. Riggi, Exptl.Mol.Pathol. Suppl., 1:83, 1963.
19. N.K. Salky, D. Mills, and N.R. DiLuzio, J.Lab.Clin.Med., 86:952, 1965.
20. N.R. Salky, N.R. DiLuzio, D.B. P'Pool, and A.J. Sutherland, "Evaluation of reticuloendothelial function in man," J.Am.Med.Assoc., 187:744, 1964.
21. G.S. Boyd, in: J.K. Grant, Ed., The Control of Lipid Metabolism. New York, Academic Press, 1963, p. 79.
22. G.S. Boyd, in: J.K. Grant, Ed., The Control of Lipid Metabolism. New York, Academic Press, 1963, p. 79.
23. R.E. Bases, I.H. Krakoff, and R.R. Ellison, Proc.Am.Assoc. Cancer Res., 3:208, 1961.
24. S.J. Riggi and N.R. DiLuzio, J.Lipid Res., 3:339, 1962.
25. A.J. Day, J.Atherosclerosis Res., 4:117, 1964.
26. J.E. French and B. Morris, J.Pathol.Bacteriol., 76:11, 1960.
27. A.J. Day and J.E. French, J.Pathol.Bacteriol., 81:247, 1961.
28. A.J. Day, Brit.J.Exptl.Pathol., 41:112, 1960.
29a. D.B. Zilversmit, M.L. Shore, and R.F. Ackerman, Circulation, 2:581, 1954.
29b. D.B. Zilversmit, and E.L. McCandless, J.Lipid Res., 1:118, 1959.
30. A.J. Day, P.R.S. Gould-Hurst, and G.K. Wilkinson, J.Atherosclerosis Res., 4:497, 1964.
31. E.H. Ahrens, Jr. and H.G. Kunkel, J.Exptl.Med., 90:409, 1949.
32. E.H. Tompkins, Arch.Pathol., 42:299, 1946.
33. A.J. Day and J.E. French, Quart.J.Exptl.Physiol., 44:239, 1959.
34. A.F. Whereat and E. Staple, Arch.Biochem.Biophys., 90:224, 1960.
35. A.J. Day, P.R.S. Gould-Hurst, and M.L. Wahlquist, J.Reticuloendothelial Soc., 1:40, 1964.
36. K.C. Dixon, Quart.J.Exptl.Physiol., 43:139, 1958.
37. A.J. Day, P.R.S. Gould-Hurst, R. Steinhorner, and M.L. Wahlquist, J.Atherosclerosis Res., 5:466, 1965.
38a. D. Kritchesky, E. Staple, and M.W. Whitehouse, J.Clin.Nutr., 8:411, 1960.
38b. F.J. Schilling, G.J. Christakis, N.J. Bennet, and J.F. Coyle, Ann. J.Public Health, 54:461, 1964.
39. J.H. Heller, in: J.H. Heller, Ed., Reticuloendothelial Structure and Function. New York, Ronald Press, 1958, p. 189.

Arteriopathy Induced By Reticuloendothelial Blockade*

P. R. Patek, S. Bernick, and V. A. de Mignard

Department of Anatomy, School of Medicine
The University of Southern California
Los Angeles, California

To have a better comprehension of vascular changes resulting from reticuloendothelial blockade, it is necessary to understand the long-term effect of blockade of reticuloendothelial cells which undoubtedly interferes with their normal function. These functional disturbances can be readily observed in the phagocytic cells of the liver after parenteral administration of foreign material. Extensive reviews of early studies have been reported by Jaffe [1], Halpern [2], and Brauer [3]. These studies have been concerned with the classification of reticuloendothelial cells and a study of their functions. Other studies have been directed toward a quantitative approach in which blood-clearance measurements were determined as an index of phagocytic activity (Benacerraf et al. [4], Dobson [5], DiLuzio [6], and others).

Since the rat is a common experimental animal used in the studies of vascular disease and cholesterol metabolism, as well as immunologic and other metabolic processes, this study was undertaken to add further knowledge about the long-term response and function of the reticuloendothelial system to foreign particles in this particular species of animal.

MATERIALS AND METHODS

The animals used in this study [7, 8] were two-month-old male and female rats of Holtzman strain. Each animal was injected intravenously with a single dose of colloidal carbon [Higgins commercial India ink, Gunther-Wagner colloidal carbon or thorium dioxide (Thorotrast)] in amounts of 5

*This research was supported by grants H 4876, H 4510, A 2549, and AM 8275 from National Institutes of Health, U.S. Public Health Service.

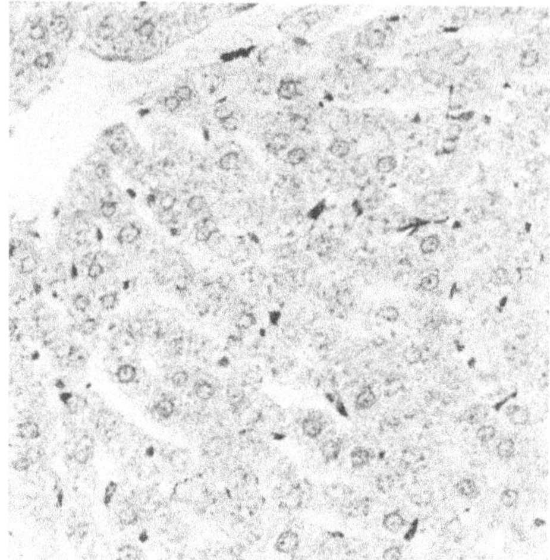

Fig. 1. Carbon-laden macrophages lining hepatic sinusoids 30 min after carbon injection. Hematoxylin and eosin. x 300. Reduced 17% for reproduction.

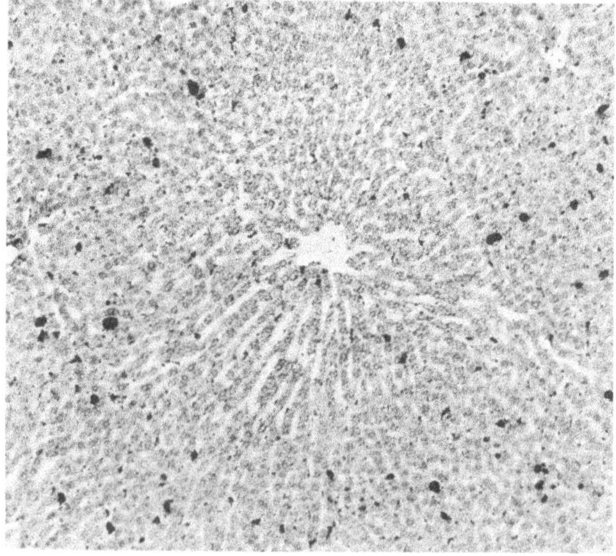

Fig. 2. Peripheral lobular distribution of macrophage conglomerates and giant cells one month after carbon injection. Hematoxylin and eosin. x 125. Reduced 17% for reproduction.

mg/100 g body weight. The animals were maintained on Purina Laboratory Chow, a natural stock ration, for the duration of the experiment. Animals were autopsied at 24, 48, and 96 hr, one, two, and three weeks, and then monthly through 14 months following injection. Specimens were fixed with cold alcohol-formaldehyde–acetic acid and prepared for paraffin and celloidin embedding in the conventional manner. Paraffin sections were cut at 7 μ and celloidin sections at 15 and 20 μ. Alternate cut sections were stained with hematoxylin and eosin, methyl green-pyronin, periodic acid-Schiff (PAS), and Verhoeff's iron-hematoxylin. Serial sections were also prepared.

OBSERVATIONS

Twenty-four hours following the carbon injection, fine carbon aggregates were observed in the reticuloendothelial cells lining the sinusoids of the hepatic lobule. These carbon-laden macrophages were not only distributed uniformly in the hepatic lobule, but all lobules throughout the liver showed the same degree of phagocytic activity (Fig. 1). In addition, migration of carbon-laden macrophages from the hepatic lobule was evident by the presence of carbon-laden cells in the lumina of central and hepatic veins.

At the end of 48 hr, the volume of carbon increased within the hepatic lobule. This was the result of an increased uptake of carbon by the individual reticuloendothelial cells. At the same time, macrophages appeared to group together in the sinusoids.

Two weeks following the carbon injection, the appearance of the liver was predominantly characterized by the presence of large aggregates of reticuloendothelial cells. These swollen conglomerates appeared to be mainly localized at the peripheral third of the hepatic lobule. In addition, there was an increase in the number of carbon-laden macrophages observed in the central veins.

By the end of the one-month period, there was a relative decrease in the number of demonstrable individual carbon-laden macrophages lining the sinusoids with a relative increase in the number of large aggregates of macrophages (Fig. 2). Many of the large conglomerates consisted of multinucleated giant cells in which the nuclei were masked by the accumulation of carbon. These large cells appeared to occlude the sinusoids (Fig. 3).

Small carbon granules, either free or in tissue macrophages, were seen in the periportal connective tissue as early as two days after the carbon injection. These macrophages increased in number and even became giant cells by the end of the first month. Three months after the carbon injection, the carbon pattern in the liver lobule had not changed perceptibly from the one-month specimen. Although most of the carbon-laden giant cells still exhibited their cellular components, a few showed evidence of lysis of cellular components.

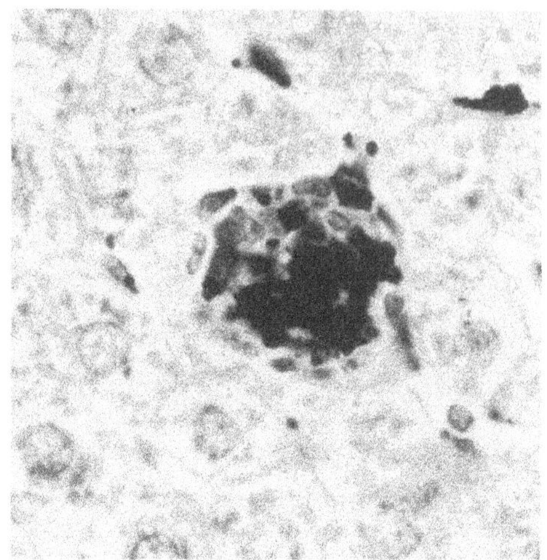

Fig. 3. Carbon-laden giant cell in hepatic sinusoid. Hematoxylin and eosin. × 850. Reduced 17% for reproduction.

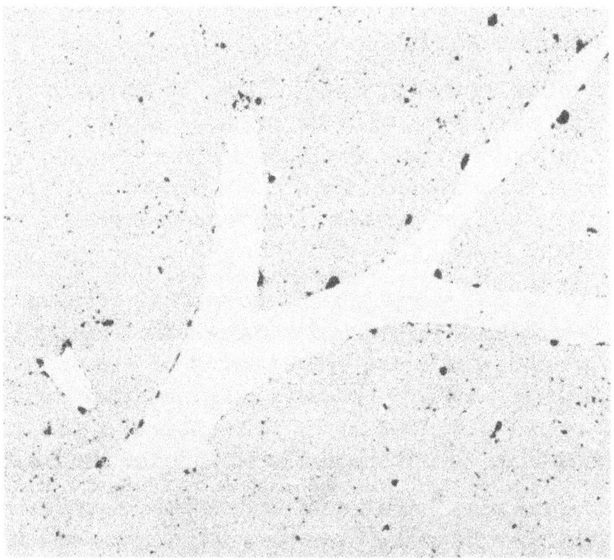

Fig. 4. Noncellular carbon masses related to wall of hepatic vein one year after carbon injection. Note relative absence of carbon in lobule periphery as seen earlier in Fig. 2. Hematoxylin and eosin. × 35. Reduced 17% for reproduction.

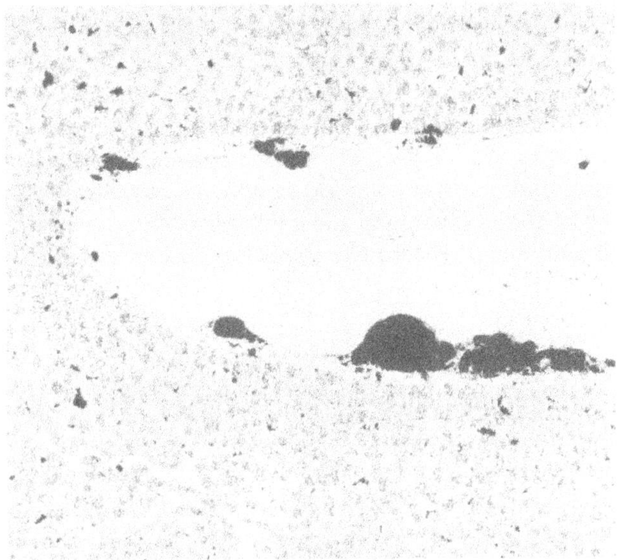

Fig. 5. Carbon masses encapsulated and projecting into hepatic vein one year after carbon injection. Note free carbon in lumen of vein. Hematoxylin and eosin. x 125. Reduced 17% for reproduction.

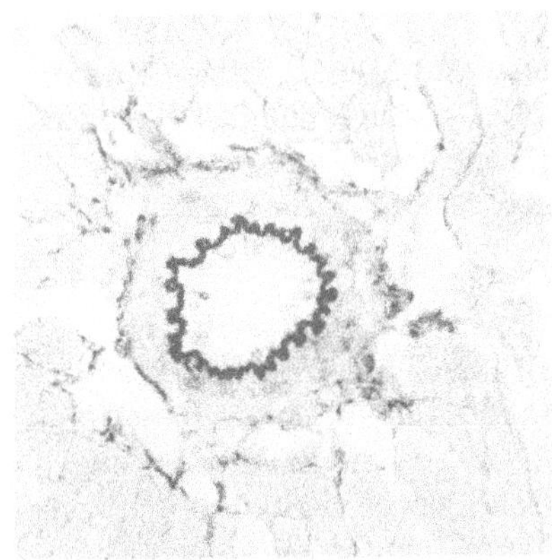

Fig. 6. Typical small coronary artery from control animal. The internal elastic membrane is prominent, smooth, and uninterrupted. Aldehyde–fuchsin. x 500. Reduced 17% for reproduction.

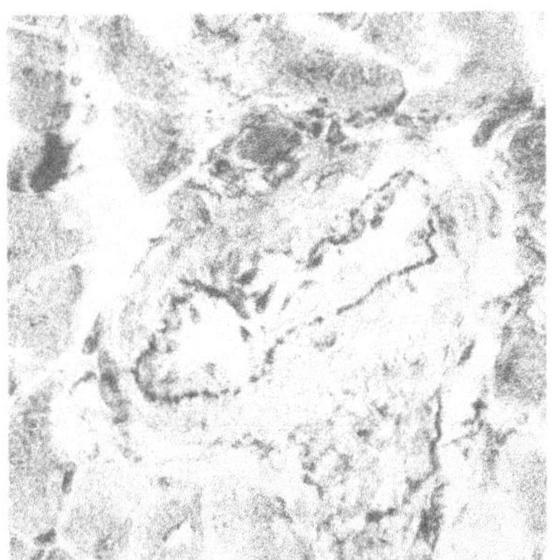

Fig. 7. Coronary artery five months after carbon injection. The internal elastic membrane is fragmented and the intima is thickened. Aldehyde–fuchsin. x 500. Reduced 17% for reproduction.

After one year the number of individual carbon-containing sinusoidal cells had considerably decreased. However, there were many which contained fine granules of injected carbon. Large masses of noncellular carbon, formerly the ingested content of giant cells, were now seen in the vicinity of, or in the walls of, the large sublobular and hepatic veins. Very few remained in the region of the lobular triads (Fig. 4). The carbon masses related to the large veins appeared to fill a perivenous space or were encapsulated by the venous adventitial connective tissue cells. Many of these encapsulated masses had bulged into the venous lumina, and others showed rupture of the capsule and the adjacent venous endothelium. The carbon content was expelled into the vascular lumina where it disintegrated (Fig. 5).

DISCUSSION

The functional interpretation of this study of tissue sections indicates a nonstatic phagocytosis and recirculation of carbon. Following the initial injection of the carbon and its ingestion by hepatic macrophages, many of these cells desquamate from the sinusoidal wall. These, as dead or dying cells, are then swept into the blood stream and the carbon is recirculated. Other macrophages, which have desquamated, unite with each other to produce giant cells which migrate to the lobule periphery. The giant cells then die and are themselves ingested by macrophages. The remaining noncellular carbon masses are forced through the sinusoids (probably by intra-abdominal pressure changes) to the sublobular and hepatic veins where they are encapsulated and then through rupture of the capsule and venous endothelium the carbon is returned to the circulation. The cycle is thus repeated.

Whatever effect the blocking of reticuloendothelial cells has upon the architecture of arteries, this effect is not that of a single assault but of repeated assaults. Hence, a single injection of a colloidal suspension may stimulate an activity which persists throughout the life of the animal.

Arterial Lesions

Atherosclerotic lesions have with difficulty been produced in rats by the feeding of large quantities of fats and cholesterol alone or in combination with choline, sodium cholate, thiouracil, and/or hypertensive regimen. Wissler and his associates [9] produced atherosclerotic lesions in rats with diets containing a high percentage of lard, casein, and small amounts of choline. Fillios and his group [11] fed their rats fat, cholesterol, sodium cholate, and thiouracil. Hartroft [12], on the other hand, produced lesions in rats on a choline-deficient diet. Malinow [13] obtained lesions by means of cholesterol, thiouracil, and/or by cellophane-induced perinephritis. Bragdon and Mickelsen [14] produced atheromatous lesions in the rat by injecting serum from hypercholesteremic rabbits.

The experimental production of arteriosclerosis in animals by the administration of colloidal suspensions or high-molecular weight substances other than cholesterol has been accomplished by Hueper [15], Lautsch et al. [16], Shimamoto [17], and Patek and Bernick [18].

Previously it had been reported [19] that rats which received a single injection of carbon (5 mg/100 g) did not show any coronary lesions until the fifth month after the carbon injection. After this time period, a few coronary arteries in each animal demonstrated an early structural alteration involving fragmentation of the internal elastic membrane and a slight thickening of the intima (Fig. 6). Stainable lipid could not be demonstrated in these vascular lesions. The frequency and severity of the coronary arterial lesions increased proportionately with the extension of the experimental time period.

Rats which received a standard synthetic diet, to which 1% cholesterol and 5% fat (cottonseed oil) was added, demonstrated no vascular lesions even after 7 months on this diet. However, rats which were placed on the cholesterol-fat diet three days after the carbon injection exhibited atherosclerotic lesions in their coronary arteries as early as two months after the beginning of the cholesterol feeding (Fig. 8). The artery in this illustration shows fragmentation of the internal elastic membrane and varying degrees of thickening of the intima. In addition, lipid droplets are observed in the intima and media. The vascular lesions became progressively more severe the longer the rats were maintained on the cholesterol-fat diet. For example, the coronary vessels from animals killed five months after the start of the cholesterol-fat feeding showed not only a splitting and reduplication of the internal elastic membrane, but a thickened proliferative intima. This intimal proliferation is composed of an increased number of cells, fine elastic fibers, and collagenous elements.

Beginning at the end of the second month following the carbon injection and the cholesterol-fat feeding, and continuing throughout the experiment, aortic lesions of varying degrees of severity were observed in all the experimental animals of this series. These lesions, for the most part, were limited to the base of the ascending aortas. The most common lesion observed consisted of a thickened intima which resulted from increased amounts of mucoid ground substance in the subendothelial region (Fig. 9). In addition there was rupture, fragmentation, and fraying of the internal elastic membrane. Small amounts of stainable lipid were demonstrated in the subendothelial ground substance and also in macrophages.

If the cholesterol-fat diet was initiated following periods longer than three days after the carbon injection, the time required for the development of coronary arterial atherosclerosis was markedly reduced. For example, those animals which received a single carbon injection and seven months later were placed on the cholesterol-fat diet, demonstrated lipomatous le-

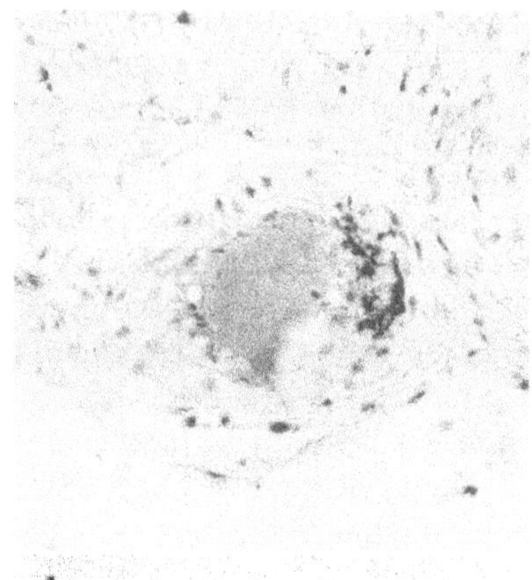

Fig. 8. Coronary artery of rat which received a carbon injection and three days later was placed on a diet containing 1% cholesterol-5% fat for two months. Lipid is stained in ground substance and macrophages of the thickened intima. Oil red O. × 250. Reduced 17% for reproduction.

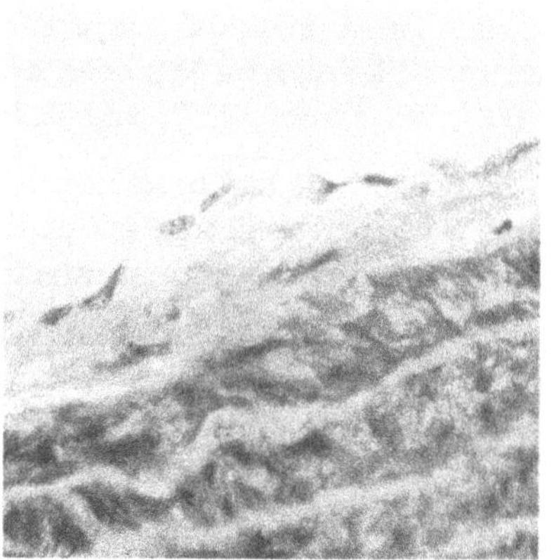

Fig. 9. Aorta of rat which received an injection of carbon and three days later was placed on a diet containing 1% cholesterol-5% fat for five months. The intima is considerably thickened by increased mucoid ground substance. Periodic acid-Schiff (PAS). × 500. Reduced 17% for reproduction.

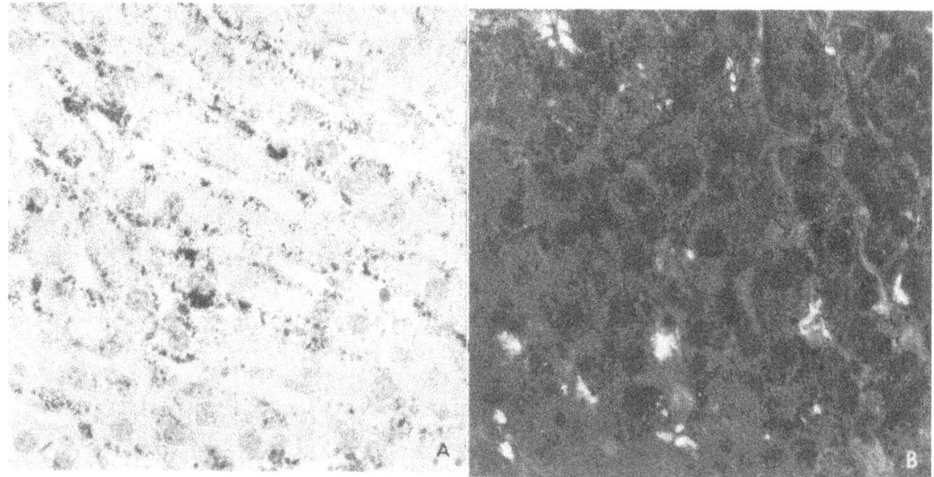

Fig. 10. Frozen section of liver from rat maintained on diet containing 1% cholesterol-5% fat for three days. Oil red O. × 450. Reduced 17% for reproduction. A. Lipid droplets are in reticuloendothelial cells and in hepatic cells adjacent to cell membranes. B. Under polarized light a few refractile granules (presumably cholesterol) are seen in the reticuloendothelial cells.

sions of the same type and frequency only 10 days after the beginning of the cholesterol-fat diet.

In another series of experiments, rats were maintained on 1% cholesterol-5% fat diet for five months. Each was then given a single injection of carbon (5 mg/100 g). These animals exhibited typical coronary arterial atherosclerotic lesions as early as 21 days after the carbon injection. In addition to the thickened intima and fragmentation of the internal elastic membrane, lipid droplets were observed in the intima and media. These droplets were lying free or in macrophages.

Lipid Study

Biggs, Friedman, and Byers [20] and Chaikoff et al. [21] have demonstrated that all absorbed cholesterol enters the blood via the thoracic duct as part of the chylomicrons. These relatively large particles appear to stimulate activity in a manner similar to the injected colloidal suspensions. They are picked up by macrophages of the reticuloendothelial system in a manner similar to the phagocytosis of carbon or thorium dioxide [22, 23], and could be thought of as at least transient "blocking agents" of the reticuloendothelial system. Also, both the injection of carbon and the feeding of cholesterol to rats cause the thyroid gland to become hyperplastic and stimulate an increase in the hypophyseal thyrotropic cells [24].

In order to better understand the effects of lipid and cholesterol feeding on the reticuloendothelial system, rats were maintained on a standard synthetic diet to which 1% cholesterol-5% cottonseed oil were added for five months [25].

In the earlier stages of the experiment, the cholesterol was demonstrated in the form of small refractile granules by the polarizing microscope and was found predominantly in the reticuloendothelial cells (Fig. 10). However, with the extension of the experimental period up to five months, these granules progressively infiltrated into the parenchymal cells. In the parenchymal and reticuloendothelial cells the birefringent granules soon aggregated into the typical needlelike crystals characteristic of cholesterol, which became elongated until they appeared to extend over two, three, or more cells (Fig. 11). It is of further interest to note that this deposition of lipids and cholesterol in the reticuloendothelial and parenchymal cells was transitory in nature. When the animals were placed on the standard stock diet after their exposure to cholesterol for long periods, the large lipid droplets, as well as the needlelike crystals disappeared. Only a few uniformly-sized lipid globules and associated refractile granules remained. Thus it may be assumed that free cholesterol disappeared and the lipid globules and the associated refractile granules that remained may be classified as cholesterol esters.

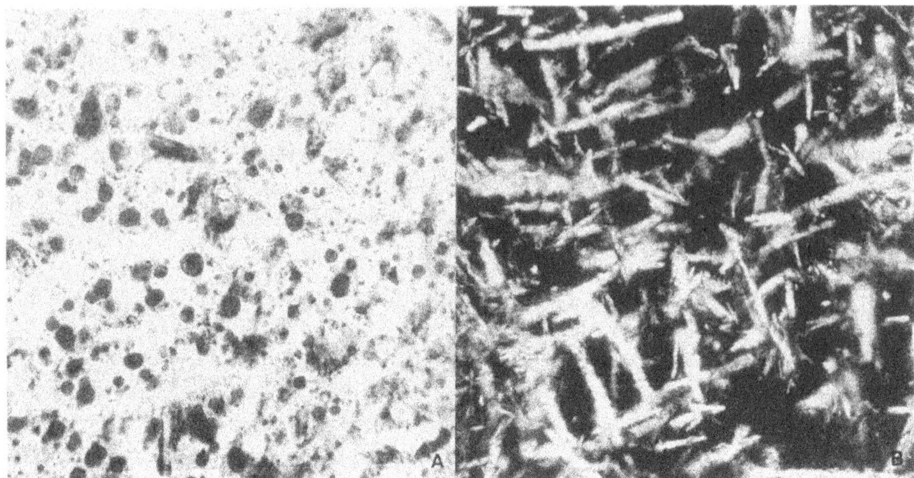

Fig. 11. Frozen section of liver from rat maintained on diet containing 1% cholesterol-5% fat for five months. Oil red O. × 450. Reduced 17% for reproduction. A. Large lipid globules are in hepatic and reticuloendothelial cells. B. Under polarized light large needlelike crystals have tremendously distended the hepatic cells.

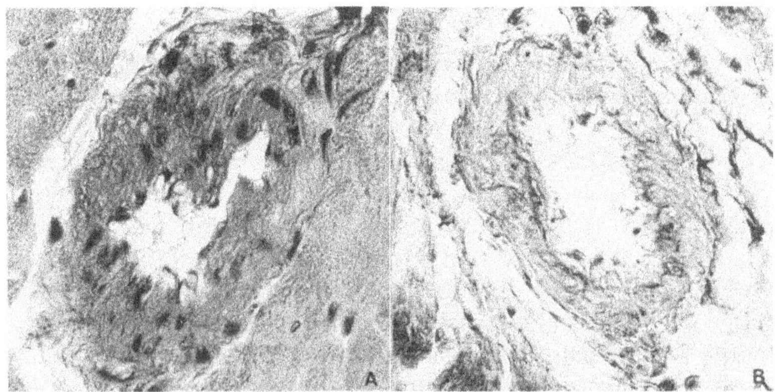

Fig. 12. A. Coronary artery of a carbon-injected parabiont six months after parabiosis. This artery demonstrates a considerably thickened, fibrous, and cellular intima. Hematoxylin and triosin. × 350. B. Coronary artery of noninjected parabiont six months after parabiosis. This artery also shows a thickened intima as well as an irregular, fragmented internal elastic membrane. Aldehyde-fuchsin stain. × 350. Reduced 17% for reproduction.

From the data derived from this project, it is obvious that one cannot separate the process of the removal of cholesterol from the plasma without at the same time considering the simultaneous removal of lipids. This is based on the findings that the lipids were demonstrable in the reticuloendothelial and hepatic cells before these phagocytic cells ingested cholesterol. As the experimental periods were prolonged, lipid droplets were always present in the various cellular components of the liver in greater quantity than was the cholesterol.

Parabiosis Study

The technique of parabiosis was used to investigate the hypothesis that reticuloendothelial system blockade by an inert colloidal suspension causes production of a humoral substance which is injurious to arteries. In this study, rats receiving colloidal carbon intravenously were united to non-treated rats following the time necessary for removal of free-circulating carbon particles from the blood stream. Thus, neither the hepatic cells nor the reticuloendothelial cells of the noninjected parabionts could be influenced directly by the carbon particles.

Twenty-six Holtzman strain male rats each received a single intravenous injection of colloidal carbon (5 mg/ 100 g body weight). Three days later the injected animals were united by parabiosis to noninjected animals of the same sex, weight, and genetic strain.

Carbon granules were found in the reticuloendothelial cells of injected rats, but few or no granules were found in reticuloendothelial cells of their noninjected parabiotic partners. Coronary arteries of both injected and noninjected animals showed thickening and fragmentation of the internal elastic membrane after two months. After four to six months the lesions included degenerative changes of smooth muscle cells just external to the internal elastic membrane and thickening of the intima (Fig. 12). Hyperplasia of the thyroid was found in both parabionts.

Addition of 1% cholesterol-5% fat to the diet caused deposition of lipid in endothelial cells and intimal macrophages of the damaged arteries of both parabionts. Distribution of lipid within the hepatic parenchymal cells was also altered in the experimental animals but not in controls.

It is suggested that uptake of particulate matter by cells of the RES causes them to release a substance capable of producing arterial lesions.

REFERENCES

1. R.H. Jaffe, "The reticuloendothelial system," in: H. Downey, Ed., Handbook of Hematology. New York, P.B. Hoeber, 1938, pp.974-1271.
2. B.N. Halpern, Ed., Physiopathology of the Reticuloendothelial System – A Symposium. Oxford, Blackwell Scientific Publications, 1957.

3. R.W. Brauer, A Symposium on Approaches to the Quantitative Description of Liver Function. Washington, D.C., American Institute of Biological Sciences, 1958.
4. B. Benacerraf, G. Biozzi, B.N. Halpern, and C. Stiffel, "Physiology of phagocytosis of particles by the RES," in: B.N. Halpern, Ed., Physiopathology of the Reticuloendothelial System – A Symposium. Oxford, Blackwell Scientific Publications, Ltd., 1957, pp. 52-79.
5. E.L. Dobson, "Factors controlling phagocytosis," in: B.N. Halpern, Ed., Physiopathology of the Reticuloendothelial System – A Symposium. Oxford, Blackwell Scientific Publications, Ltd., 1957, pp. 80-115.
6. N.R. DiLuzio, "Lipid composition of Kupffer cells," Am.J. Physiol., 196 : 884-886, 1959.
7. H.H. Frankel, P.R. Patek, and S. Bernick, "Long-term studies of rat reticuloendothelial system and endocrine gland responses to foreign particles," Anat. Record, 142 : 359-374, 1962.
8. V.A. de Mignard, P.R. Patek, and S. Bernick, "Nonsinusoidal removal of foreign material by direct extrusion into large hepatic veins," Anat. Record., 154 : 337, 1966.
9. R.W. Wissler, M.L. Eilert, M.A. Schroeder, and L.A. Cohen, "Production of lipomatous and atheromatous arterial lesions in the albino rat," Arch. Pathol., 57 : 333-351, 1954.
10. R.J. Jones, R.W. Wissler, and S. Huffman, "Certain dietary effects on the serum cholesterol and atherogenesis in the rat," 63 : 593-601, 1957.
11. L.C. Fillios, S.B. Andrus, G.V. Mann, and F.J. Stare, "Experimental production of gross atherosclerosis in the rat," J. Exptl. Med., 104 : 539-554, 1956.
12. W.S. Hartroft, J.H. Ridout, E.A. Sellers, and C.H. Best, "Atheromatous changes in aorta and coronary arteries of choline-deficient rats," Proc. Soc. Exptl. Biol. Med., 81 : 384-393, 1952.
13. M.R. Malinow, D. Hojman, and A. Pellegrino, "Different methods for the experimental production of generalized arteriosclerosis in the rat," Acta Cardiol., 9 : 480-499, 1954.
14. J.H. Bragdon and O. Mickelsen, "Experimental atherosclerosis in the rat," Am. J. Pathol., 31 : 965-973, 1955.
15. W.C. Hueper, "Experimental studies in cardiovascular pathology. III. Polyvinyl alcohol atheromatosis in the arteries of dogs," Arch. Pathol., 31 : 11-24, 1941.
16. E.V. Lautsch, G.C. McMillan, and G.L. Duff, "Atherosclerosis in rabbits after intravenous injection of colloidal solutions," Arch. Pathol., 65 : 40-46, 1958.
17. T. Shimamoto, Arteriosclerogenic Substances and Arteriosclerosis by These Substances. Tokyo, Tokyo Medical and Dental University Press, 1959.

18. P.R. Patek and S. Bernick, "Experimental arterial lesions produced by reticuloendothelial blocking agents," Arch. Pathol., 69:35-43, 1960.
19. P.R. Patek, S. Bernick, and H.H. Frankel, "Arterial lesions in rats by reticuloendothelial blocking agents," Arch. Pathol., 72:70-78, 1961.
20. M.W. Biggs, M. Friedman, and S.O. Byers, "Intestinal lymphatic transport of absorbed cholesterol," Proc. Soc. Exptl. Biol. Med., 78:641-643, 1951.
21. I.L. Chaikoff, B. Bloom, M.D. Siperstein, D.Y. Kiyasu, W.O. Reinhardt, G.W. Dauben, and J.R. Eastham, "^{14}C Cholesterol: Lymphatic transport of absorbed cholesterol-4-^{14}C," J. Biol. Chem., 194:407-412, 1952.
22. M. Friedman, S.O. Byers, and R.H. Rosenman, "Observations concerning the production and excretion of cholesterol in mammals. XII. Demonstrations of the essential role of the hepatic reticuloendothelial cell (Kupffer cell) in normal disposition of exogenously derived cholesterol," Am. J. Physiol., 177:77-83, 1954.
23. T. Neveu, G. Biozzi, B. Benacerraf, C. Stiffel, and B.N. Halpern, "Role of reticuloendothelial system in blood clearance of cholesterol," Am. J. Physiol., 187:269-274, 1956.
24. S. Bernick and P.R. Patek, "Effect of cholesterol feeding on selected endocrine glands," Arch. Pathol., 72:321-330, 1961.
25. S. Bernick and P.R. Patek, "Effect of cholesterol feeding on rat reticuloendothelial system," Arch. Pathol., 72:310-320, 1961.
26. P.R. Patek, S. Bernick, and D.K. MacCallum, "Production of arterial lesions by a humoral factor in parabiotic rats," Circulation Res., 12:291-297, 1963.

A Form of Immunological Atherosclerosis

Louis Levy

Riker Laboratories
Northridge, California

During the last two decades, the literature on atherosclerosis has become overwhelming. Not only have there been many original scientific contributions, but the subject has been discussed extensively in review articles and books. The pathology observed in human coronary atherosclerosis appears to be unique but does bear some resemblance to certain phases of both induced and spontaneous atherosclerosis in animals. Factors that appear to contribute to both human and animal vascular derangement embrace a wide diversity of stimuli. Dietary components such as lipids have been, and still are, fashionable as pathogenic agents [1]. There is a strong school of thought that believes the early formation of thrombi is of paramount importance in the human disease [2]. The rheologists believe that the turbulence and flow through vessels of certain sizes contribute profoundly to the pathogenesis of atherosclerosis [3]. Other investigators believe that prospective coronary artery disease patients can be found using personality test interviews [4]. Correlations have been found relating coronary heart disease with hypertension, obesity, cigarette smoking, circulating catecholamines, and heredity [5]. It is obvious from the numerous studies by reputable investigators that the formation of the ultimate vascular change called "atheroma" is probably a common result of a variety of stimuli. Not only do these multiple etiologic factors have a similar pathologic manifestation, but also there must be a receptive vessel in an appropriately receptive individual for the formation of an atheromatous lesion.

The histologic morphology of the experimental and spontaneous atherosclerotic lesion has also been the subject of much controversy. The primary lesion has been thought to be in the intima, the elastic membrane, or the media by different workers. Variabilities in experimental design and observations such as the age of the lesion or the means used for inducing the lesion, as well as in the species under study, have contributed to these different opinions [6].

Our interest is in the relationship of vascular hypersensitivity to atherosclerosis. It had been shown that arterial lesions similar to those seen in humans could be induced in rabbits by immunologic means [7]. The unique localization of the vascular lesion in the arterial tree in experimentally induced serum sickness indicated that the large coronary arteries and the aorta are the prime sites for vascular damage [8, 9]. There have been few studies reported in which high blood cholesterol levels have been superimposed on immunologically induced vascular lesions. Serum sickness was induced in rabbits both on normal diets and cholesterol-supplemented diets, and observations were made on the hearts and aortas. The microscopic observations of these hearts and aortas are the subject of this report.

METHODS

Male New Zealand albino rabbits of approximately 2 kg body weight were obtained locally and used throughout these experiments. A total of 80 rabbits was studied using four different treatments. One group of rabbits was given a single intravenous injection of physiological saline solution and regular rabbit diet (Purina). Another group was given the same i.v. saline injection but also placed on regular feed containing 1% cholesterol. A third group received a single i.v. injection of 250 mg/kg bovine serum albumin (BSA)* plus regular feed. A fourth group received 250 mg/kg of BSA i.v. plus regular feed containing 1% cholesterol. Groups of rabbits were sacrificed at either 2 or 3 weeks from the date of i.v. injection and organs were removed. Gross examinations of the heart, aorta, and kidneys were made at the time of sacrifice and these tissues were fixed in Bouin's solution or 10% neutral formalin for subsequent histological study. Serial sections of either 6 or 20 μ were made of the hearts and aortas. Approximately 300 sections were made of each heart. Some sections were stained with hematoxylin and eosin (H and E), others with Sudan IV for fat, and another group with Weigert—Von Giesen stain for elastic tissue.

RESULTS

The main object of this study was to determine the existence of a phenomenon, and the data will be described and illustrated. Three general types of lesions were observed, depending on the treatment given the animals. Those animals that received the 1% cholesterol diet had a very low frequency of almost pure foam cell growths that occurred exclusively in the aorta. In the group that received the BSA without the cholesterol, about 20% of the animals had endothelial proliferation without discernible amounts

*Nutritional Biochemicals, 2× recrystallized.

Fig. 1. Foam cell plaque in coronary artery of rabbit No. 51. Hematoxylin and eosin preparation from Bouin's-fixed tissue (x 100). The animal received a single injection of 250 mg/kg of BSA and a 1% cholesterol diet for 2 weeks, after which it was sacrificed.

Fig. 2. Marked proliferation in coronary artery of rabbit No. 101. Hematoxylin and eosin preparation from formalin-fixed tissue and cut by frozen section (x 100). The animal received a single injection of 250 mg/kg BSA and a 1% cholesterol diet for 2 weeks, after which it was sacrificed.

Fig. 3. Sudanophilic material below the proliferative area in a coronary artery from rabbit No.101. Sudan IV preparation from formalin-fixed tissue and cut by frozen section (x 100). The animal received a single injection of 250 mg/kg BSA and a 1% cholesterol diet for 2 weeks, after which it was sacrificed.

Fig. 4. Mitotic figure observed in aortic valvular area of rabbit No. 1. Hematoxylin and eosin preparation from Bouin's-fixed tissue (oil immersion, x 1000). The animal received a single injection of 250 mg/kg BSA and a 1% cholesterol diet for 2 weeks, after which it was sacrificed.

Fig. 5. Foam cell accumulation at the point of branching off the aorta of rabbit No. 77. Hematoxylin and eosin preparation from Bouin's-fixed tissue (x 40). The animal received a single injection of 250 mg/kg BSA and a 1% cholesterol diet for 2 weeks, after which it was sacrificed.

Fig. 6. Foam cells in the artery of the aorta of rabbit No. 77 beyond the branching as seen in Fig.5. Hematoxylin and eosin preparation from Bouin's-fixed tissue (x 40).

Fig. 7. Greater magnification of foam cells seen in Fig. 6 of the vessel beyond the branch in the aorta. Hematoxylin and eosin preparation from Bouin's-fixed tissue (x 100).

Fig. 8. Sudan stain seen at a branch in the aorta of rabbit No. 92. Sudan IV preparation from formalin-fixed tissue and cut by frozen section (x 100). The animal received a single injection of 250 mg/kg BSA and a 1% cholesterol diet for 2 weeks, after which it was sacrificed.

Fig. 9. Small breaks in the internal elastica of a coronary artery directly beneath small foam cell plaques in rabbit No. 4. Weigert–Von Giesen stain from Bouin's-fixed tissue (x 450). The animal received a single injection of 250 mg/kg BSA and a 1% cholesterol diet for 2 weeks, after which it was sacrificed.

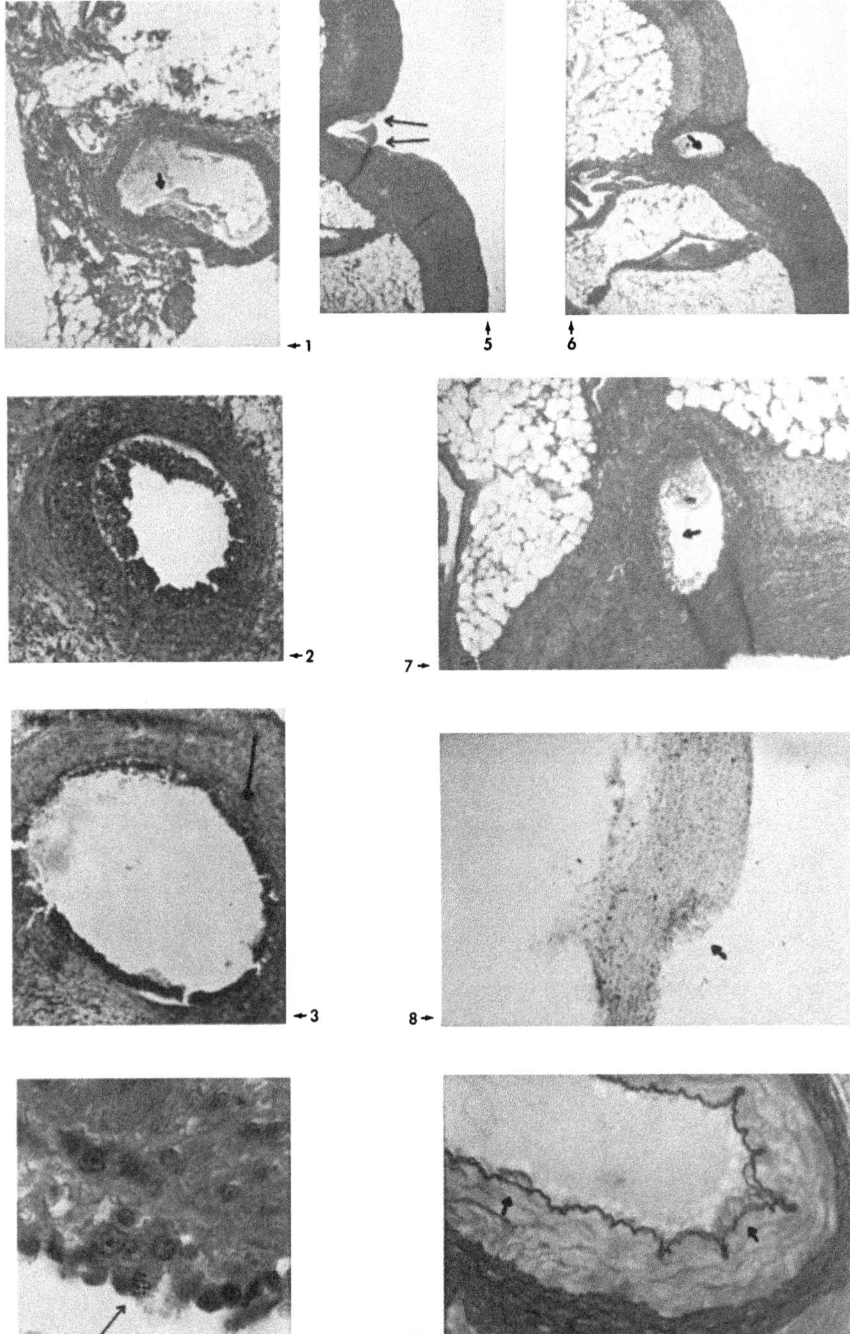

1
5
6
2
7
3
8
4
9

of foam cells in the aorta, valvular areas, or coronary arteries. When both BSA and cholesterol were administered, about 50% of the animals had endothelial proliferation with foam cells also present. None of the saline control animals showed any changes. No gross pathology was observed at autopsy in the heart, aorta, or kidneys in any of the four groups of animals.

General Locations of Lesions

In all cases where lesions were observed in the heart, they were in areas of the aortic valves and the coronary artery outflows from the aorta. Those parts of the aorta that showed changes were primarily at branches coming off the aorta.

Histological Description

Three general types of lesions were observed. Some showed only a proliferation, whereas others appeared to be comprised of foam cells. A third group contained a mixture of foam cells and proliferation. In Fig. 1, a coronary vessel can be seen with an intimal growth identified as foam cells. Figure 2 illustrates a coronary artery with marked endothelial or intimal proliferation. The tissue in Fig. 2 was also stained for fat, and Fig. 3 illustrates sudanophilic material in the proliferative area. Figures 2 and 3 were made from thick (20 μ) frozen sections. Figure 4 illustrates the process of mitosis in the proliferative area. It can be seen from these illustrations that the alterations observed are in the endothelium with no apparent involvement of the media.

In the aorta, foam cells appeared at the branches, as can be seen in Fig. 5. The proliferation continued in the branch beyond the aortic orifice, as can be seen in Figs. 6 and 7. Areas of aortic branches stained for fat contained sudanophilic material, as seen in Fig. 8. Figure 9 is a vessel examined with Weigert stain, showing the internal elastic membrane. Small breaks are noticeable in the membrane directly under the growth points.

DISCUSSION

Numerous theories have been put forth to explain the pathogenesis of atherosclerosis. From the morphological point of view, it is generally agreed that the areas of high blood pressure and great turbulence are the most susceptible to injury. This is consistent with our and other findings, that most lesions are found in the larger coronary arteries, directly off the aortic valves, and in the branches off the aorta, primarily near the arch. In addition to the physical aspects of pressure and turbulence, injury to the vessels and high blood lipid levels are the other members of the "troika" considered necessary parts of the optimal environment for the occurrence of the lesions. The mild injury induced by serum sickness in the presence of high lipid levels appeared to be capable of predisposing a vascular site for experimental atherosclerosis. The accompanying illustrations indicate that some lesions have been obtained superficially resembling early atherosclerosis. In the series of animals receiving both BSA and cholesterol, approximately 50% showed lesions. Those with BSA alone showed a 20% incidence, and in the cholesterol or saline control groups no lesions were seen in the heart.

Living systems are exposed to a hostile environment that includes immunological sensitization. This sensitization is at times acutely life-threatening, as in the case of anaphylactic shock, or life-sparing, as when there are circulating protective antibodies. It is reasonable to conceive of a condition which is not acute but can occur over many years, in which an individual episodically builds up circulating antibodies to circulatory antigens causing a mild, subclinical form of serum sickness. If these antigen–antibody complexes are formed in an environment of high blood lipids, the vascular damage can be self-perpetuating. Under these circumstances, the lipid incorporated in the intimal tissue can act as an injury (or irritant) to sustain the lesion. Under normal circumstances, serum thickness heals and leaves little or no residual damage. However, the inclusion of lipid may contribute to the preparation of a focal site for continued and future damage. Hypertension may be another synergistic factor in preparing the vascular bed for the ultimate atherosclerosis, since Wilens [10] showed that serum sickness is enhanced by elevated blood pressure. Small molecular substances acting as haptens can also cause immunological injury to the coronaries and the aorta [11].

If continued exposure to immunological insult leads to vascular damage, this offers some therapeutic opportunities. Since antigen–antibody complexes are localized in discrete areas, presumably by phagocytic mechanisms as some authors believe [9], we might alter the course of the reaction by pharmacologically influencing the reticuloendothelial system (RES) and phagocytic cells to remove these complexes. Indeed, some investigators are already looking into the problem of the role of the RES in systemic immunological reactions [12, 13].

Second, it is believed that leucocytes are instrumental in the phagocytic process, and may release chemical mediators that cause the inflammation or proliferation [14]. The use of antagonists to these chemical mediators might abort the pathological processes leading to atherosclerosis. Some evidence has already been obtained indicating that certain monoamine oxidase inhibitors [15], antihistaminics [16], antibradykinin agents [17], and cortisone [18] are capable of altering either serum sickness or experimental atherosclerosis.

In the light of the above argument, it is believed that ultimate decreased morbidity and mortality can be achieved. Pharmacologically, it is now possible to alter the blood pressure to decrease the risk from changes in cardiovascular dynamics. Either diet or drugs like heparin or heparinoids

[19, 20] can lower lipemia and thereby decrease added stress to the vessels. The probability of thrombus formation can be attacked from two major areas. If thrombus formation is believed to be independent of injury to the vessel, then anticoagulant agents or fibrinolytic agents can be used. However, if thrombus formation is part of the sequelae of injury, then certain types of anti-inflammatory agents should suppress the process. It is to this latter phenomenon that this investigation has been directed. Injury has been induced by mild immunological means and lipid has appeared to be incorporated into this inflamed area. When the mediator or mediators that are responsible for the injury have been found, then appropriate pharmacological depressants should be capable of reducing the morbidity and mortality from atherosclerotic heart lesions.

SUMMARY

Serum sickness was induced in hypercholesterolemic rabbits by a single i.v. injection of bovine serum albumin. After two or three weeks, the animals were sacrificed and serial sections were made of the heart and aorta. It was found that the animals on a cholesterol diet and with serum sickness had a high incidence of vascular damage at the aortic valves, coronary arteries, and the branches at the arch of the aorta.

ACKNOWLEDGMENTS

The author wishes to thank J.K. Smith, R. Gayek, L. Seifert, M. von Diepow, and P. Cohen for their help on this study.

REFERENCES

1. H.F. Watts, "The mechanism of arterial lipid accumulation in human coronary artery atherosclerosis," in: W. Likoff and J.F. Moyer, Eds., Coronary Heart Disease. New York, Grune & Stratton, 1963.
2. G. Pickering, "Pathogenesis of myocardial and cerebral infarction: modular arteriosclerosis," Brit.Med.J., 1:517, 1964.
3. M. Texon, "The role of vascular dynamics in the development of atherosclerosis," in: M. Sander and C.H. Bourne, Eds., Atherosclerosis and Its Origin. New York, Academic Press, 1963.
4. R.H. Rosenman and M. Friedman, "Behavior patterns, blood lipids, and coronary heart disease," J.Am.Med.Ass., 184:934, 1963.
5. J.W. Gofman, Coronary Heart Disease. Springfield, Illinois, Charles C. Thomas, 1959.
6. J.C. Roberts and R. Strauss, Eds., Comparative Atherosclerosis. New York, Hoeber Medical Div. of Harper & Row, 1965.
7. O. Saphir, D. Stryzak, and L. Ohringer, "Hypersensitivity changes in coronary arteries of rabbits and their relationship to arteriosclerosis," Lab.Invest., 7:434, 1958.

8. F.G. Germuth, Jr., "A comparative histologic and immunologic study in rabbits of induced hypersensitivity of the serum sickness type," J.Exptl.Med., 97:257, 1953.
9. W.T. Kniker and C.G. Cochrane, "Pathogenic factors in vascular lesions of experimental serum sickness," J.Exptl.Med., 122:83, 1965.
10. S.L. Wilens, "Enhancement of serum sickness lesions in rabbits with pressor agents," Arch. Pathol., 80:590, 1965.
11. O. Saphir, M. Telischi, and L. Ohringer, "Rabbit sulfa drug hypersensitivity and lesions resembling arteriosclerosis," Arch. Pathol., 73:414, 1962.
12. D.A. Blickens and N.R. DiLuzio, "Induction of phagocytic inhibition and the generalized Shwartzman phenomena by the administration of plasma from reticuloendothelial hypofunctional mice," J. Reticuloendothelial Soc., 2:187, 1965.
13. P.D. Mott and S.M. Wolff, "The association of fever and antibody response in rabbits immunized with human serum albumin," J. Clin. Invest., 45:372, 1966.
14. W.T. Kniker and C.G. Cochrane, "Localization of circulating Ag—Ab complexes in serum sickness," Federation Proc., 25:474, 1966.
15. T. Shimamoto, "The relationship of edematous reaction in arteries to atherosclerosis and thrombosis," J. Atherosclerosis Res., 3:87, 1963.
16. D. Harman, "Inhibiting effect of an antihistaminic drug, chlorphenir-amine," Circulation Res., 11:277, 1963.
17. T. Shimamoto, F. Numano, and T. Fujita, "Atherosclerosis-inhibiting effect of an antibradykinin agent, pyridanolcarbamate," Am. Heart J., 71:216, 1966.
18. M. Friedman, S. Byers, and S. St. George, "Cortisone and experimental atherosclerosis," Arch. Pathol., 77:56, 1964.
19. L. Levy and G. Cronheim, "Blood levels and clearing activity of a synthetic heparinoid," Biochem. Pharmacol., 7:27, 1961.
20. L. Levy and F.J. Petracek, "Chemical and pharmacological studies on N-resulfated heparin," Proc. Soc. Exptl. Biol. Med., 190:901, 1962.

Synthetic Cholesterol-Ester Antigens in Experimental Atherosclerosis*

J. Martyn Bailey and Jean Butler

Department of Biochemistry
George Washington University School of Medicine
Washington, D. C.

It seems fairly well established, as the result of previous reports [1, 2, 3] and of work reviewed elsewhere in this symposium, that stimulation of the RES can influence some aspects of lipid metabolism. Early work by Weinhouse and Hirsch [4] on the composition of atherosclerotic plaques showed that the principal sterol fraction was the esterified form. In a similar study we found that the progression of atherosclerotic lesions in the thoracic aorta of cholesterol-fed rabbits was much more closely linked to increases in tissue cholesterol esters than to free cholesterol itself. Thus, after 12-14 weeks on cholesterol diets, when the plaques covered from 50-100% of the surface of the aorta, the ester cholesterol content of the aorta had increased to 23 times the normal levels as compared to only 2- to 3-fold increase in the free cholesterol content (Table I). It was of interest, therefore, to study the influence on the atherosclerotic process of immunization with antigens directed specifically against the cholesterol ester fraction of the serum lipoproteins. The feasibility of coupling steroid-type molecules as haptens to specific carrier proteins has been demonstrated for progesterone, desoxycorticosterone, and estrone by Erlanger and Borek et al. [5].

SYNTHESIS OF CHOLESTEROL–SEBACATE ANTIGENS

These syntheses were accomplished by the general procedure outlined in Scheme 1 on the following page.

Cholesterol-4-^{14}C powder (10 g, 20 μc) was dissolved in warm sebacyl dichloride (10 ml), pyridine was added as catalyst, and the mixture was

* The work described here was supported by U.S. Public Health Service grants Nos. HE 05062 and 1K3 Ca 16730.

Table I. Free and Ester Cholesterol Content of Rabbit Aorta During Developing Atherosclerosis

Weeks on diet†	Severity of atherosclerosis range (%) ‡	Aorta cholesterol content mg/100 g wet wt. *		Relative increase above normal	
		Free	Ester	Free	Ester
0	0	100 ± 10	10 ± 3	0	0
6	5-15	121 ± 11	35 ± 6	0.21	2.5
9	15-30	145 ± 36	44 ± 7	0.45	3.4
12	30-50	243 ± 29	193 ± 29	1.43	18.3
14	50-100	287 ± 21	243 ± 42	1.87	23.3

*Mean ± S.E.

†Diet of commercial rabbit pellets supplemented with 1% cholesterol.

‡Expressed as percentage of aorta surface involved with atherosclerotic plaques.

Table II. Lipid Levels in Serum of Normal and Immunized Rabbits Following Cholesterol Feeding

Group No. and treatment	Number of rabbits	Total lipid (mg/100 ml)*	Total cholesterol (mg/100 ml)*	Ratio ester/free cholesterol*	Plaque grade (%)*
I Normal diet, 21 weeks	3	310 ± 93	32 ± 5	1.4 ± 0.2	0
II Immunized, 6 weeks; normal diet, 21 weeks	4	260 ± 44	41 ± 6	2.0 ± 0.1	0
III Normal diet, 6 weeks; 1% cholesterol, 15 weeks	5	4497 ± 348	1362 ± 42	1.8 ± 0.4	66 ± 16
IV Immunized, 6 weeks; 1% cholesterol, 15 weeks	8	2682 ± 210	1020 ± 46	2.2 ± 0.2	30 ± 6
Group III vs Group IV		P < 0.001	P < 0.001	P > 0.05	P < 0.05

Groups II and IV animals were immunized twice weekly for six weeks with synthetic antigen. Groups I and III were maintained as unimmunized controls. Rabbits in groups III and IV were then placed on 1% cholesterol diet for 15 weeks. Values given are for plasma lipid levels after 21 weeks, preceding death and examination of aortas for atherosclerotic plaques. Plaque grade represents the mean percentage of the aorta surface covered with atherosclerotic plaques.

*Mean ± S. E.

SCHEME I

R−OH (Cholesterol)	+	$ClCO(CH_2)_8COCl$ (sebacyl dichloride)	--------→	$ROCO(CH_2)_8COCl$ (Cholesterol sebacyl monochloride)
+ Protein−NH_2		----------→		Protein−$NHCO(CH_2)_8COOR$ (Protein−cholesterol sebacate antigen)

heated at 120° for 1 hr. Excess sebacyl dichloride was distilled off in vacuo (2 mm Hg, 162°). The residue of cholesterol sebacyl chloride and inert dicholesterol sebacate was dissolved in warm dioxane (1 L) and added slowly to an ice cold solution of bovine albumin (10 g fraction V) in isotonic saline (1 L). The pH was maintained at 8.3 by dropwise addition of sodium hydroxide. Pyridine was added and the mixture stood overnight at 4°. The product, precipitated by addition of one volume of acetone−alcohol (1:1), was filtered, washed repeatedly with ethanol−ether (1:1), and air dried. The resulting powder was refluxed in a Soxhlet apparatus with ethanol−ether (1:1) to constant specific activity. Yield was 9.5 g of a pale yellow powder having 9.5 moles of bound ^{14}C-cholesterol per 50,000 g albumin. In later experiments human β-lipoprotein was used in place of bovine albumin as the carrier protein (see below). The general procedure used was the same as that described here for bovine albumin and gave a similar relative degree of substitution with ^{14}C-cholesterol sebacate. These products were dispersed in dilute alkali, saturated alum solution was added, and the precipitates were suspended in isotonic saline (containing merthiolate as preservative) for injection.

ANTIGENS WITH BOVINE ALBUMIN AS THE CARRIER PROTEIN

The first experiments were carried out with an antigen in which crystalline bovine serum albumin was the carrier protein, substituted with an average of 9.5 moles of covalent-linked cholesterol sebacate per 50,000 g protein.

Twenty New Zealand White male rabbits were divided into four groups, as outlined in Table II. Two groups (II and IV) were immunized intramuscularly twice weekly for six weeks with 25 mg antigen protein until the mean antibody titer measured by an interfacial precipitation technique was 1:7000. At this time rabbits in group III (unimmunized control) and group IV (immunized) were transferred to a diet supplemented with 1% cholesterol. Plasma lipid levels were measured biweekly and booster shots of antigen were given to groups II and IV animals at similar intervals. Groups I and II were maintained on normal diet throughout the experiment. Intake of food and average gain in weight were the same in all four groups.

After 15 weeks on the experimental diet, all animals were killed and the thoracic aortas were examined for atherosclerotic plaques. By projec-

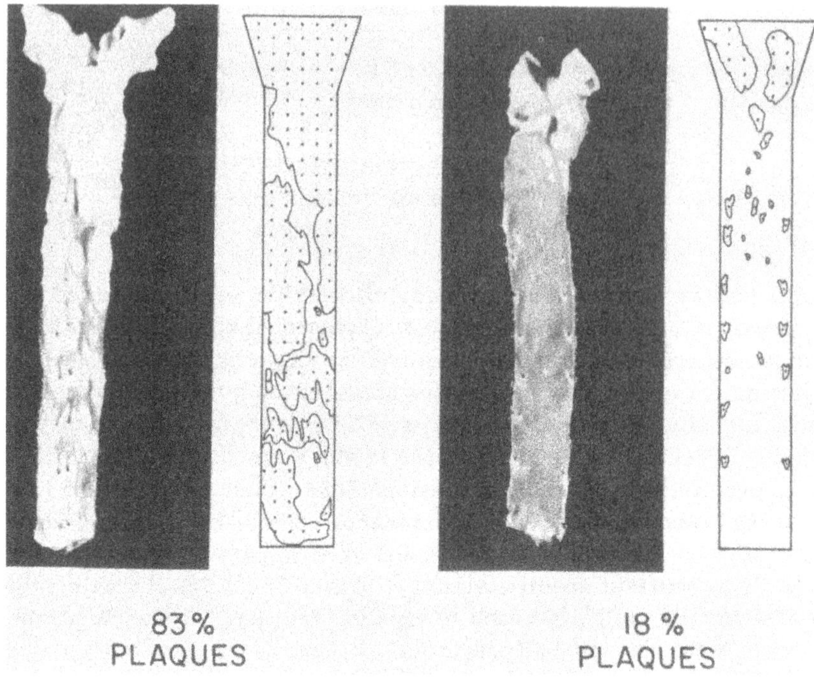

Fig. 1. Planimetry of atherosclerotic plaques.

tion of the plaques onto a standardized grid stencil, the intensity of atherosclerosis was scored as percentage involvement of the aorta surface. For an illustration of an application of the technique, see Fig. 1. No plaques were observed in either normal or immunized animals on the standard diet (groups I and II). Intensity of plaques in the immunized group fed cholesterol (30%) was significantly less than in control animals (66%) maintained on the same diet. Both total lipids and total cholesterol were significantly lower in plasma of the immunized group. The ratio of esterified to free cholesterol was not significantly altered (Table II).

In a second experiment using the bovine albumin, in contrast to immunizing for six weeks before beginning the cholesterol feeding, the efficacy of beginning the cholesterol feeding simultaneously with the immunization was tested. After 13 weeks the control animals fed 1% cholesterol had plaque intensities of 41 ± 4% compared to the average intensity of only 17 ± 13% in the immunized group (Table IV). It was concluded, therefore, that a preimmunization period was of no special advantage, and in all subsequent experiments the immunization procedure and cholesterol feeding were begun at the same time.

The presence of antibodies against the cholesterol ester as a hapten in serum of animals immunized with the bovine albumin synthetic antigen was demonstrated by cross reaction of the bovine specific antiserum with a synthetic egg albumin–cholesterol sebacate. Experiments in which rabbits were immunized with nonspecific antigens including unsubstituted β-lipoproteins or polysaccharide antigens (yeast zymosan) or with the saline-phenol merthiolate and alum mixture used in preparing the antigens for injection, produced no significant change in the serum lipid levels or in the intensity of plaques in the aorta of cholesterol-fed rabbits. In earlier experiments in which unmodified cockerel β-lipoproteins were used as antigens, some change in the distribution of cholesterol in the various protein factors in rabbit serum was found [6]. Significant increase in cholesterol content of the γ-globulin fraction (isolated by chromatography on DEAE cellulose) was not however observed in animals immunized with either the albumin–cholesterol sebacate or the human β-lipoprotein cholesterol–sebacate antigens.

ANTIGENS WITH HUMAN β-LIPOPROTEIN AS THE CARRIER PROTEIN

Because of the favorable results using the bovine albumin carrier, attempts were made to design an antigen which would resemble more closely the "target" lipoproteins in rabbit serum. As a working hypothesis the mechanism of the protective effect is considered to involve production of antibodies which interact with host lipoproteins. Immunization with a protein antigen carrying a cholesterol ester as a hapten would thus produce antibodies capable of interacting with those host serum lipoproteins which contain cholesterol esters. It was reasoned, therefore, that by also using a carrier protein more closely related to the host lipoprotein an even more specific antigen may result.

An antigen having human β-lipoprotein as the carrier was synthesized by the general method outlined in Scheme 1. The product (4.3 g from 5 g human β-lipoprotein) had 70 moles of covalent-bound cholesterol per 250,000 g protein. The antigenicity of this product in the rabbit, as measured by the quantitative precipitation reaction, was considerably less than that of the bovine albumin product (Fig. 2). When rabbits immunized with this material, however, were placed on the cholesterol diet for 12 weeks, an enhanced effect both on the reduction of serum lipid levels and on the intensity of atherosclerotic plaques was obtained (Table III). After 12 weeks, 9/10 control animals had plaques of average grade 24 ± 4%. Only 3/13 of the immunized group developed plaques of average grade for the group of 3 ± 1% (Fig. 3).

DURATION OF THE PROTECTIVE EFFECT

It is well known that the development of atherosclerotic lesions in rabbit aorta is a function both of the absolute serum cholesterol level and also

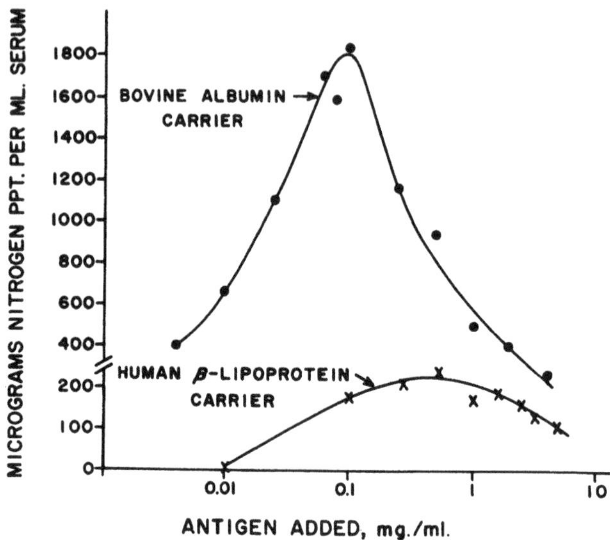

Fig. 2. Quantitative preciptin curves for rabbit antisera.

Table III. Influence of Immunization with Synthetic Human Beta-Lipoprotein Antigen on Experimental Atherosclerosis in Rabbits

	Controls	Immunized
Plasma total lipids*	2487 ± 385	1206 ± 127
Plasma cholesterol*	1037 ± 166	673 ± 95
Plaque grade % *	24 ± 4	3 ± 1
Number of animals with plaques	9/10	3/13

*Mean ± S. E.

All animals were fed a 1% cholesterol diet for 12 weeks. The experimental groups were immunized weekly for the first six weeks with 2-mg doses of a synthetic human beta-lipoprotein cholesterol sebacate antigen given intramuscularly. Two booster shots were given at 2- and 3-week intervals. Values given are for final serum lipid levels following sacrifice of the animals.

Table IV. Protective Effect of Immunization Procedure as a Function of the Duration of Cholesterol Feeding

Duration of experiment (weeks)	Antigen	Controls		Immunized	
		No. of animals	Plaque grade, %*	No. of animals	Plaque grade, %*
12	β lip.	10	24 ± 4	13	3 ± 1
13	Alb.	5	41 ± 4	4	17 ± 13
15†	Alb.	5	66 ± 16	8	30 ± 6
24‡	β lip.	19	54 ± 7	9	41 ± 8
36 **	β lip.	7	66 ± 6	6	63 ± 10

*Mean ± S.E.

†Immunized for six weeks before cholesterol feeding was begun. For all others, immunization was begun at the same time as cholesterol feeding.

‡Cholesterol fed only for first 12 weeks.

**Fed 0.2% cholesterol for six months and 1% cholesterol for final three months.

the duration of the hypercholesterolemia [7]. Some measure of the duration of the protective effect of the immunization procedure was obtained by using more prolonged experimental periods of six and nine months. In these experiments the same schedule of immunization was used for the first six weeks followed by booster shots at 3- to 4-week intervals. In the nine-month experiment, to overcome the lethal effects of prolonged feeding of 1% cholesterol [8], the diet consisted of 0.2% cholesterol in both control and immunized animals for the first six months followed by a final three months of 1% cholesterol diet. In Table IV are collected the results of all our experiments to date in which the protective effect of the immunization may be compared to the duration of the experiment. A significant reduction in intensity of atherosclerosis was found over all experimental periods of up to six months duration. The magnitude of the protective effect decreases with increasing time of exposure to the hypercholesterolemia. For the nine-month experiment, due to the more prolonged period of hypercholesterolemia, the severity of atherosclerosis was not significantly less in the immunized group. Serum cholesterol levels in immunized animals remained lower than controls over the entire period of cholesterol feeding (Fig. 4).

SUMMARY

Antigens having an analog of serum cholesterol esters as a haptenic group were synthesized by coupling ^{14}C-cholesterol sebacyl chloride to either bovine albumin or human β-lipoprotein as carrier proteins.

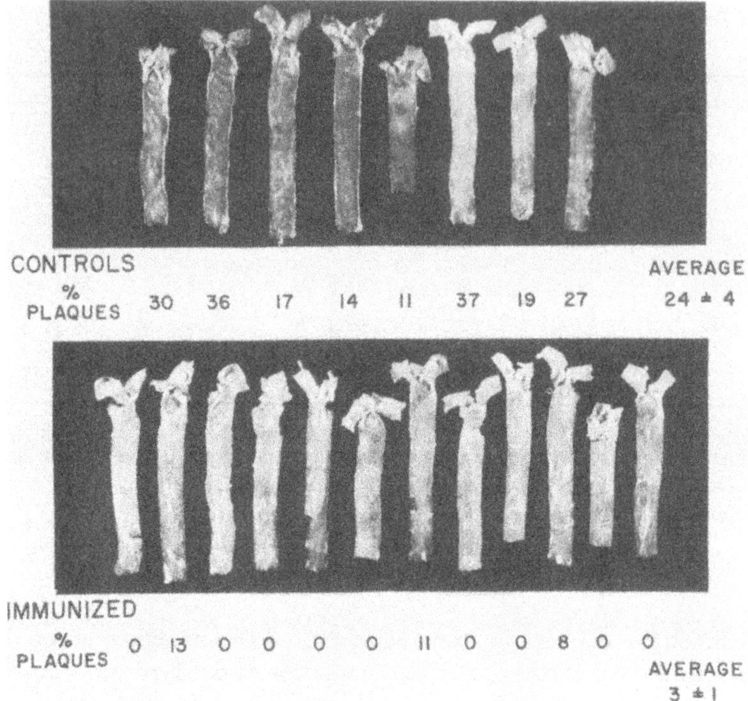

Fig. 3. Atherosclerosis in rabbits immunized with human β-lipoprotein synthetic antigen.

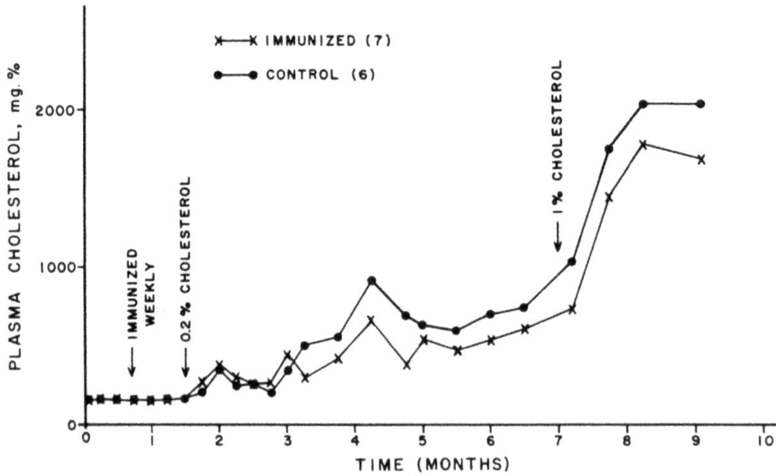

Fig. 4. Plasma cholesterol levels in control and immunized rabbits during prolonged cholesterol feeding.

Following immunization with these products, significant decreases in serum cholesterol levels in cholesterol-fed rabbits were observed for experimental periods of up to nine months. A significant reduction in the severity of atherosclerotic lesions in the thoracic aorta was also obtained for periods of up to six months on the hypercholesterolemic diets. These results demonstrate the feasibility of immunological manipulation of serum lipid levels and of host response to hypercholesterolemia by use of antigens directed against specific serum lipoprotein constituents.

REFERENCES

1. S. Gero, J. Gergely, L. Jakab, J. Szekely, S. Virag, K. Farkas, and A. Czuppon, Lancet, 1119, 1961.
2. S.J. Riggi and N.R. DiLuzio, J.Lipid Res., 3:339, 1962.
3. J.M. Bailey, R. Bright, and R. Tomar, Nature, 201:407, 1964.
4. S. Weinhouse and E.F. Hirsch, Arch. Pathol., 29:31, 1940.
5. B.F. Erlanger, F. Borek, S.M. Beiser, and S. Lieberman, J.Biol. Chem., 234, 1090, 1959.
6. J.M. Bailey and R. Tomar, J. Atherosclerosis Res., 5:203, 1965.
7. P. Constantinides, Experimental Atherosclerosis. Amsterdam, Elsevier, 1965, p. 42.
8. P. Constantinides, Experimental Atherosclerosis. Amsterdam, Elsevier, 1965, p. 43.

Atherosclerosis Induced Experimentally By Repeated Intravenous Administration of Hypercholesterolemic Serum and of Lipoproteins

A. N. Klimov, L. G. Petrova-Maslakova,
L. P. Rodionova, and T. A. Sinitzina

Laboratory of Lipid Metabolism
Institute of Experimental Medicine
Leningrad, USSR

ABSTRACT. Serum from rabbits rendered hypercholesterolemic by dietary supplement was administered intravenously daily in 10-ml aliquots to four recipient rabbits: one for 5 months (total cholesterol 13.7 g), three for 6-7 months (total cholesterol 22-23 g). All animals showed marked elevation of serum cholesterol and serum β-lipoproteins. The rabbits treated for 6-7 months which received high quantities of cholesterol developed atherosclerotic plaques in the aorta, carotid, and cardial arteries.

The next step included the separation of serum into chylomicrons and lipoproteins and their intravenous injection into other recipient rabbits, for 6 months. Atherosclerosis was induced only in the case when lipoproteins (total cholesterol 24-25 g) were injected.

These data prove directly the atherogenic action of lipoproteins.

* * *

As is well known, all cholesterol in plasma is present in lipoproteins of different density and in chylomicrons.

Gofman et al. [1] and some other authors have suggested that lipoproteins of low density having Sf 12-20 may penetrate the endothelium of the aorta and remain deposited in the intima. Identity of lipoproteins of low density in the serum and aorta was shown by immunological investigations [2].

Investigations with the labeled lipoproteins in the protein part of the molecule have shown that when such lipoproteins were injected intravenously, radioactivity was found in the proteins of the aorta [3].

Another point of view has been suggested by Gordon [4]. He supposes that only chylomicrons can deposit on the intima of the vessel.

There is also an interesting report by Friedman and Byers [5] who injected in vivo the following forms of cholesterol into the ligated part of the carotid artery of rabbits: the serum with a high concentration of cholesterol, the solution of low-density lipoproteins, chylomicrons, and the suspension of cholesterol. Lesions in the artery were found only following the injection of chylomicrons or of the suspension of cholesterol.

So there are different points of view and different experimental data about the form of cholesterol responsible for the experimental development of atherosclerosis.

Three years ago, it was demonstrated in our laboratory that the greatest part of cholesterol in the aorta of normal rabbits or of rabbits with experimental atherosclerosis was in lipoproteins [6, 7]. Using several water solutions including a veronal buffer solution, we extracted 80-90% of the total cholesterol from the homogenized aorta.

Then we applied Burstein's method [8] for determination or isolation of β-lipoproteins in the aorta. This method is based on the capacity of heparin to precipitate the lipoproteins having density 1.06 and below in the presence of calcium ions. By this method we were able to show that in rabbits with experimental atherosclerosis the content of low-density lipoproteins precipitated by heparin was greatly increased, not only in the serum, but also in the wall of the aorta.

It can be supposed that cholesterol infiltrates the aortic wall mostly in the form of lipoproteins, mainly low-density β-lipoproteins, in many respects analogous to the lipoproteins found in blood. Our own findings, as well as data from the literature, suggest the β-lipoproteins of human plasma are able to penetrate and become deposited in the arterial wall.

If this is the case, infusion of a large amount of β-lipoproteins or serum from animals with hypercholesterolemia or hyper-β-lipoproteinemia should enhance the development of atherosclerosis.

The purpose of the present work was to ascertain whether it is possible to induce marked atherosclerosis in healthy rabbits by repeated administration of serum with a high cholesterol content and of serum containing a high concentration of lipoproteins (without chylomicrons).

Table I. The Content of Cholesterol and β-Lipoproteins in Serum and Aorta of Different Groups of Rabbits and the Degree of Atherosclerotic Lesions in Their Aorta

No.	Injected material	No. of injections	Quantity of injected cholesterol, g	Serum		Aorta		Degree of atherosclerotic lesions in the aorta
				Cholesterol, mg%	β-lipoproteins, mg%	Cholesterol, mg%	β-lipoproteins, mg%	
1	Serum	124	13.7	89	170	336	510	None
2	Serum	187	22.1	380	1375	940	880	Heavy
3	Serum	142	21.2	621	1720	290	351	Slight
4	Serum	152	23.1	511	1420	702	626	Heavy
5	Lipoproteins	156	24.5	1104	3760	440	395	Intermediate
6	Lipoproteins	156	24.8	976	3245	830	780	Very heavy
7	Chylomicrons	156	2.3	108	247	293	280	None
8	Chylomicrons	156	3.1	117	312	350	288	None
9	Physiological saline	192	–	58	110	325	180	None
10	Control	–	–	44	135	375	298	None
11	Control	–	–	56	115	500	300	None
12	Control	–	–	60	210	441	280	None
13	Control	–	–	72	170	426	218	None

METHODS

One hundred and fifty donor rabbits were fed a standard laboratory diet supplement by 1 g cholesterol daily for a period of 2-4 months. At the end of this period, serum cholesterol level was 580-1600 mg%, while serum β-lipoproteins level was 1650-4000 mg%.

Four healthy rabbit recipients weighing about 2.5 kg were injected daily (except Sundays) with 10 ml of serum collected from donor animals. The donor animals were rotated so that the same animals were not used on two consecutive days.

Two other healthy recipients were injected daily with 10 ml serum after separating the chylomicrons. In this case the recipients received cholesterol in the form of lipoproteins only. The last two recipients were injected daily with 10 ml emulsion of chylomicrons in physiological saline prepared by centrifugation of hypercholesterolemic serum at 40,000 rpm for 40 min. A ninth animal served as a control and received 10 ml physiological saline for a period of eight months on the same schedule.

Data illustrating the experimental conditions are in Table I. The cholesterol and β-lipoprotein content in each portion of serum, lipoproteins or chylomicrons administered, was assessed every day. The blood level of cholesterol and β-lipoproteins in the recipient animals were measured periodically.

Recipient animals were killed at the end of the infusion period. Aorta and other vessels were examined by histochemical and biochemical methods. Serum and aorta cholesterol were measured according to the method of Neuschloss [9]. The content of lipoproteins in serum and aorta was estimated by the method of Burstein in our modification [10].

RESULTS

The content of cholesterol and β-lipoproteins of the serum of the control animal receiving the physiological saline was within a normal range throughout the course of the experiment. Necropsy failed to reveal any pathological changes. Histological examination of the aorta, cardiac, and cerebral arteries was also negative. Cholesterol and β-lipoprotein content of the aortic wall was within normal limits.

Figure 1 illustrates the changes in serum cholesterol in the rabbit receiving the hypercholesterolemic serum for a 5-month period. A twofold increase in serum cholesterol and in lipoprotein levels is apparent after 5-6 weeks, but subsequently the levels decline, so that at the end of 5 months they were approximately equal to those found at the onset of the experiment. Macroscopic and histological examinations failed to reveal marked atherosclerotic changes in the aorta of the animal. Thus, atherosclerosis was not

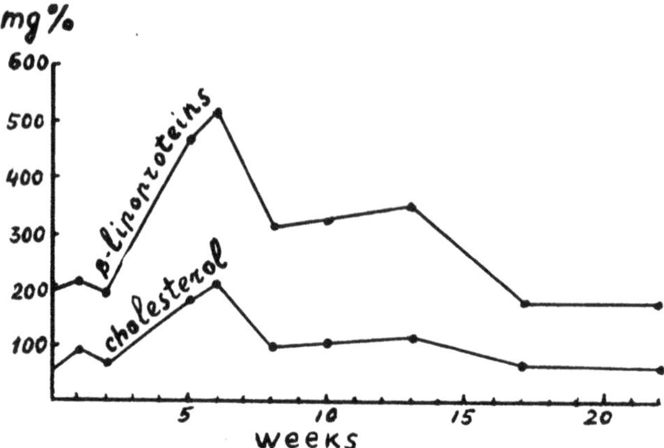

Fig. 1. Cholesterol and β-lipoprotein content in serum of one recipient (rabbit No. 1) after daily intravenous administration of hypercholesterolemic serum for five months.

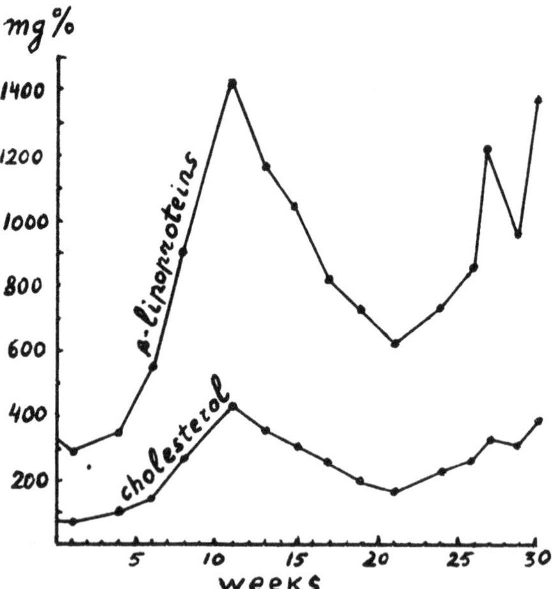

Fig. 2. Cholesterol and β-lipoprotein content in serum of one recipient (rabbit No. 2) after daily intravenous administration of hypercholesterolemic serum for 7½ months.

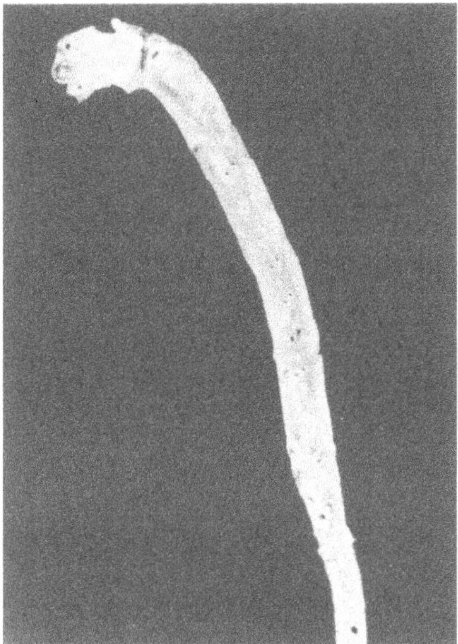

Fig. 3. Atherosclerotic lesions in the aorta of one recipient (rabbit No. 2).

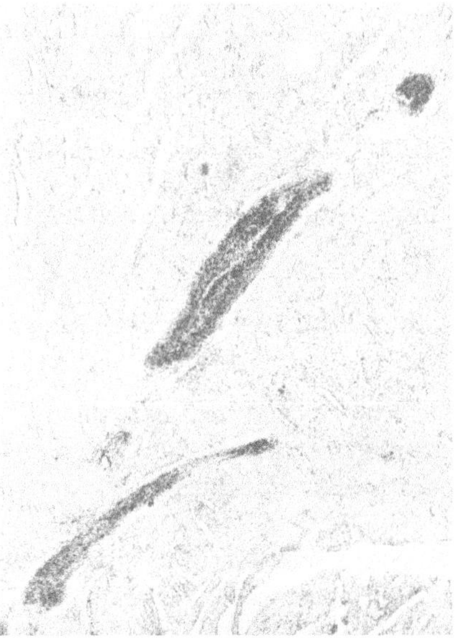

Fig. 4. Atherosclerotic plaque with a great number of large lipid particles in intracardiac artery of one recipient (rabbit No. 2). Stained with Sudan III. × 450.

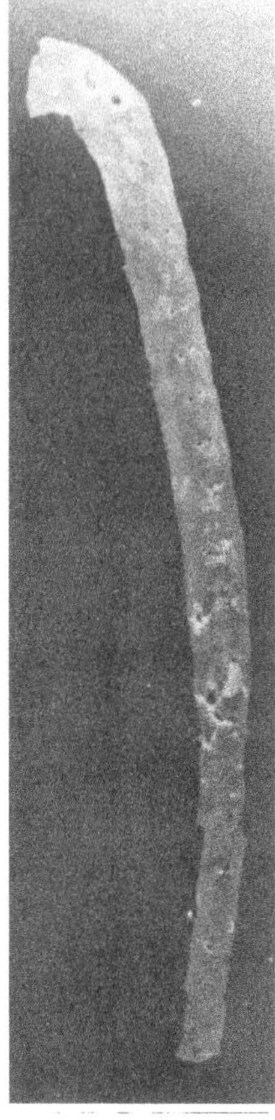

Fig. 5. Atherosclerotic lesions in aorta of one recipient (rabbit No. 6) after daily intravenous administration of serum lipoproteins for 6 months.

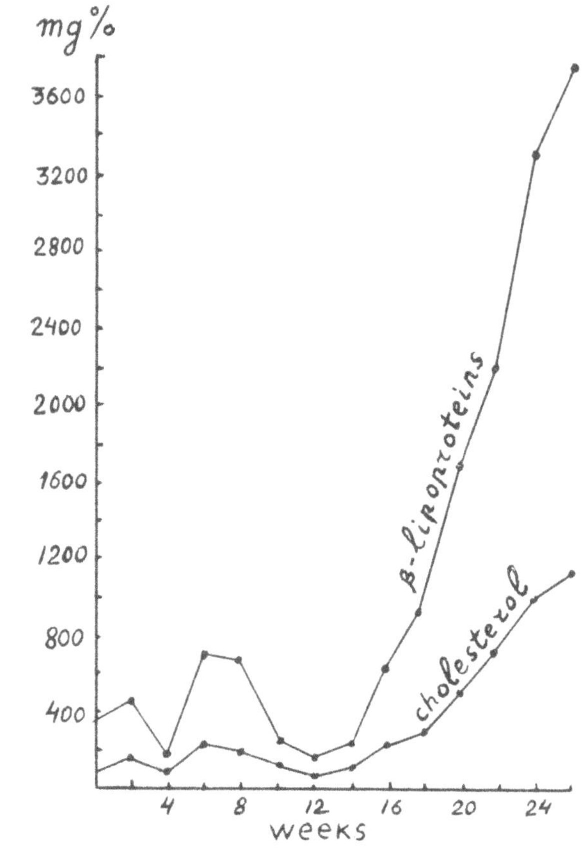

Fig. 6. Cholesterol and β-lipoprotein content in serum of one recipient (rabbit No. 5) after daily intravenous administration of serum lipoproteins for 6 months.

induced by protracted administration of hypercholesterolemic serum over a five-month period.

Figure 2 shows the changes in blood cholesterol and lipoproteins in the animal receiving hypercholesterolemic serum for a 7.5-month period. Cholesterol and β-lipoproteins rose markedly during the first 11 weeks to a value five times above the initial levels. During the subsequent 10 weeks these values declined despite continued administration of serum. This decline was followed by a second increase to a value of 1385 mg% β-lipoproteins and 380 mg% cholesterol at the termination of the experiment.

The same picture was observed in two other rabbits with repeated intravenous administrations of serum for six months.

It is difficult to explain why a marked drop in serum cholesterol and β-lipoproteins occurred in the experimental animals despite the continuing regimen of hypercholesterolemic infusion. This may have been due to the deposition of β-lipoproteins and cholesterol in organs and tissues, to an increased metabolic turnover of cholesterol (e.g., its oxidative transformation into bile acids in the liver), or to a combination of both these factors. The possible influence of other factors, e.g., immunological ones, cannot be ruled out. It is important to emphasize that there was a striking increase in serum cholesterol and β-lipoproteins during infusion. The curves of serum content of both components are almost parallel in all experimental animals. This suggests that β-lipoproteins are the basic carriers of cholesterol in hypercholesterolemia.

Typical multiple atherosclerotic plaques in the aortic wall (Fig. 3) were found in three animals (Nos. 2, 3, 4 in Table I) injected with serum containing a large quantity of cholesterol (22-23 g altogether). Histological examination revealed also atherosclerotic lesions in the carotid artery and the coronary arteries (Fig. 4).

On the basis of our experiments it is difficult to prove whether lipoproteins or chylomicrons are responsible for the development of atherosclerosis. The serum which we injected intravenously contained both lipoproteins and chylomicrons.

In order to solve this question, we carried out the following experiment. The serum from rabbit donors was separated into chylomicrons and lipoproteins. Chylomicrons were then injected into two rabbit recipients,

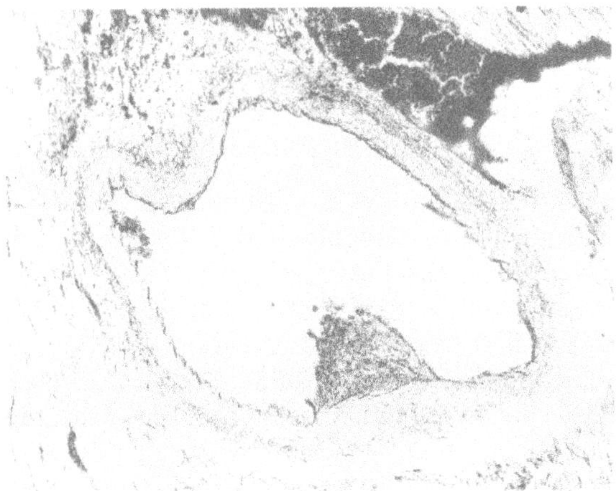

Fig. 7. Atherosclerotic plaque in subepicardial vessel of the left coronary artery of one recipient (rabbit No. 6) after daily intravenous administration of serum lipoproteins. Stained with Sudan III + hematoxylin. × 71.

and lipoproteins were injected into two other rabbits for six months.

A marked atherosclerosis was induced in both animals to whom lipoproteins were injected (Fig. 5). These animals showed significant elevation of serum cholesterol and β-lipoproteins (Fig. 6). One of them had a very high concentration of these components in the aorta (see Table I). Microscopic examinations revealed marked atherosclerotic lesions in the coronary arteries. In the majority of intramuscular branches the plaques led to partial stenosis. The plaques showed a lipid infiltration of Sudan staining. Significant lesions were found also in some subepicardial vessels predominantly of the left coronary artery (Fig. 7). Small foci of lipid myocardial degeneration were common. Lumina of many small arteries and capillaries were filled with lipids. There was a marked lipid infiltration of the liver. Hypertrophy of the wall of arteries in the Malpighian bodies in the spleen was found. A considerable lipid infiltration was found in the wall of the arteries as well as in the capsule and in the reticuloendothelial cells of the spleen.

It is necessary to mention that the administration of chylomicrons to rabbits did not produce atherosclerosis. Only a slight elevation of the concentration of cholesterol and lipoproteins in serum occurred.

The quantity of cholesterol administered with isolated chylomicrons was small in comparison with that of serum or lipoproteins (see Table I). However, chylomicrons administered to rabbit recipients were prepared from the same volume (10 ml) of hypercholesterolemic serum which, when administered to other rabbit recipients, produced atherosclerosis. Lipoproteins showing the atherogenic action were prepared also from the same volume of hypercholesterolemic serum. From this, one may conclude that chylomicrons in themselves, are not atherogenic.

REFERENCES

1. J. W. Gofman, F. Lindgren, et al., Science, 111: 166, 1950.
2. H. Ott, F. Lohss, and J. Gergely, Klin. Wochschr., 36: 383, 1958.
3. T. Okishio, Med. J. Osaka Univ., 11: 367, 1961.
4. J. Gordon, J. Atherosclerosis Res., 3: 1, 1963.
5. M. Friedman and S. Byers, Am. J. Pathol., 45: 825, 1964.
6. A. Klimov, Tezis. Dokl. Vses. Biokhim. S'ezda, 2: 161, 1963.
7. T.N. Lovyagina and E.B. Ban'kovskaya, Vopr. Med. Khim., 11: 17, 1965.
8. M. Burstein and J. Samaille, Presse Med., 1: 59, 1962.
9. S.M. Neuschloss, Biochem. Z., 225: 115, 1930.
10. A.N. Klimov, T.N. Lovyagina, and E.B. Ban'kovskaya, Lab. Delo, 5: 276, 1966.

Experimental Arteriopathy Induced in the Rabbit Through Rat Aorta Homogenate Injections: A Study of the Aortic Tissue Specificity

L. Scebat, J. Renais, N. Groult, and J. Lenegre

Centre de Recherches Cardiologiques
Hospital Boucicaut
Paris, France

ABSTRACT. An arteriopathy may be induced in the rabbit by an injection of homologous or heterologous aorta homogenates [1]. Such lesions coincide with the presence of circulating antibodies and of a delayed hypersensitivity reaction toward the injected antigen. In particular, rat aorta homogenate injections [2] are those which induce most constantly extensive and damaging lesions, and also the highest levels of circulating antibodies. It has been considered necessary to check whether this arteriopathy is specifically connected with the aorta homogenate injection, or whether, on the contrary, it may be merely a nonspecific answer taking place in the course of tissue or nontissue immunization.

MATERIAL

Eighty-four Vendee strain white rabbits, of both sexes, with an average weight of 3.5 kg, were used. Before being subjected to our experiments these animals were kept in our animal room for one month.

METHODS

Preparation of the Antigens

The following antigens were used: aorta, liver, heart and rat serum, rabbit serum, bovine albumin. The technique used for the tissue antigen preparations has already been described [1]. It consists in pounding the tissues with an "ultraturax" into physiologic serum, and in distributing them in vials for lyophilization. At the moment of use the suspension is brought back to its initial volume with an addition of distilled water. One ml of suspension contains 0.5 mg proteins or 80 gammas of nitrogen, assayed by the microkjeldahl method.

The rat or the rabbit sera are withdrawn at the moment of injection.

Rabbit Immunization

The rabbits were divided into seven groups:

Group	No. of Animals	Antigens
I	15	Rat aorta
II	15	Rat heart
III	8	Rat liver
IV	8	Rat serum
V	8	Bovine albumin
VI	5	Rabbit serum
VII	25	Controls, two of which were given injections of saline isotonic serum

The same technique was used for all the injections, i.e., twice weekly, alternatively intramuscular: at the root of the limbs, and into the ball of the paw, for five weeks.

Each injection of these tissue homogenates consists of a mixture of 1 ml of Freund's adjuvant and 1 ml of homogenate suspension containing 0.08 mg nitrogen. The bovine albumin dose equals 80 gammas of nitrogen (0.5 mg albumin). The quantity of serum injected is 1 ml, corresponding to 70 mg total protein.

Testing the Immunization

Immunization was tested by detecting the circulating antibodies and studying the intradermal reaction. For these tests, the antigen used was the supernatant of the tissue homogenate centrifuged five minutes at 3000 rpm. Two different techniques were adopted for the investigation of the circulating antibodies:

1. Immunodiffusion in agar gel.

2. Passive hemagglutination according to Boyden's technique [3] modified by the use of a tannin solution at $^1/_{300,000}$. The tanned red blood cells are labeled with the antigen up to 0.5 mg proteins for 2 ml tanned red blood cells suspension at 2.5%. The inverse of the weakest solution giving an agglutination was expressed as the titer.

The intradermal reaction was made in the previously shaved dorsal skin. The quantity of injected antigen corresponded to 5 gammas protein. The reactions were read at once, and 3, 24, and 48 hr after the injection. Diameter, thickness, and color of the papule examined, whenever one is formed, were taken into account. A reaction is termed "negative" when the papule diameter is under 6 mm. The antigens used for the controls were, beside the antigen used for the immunization, the rabbit aorta and heart, and the rat aorta.

Protocol of the Experiment

The animals subjected to the same microclimate conditions were fed a diet currently found on the market, and given tap water. A blood sample was withdrawn to detect its circulating antibodies before starting immunization.

The first checkup was made 30-40 days after the first injection, followed by others after the 60th and 90th days, and then monthly until the sacrifice of the animal. The intradermal reaction was carried out 48 hr before the sacrifice of the animal. Animals were systematically sacrificed during the seventh month. An exception was made, however, and the sacrifice took place earlier, when the health of the animal was deteriorating, or when casual handling caused an accident with a resulting paralysis of the hind legs.

At autopsy, the aorta was removed completely with its branches dissected as far as possible. The aorta was then opened longitudinally and examined by the naked eye, and then with a binocular magnifying lens. Fragments of aorta and myocardium were put into paraffin and cut and stained with hematin eosin, Masson's trichromium, and Alcian Blue.

RESULTS

I. Immunological Reactions

The results obtained with the two immunodiffusion and passive hemagglutination techniques were identical except that for hemagglutination levels under 1000, the precipitation lines no longer appeared.

We shall therefore take into account only those results which were obtained with passive hemagglutination. This offers the advantage of supplying a quantitative estimation of the circulating antibodies.

Group I – Rat Aorta (Table I)

Against the rat aorta the highest levels were obtained 8-10 days after the end of the immunization, i.e., 30-40 days after the first injection. These levels decreased progressively, but the reaction may be observed until the end of the test. Crossreactions were observed at lower levels with the serum and heart of rat. There was no crossreaction with the rabbit aorta or its heart.

It was possible to obtain an intradermal reaction in 10 animals. When positive, the reaction did not occur before the third hour. The papule became fully developed at the 24 hr only, and disappeared at around 48 hr. The reaction was markedly positive in nine cases with the rat aorta, and in three cases its diameter exceeded 15 mm. It was always positive with the rabbit aorta, and in two cases the diameter exceeded 15 mm. With the rat heart, the reaction was positive in five cases, and its diameter less than 10 mm. The reaction always remained negative with the rabbit heart.

Group II – Rat Heart (Table II)

Passive hemagglutination was positive against the rat heart as soon as the immunization process was over, and reached its peak toward the second or third month after the first injection. Then the levels showed a tendency to decrease, and became very low or even negative during the fourth month.

A "booster injection" administered at that time to five animals provoked a remarkable increase of the antibody levels on the fourth day. This increase lasted or was further accentuated for a whole month. With the rat aorta, or the rabbit heart, a crossreaction was observed at a much lower level. The reaction toward the rabbit aorta remained negative. The intradermal reaction was positive on the 24th hr toward the rat heart, and the papule diameter exceeded 20 mm in four cases out of 12. It was posi-

Table I. Summary of Observations on 15 Rabbits Treated by Rat Aorta Homogenate Injections

Rabbit No.	Duration, days	Passive Hemagglutination		Intradermoreaction				Macroscopic Lesions
		30 days	90 days	RA	RbA	RH	RbH	
1549	43			"	"	"	"	++
1546	79	2.560	640	"	"	"	"	±
1521	90	2.560	120	0	0	0	0	+++
1523	98	1,280	120	0	0	0	0	+++
1525	98	640	60	0	0	0	0	+++
1545	115	5,120	1280	"	"	"	"	+
1527	121	10,240	240	"	"	"	"	++
1528	164	5,120	240	"	"	"	"	0
1548	180	2,560	160	00	0	0	0	0
1544	185	2,560	320	0	0	0	0	++
1547	185	–	160	0	00	0	0	++
1550	185	10,240	80	0	0	0	0	+++
1522	186	10,240	80	00	0	0	0	0
1524	186	1,280	60	00	0	0	0	+
1526	186	5,120	120	0	00	0	0	+++

RA = rat aorta; RbA = rabbit aorta; RH = rat heart; RbH = rabbit heart.
+++ = generalized lesions; ++ = bipolar lesions; + = confluent lesions; ± = minor lesions. (Lesions are of the ascending aorta and the arch of the aorta.)
0 = negative reaction; 0 = papule less than 10 mm; 0 = papule 10-15 mm; 00 = papule 15-20 mm; 000 = papule over 20 mm.

Table II. Summary of Observations on 15 Rabbits Treated with Rat Heart Homogenate Injections

Rabbit No.	Duration, days	Passive Hemagglutination		Intradermoreaction				Macroscopic Lesions
		40 days	90 days	RA	RbA	RH	RbH	
1600	36	"	"	"	"	"	"	±
1568	83	1,280	40.000	"	"	"	"	±
1562	101	1,280	40.000	"	"	"	"	0
1565	103	1,280	1.280	0	0	000	0	±
1560	194	2,560	2,560	0	0	0	0	++
1561	194	5,120	60	0	0	00	0	±
1564	197	15.000	2.560	0	0	00	0	±
1566	197	2.560	640	0	0	000	0	±
1567	197	1,280	120	0	0	000	0	±
1569	207	1,280	5,120	00	00	000	0	±
1571	207	10.240	5,120	0	00	00	0	±
1572	207	10.240	5,120	0	0	00	0	±
1599	209	2,560	5,120	0	0	0	0	++
1601	209	2,560	20.000	0	0	00	0	±
1603	209	10.240	80.000	0	0	00	0	±

RA = rat aorta; RbA = rabbit aorta; RH = rat heart; RbH = rabbit heart.
+++ = generalized lesions; ++ = bipolar lesions; + = confluent lesions; ± = minor lesions.
(Lesions are of the ascending aorta and the arch of the aorta.)
0 = negative reaction; 0 = papule less than 10 mm; 0 = papule 10-15 mm; 00 = papule 15-20 mm; 000 = papule over 20 mm.

Table III. Summary of Observations on Eight Rabbits Treated with Liver Tissue Homogenate Injections

Rabbit No.	Duration, days	Passive Hemagglutination		Intradermoreaction				Macroscopic Lesions
		40 days	90 days	RA	RbA	RH	RL	
1553	8	"		"	"	"	"	±
1555	58	"		"	"	"	"	±
1552	205	2,560	240	"	"	"	"	0
1554	206	2,560	0	0	0	0	0	+++
1556	206	2,560	240	0	0	0	0	0
1557	207	1,280	240	0	0	0	0	0
1558	207	20.000	640	0	0	0	0	+++
1559	207	640	0	0	0	0	0	0

RA = rat aorta; RbA = rabbit aorta; RH = rat heart; RL = rat liver.
+++ = generalized lesions; ++ = bipolar lesions; + = confluent lesions; ± = minor lesions.
(Lesions are of the ascending aorta and the arch of the aorta.)
0 = negative reaction; 0 = papule less than 10 mm; 0 = papule 10-15 mm; 00 = papule 15-20 mm; 000 = papule over 20 mm.

Table IV. Summary of Observations on Eight Rabbits Treated with Rat Serum Injections

Rabbit No.	Duration, days	Passive Hemagglutination		Intradermoreaction				Macroscopic Lesions
		40 days	90 days	RA	RbA	RbH	RS	
1583	25	"		"	"	"	"	+
1604	66	5,120	"	"	"	"	"	±
1589	116	5,120	40.000	"	"	"	"	±
1584	144	5,120	60.000	"	"	"	"	±
1585	197	2,560	150.000	0	0	0	000	0
1586	197	5,120	150.000	0	0	0	000	+
1588	197	2,560	100.000	0	0	0	000	0
1590	197	5,120	250.000	"	"	"	"	0

RA = rat aorta; RbA = rabbit aorta; RS = rat serum; RbH = rabbit heart.
+++ = generalized lesions; ++ = bipolar lesions; + = confluent lesions; ± = minor lesions.
(Lesions are of the ascending aorta and the arch of the aorta.)
0 = negative reaction; 0 = papule less than 10 mm; 0 = papule 10-15 mm; 00 = papule 15-20 mm; 000 = papule over 20 mm.

Table V. Summary of Observations on Eight Rabbits Treated with Bovine Albumin Injections

Rabbit No.	Duration, days	Passive Hemagglutination			Intradermoreaction				Macroscopic Lesions
		40 days	60 days	90 days	RA	RbA	RbH	ALB	
1591	208	480	30.000	0	0	0	0	00	0
1592	208	"	15.000	0	0	0	0	00	±
1593	205	"	15.000	0	0	0	0	00	±
1594	205	15.000	40.000	0	0	0	0	000	±
1595	205	"	15.000	0	0	0	0	0	+
1596	205	480	40.000	0	0	0	0	00	++
1597	205	15.000	30.000	0	0	0	0	000	0
1602	205	240	0	0	0	0	0	000	±

RA = rat aorta; RbA = rabbit aorta; ALB = bovine albumin; RbH = rabbit heart.
+++ = generalized lesions; ++ = bipolar lesions; + = confluent lesions; ± = minor lesions.
(Lesions are of the ascending aorta and the arch of the aorta.)
0 = negative reaction; 0 = papule less than 10 mm; 0 = papule 10-15 mm; 00 = papule 15-20 mm; 000 = papule over 20 mm.

tive in nine out of 12 cases against the rabbit aorta. In two cases the papule diameter exceeded 15 mm. It was positive in four out of 12 cases against the rat aorta, and was always negative with the rabbit heart.

Group III – Rat Liver (Table III)

The passive hemagglutination reaction was positive against the rat liver as soon as the immunization ended, at which time it reached its maximum level. The latter decreased very rapidly, to become very low or cease altogether during the third month, or at times as early as the second month. Crossreactions were observed with the rat serum and heart, but none with the aorta of rat or rabbit. The delayed intradermal reaction was always positive when rat liver was used. Crossreactions were observed with the aorta and heart of rat, as well as with the aorta of rabbit, although less constantly with the latter.

Group IV – Rat Serum (Table IV)

The antibody rate toward the rat serum, evaluated by passive hemagglutination, increased progressively during the months following immunization, and reached very high levels during the third month. In two animals the rate decreased or disappeared altogether during the sixth month (1584 and 1589). In three others it remained very high. No crossreaction was observed during the utilization of other rat tissues or of rabbit aorta. In the three animals in which the intradermal reaction with the rat serum was observed, it gave a highly significant positive answer, and showed a necrotic trend of the papule center. In only one of these rabbits (1585) a crossreaction was observed with rabbit aorta.

Table VI. Summaries of Observations on Five Rabbits Treated with Normal Rabbit Serum Injections

Rabbit No.	Duration, days	Passive Hemagglutination		Intradermoreaction				Macroscopic Lesions
		40 days	90 days	RA	RbA	RbH	RbS	
1490	180	60	0	"	"	"	"	0
1491	180	0	0	0	0	0	0	±
1414	270	0	0	0	0	0	0	0
1415	270	0	0	0	0	0	0	0
1418	270*	0	0	0	0	0	0	±

RA = rat aorta; RbA = rabbit aorta; RbH = rabbit heart; RbS = rabbit serum.
+++ = generalized lesions; ++ = bipolar lesions; + = confluent lesions; ± = minor lesions. (Lesions are of the ascending aorta and the arch of the aorta.)
0 = negative reaction; 0 = papule less than 10 mm; 0 = papule 10-15 mm; 00 = papule 15-20 mm; 000 = papule over 20 mm.

Group V — Bovine Albumin (Table V)

The passive hemagglutination reaction toward bovine albumin was precociously positive, reaching its highest level during the second month following the first injection. It became negative toward the end of the third month. There was no crossreaction with the aortic or heart tissues of the rat or the rabbit.

The intradermal reaction was always highly significantly positive toward bovine albumin. In three cases the papule center appeared necrotic. Crossreactions with rat or rabbit aorta were observed in five animals.

Table VII. Summary of Observations Carried Out on 25 Rabbits Kept in the Laboratory during the Experiment

Rabbit No.	Duration, days	Passive Hemagglutination		Intradermoreaction				Macroscopic Lesions
		40 days	90 days	RA	RbA	RH	RbH	
1681	120	"	"	"	"	"	"	0
1689	135	"	"	"	"	"	"	0
1607	180	0	0	"	"	"	"	0
1608	180	0	0	0	0	0	0	±
1609	180	0	0	0	0	0	0	±
1610	180	0	0	0	0	0	0	0
1611	190	0	0	0	0	0	0	±
1612	190	0	0	0	00	0	0	++
1613	190	0	0	0	0	0	0	0
1614	190	0	0	"	"	"	"	±
1605	200	0	0	"	"	"	"	±
1606	200	0	0	"	"	"	"	0
1675	200	0	0	0	0	0	0	±
1676	207	0	0	0	0	0	0	0
1677	207	0	0	0	0	0	0	±
1678	207	0	0	0	0	0	0	±
1679	208	0	0	0	0	0	0	0
1680	214	0	0	0	0	0	0	0
1681	220	0	0	0	0	0	0	+++
1682	221	0	0	0	0	0	0	0
1684	221	0	0	0	0	0	0	0
1685	229	0	0	0	0	0	0	0
1690	229	0	0	0	0	0	0	±
1421 *	180	0	0	0	0	0	0	0
1423 *	180	0	0	"	"	"	"	±

RA = rat aorta; RbA = rabbit aorta; RH = rat heart; RbH = rabbit heart.

+++ = generalized lesions; ++ = bipolar lesions; + = confluent lesions; ± = minor lesions. (Lesions are of the ascending aorta and the arch of the aorta.)

0 = negative reaction; 0 = papule less than 10 mm; 0 = papule 10-15 mm; 00 = papule 15-20 mm; 000 = papule over 20 mm.

* These two animals received injections of physiological serum.

Their intensity was low, and the papule diameter never exceeded 10 mm. No crossreaction was observed with the rabbit heart.

Group VI – Rabbit Serum (Table VI)

No passive hemagglutination reaction was observed in the five rabbits of this group, either toward the rabbit serum used for the immunization, or toward the other tissue antigens. The intradermal reaction was positive toward the rabbit aorta in two cases out of the four which could be observed.

Group VII – Controls (Table VII)

In 25 rabbits, no circulating antibody was ever detected against the antigens used in the present study. In 17 rabbits subjected to an intradermal reaction, a positive reaction was obtained in 10 cases against the rabbit aorta.

II. Anatomic Lesions

A. Macroscopic Appearance of Arterial Lesions

Group I – Rat Aorta (Table I). Of 15 animals in this group, 12 had macroscopic lesions of the aorta. In five, these lesions affected the whole trunk and its branches (1521, 1523, 1525, 1550, and 1526). In four others, the lesions, although widespread, left large areas of the wall apparently undamaged (1549, 1527, 1544, and 1547). In two others the whole of the aortic arch showed damage. Two small papules, protruding slightly and with a wrinkled surface, were observed in the last animal.

These lesions are identical to those previously described [1]. They mutilated the vessel, which became irregularly dilated, sinuous, and wrinkled. Its wall was obviously calcified (Fig. 1). Its endothelium appeared very irregular, filled with spiculae (Fig. 2), and in some areas it seemed armored with large, hard plates.

Group II – Rat Heart (Table II). Of the 15 animals of this group, 14 showed lesions macroscopically visible. No generalized alterations appeared in any of them, and the external aspect of the vessel was normal. Two of the animals (1560 and 1599) showed bipolar lesions (Fig. 3) affecting both the ascending aorta and the origin of the abdominal aorta. Such lesions are papular, vesicular, bullate or striated, isolated or confluent, with calcified areas and small aneurisms. In all the others, the lesions were very slight, with one or more papules of reduced diameter. They were located only at the root of the aorta or around the origin of the brachiocephalic vessels.

Group III – Rat Liver (Table III). Four animals out of eight had arterial lesions visible to the naked eye. In two of these (1554 and 1558), the lesions were generalized (Fig. 4) and comparable to those already described in the animals of Group I.

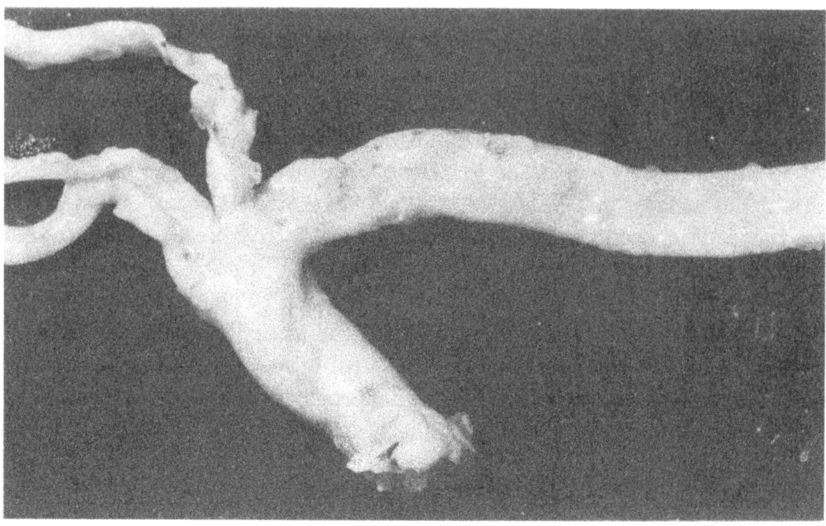

Fig. 1. Thoracic aorta of rabbit treated with rat aorta injections.

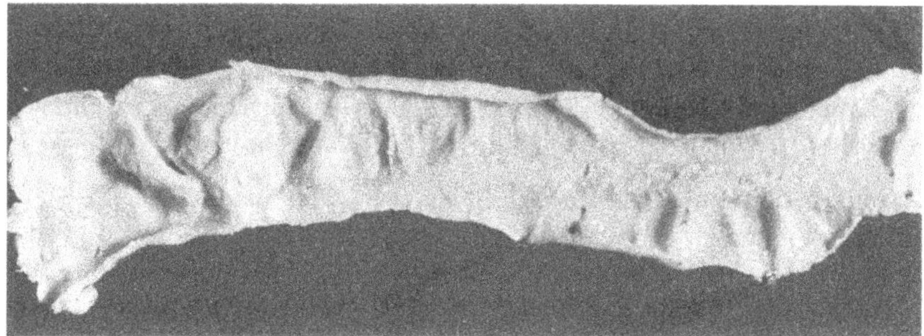

Fig. 2. Thoracic aorta of rabbit treated with rat aorta injections, and divided longitudinally.

In the other two animals, the lesions were localized and situated around the root of the aorta. They were mild.

Group IV – Rat Serum (Table IV). Of these eight rabbits, five showed aortic macroscopic lesions. In all the animals they were localized into the ascending aorta. In two cases (1583 and 1586) the lesions were confluent and covered practically all the origin of the vessel. In the other three observations the lesions were mild and papular.

Group V – Bovine Albumin (Table V). Six of these eight rabbits had macroscopic lesions of the aorta. In one rabbit (1596) they were bipolar, affecting the ascending aorta and the origin of the abdominal aorta. In another (1595), they involved the whole circumference of the root of the aorta. In the others the lesions were slight and papular.

Group VI – Rabbit Serum (Table VI). Two animals showed mild papular lesions at the root of the aorta.

Group VII – Controls (Table VII). Of this group of 25 control rabbits, 12 showed macroscopic lesions. In 10 of these the alterations were mild, with one or two papular elements on the ascending aortà or the aortic arch.

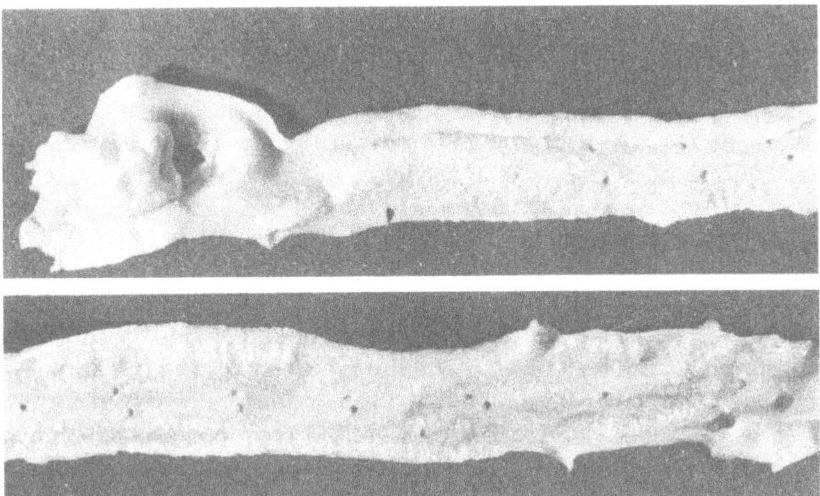

Fig. 3. Aorta of rabbit treated with rat heart injections, showing a fragment of the thoracic and abdominal aorta.

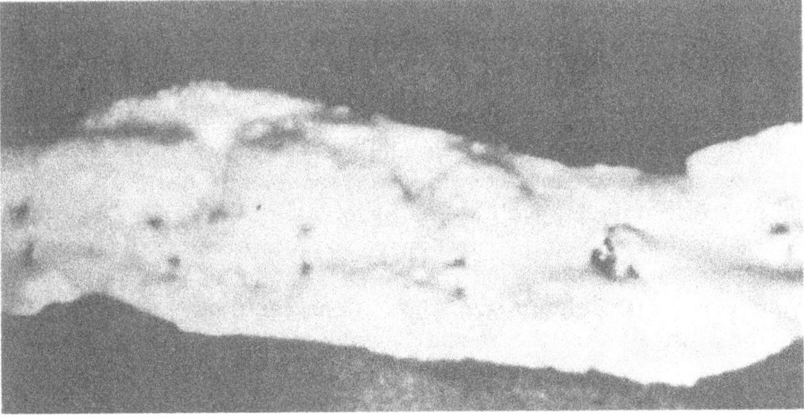

Fig. 4. Aorta of rabbit treated with liver injections.

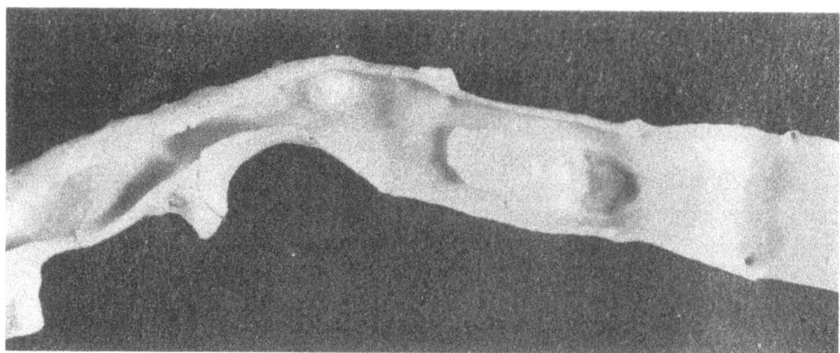

Fig. 5. Aorta of control rabbit showing aneurism of the abdominal aorta.

In rabbit 1612 (Fig. 5), these papular lesions were more confluent and involved a greater surface of the vessel at its root. They coincided with an aneurism of the abdominal aorta. In the last animal (1691), the lesions involved the whole vessel.

B. Histologic Lesions

Histologic lesions were found in all the animals treated with rat aorta, even if none of these lesions were visible macroscopically. But, on the other hand, in the control animals, or in the rabbits immunized with the other antigens, the histologic lesions were far from constant when macroscopic lesions were lacking. This was the case with animals treated with rat serum or heart, with rabbit serum, and with bovine albumin. In three animals treated with liver homogenates, however, microscopic lesions were found only in the aorta (1556 and 1559), or in one coronary artery (1552).

The elementary histologic changes which form these lesions, both in the immunized animals and in the controls, were found to be the same in all the groups, and may be described together, although they differ considerably in extent or in their destructive character.

Aortic Lesions. The simplest lesions consisted of infiltration of the intima by an edema stained with Alcian Blue. At times it was the sole anomaly observed in areas otherwise macroscopically healthy. Collagenous and elastic fibrils, as well as the fibroblasts, were increased in number in these lesions. This process ended in an intimal thickening which protruded into the vessel lumina. At an early stage these elastic fibrils became covered with calcium granules. Concommitantly with the intimal lesions, or a little later, the media become edematous, with disruption of the elastic lamina and alteration of the direction of the muscular fibers which became homogenized, vacuolated, and finally turned necrotic.

The more or less extensive necrotic foci may cover the whole circumference of the vessel and spread along a very great length. Collagenous fibers are numerous in this necrotic mash, becoming sclerotic and finally calcified, with all this taking place at a more or less early phase. At times these calcifications spread all over to the point of provoking a real dissection.

There were no alterations in the adventitia, or lesions of the vasa vasorum, or cell infiltrations. In lesions which are not extensive, such as those observed in the control animals, everything may be restricted to a degeneration of the myocytes accompanied by a proliferation of a sclerotic tissue, more or less laden with calcium, and covered by a fibrous thickening of the intima.

Tissue Lesions. The same elementary lesions, but grouped in different ways according to their importance, may be observed in the arteries or arterioles of the various renal, hepatic, muscular, and cardiac tissues. The adventitia are always spared, and so are the capillaries, veinules, and the veins. Usually the parenchyma remained intact, except in renal tissue, where an intratubular calcinosis was observed.

DISCUSSION

Two preliminary observations should be made. First is the unusual frequency of the spontaneous lesions in control animals (14 animals out of 30, including the animals treated by injections of normal rabbit serum). In the series previously studied in our laboratory, the ratio of spontaneous lesions ranged between 8 and 30% [1]. A careful investigation of such lesions, carried out with a powerful binocular lens, elucidates this high frequency to only a small extent. No epizootic broke out in our animal room, and the spontaneous death rate was particularly low.

On the whole, these lesions were mild and strictly localized at the aortic root, except in two rabbits (1612 had an abdominal aorta aneurism; 1691 showed destructive, calcified lesions spreading all over the vessel). This is the only observation of this kind made in our laboratory among a few hundred control rabbits sacrified in recent years.

The second point concerns the fact that spontaneous lesions usually coincide with positive intradermal reactions. Of 16 control animals on which we performed an intradermal reaction, eight showed lesions. These eight animals all had a positive and delayed intradermal reaction. Rabbit 1676, however, which had neither macroscopic nor microscopic lesions, nevertheless reacted as positive. In none of these control animals were circulating antibodies evidenced against the rabbit aorta, or any other aortic tissue. These observations have already been reported [1]. They may be interpreted as the immunologic response to an arterial injury of an undefined nature. They reveal the presence of antibodies bearing witness to the injury.

The present work confirms observations already published [1], that repeated rat aorta injections associated with Freund's total adjuvant induce a fairly regular development of widely spread and destructive lesions of the aorta.

Such lesions coincide with the presence of circulating antibodies evidenced by passive hemagglutination or immunodiffusion. These antibodies react directly with the rat aorta, and give a crossreaction with the serum and heart of rat, while they never react toward the rabbit aorta. There is no parallelism between the intensity of such lesions and the antibody levels detected by passive hemagglutination. In Group I, all the rabbits that showed lesions evidenced a delayed response to the intradermal reaction. There is some parallelism between the intensity of the lesions and the importance of the reaction.

These findings, when compared with those we previously reported [1], support the hypothesis that these lesions are of an immunologic nature.

The scope of the present work was to check the specificity of aortic tissue in the genesis of such lesions. The observations on the control animals, however, in which lesions were often found, lead to a cautious interpretation of the results. Among the lesions, only those which are widespread or confluent should be taken into account, since they are hardly ever observed in the control animals.

Table VIII. Comparative Frequency of Lesions in Different Groups (Animals belonging to Groups VI and VII are included in the controls)

	No. of animals	Number and percentage of animals bearing macroscopic lesions			
		Generalized		Very small	
Controls	30	2	(6.6%)	12	(40%)
Rat aorta	15	11	(73.3%)	1	(6.6%)
Rat heart	15	2	(13.3%)	12	(80%)
Rat liver	8	2	(25%)	2	(25%)
Rat serum	8	2	(25%)	3	(37.5%)
Bovine albumin	8	2	(25%)	4	(50%)

In Table VIII the lesions found are classified in two groups. In the first are the following lesions: generalized or bipolar, affecting the arch and the abdominal aorta simultaneously, or localized at the aortic arch but confluent. In the other are included the small, pinpoint lesions strictly localized within the ascending aorta.

Study of this table shows the marked frequency of widespread lesions in animals treated with rat aorta, 73.3% as compared with the frequency, which may be observed in the other groups of immunized rabbits. This frequency is identical with the one previously observed in another study [2] where, out of 20 rabbits having received the same treatment with rat aorta, 16 showed widespread aortic lesions, i.e., an 80% ratio.

But, in the animals of Groups II, III, IV, and V it has been ascertained that the frequency of widespread lesions was higher than in the control animals. The destructive generalized lesions occurred less frequently, however, and were observed in only two of the eight rabbits treated with injections of liver tissue. With the rat myocardium or serum, or even with bovine albumin, only confluent lesions of the aortic arch or bipolar ones are observed.

Antirat aorta circulating antibodies are found only in the rabbits of Groups II, III, and IV. Their levels are very low (under 160). Besides, the intradermal reaction was positive against rat or rabbit aorta, or both, in a large number of animals belonging to Groups II, III, IV, and V, which all had lesions. Three animals were exceptions (1586, treated with rat serum, and 1596 and 1602, treated with bovine albumin) as their reactions against aortic antigen were negative in spite of the presence of lesions. These reactions of delayed hypersensitivity toward the aortic tissue bear witness to the presence of antibodies which may result from or produce the lesion itself.

It does not appear that the mechanism by which these various nonaortic antigens provoke the aortic lesions associated with a delayed reaction of hypersensitivity is univocal. It seems unlikely that antigenic motives common to rat tissues may be responsible for these lesions. In that case it would be difficult to explain why such lesions are not just as frequent as they are with aortic tissue. This explanation would hardly apply when bovine albumin is used.

It may be that in the myocardium and liver tissues a certain amount of arterial tissue is included and which cannot be eliminated, and must be held responsible for the genesis of arterial lesions. But, here again, this would not apply either to the rat serum or to the bovine albumin.

A hypothesis might be put forward about these two antigens. It is known that a single injection into the rabbit of bovine albumin induces histologic arterial lesions which may be detected from the 12th day onward, and which disappear toward the 30th day [3,4]. In serum sickness similar alterations are observed. Such lesions modify the structure of the arterial tissue which would turn into an autoantigen, at least during the pathologic period. In the present investigation, repetition of injections might lengthen the production time of this hypothetical autoantigen, while repeated injections of Freund's total adjuvant would stimulate against this autoantigen an increased production of antibodies which would therefore become an autoantibody.

Control experiments are still necessary to support the above concept, and they are now under way in our laboratory.

SUMMARY

1. Eighty-four rabbits were used in this experiment. Fifteen animals were injected with rat aorta homogenate associated with Freund's adjuvant, at the rate of two injections weekly for five weeks.

2. Thirty-nine animals were given injections of rat heart or liver homogenate, rat serum or bovine albumin, following the same experimental protocol.

3. Thirty rabbits were used as controls, either receiving no treatment, or subjected to an injection of physiological serum, or one of rabbit serum.

4. Of the animals treated with rat aorta, 73.3% showed widespread and destructive lesions of their aorta and its branches.

5. Of the animals treated with other antigens, 20.5% showed widespread aortic lesions, although less extensive than in the rabbits treated with the aortic tissue.

6. Of the control animals, 6.6% had a widespread arteriopathy.

7. In all the animals showing lesions, a positive reaction of delayed hypersensitivity against the rabbit aorta, or the rat aorta, or both, was detected.

8. These experiments confirm our previous investigations on the pathogenic capacity of aortic tissue injections.

9. They are evidence of aortic tissue specificity in the genesis of this type of lesion, which is much more severe and frequent with this antigen than with any other tissue. They therefore further support the hypothesis of an immunologic mechanism in this arteriopathy.

The mechanism through which the injection of other antigens may induce severe lesions in a small proportion of cases is also discussed.

ACKNOWLEDGMENT

The present study was carried out jointly by the Centre de Recherches Cardiologiques de l'Association Claude Bernard and the RCP 96 (C.N.R.S.), France.

REFERENCES

1. L. Scebat, J. Renais, N. Groult, and J. Lenegre, Rev.Athero-sclerose. Suppl. *l*:56 1966.
2. L. Scebat, J. Renais, N. Groult, and J. Lenegre, Rev.Franc.Etudes Clin.Biol. 11:806 1966.
3. S.V. Boyden, J.Exptl.Med., 93:107, 1951.
4. F.G. Germuth, J.Exptl.Med., 97:257, 1953.
5. C.V. Hawn and C.A. Janeway, J.Exptl.Med., 97:571, 1947.

Enzymatic Activity of the Serum and the Aortic Wall in Animals Immunized by Homologous and Heterologous Aortic Extracts*

M. Dallocchio, R. Crockett, G. Razaka, F. A. Gandji, H. Bricaud, R. Pautrizel, and P. Broustet

Unité de Recherches de Cardiologie de l'I.N.S.E.R.M.
Hôpital du Tondu
Bordeaux, France

By injecting animals' aorta homogenates it has been found possible to induce in them extensive and specific aortic lesions. This was shown by Scebat in 1964.

Within the framework of an established plan, we resumed his experimentation by immunizing rabbits, either with heterologous horse aorta extracts (intima + media) or homologous aortic extracts (rabbit aorta). Taking into account the anatomic lesions engendered by immunization, we studied more particularly the immunological, biochemical, and enzymological behavior of the animals thus treated.

* * *

The first series of our experiments was carried out with a heterologous aortic extract, using the horse-aorta antigen.

From eight different litters, 39 young rabbits were equally distributed and divided at birth into two groups (A = 21 young rabbits, B = 18 young rabbits).

The young rabbits in Group A (distinguished by a cut at the right auricle level) were exposed to the antigen in the first hours following their birth.

* Report from the "Unités de Recherches d'immunologie parasitatre (Faculté de Médecine de Bordeaux: Dr. Prof. R. Pautrizel) et de Cardiologie (U8; Hôpital du Tondu-Bordeaux, Drs: Prof. P. Broustet and H. Bricaud) of the I. N. S. E. R. M." as part of the "Recherche concertee sur programe (RCP 96)" of the C. N. R. S. (Director: L. Scebat). Technicians: Mrs. C. Bacquey, M. Bourges, and F. Lefebvre.

After they were born, and for five days, they received daily a subcutaneous injection of a horse aorta extract (2.5 mg total proteins by injection).

Monthly, up to their fourth month, these animals received a subcutaneous or intramuscular booster injection of 5 mg total proteins from a horse aorta extract. From their fourth to their sixth month the Group A rabbits were not given any antigenic injection.

The animals of Group B did not receive any antigen injection between birth and the time they were six months old, but their ambient conditions were the same as the animals of Group A, since they belonged to the same litters.

During their sixth month, all animals (Groups A and B) were subjected to a hyperimmunization for five weeks, at the rate of three injections of antigen weekly (subcutaneous and intramuscular). Different points were selected for these injections, each supplying the animals with 5 mg total protein from horse aorta extracts. When this hyperimmunization ended, the animals of both groups were seven months old.

No antigen injections were administered to the animals from their seventh to their ninth month.

At nine months, i.e., two months after the end of the hyperimmunization carried out during their sixth month, the surviving animals were sacrificed. There were nine from Group A and six from Group B (seven males and eight females).

During the whole experimental period five biological withdrawals were made in both groups:

(1) At six months, immediately before hyperimmunization.

(2) During hyperimmunization.

(3) Immediately after hyperimmunization (five days after hyperimmunization was suspended).

(4) Thirty days after hyperimmunization was suspended.

(5) Sixty days after hyperimmunization was suspended.

After each biological withdrawal the following assays were carried out:

(1) Biological tests: total lipids, total cholesterol, phospholipids, Burstein's test (selective analysis of the serum beta-lipoproteins), and total proteins.

(2) Enzyme determination. Two dehydrogenases: lactic dehydrogenase (L.D.H.), and the alpha-hydroxybutyric dehydrogenase (alpha-H.B.D.H.). Two transaminases: glutamic oxalacetic transaminase (G.O.T.) and glutamic pyruvic transaminase (G.P.T.). Two phosphatases: a nonspecific

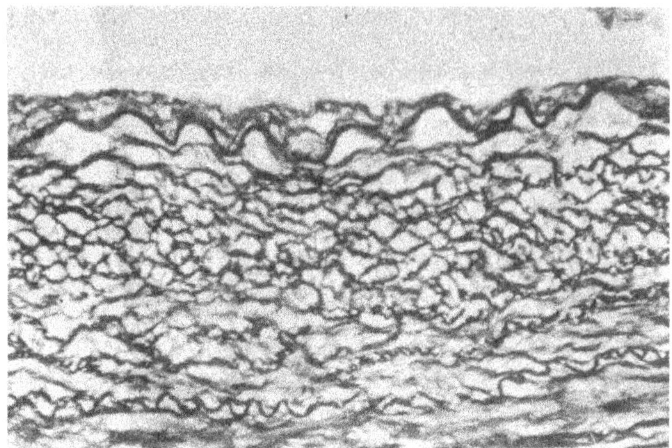

Fig. 1. Thoracic aorta of a rabbit immunized by horse aorta homogenate. Note disruption of the elastic structure (Weigert stain).

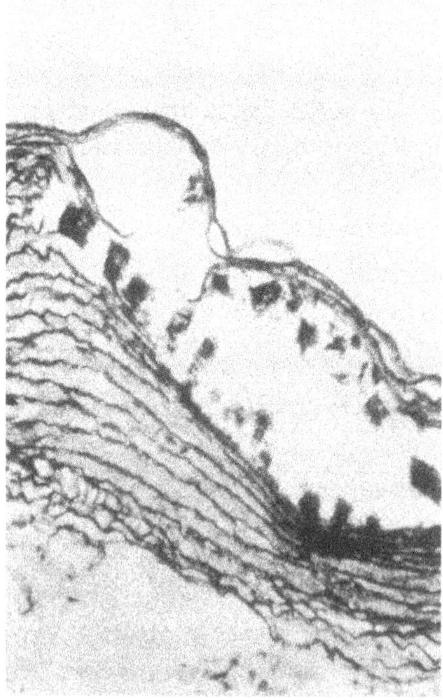

Fig. 2. Thoracic aorta of rabbit immunized by horse aorta homogenate. Subintimal necrosis of the media with alteration of the elastic structures on the entire width of the wall (Weigert stain).

phosphatase : alkaline phosphatase or phosphomonoesterase I (Phse Alk.), and a specific phosphatase : adenosine triphosphatase or adenyl pyrophosphatase (ATpase).

(3) Antiaorta sero-antibodies titration (using Boyden's technique of passive hemagglutination).

Just before sacrificing the rabbits (after the last biological withdrawal) an intradermal reaction is conducted using the horse aortic antigen.

Immediately after sacrifice, the aortas of all immunized animals were removed (Groups A and B).

These aortas were subjected to an anatomical observation (macroscopic and microscopic), and then to a study of their enzymes. Particular attention was given to the thoracic aorta (intima + media) enzymatic activity. Our assays were made on five enzymes: two dehydrogenases (L.D.H. and alpha-H.B.D.H.), two transaminases (G.O.T. and G.P.T.), and one phosphatase (the ATpase).

AORTIC LESIONS

Fifteen rabbits were sacrificed when they reached their ninth month, 60 days after the end of hyperimmunization. Lesions almost always situated at the thoracic aorta level were observed in these animals. Both the macroscopic and the microscopic lesions were found with equal frequency in animals exposed to the antigen immediately at birth (Group A) and in those immunized from the sixth month onward (Group B).

Aortic lesions were, in fact, present in two-thirds of the cases, a ratio similar to that reported by Scebat, who observed aortic damage in 70% of the rabbits immunized by heterologous aortic extracts.

Macroscopic lesions consisted of nacreous stains, in calcareous plates which, at times, alternated with more or less diffused ulcer-shaped areas wherein the now thinner aortic wall assumed a puffed "lacelike" appearance.

Microscopic lesions evidenced by the histologic assay were extremely interesting (Figs. 1, 2, 3).

Most of them showed a precocious rupture of the elastic structure with a necrosis forming more or less confluent islets. The diseased areas were either located just underneath an often thickened intima, or else right in the center of the media.

In the vicinity of these necrotic islets, and recalling at times the pictures of a media necrosis, were found the mucopolysaccharide deposits (mucopolysaccharide acids) which, in the incipient stage of the lesion, formed genuine "patches" drawing apart and dislocating the elastic fibers.

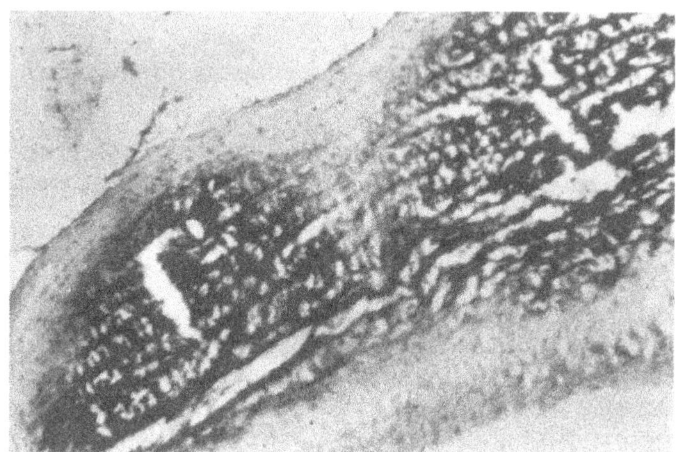

Fig. 3. Thoracic aorta of a rabbit immunized by horse aorta homogenate. Note wall calcification (Von Kossa stain).

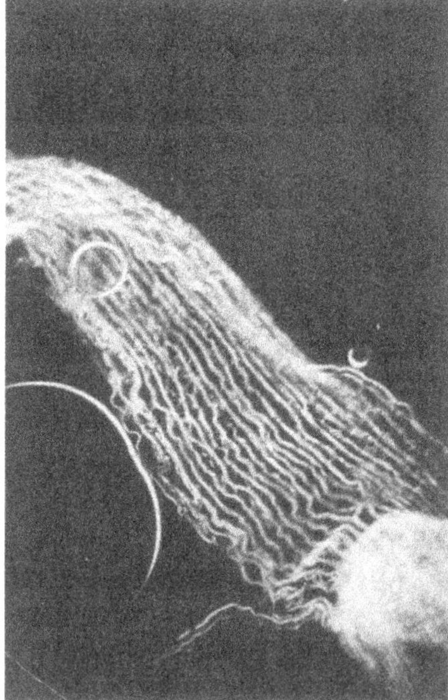

Fig. 4. Thoracic aorta of a rabbit immunized by rabbit aorta homogenate plus nonimmunized control rabbit serum plus fluorescein-labeled antiglobulin serum of rabbit. Negative reaction.

At a later stage, massive calcifications often appeared which, at times, might be comparable to those of Mönckeberg's media-callus because of their circular arrangement within the media. They were more particularly evidenced by Von Kossa's silver nitrate stain.

IMMUNOLOGICAL ASSAY

Antiaorta Sero-Antibodies

We made a comparative study of the evolution of the horse antiaorta antibodies level (Table I) in the serum of Group B rabbits (immunized at 6 months) and that of Group A rabbits (immunized at birth). At six months, before hyperimmunization, Group A animals already showed a high level of antibodies ($^1/_{800}$ on an average), while in animals of Group B the antibody level was less than $^1/_{10}$ in all cases.

Under the stimulus of hyperimmunization by the horse aortic antigen, the horse antiaorta antibody level increased markedly in both groups of rabbits. Its maximum was reached at the end of hyperimmunization, and then gradually decreased.

The horse antiaorta antibody level was always found higher in Group A animals than in those of Group B, but, on the whole, the two curves are practically parallel.

Table I. Evolution of the Horse Antiaorta Antibody Level in the Animals of Groups A and B.

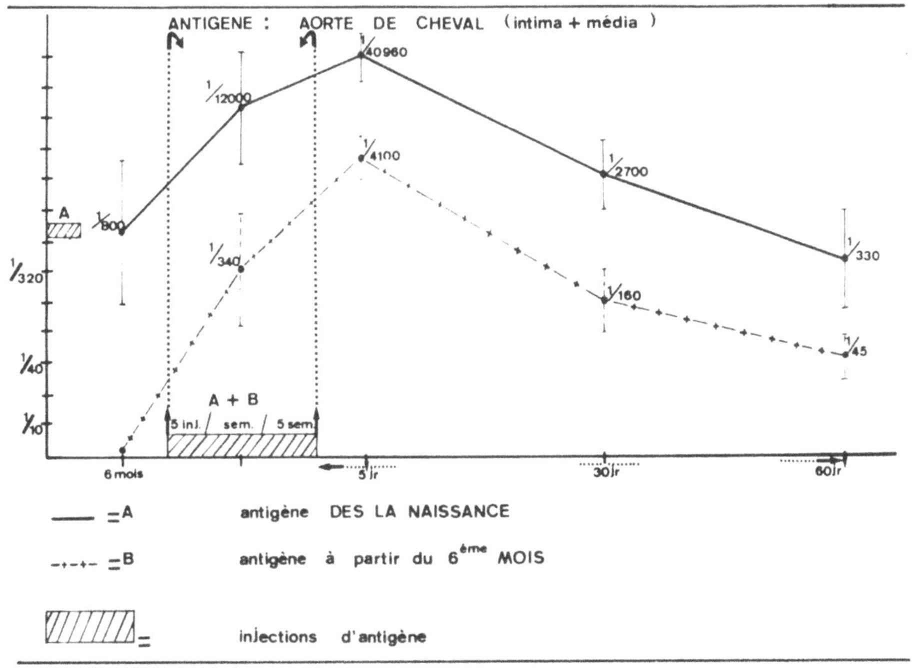

One finding is worth mentioning: in rabbits immunized by horse aorta we detected the presence of rat antiaorta sero-antibodies at levels which remained always inferior to the titrations in horse antiaorta antibodies.

This tends to prove the existence of common antigenic factors in different species of mammals.

It should nevertheless be underlined that we never found any rabbit antiaorta antibodies in the animals of either Groups A or B.

We compared the levels observed in the horse antiaorta antibodies in animals showing aortic lesions, and in those with no aortic lesions. No significant difference was found in the two lots of rabbits. In fact, five days after hyperimmunization, the horse antiaorta antibody level was at $^1/_{17,000}$ in the animals showing aortic lesions, and at $^1/_{28,000}$ in the others which were free from lesions. Sixty days after hyperimmunization, at the end of the experiment, the horse antiaorta antibody level was at $^1/_{540}$ in the

Table II. A Summary of the Main Biological Variations Observed in Rabbits of Groups A and B During the Hyperimmunization Phase

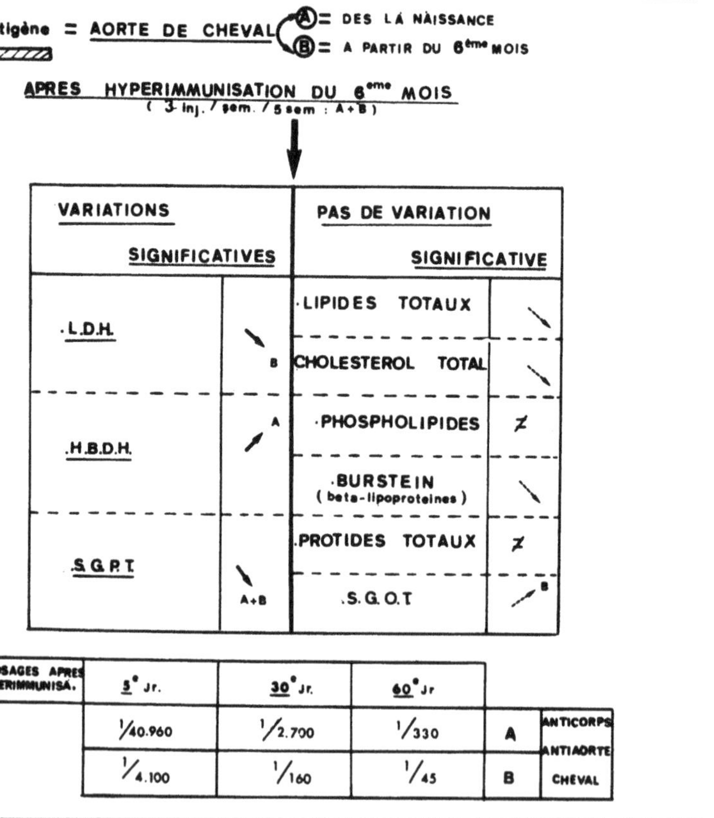

Antigène = AORTE DE CHEVAL — (A) = DES LA NAISSANCE ; (B) = A PARTIR DU 6ème MOIS

APRES HYPERIMMUNISATION DU 6ème MOIS
(3 inj. / sem. / 5 sem : A+B)

VARIATIONS SIGNIFICATIVES		PAS DE VARIATION SIGNIFICATIVE	
.L.D.H.	↘ B	.LIPIDES TOTAUX	↘
		CHOLESTEROL TOTAL	↘
.H.B.D.H.	↗ A	.PHOSPHOLIPIDES	↗̸
		.BURSTEIN (beta-lipoproteines)	↘
.S.G.P.T	↘ A+B	.PROTIDES TOTAUX	↗̸
		.S.G.O.T	↗ B

DOSAGES APRES HYPERIMMUNISA.	5e Jr.	30e Jr.	60e Jr.		
	1/40.960	1/2.700	1/330	A	ANTICORPS ANTIAORTE CHEVAL
	1/4.100	1/160	1/45	B	

rabbits with aortic lesions, and at $^1/_{40}$ in those without aortic lesions. Such divergences are in no way significant.

Intradermal Reaction

When made at the end of the experiment, the intradermal reaction to the horse aortic antigen was found to be positive (at the 24th hr) in six cases out of ten for the rabbits showing aortic lesions.

On the contrary, it remained constantly negative in animals free of aortic lesions.

Such a finding supports Scebat's own observations, in which he found that, if the aortic lesion was lacking, there never was any positive intradermal reaction to the aortic antigen used for immunizing the animals.

BIOCHEMICAL AND ENZYMOLOGICAL ASSAYS ON THE SERUM

Before considering the evolution of the various elements under assay in detail, we summarized (Table II) the statistically significant variations, and those which had no statistical significance, during and after hyperimmunization period of the sixth month for both the A and B groups of rabbits.

Table III. Assay of Total Lipids Before, During, and After Hyperimmunization (Antigen: Horse Aorta Homogenate)

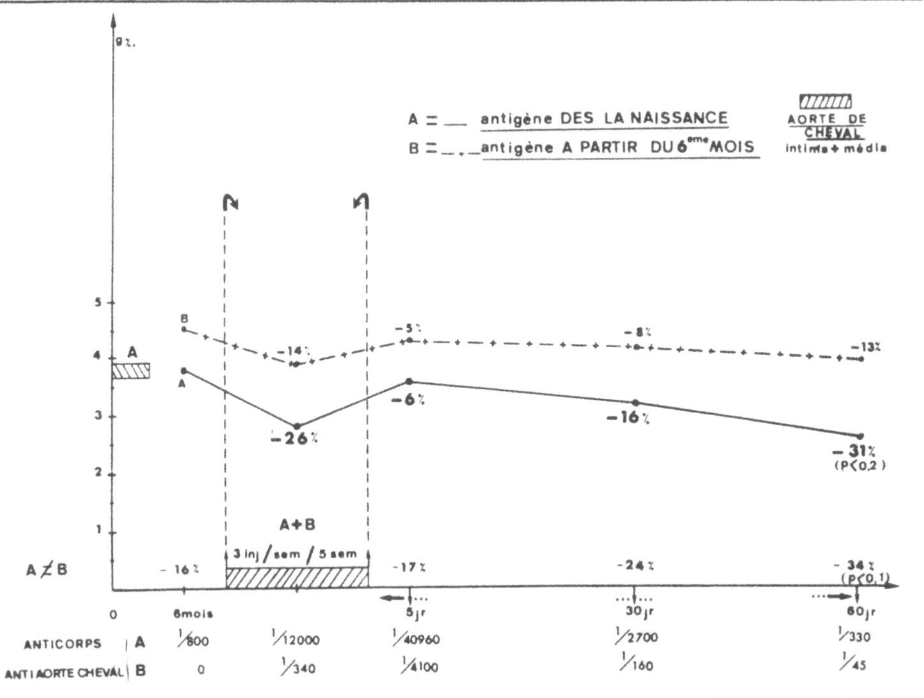

We thus observed that after hyperimmunization there were statistically significant variations in the serum of the lactic dehydrogenase level (decreasing in animals of Group B), of the alpha-hydroxybutyric dehydrogenase (increasing in animals of Group A), and of pyruvic glutamic transaminase (whose concentration in the serum decreases in both Groups A and B).

For all these animals (A and B groups), where were no statistically significant changes in total lipids, total cholesterol, phospholipid concentration, Burstein test, total protein, and oxalacetic glutamic transaminase. In fact, while a number of these components (phospholipids and total proteins) remained utterly unchanged, others (total lipids, total cholesterol, and Burstein test) showed a tendency to decrease after hyperimmunization, but oxalacetic glutamic transaminase tended to increase (especially in Group B).

Some of these biological modifications were then examined in detail.

Total lipids decreased in both groups. However, although it reached 31% (in Group A animals, for example), this fall was not statistically significant. We also observed, during the whole experiment, the lack of a significant difference between the total lipid level in Groups A and B (Table III).

Table IV. Assay of the Total Cholesterol Before, During, and After Hyperimmunization (Antigen: Horse Aorta Homogenate)

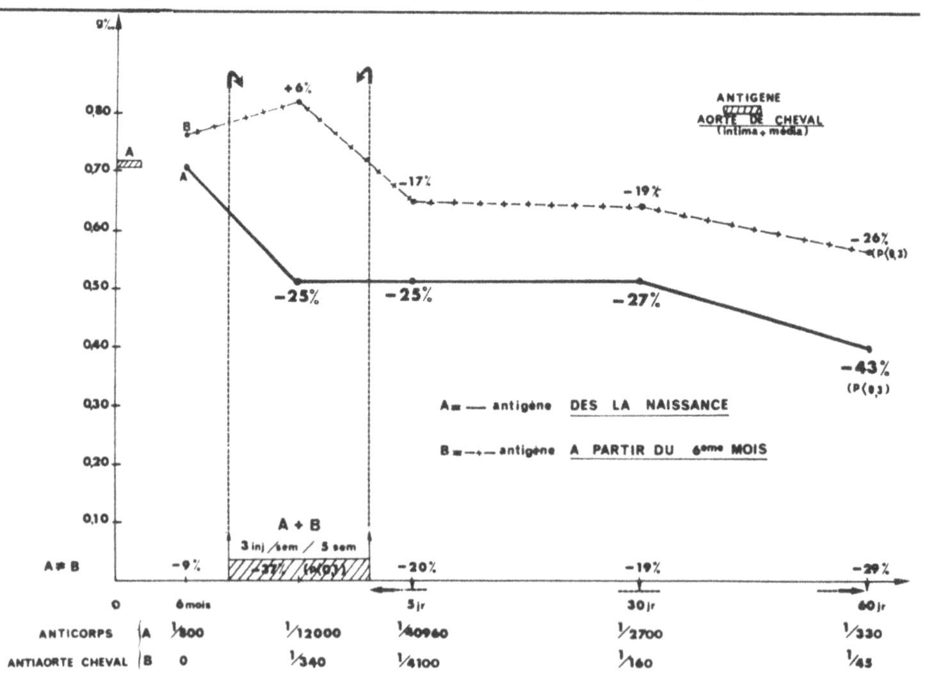

Total cholesterol development was similar. No statistically significant differences were observed at any time between the two animal groups. In spite of a 26% decrease, two months after hyperimmunization in Group B animals, and of a 43% decrease in the same period in those of Group A, we considered these variations were equally without statistical significance (Table IV).

On the whole, the Burstein test showed a similar trend in both the A and B groups. It decreased after hyperimmunization (about 30%, on the average).

Under the Influence of Hyperimmunization What Were the Enzymologic Findings?

As regards lactic dehydrogenase, prior to hyperimmunization, the level was lower in Group A then in Group B, but this divergence was not significant. Under the influence of hyperimmunization, there was a marked and significant decrease of the L. D. H. concentration in Group B. After hyperimmunization, the lactic dehydrogenase level showed a tendency to become almost even in both groups of animals.

The alpha-hydroxybutyric dehydrogenase showed a clearly lower concentration in Group A prior to hyperimmunization. Here the difference was clearly significant. After hyperimmunization it increased in Group A, to the extent that the levels became almost comparable in both the A and B groups after a certain lapse of time.

Oxalacetic glutamic transaminase, the levels of which were comparable in the animals of both groups prior to their hyperimmunization, varied in a slightly different manner. While its concentration remained more or less stable in Group A animals, it suddenly increased in Group B, 60 days after hyperimmunization. It was as if, at that particular time, the animals showed anatomic alterations which had long since existed in the animals of Group A exposed to the antigen at birth.

Pyruvic glutamic transaminase (Table V) concentration decreased likewise in the serum of both groups. Sixty days after hyperimmunization, the average fall was 36% in Group A animals and 29% in Group B animals (the probability indices which characterized such decreases were highly significant).

Upon concluding this experiment, we assayed the alkaline phosphatase and the adenosine triphosphatase levels in the animals' serum. In both groups the concentration of the two enzymes was very much the same. But, if we compared the levels assayed in the immunized animals (Groups A and B) with those of the control animals of the same age but not immunized, we found the values were considerably lower in the immunized animals. The differences ranged between 50% and 70%, for alkaline phosphatase and adenosine triphosphatase alike, lower than the values found for the nonimmunized controls (Table VI).

It should also be noted that at the end of the assay there were no significant differences in the serum concentration of the various enzymes observed in the immunized rabbits whether these animals showed aortic lesions or were free from any anatomic damage.

A comparison of the enzymatic activity, however, between the sera of the A and B groups of animals, all of them immunized, and those of the control animals of the same age but not immunized, showed significant differences:

(1) For the two dehydrogenases (lactic dehydrogenase and alpha-hydroxybutyric dehydrogenase) there was a marked increase in the immunized animals.

(2) For the oxalacetic glutamic transaminase there was more activity (48-56%) in the immunized animals (mostly in Group B rabbits immunized at six months).

Table V. Pyruvic Glutamic Transaminase Variations (SGPT) in the Rabbits of Groups A and B

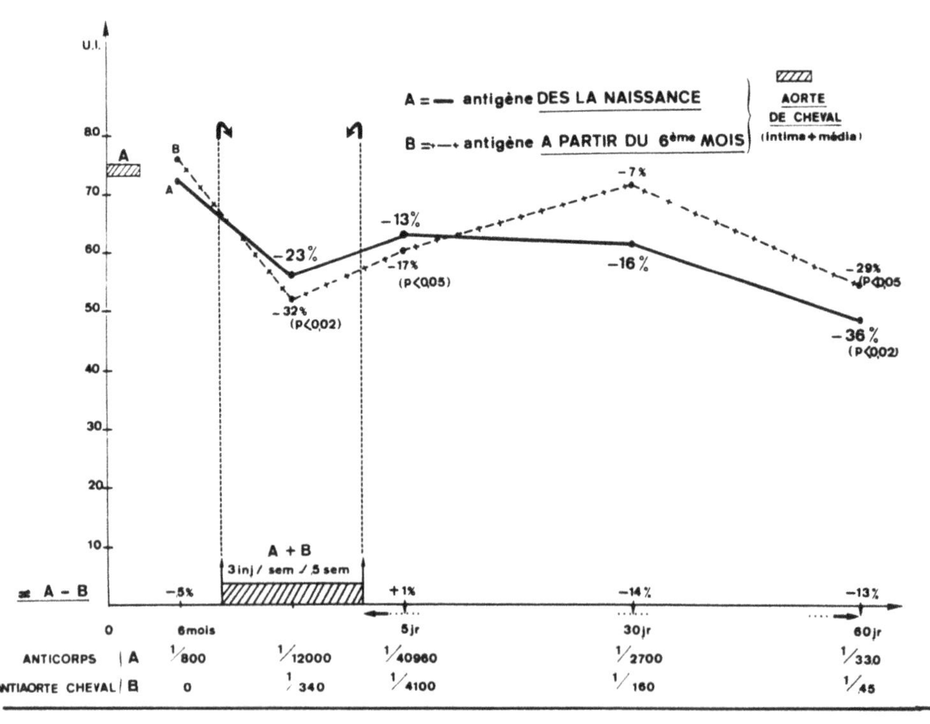

Table VI. Comparative Study of the Serum Concentration of the ATpase and the Phtse Alk. in the Nonimmunized Control Rabbits (N) and in the Immunized Rabbits (Groups A and B) by a Horse Aorta Extract. The ATpase and the Phtse Alk. Decreases in the Immunized Rabbits (A and B) Compared to the Nonimmunized Control Rabbits. There Is No Significant Difference Between the Immunized Rabbits of Groups A and B

.N = LAPINS TEMOINS NON IMMUNISES

ANTIGENE = AORTE DE CHEVAL (intima+média)
.A = LAPINS IMMUNISES DES LA NAISSANCE
.B = LAPINS IMMUNISES A PARTIR DU 6° MOIS

	ATpase		Phtse-Alc.	
N	20,8±3	$p < 0{,}01$	34,6±7	$p < 0{,}01$
A	6,8±0,9	-67% / $p < 0{,}001$	15,9±0,6	-54% / $p < 0{,}001$
B	4,9±1,7	-77% / $p < 0{,}001$	16,3±1,3	-53% / $p < 0{,}01$
A ≠ B	+39%	$0{,}1 < p < 0{,}2$	-3%	$0{,}6 < p < 0{,}7$

-N,A,B = AGE DES LAPINS (9 mois)
-A,B = 2 mois APRES ARRET DE L'IMMUNISATION

(3) In the immunized animals, we observed, on the contrary, a clearly decreased concentration of the two phosphatases (alkaline phosphatase or phosphomonoesterase I and adenosine triphosphatase or adenyl pyrophosphatase). The decreases, respectively, were 70% and 50% in the immunized animals (as compared with the nonimmunized control animals of the same age).

Table VII. Enzymatic Activity of the Thoracic Aorta Wall (Intima + Media) in Rabbits Immunized and Belonging to Groups A and B. There Is No Statistically Significant Difference Between Groups A and B

LAPINS IMMUNISES PAR DE L'AORTE DE CHEVAL (intima+média)

A = DES LA NAISSANCE B = A PARTIR DU SIXIEME MOIS

	L.D.H	H.B.D.H	G.O.T	G.P.T	AT pase
A	1051	816	873	118	79
B	1580	1184	759	83	72
≠(A/B)	− 33%	−31%	+ 15%	+ 43%	+ 10%
P	0,05 < p < 0,1	0,1 < p < 0,2	0,5 < p < 0,6	0,2 < p < 0,3	0,6 < p < 0,7

– LDH, HBDH, GOT, GPT = U.CONV/mg . prot.

– ATpase = U.I/g.prot

ENZYMATIC ACTIVITY OF THE THORACIC AORTA WALL

We also studied the activity of five enzymes at the level of the thoracic aorta wall (intima + media), the aorta having been removed immediately after sacrificing each animal.

In the rabbits of Groups A and B there was no difference in dehydrogenase, transaminase, and adenosine triphosphatase activity at the thoracic aorta level (Table VII).

No statistically significant difference was observed in the enzymatic activity (dehydrogenase, transaminase, adenosine triphosphatase) of thoracic aortas which were obviously diseased and of those of the hyperimmunized rabbits free of lesions.

In comparing the thoracic aortas (whether or not diseased) of these hyperimmunized rabbits with the thoracic aortas of nonimmunized control rabbits of the same age, two essential differences were found, and which appeared significant, at the level of the aortic wall in the immunized rabbits:

1. Increase in pyruvic glutamic transaminase activity.
2. Decrease in adenosine triphosphatase activity.

Therefore, the immunologic aggression represented by repeated injection of horse aorta extracts in the rabbit provoked the development of aortic lesions.

This phenomenon was accompanied by enzymologic alterations at the serum and at the thoracic aorta wall levels:

1. At the serum level, an increase in the concentrations of the dehydrogenases, oxalacetic glutamic transaminase, and a decrease in the phosphatase concentration.
2. At the thoracic aorta wall level (intima + media), a higher concentration of pyruvic glutamic transaminase, and a decrease of adenosine triphosphatase concentration.

One feature common to the serum and the aortic wall was the decreased activity of adenosine triphosphatase.

Our second experiment shall merely be mentioned here.

Rabbits were immunized either at birth, or later, with an autologous aortic extract, i.e., with the rabbit aorta (intima + media).

This assay is still under way.

No rabbits have yet been purposely sacrificed. Those, however, which died spontaneously had aortic lesions comparable to those observed in rabbits immunized by heterologous aortic extracts (horse aorta).

Before and after hyperimmunization by the rabbit aorta extract, we also found biochemical and enzymologic sero-modifications which, on the whole, compared to those found in rabbits hyperimmunized with horse aorta extracts.

The immunologic behavior of rabbits immunized by rabbit aorta, on the contrary, appeared slightly different. In fact, through the passive hemagglutination technique, we never could show rabbit antiaorta antibodies in these animals. At most, traces of transient horse antiaorta antibodies could be detected immediately after hyperimmunization. But, five days after suspending the hyperimmunization phase, the intradermal reaction to the rabbit aortic antigen was positive in 75% of the cases (at the 24th hr).

In these animals, therefore, there existed an immunologic conflict which could not be evidenced directly at the aortic tissue level.

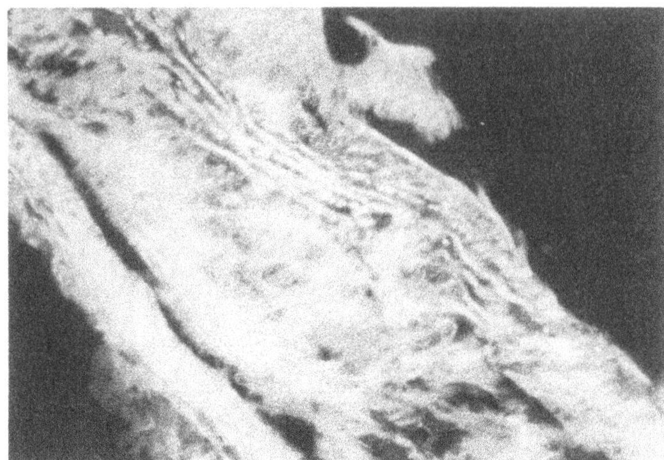

Fig. 5. Thoracic aorta of a rabbit immunized by rabbit aorta homogenate plus rabbit antiaorta immune serum plus fluorescein-labeled rabbit antiglobulin serum. Positive reaction.

Away from the diseased area, a fragment of rabbit aorta immunized by rabbit aorta was removed.

This aorta fragment was first exposed to serum from a normal rabbit, and then to an antiglobulin serum from a fluorescein-labeled rabbit. The rabbit antiglobulin serum was not fixed at the rabbit aorta level. The reaction was negative (Fig. 4).

In a second assay, the rabbit aorta immunized by rabbit aorta was exposed to the serum of that rabbit, i.e., the rabbit antiaorta immune serum. It was then observed that the fluorescein-labeled antiglobulin serum of rabbit was fixed at the level of the immunized rabbit aorta (when the rabbit was immunized by a rabbit aorta homogenate) (Fig. 5). This indicated clearly that the rabbit antiaorta immune serum was fixed at the level of the rabbit aorta immunized by rabbit aorta. The massive nature of the fluorescence proved that there was a fixation of rabbit antiaorta antibodies at the level of this aortic wall.

Therefore, an immunologic conflict occurred between the aortic wall and the rabbit antiaorta immune serum in those rabbits which were previously immunized by rabbit aorta.

CONCLUSIONS AND SUMMARY

Injection of homologous and heterologous aortic extracts induced thoracic aorta lesions in rabbits with a frequency clearly higher than the spontaneous aortic lesions usually documented in this animal species. These spontaneous aortic lesions, as far as we are concerned, were observed only in 2-3% of our cases, out of a series of more than 100 control rabbits sacrificed for the preparation of aortic extracts.

These aortic lesions were specific. This fact seemed evidenced by the immunofluorescence which enabled an observation of the rabbit antiglobulin serum fixation to the rabbits' aortas (immunized by rabbit aorta) against the rabbit antiaorta immune serum.

As a matter of fact, the aortic antigens utilized for these experiments were not wholly pure (this was confirmed by the crossreactions obtained with other aortic antigens in animals immunized by horse or rabbit aorta). This factor might explain why it was found impossible to induce a state of "immunologic tolerance" in the young rabbits treated immediately at birth.

Our observations seemed to prove that the immunologic conflict between the aortic antigen and the aortic wall of the receiving rabbit was accompanied by enzymologic modifications in the serum and the thoracic aorta wall. The more constant common denominator of this was a decrease in adenosine triphosphatase activity.

Phagocytosis of Platelets by Monocytes in Organizing Arterial Thrombi

J. C. F. Poole

Sir William Dunn School of Pathology
University of Oxford
Oxford, England

ABSTRACT. The mural thrombus which initially lines fabric prostheses of the baboon aorta has been examined in the electron microscope. Evidence has been obtained that platelets undergo phagocytosis by monocytes.

* * *

Hand and Chandler [1, 2, 3] studied the fate of artificial thrombi produced by the method of Chandler [4] when injected intravenously into rabbits and when incubated at 34-37°C outside the body. They obtained histological evidence that strongly suggested that platelets underwent phagocytosis by monocytes. It appeared that subsequent changes in these monocytes led to the formation of cells morphologically indistinguishable from the "foam cells" – macrophages laden with fat droplets – which can be seen in many atherosclerotic plaques. There is now general agreement that organization of mural thrombi in arteries plays an important part in the pathogenesis of atherosclerosis, and there is experimental confirmation of the fact that such thrombi ultimately develop into lesions closely resembling the fibrous plaques of atherosclerosis (see Crawford [5] and Poole and French [6] for reviews of the evidence). Much remains to be learned about the details of the sequence of events whereby a mural thrombus changes into a fibrous plaque. Among other things, the origin of the small amount of fat to be seen even in predominantly fibrous lesions has hitherto been somewhat of a mystery. Hand and Chandler's studies suggested a possible mechanism (not necessarily the only mechanism) by which this fat might appear in the lesions. Electron microscopical confirmation that platelets can be engulfed by monocytes has been provided by David, Hackensellner, and Wolf [7] and by Movat, Weiser, Glynn, and Mustard [8]. The present investigation was undertaken because it seemed at least possible that phagocytosis of platelets by monocytes is a matter of importance in the pathogenesis of atherosclerosis and that therefore further information about the phenomenon is to be desired. A fuller account of this work, with a number of illustrations, has been published elsewhere [9].

In the course of a study of the regeneration of aortic tissues in fabric prostheses of the baboon aorta [10, 11, 12], it was observed that during the first week after operation the prosthesis was lined by a thin layer of material which had the histological and electron microscopical appearances characteristic of a mural thrombus in an artery: it consisted of agglutinated platelets and leucocytes with fibrin and trapped red blood corpuscles. If platelets underwent phagocytosis by monocytes in such a thrombus, it seemed likely that evidence of their so doing might be obtained by examining sections of the deeper parts of the thrombus about one week after operation. Material from the deeper layers had been imbedded for electron microscopy at the time of the experiments but had not so far been examined.

The expectations were fulfilled. Most of the monocytes seen in the sections contained inclusion bodies of some kind. In some cases these were round objects bounded by a double membrane whose internal structure was that characteristic of platelets, as described by various workers (see French and Poole [13]). In a few cases it was possible to observe platelets which had been almost, but not completely, engulfed. It is to be expected that platelets after phagocytosis would not long remain intact but would begin to disintegrate. It was therefore not surprising to find rather more numerous inclusion bodies in the monocytes which showed partial loss of boundary membranes and less distinct outlines of organelles, but which nevertheless retained sufficient details of fine structure to make it reasonably certain that they were platelets undergoing the early stages of disintegration. Still more common were round inclusion bodies about the size of platelets but with an internal structure no longer identifiable as that of a platelet. It seems likely, but by no means certain, that these represent a later stage in platelet disintegration. Yet other inclusion bodies were seen which were smaller, irregularly shaped, and devoid of internal structure. Whether or not these were originally derived from platelets is at present unknown.

With two exceptions, all the cells containing inclusion bodies that were probably or possibly platelets were monocytes. One of the two exceptions was a neutrophil, the other possibly a basophil. Since the vast majority of the leucocytes in this thrombus were granulocytes, this fact provides good supporting evidence for the belief that the inclusion bodies were really inside the monocytes and not merely denting their surfaces. Indeed, with the two exceptions already mentioned, nothing was seen in any granulocyte that could reasonably be supposed to be material taken up by phagocytosis.

Electron micrographs illustrating the appearances of these inclusion bodies have already been published [9]. Further examples are given in Figs. 1 and 2.

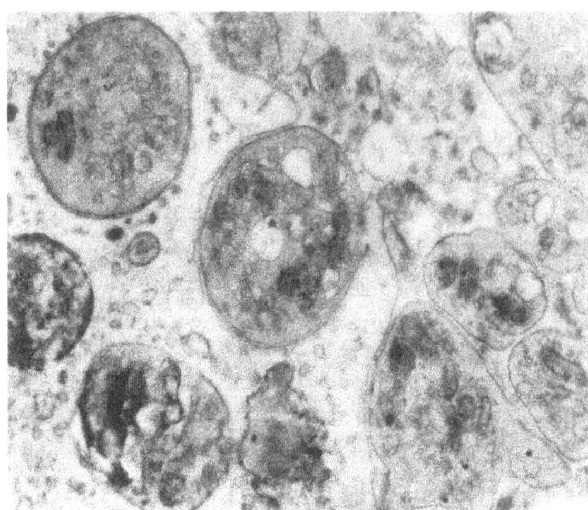

Fig. 1. Electron micrograph of a section showing part of a monocyte (left) and neighboring platelets (right). In the center of the field is a platelet which has been partly engulfed. Another platelet (upper left) appears to be wholly inside the monocyte. The other inclusion bodies seen are possibly platelets in various stages of disintegration. Araldite section stained by uranyl acetate and lead citrate. × 24,000. Reduced 50% for reproduction.

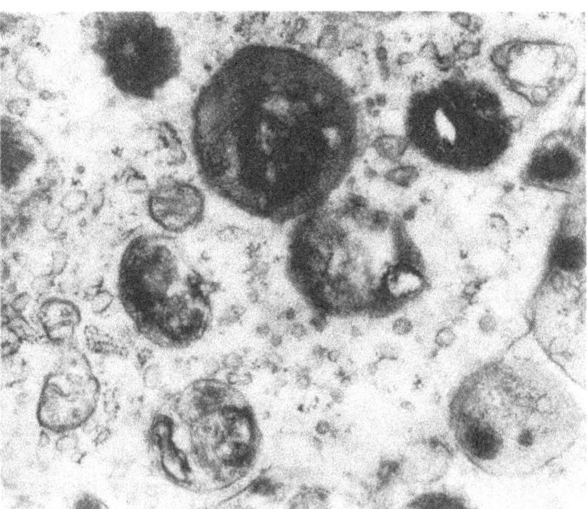

Fig. 2. Electron micrograph of a section showing part of a monocyte with various inclusion bodies. The large one in the upper part of the field is possibly a disintegrating platelet. The nature of the others is uncertain. Araldite section stained by uranyl acetate and lead citrate. × 34,000. Reduced 50% for reproduction.

These findings, taken in connection with those of the other studies referred to above, make it reasonably certain that platelets can undergo phagocytosis by monocytes. It is not yet possible to say that this happens in every organizing thrombus, but in view of the diversity of experimental systems in which the phenomenon has so far been observed, it may well be a common, if not a universal, occurrence. These findings do not, of course, add anything to the evidence provided by Chandler and Hand that monocytes having engulfed platelets later become foam cells. Moreover, it is quite possible that fat could be incorporated in fibrous plaques of atherosclerosis in other ways. For example, Friedman and Byers [14] have demonstrated incorporation of dietary cholesterol into organizing arterial thrombi, a finding which seems to point to an entirely different mechanism contributing to fat deposition. Nevertheless, the phagocytosis of platelets by monocytes, at least under certain conditions, now seems to be well established.

REFERENCES

1. R.A. Hand and A.B. Chandler. Cited by Chandler and Hand, 1961.
2. R.A. Hand and A.B. Chandler, Am.J.Pathol., 40:469, 1962.
3. A.B. Chandler and R.A. Hand, Science, 134:946, 1961.
4. A.B. Chandler, Lab.Invest., 7:110, 1958.
5. T. Crawford, J. Atherosclerosis Res., 1:3, 1961.
6. J.C.F. Poole and J.E. French, J. Atherosclerosis Res., 1:251, 1961.
7. H. David, H.A. Hackensellner, and W. Wolf, Frankfurter Z.Pathol., 72:548, 1963.
8. H.Z. Movat, W.J. Weiser, M.F. Glynn, and J.F. Mustard, J.Cell Biol., 27:531, 1965.
9. J.C.F. Poole, Quart.J.Exptl.Physiol., 51:54, 1966.
10. H.W. Florey, S.J. Greer, J.C.F. Poole, and N.T. Werthessen, Brit.J.Exptl.Pathol., 42:236, 1961.
11. H.W. Florey, S.J. Greer, J. Kiser, J.C.F. Poole, R. Telander, and N.T. Werthessen, Brit.J.Exptl.Pathol., 43:655, 1962.
12. J.C.F. Poole, Symp.Zool.Soc.Lond., 11:131, 1964.
13. J.E. French and J.C.F. Poole, Proc.Roy.Soc.(London), Ser.B., 157:170, 1963.
14. M. Friedman and S.O. Byers, Brit.J.Exptl.Pathol., 46:1, 1965.

Platelets, Atherosclerosis, and Lipid Metabolism

Giorgio Ballerini

Department of Medical Clinics
University of Ferrara
Ferrara, Italy

ABSTRACT. The role of platelets in the pathogenesis of atherosclerosis is reviewed. In particular, the results of researches on the platelet anti-"clearing" activity in atherosclerosis and other vascular diseases are illustrated.

* * *

The role of platelets in the pathogenesis of atherosclerosis is complicated and not yet completely clarified. First of all, they influence the so-called "thrombophilic diathesis" of the disease through their procoagulant activity. An increased thromboplastic function and adhesiveness has been described in atherosclerosis [1, 2]. In recent years, the hypothesis of Rokitansky, that atheromatous lesions can be induced by microthrombi from circulating blood has been supported by several authors [3-6]. Actually, after the recent researches of Murphy and Mustard [3], the mean platelet survival was shorter and the mean platelet turnover was greater in the atherosclerotic subjects than in normals. The second step is the organization and recanalization of the thrombi through the phagocytic activity of monocytes in the lipid-rich platelet material. It is to be underlined that the lipid content of platelets is very high compared with that of the red cells, so that it can be determinant in the origin of lipid deposits in the atheromatous plaques [7].

The platelet influence on atherosclerosis can be supported by the study of another platelet function, the so-called anti-"clearing" activity, that interferes with lipid metabolism. Since 1961, we demonstrated that the platelet factor 4 or antiheparin factor is responsible for the anti-"clearing" activity of normal platelet-rich plasma [10, 11]. The influence of platelets on lipid metabolism can be summarized according to the scheme on page 489.

Our results have been subsequently confirmed, although some attempt has been made to differentiate the antiheparin factor from the anti-"clear-

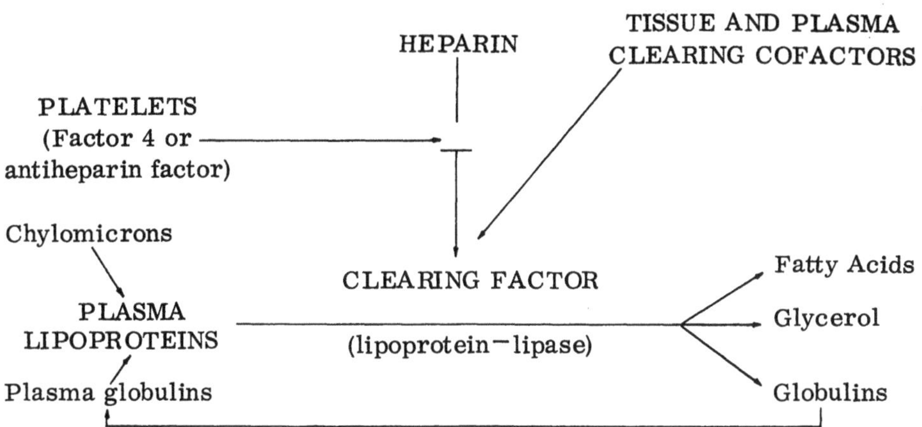

Table I. Lipid Content of Platelets and Red Cells (% of dry weight) after Barkhan and Maupin [8, 9]

Fraction	Platelets	Red Cells
Total lipids	17.0-19.0	1.26
A. Phospholipids	13.3-13.8	0.85
B. Nonphospholipids	4.2- 5.2	0.35

Table II. Platelet Anti-"Clearing" Activity of Control and Dyslipidemic Subjects

Subjects	No.	Platelet Anti-"Clearing" Activity		
		Normal	Decreased	Increased
Diabetics	28	5	21	2
Cirrhotics	10	2	8	–
Atherosclerotics	20	4	10	6
Controls	30	30	–	–

ing" activity of platelets [12]. In the course of researches on acquired thrombopathies, we observed that the anti-"clearing" activity of platelets in dyslipidemic states such as liver cirrhosis and diabetes was often diminished [13]. We extended the study on atherosclerosis with hypercholesterolemia, altered alpha-beta-lipoprotein ratio, and hypertension.

For the determination of the anti-"clearing" activity of platelets in these cases, the incubation mixture was composed as follows:

(1) Normal platelet-free postheparin plasma (pooled from normal subjects 20 min after i.v. injection of 300 U heparin).

(2) Homogenized and stabilized coconut oil suspension (Ediol, Schenley).

(3) Platelet suspension (or saline as control of the "clearing" activity of the postheparin plasma).

The turbidimetric determination was done every 10 min, after incubation, up to 60 min at 37°C.

The results obtained in this study are summarized in Table II.

Our study points out the presence of a thrombocytopathic situation even in several cases with atherosclerosis: there is a deficiency in the anti-"clearing" activity of platelets. This platelet defect can be of great importance in the pathogenesis of the lipidic alterations reported, as well as in basal conditions as after fatty meals, in the atherosclerotic serum [14-16].

However, at present it is still impossible to state if the anomalous behavior of the anti-"clearing" platelet activity in atherosclerosis is one of the causes and not a direct consequence of the peculiar dyslipidemia of the disease itself.

REFERENCES

1. L. McDonald, Lancet, 2:457, 1957.
2. J.F. Mustard, Can.Med.Ass.J., 79:554. 1958.
3. E.A. Murphy and J.F. Mustard, Circulation, 25:114, 1962.
4. J.F. Mustard, H.G. Downie, E.A. Murphy, and H.C. Rowsell, Lipids, Platelets, and Atherosclerosis. in: Henry Ford Hospital International Symposium, "Blood Platelets." Boston, Little, Brown & Co., 1961, pp. 191-204.
5. H.Z. Movat, M.D. Haust, and R.H. More, Am.J.Pathol., 35:93, 1959.
6. J.B. Duguid, J.Pathol.Bacteriol., 60:57, 1948.
7. R.A. Hand and A.B. Chandler, Am.J.Pathol., 40:469, 1962.
8. P. Barkhan, M.J. Silver, and L.M. O'Keefe, The Lipids of Human Erythrocytes and Platelets and Their Effect on Thromboplastin Formation. in: Henry Ford Hospital International Symposium, "Blood Platelets." Boston, Little, Brown & Co., 1961, pp. 303-318.
9. B. Maupin, Les Plaquettes Sanguines de l'Homme. Paris, Masson, 1954, p. 102.
10. G. Ballerini and S. LaPaglia, Boll.Soc.Ital.Biol.Sper., 37:289, 1961.
11. G. Ballerini and S. LaPaglia, Schweiz.Med.Wochschr., 91:1141, 1961.
12. A. Poplawski and S. Niewiarowski, Biochim.Biophys.Acta, 90:403, 1964.
13. A. Baserga and G. Ballerini, Les Défauts Plaquettaires Acquis. in: Proc. 9th Congr.Europ.Soc.Hematol., Lisbon, 1963. Basel-New York, S. Karger, 1963, pp. 1213-1221.

14. F. Conconi, F. Manenti, A. Torri, and C. Nava, Acta Vitaminol., 18: 13, 1964.
15. G. Pasero and M. Manca, Giorn. Gerontol., 9: 173, 1961.
16. P. DeNicola, Giorn. Gerontol., 9: 143, 1961.

Plasma Clearance of Products of Fibrinolysis

M. I. Barnhart* and D. C. Cress

Department of Physiology and Pharmacology
Wayne State University School of Medicine
Detroit, Michigan

Alterations in fibrinogen metabolism frequently occur in physiologic adaptations to stress and also accompany many pathologic states. Unfortunately, the significance of such alterations remains unknown. However, fibrin deposits can impair organ function and are likely to be major contributors to the debilitation eventuating with numerous diseases of unrelated etiologies. Fibrin deposition and its removal are recognized problems in the thrombotic diseases such as myocardial infarction and cerebrovascular thrombosis. But only recently has fibrin deposition alone and in association with immunologic diseases been considered of consequence in renal dysfunction [1]. Even more recent is the still limited appreciation of the role of fibrin deposits in perpetuating and recycling joint inflammations occuring in rheumatoid diseases [2, 3]. Of obvious value is the further identification and improved understanding of the mechanisms available for resolving the problems of fibrinogen metabolism and fibrin deposition and degradation. The purpose of this communication is to report on the cellular mechanisms for eliminating altered fibrinogen and fibrin and their degradation products from the circulation.

Two cellular degradation depots for fibrin, the reticuloendothelial (RE) cells and neutrophils, have been implicated by previous immunofluorescent work here and in other laboratories. However, the relative importance of these two cellular mechanisms in handling fibrin, fibrinogen, or their degradation products has not been reported until now.

Lee and McCluskey [4] reported in 1962 that RE cells of liver and spleen phagocytized circulating fibrin aggregates formed by infusion of either thrombin or endotoxin into rabbits. They suggested that the reticuloendothelial system removed the bulk of fibrin formed during low grade intravascular coagulation.

* Supported by research grant HE 04712 of the National Institutes of Health, U.S. Public Health Service and the Michigan Heart Association.

Since 1963, our group in Detroit has emphasized that neutrophils under certain circumstances contain some molecules immunologically related to fibrin. These neutrophil responses were reported in dogs undergoing intravascular thrombosis initiated by thrombin [5, 6] and also occurred in sterile inflammatory sites [7]. Some evidence of neutrophil phagocytosis of fibrin-related material was observed in humans with cerebrovascular thrombosis and myocardial infarction [5], and in thrombotic thrombocytopenia purpura [8]. From the studies on inflammation it was clear that neutrophils actually phagocytized fibrin [7]. However, the neutrophil response induced in the examples of thrombosis might have reflected phagocytosis with intracellular digestion or even the uptake of degradation products of fibrin or fibrinogen [5].

EXPERIMENTAL MICROTHROMBOSIS

A valuable method for inducing in vivo fibrin is to produce generalized intravascular coagulation in the microcirculation by a slow infusion of thrombin. Sequence studies of the cellular uptake of protein as assessed by the fluorescent antibody technique coupled with measurements of the changes in plasma proteins can be instructive (Fig. 1). The effectiveness of thrombin in eliciting fibrin deposition was demonstrated by the decrease in plasma fibrinogen. There was loss of both properties ordinarily assigned to native and unaltered fibrinogen: clottability with thrombin [9] and heat precipitability at 56°C [10].

Prothrombin declined, and the platelets also dropped, to signal that coagulation mechanisms had produced fibrin deposits. Peripheral blood neutrophils that were unreactive with fluorescent (rhodamine) antifibrinogen prior to the thrombin infusion began to react with the fluorescent marker (Fig. 1). There were increased numbers of fluorescent neutrophils. Also, the brilliance of cytoplasmic fluorescence was enhanced with time and following another fibrin deposition produced by a second infusion of thrombin. Neutrophilic fluorescence clearly signaled the intracellular presence of molecules immunologically related to fibrinogen. It is attractive to consider that this neutrophilic fluorescence reflected the phagocytosis of fibrin from thrombi or emboli lodged in the microcirculation. However, it is not necessarily the correct, or the only, conclusion to be drawn from these data.

Interpretation of the immunofluorescent data is made difficult by both limitations of immunology and additional complications in the experimental model of microthrombosis. Although immunofluorescent tools have great value, they cannot distinguish between molecules that contain identical antigenic determinants. Thus, fibrin, fibrinogen, and their proteolysis products all have common antigenic groupings to react with fluorescent antibody. Fibrinogen, at least as normal or native molecules, seems a most unlikely candidate for the observed neutrophilic fluorescence. Neither normal un-

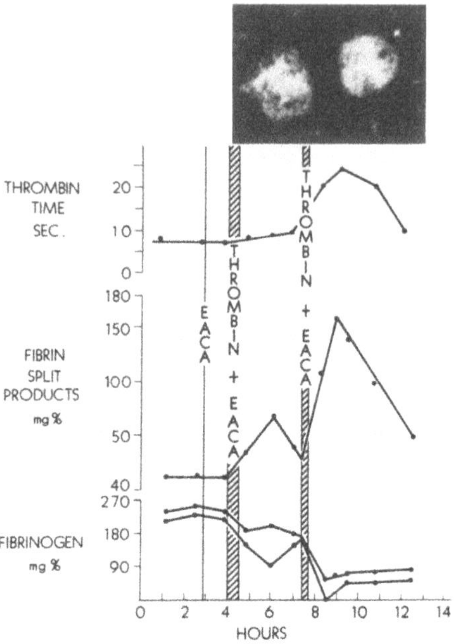

Fig. 1. Sequential analysis of neutrophil function and some plasma protein changes during experimental microthrombosis. The fluorescent micrograph illustrates the neutrophil response to applied univalent rhodamine antifibrinogen. Neutrophils picked up fibrin, fibrinogen, or their split products after infusion of thrombin (100 and 120 U/kg body weight). Episilon aminocaproic acid (15 mg EACA per kg body weight) limited plasma fibrinolysis. Probably fibrinolysis was occurring in the intravascular thrombi to account for the prolongation of thrombin time (a measure of developed anticoagulant power) and elevation in fibrin split products. Fibrinogen was assessed by its clottability with thrombin (top curve) and its heat precipitability (bottom curve).

stressed animals nor plasmapheresed ones with fibrinogen depletion exhibited neutrophilic fluorescence. The cellular synthesis of fibrinogen occurred following plasmapheresis but only involved the liver parenchymal cells [11]. Thus, the neutrophil fluorescence encountered during microthrombosis may best be explained in terms of ingestion of either fibrin or proteolysis products of fibrinolysis, or both. As activation of the fibrinolytic system is a frequent response to thrombin infusion [12] and microthrombosis [13], its occurrence only complicates interpretation of the cytofluorescent data.

We tried to inhibit fibrinolysis in these microthrombosis experiments by pretreating dogs with episilon aminocaproic acid (EACA) and also infusing it with thrombin. Although generalized plasma protein proteolysis was inhibited, a complete inhibition of fibrinolysis was not achieved by the concentrations of EACA employed. Apparently fibrinolysis of the microthombi proceeded as a consequence of activation of the profibrinolysin adsorbed on the fibrin. Either the EACA did not reach these fibrinolytic loci or the concentration was insufficient to inhibit such fibrinolysis. The appearance of a circulating anticoagulant and the increase in nonclottable fibrinogen-related molecules were sensitive indicators of existing fibrinolysis (Fig. 1). A quantitative immunoprecipitin test employing univalent antifibrinogen permitted measurement of the nonclottable fibrinogen-related molecules that developed in the serum [14]. As these molecules followed microthrombosis and fibrinolysis they are referred to as "fibrin split" products. Their disappearance from the circulation was paralleled by the increasing fluorescence of the neutrophils. Consequently, the intracellular appearance of fibrinogen-related molecules in these neutrophils could represent either products of extracellular fibrinolysis, or fibrin per se, or products of its intracellular digestion. Without additional information, a selection among these explanations is impossible.

CLEARANCE OF SOLUBLE FIBRINOLYTIC PRODUCTS

Problems in the interpretation of the cytofluorescent data from dogs with thrombin-induced microthrombosis were overcome by this new experimental design. Soluble products of fibrinolytic activity were infused into normal dogs in an attempt to define precisely the cellular fate of altered fibrinogen and degraded fibrin. Since fibrin is a polymer of molecules derived from the major portion of fibrinogen molecules, it was reasonable and more convenient to employ chemical manipulations of fibrinogen in these studies.

Proteolysis products were collected from the digest of purified fibrinogen by the enzyme fibrinolysin [14]. These products (FSP) were separated from any undigested fibrinogen, the active enzyme, and in some cases from one another by polyacrylamide gel filtration. Such molecules were then characterized by immunoelectrophoresis with univalent antifibrinogen (Fig. 2) and they corresponded to the fibrinogen derivatives D and E of Nussenzweig [15]. These molecules did not clot on addition of thrombin, so were incapable of forming fibrin. Also, they possessed anticoagulant activity. Mixtures of fibrinogen derivatives D and E or D alone were infused into normal dogs via gastrosplenic vein or femoral vein, and the plasma clearance was followed. Each dog served as his own control and was studied approximately 10 hr. The cellular fate of the infused FSP was assessed with the aid of immunofluorescent procedures applied to serial biopsies of liver and spleen taken before, during, and after infusion of FSP. Bone marrow smears were taken serially in some dogs. Terminal imprints from lung and kidney also were studied for any cellular accumulations of FSP.

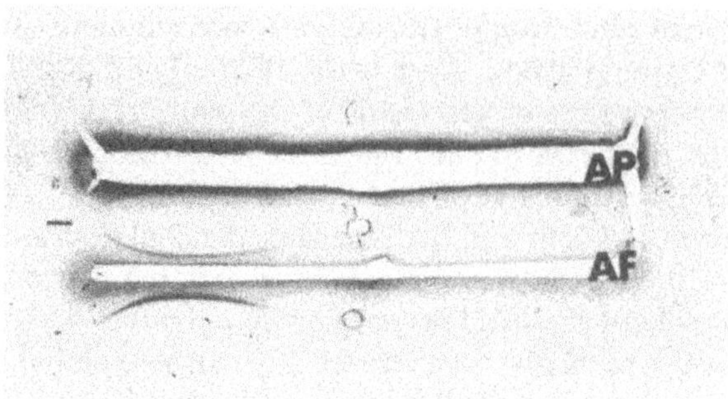

Fig. 2. Immunoelectrophoretic patterns of canine fibrinogen split products reacted with antiplasma (AP) and antifibrinogen (AF). The center segment shows purified β_2 fibrinogen derivative D, a prominent arc near the negative electrode (–). The lower segment shows a mixed product that contains two components, derivative D and derivative E.

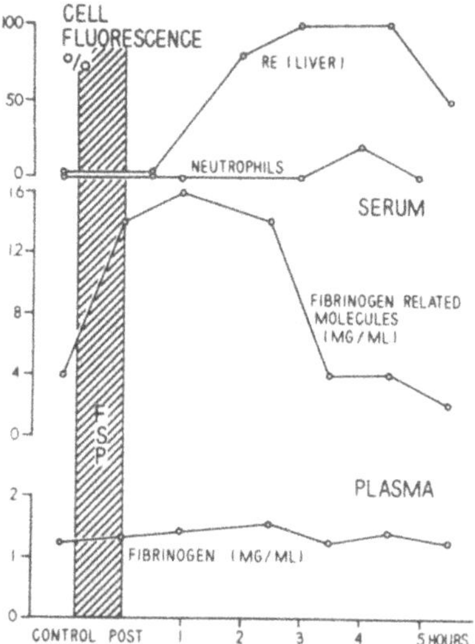

Fig. 3. Responses to infusion of bovine FSP (228 mg/kg body weight). Liver RE cells picked up the soluble FSP with 100% of the population fluorescent at 3 hr post infusion. This was paralleled by a rapid decrease in circulating nonclottable fibrinogen molecules which returned to control values by 3½ hr. Blood clotting mechanisms were not activated as the fibrinogen concentration remained near control levels.

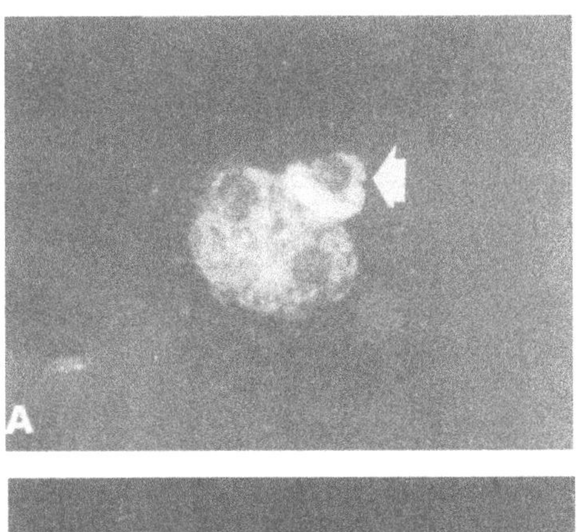

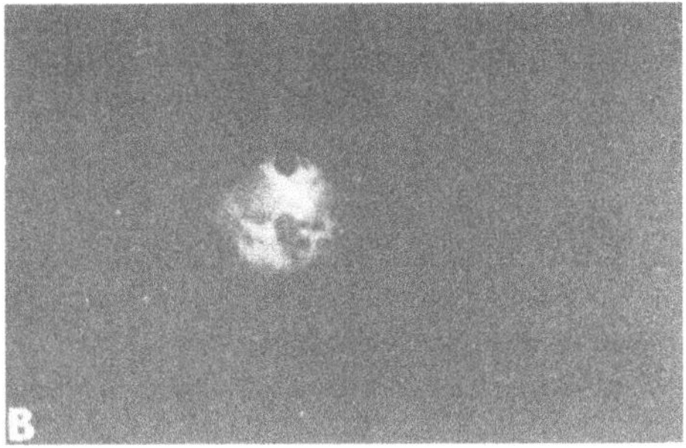

Fig. 4. Comparison of RE cell and hepatocyte fluorescence 2½ hr after infusion of FSP. Rhodamine antifibrinogen was applied to this cell imprint for 20 min. Tri-X film; exposure 1½ min; OG4 filter and forced development. A. Observe brilliant RE cell (arrow) with FSP contained in the cytoplasm. Large hepatocytes showed autofluorescence or minimal storage of fibrinogen. B. Another liver RE cell with FSP. Note vacuoles (black spaces). Digestion was complete in these intracellular sites.

Cellular Ingestion of FSP

The RE cells of the liver promptly picked up FSP and this correlated with the disappearance of FSP from serum (Fig. 3). There was essentially no activity by peripheral blood or bone marrow neutrophils. Bovine FSP (228 mg/kg body weight) was given; this dose was large and was equivalent to degrading twice as much fibrinogen as this dog actually possessed in his circulation. Although a distinct separation of the RE cell and neutrophil functions was achieved, the RE cellular localization of FSP might have been a response to the foreign bovine FSP (Fig. 3).

In six additional dogs, canine FSP was infused in doses ranging from 9-55 mg/kg. These doses simulated the conversion of each dog's own fibrinogen in amounts of 5-100%. Again, only RE cells reacted to the infused FSP and removed it from the circulation (Fig. 4). Details are presented for one dog that received 55 mg FSP/kg, which was equivalent to

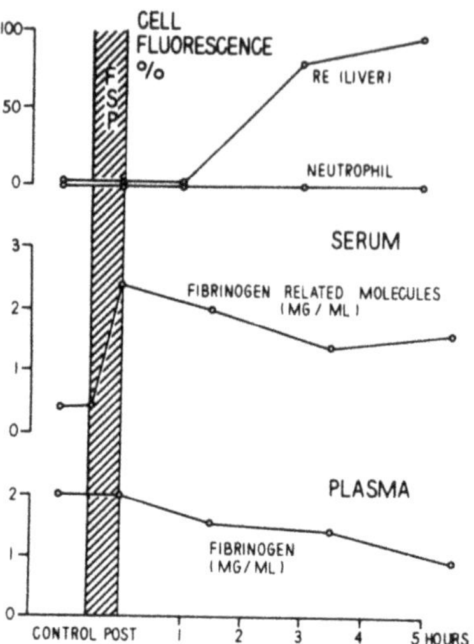

Fig. 5. Responses to infusion of purified canine FSP (55 mg/kg body weight). Liver RE cells cleared the infused FSP. Neutrophils were negative with fluorescent antifibrinogen.

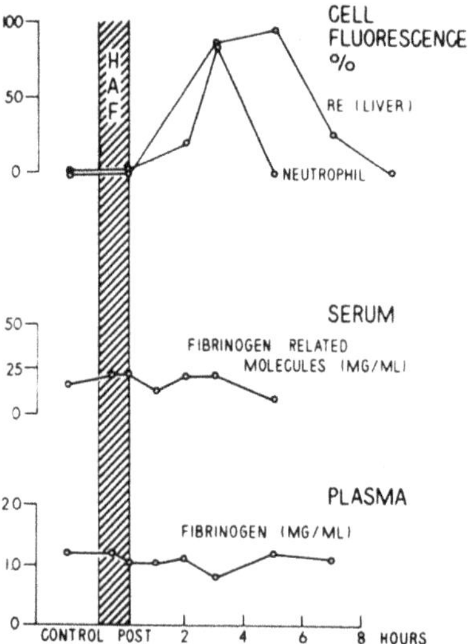

Fig. 6. Responses to infusion of heat-aggregated canine fibrinogen (HAF). Both neutrophils and liver RE cells can remove fibrinogen aggregates. Plasma fibrinogen and serum fibrinogen relatives remained near control values indicating that neither blood clotting nor plasma fibrinolytic mechanisms were initiated. Intracellular digestion of the phagocytized HAF was more rapid in blood neutrophils than in RE cells. Note that cellular digestion products (at least large ones) were not released to the circulation in measurable amounts as the serum value for immunologic relatives of fibrinogen was not elevated.

replacing 100% of his plasma fibrinogen by the degraded molecules FSP (Fig. 5). This dog showed an immediate rise in serum molecules related to fibrinogen and the concentration reached 2.4 mg/ml, which accounted for all of the FSP infused plus his control serum value. The early small clearance of FSP likely reflected adsorption of FSP onto platelet and blood cell surfaces. By 3 hr, the RE cell uptake of FSP was prominent and 90% of these cells contained some FSP at 5 hr. Neutrophils did not show any evidence of involvement with FSP throughout the experiment.

The described ingestion of FSP by liver RE cells was successfully blocked by a prior infusion with heat-denatured human albumin [16]. Very little, or no, cell fluorescence to antifibrinogen occurred in the first 5 hr. Most of the RE cells contained human albumin when checked with fluorescent antihuman albumin. The uptake of albumin by RE cells was immediate, and intracellular digestion occurred rapidly. Neutrophils did not take up the heat-denatured albumin nor did it encourage them to pick up FSP. Following albumin treatment, the FSP infusion was not picked up very readily by these RE cells. Appreciable amounts of the FSP remained in the circulation even $7\frac{1}{2}$ hr after infusion. By 5 hr, some RE cells contained FSP, but the cellular fluorescence and number of participating cells was small compared to another dog that was treated only with an equivalent dose of FSP (20 mg/kg body weight).

Clearance Time for FSP

This was assessed in two different ways. First, the anticoagulant power of the infused FSP was used as a guide to the dog's ability to handle FSP. The normalization time for six dogs averaged about $3\frac{1}{2}$ hr. The second test system employed an immunologic quantitative precipitin test for FSP in the serum [14]. On the average, about 3 hr was required for the serum fibrinogen-related molecules to reach preinfusion values. The dosage and amount of stress endured by the animal clearly influenced the clearance time. When serum values for fibrinogen-related molecules did not exceed 1.6 mg/ml, the clearance time of seven dogs was 3 hr. With values greater than 2 mg/ml, the clearance time was prolonged, as it was when RE blockade was induced with heat-denatured albumin.

The importance of the liver as a filter for altered fibrinogen was demonstrated by the prompt appearance of nonclottable fibrinogen molecules in the lymph after infusion of FSP. The control lymph did not have measurable amounts of these molecules. Within 5 min of infusion of FSP (20 mg per kg body weight) the lymph values for nonclottable fibrinogen-related molecules was 2.4 mg/ml and remained at this level for 3 hr post infusion. By 5 hr, the lymph was again negative in the quantitative immunoprecipitin test for nonclottable fibrinogen-related molecules [14]. In this dog, the plasma clearance of FSP was 4 hr for normalization according to the test for developed anticoagulant power.

The clearance time for the in vivo developed fibrinolytic products resulting from microthrombosis in response to infused thrombin (50-120 U per kg body weight) averaged 3½ hr for nine dogs. These dogs were studied pre- and post-thrombin with the aid of the immunologic assay for nonclottable fibrinogen molecules [14].

REMOVAL OF HEAT-AGGREGATED FIBRINOGEN

With convincing evidence that only the RE cells ingested soluble fibrinolytic products, we turned our attention again to the neutrophil. Were dog neutrophils capable of phagocytizing fibrinogen aggregates placed in the circulation? Following the infusion of sonified, heat-aggregated dog fibrinogen (24 mg/kg), which was equivalent to converting 32% of the dog's own fibrinogen to particulate material, both neutrophils and RE cells phagocytized the fibrinogen aggregates (Fig. 6). By 2 hr, 80% of the peripheral blood neutrophils fluoresced brightly and showed only diminished intensity approaching the normal autofluorescence at 5 hr. Although RE cells phagocytized the fibrinogen aggregates, the intensity of the response never equaled that of the neutrophils. Some cells presented well-defined phagosomes which fluoresced when the antifibrinogen marker was applied. Since serum levels of fibrinogen-related molecules were never elevated, the cellular material that appeared early in both neutrophils and liver RE cells was the infused heat-aggregated fibrinogen. As the RE cells had a chance to pick up only the fibrinogen aggregates that circulated past or lodged in the liver sinusoids, the RE function was limited. In contrast, the neutrophils had a more widespread activity in the microcirculation and likely invaded the aggregated fibrinogen deposits whenever present [21].

CONCLUSIONS

Three pathways for clearance of altered fibrinogen were investigated in dogs infused with either products of fibrinolysis or heat-aggregated fibrinogen. These routes were the peripheral blood neutrophils, the RE cells of liver, lung, or spleen, and, third, the kidney.

Liver RE cells rapidly removed soluble products of fibrinolysis and heat-denatured albumin from the circulation. Overloading the liver macrophages with denatured albumin impaired the RE cells' capacity to remove the subsequently infused FSP. Splenic RE cells, also, were involved in the clearance of FSP but were not as prominent as the liver RE cells. Neither lung nor kidney cells were marked by the immunofluorescent reagent. Thus, they appeared to be insignificant routes for clearance of FSP. Peripheral blood leucocytes did not contribute to the clearance of FSP nor were they involved in the removal of the denatured soluble albumin.

The clearance time for FSP was about 3 hr according to elimination of immunologically reactive molecules from the serum, removal of the induced anticoagulant power of serum and the cellular uptake of the altered fibrinogen, as revealed by the fluorescent antibody technique.

Insoluble protein aggregates, such as heat-denatured fibrinogen and fibrin deposition as a consequence of microthrombosis, elicited the phagocytic ability of peripheral blood neutrophils.

In the dog, two cellular mechanisms, blood neutrophils and RE cells, exist for removal of altered fibrinogen. Neutrophils provide a mobile cellular mechanism for entering, phagocytizing, and digesting aggregated fibrinogen or fibrin that may accumulate anywhere in the circulation. RE cells, when they have the opportunity, remove circulating aggregates of fibrin or fibrinogen. The RE cells of liver are especially effective in clearance of circulating soluble derivatives of fibrinogen and fibrin that can result from proteolysis.

REFERENCES

1. R.T. McCluskey, P. Vassalli, G. Gallo, and D.S. Baldwin, "An immunofluorescent study of pathogenic mechanisms in glomerular diseases," New Engl.J.Med., 274:695-701, 1966.
2. J.M. Riddle, G.B. Bluhm, and M.I. Barnhart, "Interrelationships between fibrin, neutrophils, and rheumatoid synovitis," J.Reticuloendothelial Soc., 2:420-436, 1965.
3. G. B. Bluhm, J.M. Riddle, and M.I. Barnhart, "Significance of fibrin and other particulates in rheumatoid joint inflammation," Henry Ford Hospital Med.Bull., 14:119-130, 1966.
4. L. Lee and R.T. McCluskey, "Immunohistochemical demonstration of the reticuloendothelial clearance of circulating fibrin aggregates," J.Exptl.Med., 116:611-618, 1962.
5. M.I. Barnhart, "Importance of neutrophilic leucocytes in the resolution of fibrin," Federation Proc., 24:846-853, 1965.
6. M.I. Barnhart, "Cellular fibrinogen," Thromb.Diath.Hemorrhag., 10:157-165, 1964.
7. J.M. Riddle and M.I. Barnhart, "Ultrastructural study of fibrin dissolution via emigrated polymorphonuclear neutrophils," Am.J.Pathol., 45:805-823, 1964.
8. M.I. Barnhart, S.A. McCutcheon, J.M. Riddle, and J.M. Ohorodnik, "Thrombotic thrombocytopenic purpura as a model of accelerated protein synthesis," Thromb.Diath.Hemorrhag., 12:211-231, 1964.
9. A.G. Ware, M.M. Guest, and W.H. Seegers, "Fibrinogen with special reference to its preparations and certain properties of the product," Arch.Biochem., 13:231-236, 1947.
10. R.M. Stirland, "A rapid method of estimating fibrinogen," Lancet, 1:672, 1956.
11. W.B. Forman and M.I. Barnhart, "Cellular site for fibrinogen synthesis," J.Am.Med.Ass., 187:128-132, 1964.

12. W.H. Seegers, R.H. Landaburu, and J.F. Johnson, 'Thrombin-E as a fibrinolytic enzyme," Science, 131: 726, 1960.
13. M.I. Barnhart and W.B. Forman, "The cellular localization of fibrinogen as revealed by the fluorescent antibody technique," Vox Sanguinis, 8: 461-473, 1963.
14. M.I. Barnhart, D.C. Cress, R.L. Henry, and J.M. Riddle, "Influence of fibrinogen split products on platelets," Thromb. Diath. Hemorrhag., 17: 78-98, 1967.
15. V. Nussenzweig, M. Seligmann, and P. Grabar, "Les products de degradation du fibrinogene aumain par la plasmin," Ann. Inst. Pasteur, 100: 490-508, 1961.
16. B. Benacerraf, G. Biozzi, B.N. Halpern, C. Stiffel, and D. Mouton, "Phagocytosis of heat-denatured human serum albumin labeled with ^{131}I and its use as a means of investigating blood flow," Brit. J. Exptl. Pathol., 38: 35-48, 1957.

Subject Index

Acetate-C^{14}, 41, 44, 93
Acetylcholinesterase (AChe), 122, 123
Actinomycin D, 63, 70, 72
Adenosine triphosphatase, 471, 477
Adrenal cortex, 266
Adrenal cortical trophic hormone, 233
Adrenalectomy, 275
Adventitia, 463
Aging, 404, 408
Agranulocytosis, 369
Albumin
  Bovine, 427, 436, 452
  Heat-denatured human, 499
Alveolar Macrophage(s)
  comparative properties, 133, 206
  germfree, 139
  isolation, 59, 134, 204
  origin, 58, 108
  relation to pulmonary disease, 58, 109
Anesthesia
  influence on stimulated animals, 260
Animal(s)
  germfree, 133, 139, 175
Antibody, 311
  antiaorta, 473
  natural, 286
  synthesis, 333, 345, 346
Antigen, 20, 286, 333
  cholesterol ester, 433
  polysaccharide (yeast zymosan), 437
Aorta
  calcification, 473
  foam cells, 427, 429, 484, 487
  lesions, 462, 471, 483
  thoracic, 471
Arteriopathy, 413, 451, 459
Arthritis, 357, 358
Atherosclerosis, 418, 442, 451, 488
  immunological, 426, 483
  induced by aortic extracts, 481
  induced by microthrombin, 488
Atherosclerosis (cont.)
  infiltration theory, 450
  plaques, 148, 433, 449, 484

Bacillus Calmette Guerin, 203, 256
"Binding sites," 15
Blockade, 25, 63, 68, 85, 278, 286, 387, 413
  agents, 272, 499
  susceptibility to injury, 267
Bacteriophage, 334
Blood coagulation, factor in colloid clearance, 25
Brucella abortus, 198
Burn, standard, 257
  infection, 257
Butyrylcholinesterase (BChE), 122, 123

Calcium, 25, 163, 167
  pyrophosphate, 364
Carcinogen(s), 62
Cathepsin, 134, 142
Chloramphenicol, 55, 345
Cholesterol, 197, 199, 388, 410, 433, 435, 476
  diet, 419, 487
  localization – RE cells, 421
  oleate, 188
  transport, 404
Chylomicrons, 53, 148, 383, 398, 443, 445
  fate, 389
  nonatherogenic nature, 450
  washed, 390
Colloids, 18
  carbon 1, 58, 63, 66, 86, 198, 298, 301, 413
  chromium phosphate, 287
  distribution, as a function of charge, 29
  gold, 286, 386, 405
  toxicity, 70
Colloidophagy, 147
Complement, 159, 286, 290

Cortisone, 85, 92, 225, 250, 266, 271
acetate, 86, 268
Culture
tissues, 74

Dehydrogenase
lactic, 469, 477
alpha-hydroxybutyric, 469, 477
Detoxification, 130
Dextran, 301
toxicity, 302
Diabetes
susceptibility to infection, 369
Dicumarol, 26, 28
Diethylstilbestrol, 191, 192
Diphtheria toxoid, 346
DNA-protein
complexes, 359
synthesis, 115
Desoxycorticosterone acetate (DOCA), 225

Emulsion – lipid, 383, 385
Endoplasmic reticulum, 140, 350
Endotoxin(s), 14, 71, 262, 266, 267, 277, 289
detoxifying factor, 129
enhanced sensitivity, 285
shock, 247, 257, 297, 299
tolerance, 275, 282, 285
toxemia, 311
Epinephrine, 50
Epsilon aminocaproic acid (EACA), 494
Erythrophagocytosis, 159
Escherichia coli, 133, 245, 370, 373
Esterases
endothelial, 121
macrophage, 121
nonspecific, 122
role in detoxification, 130
role in lipid metabolism, 130
Estradiol
17 Beta, 225
benzoate, 192
monobenzoate, 227
Estrogen, 191, 214, 218, 219
Estrone, 226
Ethinylestradiol, 227
Euglobulin, modification of endotoxin, 289

Fatty acids, 41, 384
Fibrin, 25, 360, 485, 492
Fibrinogen, 492, 493, 500
Fibrinolytic soluble products (FSP), 497
RE cellular ingestion, 497
Fibroblasts, 130, 462
Foam cells (see aorta)
Freund's adjuvant, 108, 109, 345, 452
Friend leukemia virus (FLV), 315, 317, 328

Gamma radiation
depression of phagocytic capacity, 1, 15
Gelatin, 26, 51, 176
antibodies, 288
poly-1-glutamyl, 26, 30
poly-1-lysyl, 26
stimulation, 183
Gland of Faussek, 150
Glucagon, 50
Glucan, 4, 14, 244, 256, 257, 260, 263, 266, 272, 387, 393
Glucose, 48, 207
Glutaraldehyde
use in cell separation, 34
Glycerol-C^{14}, 41, 44
Glyceryl trioleate, 98, 101
Glyceryl tripalmitate-C^{14}, 388
Golgi complex, 141, 350
Goodpastures syndrome, 147
Gout, 358, 361

Hemolysin, 159
Hemorrhage, 267
Hemosiderin, 147
Heparin, 26, 28, 31, 52, 287, 319, 330, 383, 430, 489
Hydrocortisone, 225
Hypophysectomy, 275
Hypotonic shock, 176
Hypoxia, 49

Immune mechanism(s), 20
Immune serum, effect on phagocytosis, 53, 276
Immunoglobulin, 333
Infarction, myocardial, 493
Inflammatory response, 221, 231
Insulin
binding by leukocytes, 378

Interferon, 315, 317, 325, 328
Intima
    infiltration, 462
Iron oxide, saccharated, 267, 272

Kinetics
    phagocytic, 1, 23
Klebsiella pneumoniae, 275, 300, 304
    clearance, 277
Kupffer cells, 20, 87, 92, 215, 218, 282, 383, 407

Lactate, 48
Lecithin, 197, 199
Leukocyte(s), 20, 67, 111, 232, 357, 369
Lipids
    total serum, 475, 476
Lipoproteins, 437, 442, 443, 489
Lipoprotein lipase, 398
Liver
    blood flow, 94
    carbon-containing phagocytes, 60
    cell suspensions, 40
    perfusion, 46
    Shark, 243
    trypsinized, source of macrophages, 79
Lymph nodes, 128
Lymphocytes, 111
Lysolecithin, 197, 199
Lysosomal enzymes, 98, 262
Lysosome, 198, 199
    synthesis, 105
Lysozyme, 134, 138

Macrophage(s)
    cadaveric, 152
    comparative morphology, 74, 81
    human, 151
    mitoses, 83, 351
    permeability, 199
    processes, 105
    tissue culture, 77
Magnesium, 163, 167
Maytenus laevis, 188
Metabolism, lipid, 130
Methyltestosterone, 228
Microscopy
    electron
        liver, 35, 85, 87, 92, 150, 218
        lung, 111, 133, 134, 205, 207, 210
        monocytes, 486
        neutrophils, 357, 361
        peritoneal cells, 101, 103, 133
        plasma cells, 350
    light, 134, 138, 357
    phase, 35, 98, 102
Mitochondria, 51, 141
Model
    mathematical, 1
    particle system, 26
Mycobacterium
    bovis, 204
    butyricum, 345
    phlei, 252
Myocardial infarction, 493

Neutrophils, 357, 371, 492, 493

Opsonin(s), 63, 66, 83, 85, 93, 147, 278, 286, 289

Palmitate
    ethyl, 188
    methyl, 53, 54
Parabiosis, 423
Parenchymal cell, 39, 46, 92, 94, 383
Particle
    charge, 18, 22
    electrophoretic mobility, 26, 172
Peritoneal
    dialysis, source of human macrophages, 153
    macrophages, 77, 98, 133, 134, 163, 165, 175, 185, 340
Pertussis vaccine, 256
Phagocytosis
    capacity 1, 6
    clearance rates, 65, 290
    depression, 232
    index, 65, 165, 170
    in vitro assay, 83, 167, 175, 302
    mathematical model, 1
    platelets, 484, 487
    reverse, 20
    saturation cells, 63, 85
    starch granules, 157, 164

Phagosomes, 357, 360
Phlobaphenes, 190
Phosphatases
 acid, 77, 98, 134, 138, 198
 alkaline, 471, 477
 nonspecific, 469
Phospholipid, 476
Phytohemagglutinin, 315, 318, 328
Pinocytosis, 93, 218
Plasma
 cells, 350
 factors in phagocytosis (see also opsonins), 25, 51
 proteins, 7
Platelets, 329, 484, 487, 489, 493
 adhesiveness, 488
 anti "clearing" activity, 488, 489
 factor-4, 488
 role in atherogenesis, 488
Pneumoconioses, 109
Pyran Copolymer, 315, 318
Polysomes, 338
Polystyrene latex particles, 18, 26, 29, 164
Prednisolone, 50
Prednisone, 225
Proferrin, 267
Progesterone, 228
Properdin, 291
Prothrombin Time, 27
Protein
 plasma, 7
 synthesis, 1, 9, 11
 total, 476
Pseudogout, 357, 358
Pseudomonas aeruginosa, 257, 300
Puromycin, 1, 63, 72
Pyrexal^{R}, 193
Pyruvate, 48

Rabbits
 cholesterol-fed, 433
Radioprotection
 effect of RE stimulants, 194
Restim, 243, 246, 256, 257
Reticuloendothelial
 depressing substance (RDS), 293, 299
 endoplasmic reticulum, 140
 stimulation (see glucan, estrogen, restim)
 test lipid emulsion, 395
Rheumatoid arthritis, 358
Rheumatoid diseases, 492
Ribosomes, 339
RNA synthesis, 340
Rous Sarcoma Virus (RSV), 246

Saccharomyces cerevisiae, 387
Salmonella
 abortus equi, 193
 enteritidis, 52, 252, 277
 typhi, 334
 typhimurium, 148, 245, 267, 300
 typhosa, 300
 typhosa endotoxin, 4, 14
Salmonella typhi lipopolysaccharide, 177
Sarcina lutea, 204
Scholler lignin, 190
Serotonin, 291
Serratia marcescens, 288
Serum
 factors (see opsonins)
 hypercholesterolemic, 442
 immune, 53
 sickness, 427
Shock
 drum, 267, 297
 endotoxin, 257, 267, 299
 hemorrhage, 267
 hypotonic, 176
 ischemic, 298
 syndrome, 299
 trauma, 267
Skin window technique, 369, 370
Sodium urate, 361
Splenomegaly
 Friend leukemia virus induced, 317
 inhibition, 323
Staphylococcus
 albus, 203
 aureus, 52, 133, 204
Statolon, 318, 328
 induction of interferon, 315
Streptococcus mastitidis, 300
Sulfobromophthalein (BSP), 387

Tailing effect of particles, 20
Testosterone, 227
Thorotrast, 61, 85, 86, 94, 214, 215, 413
Thrombocytes, 23
Thrombosis
 cerebrovascular, 493
Thrombocytopenia, 325, 329

Thrombophilic diathesis, 488
Thrombotic thrombocytopenia purpura, 493
Thrombus, 487
 formation, 431
 mural, 484
Thyroid, 147
Tissue cultures, macrophages, 74
Tolerance
 immunologic, 282, 483
 endotoxin, 285
Transaminase
 oxalacetic glutamic, 469, 476, 477
 pyruvic glutamic, 469, 477
Tri-anisyl-chloro-ethylene, 191
Triglyceride, 188, 244, 383
Triiodothyronine, 50
Triolein, 256, 388, 390
Triparanol, 55
Tritiated thymidine, 108, 110
Triton, 383
Tyrosine transaminase, 268, 271
Trypan blue, 58, 61
Tryptophan pyrrolase, 266, 272

Vasa Vasorum, 463
Vascular hypersensitivity, 427

Zeta potential, 19, 26
Zymosan, 15, 256, 266, 272, 387, 410

Author Index

(Underscored numbers indicate complete papers in this volume.)

Abelson, N. M., 367
Aberdeen, V., 403
Abramson, H. A., 33, 172, 174
Achong, B. G., 106
Ackerman, G. A., 370, 379
Ackerman, R. F., 412
Acs, G., 274
Ada, G. C., 343
Adams, C. W. M., 131
Adams, M. H., 284
Adler, F. B., 343
Adlersberg, L., 18-24
Agarwal, M. K., 266-274
Ahrens, E. H., Jr., 412
Ainsworth, E. J., 196
Alderman, J. M., 196
Alexander, A. E., 33
Allen, E. H., 355
Allison, F., 106, 171, 173, 174, 232, 240
Allman, R. M., 243
Ambrose, C. T., 57, 354
Ames, A. M., 173
Amos, H., 355
Anacker, R. L., 284
Andrus, S. B., 424
Antonini, F. M., 404-412
Antopol, W., 96
Apgar, J. M., 265
Appelmans, F., 202
Arion, W. J., 274
Armentrout, S., 355
Arredondo, M. I., 71, 73
Artuson, G., 264
Aschoff, L., 85, 96
Ashworth, C. T., 385, 402, 412
Askonas, B. A., 344
Astorgas, G., 367
Atkins, N., 131
Auerbach, V. H., 267, 274
Augustinsson, K.-B., 131
Austin, C. M., 343

Bacchus, H., 109, 119
Bach, M. K., 332
Baer, H., 255
Bailey, J. M., 433-441
Baillif, R. N., 220, 371, 379
Baker, L. A., 254, 331
Baker, N., 34-45
Baldwin, D. S., 501
Bale, W. F., 56
Ball, E. G., 377, 380
Ballantyne, B., 121-132
Ballerini, G., 488-491
Balner, H., 196
Bangham, A. D., 26, 33, 164, 166, 171, 173, 174
Ban'kovskaya, E. B., 450
Barclay, W. R., 232, 240
Barkhan, P., 490
Barnabei, O., 197, 201, 202
Barnhart, M. I., 357-368, 378, 379, 381, 492-502
Barnhart, R. J., 377, 380
Baron, S., 332
Barrnett, R. J., 45
Barth, C. L., 380
Baserga, A., 490
Bases, R. E., 412
Bass, J. A., 97
Bauer, H., 142, 145, 378, 381
Bean, M., 344
Beeson, P. B., 96, 274, 291
Behar, A. J., 118
Behnke, O., 107
Beiser, S. M., 441
Belfrage, P., 399, 401, 403
Benacerraf, B., 16, 17, 33, 62, 65, 72, 95-97, 195, 264, 267, 274, 284, 291, 301, 402, 404, 411, 413, 424, 425, 502
Bendien, W. M., 292
Benditt, E. P., 16, 33, 56, 66, 71-73, 96, 146, 290-292
Benhanon, J. P., 411
Bennet, N. J., 412
Bennett, B., 74-84
Bennett, H. S., 96
Bennett, W. E., 187
Benos, S. A., 96
Bensch, K., 45
Benson, B., 106, 144, 146, 187
Berlin, C. M., 274
Berliner, D. L., 56, 232, 240, 265, 397, 403
Berman, S. L., 46, 56, 401
Berman, L., 376, 380
Bernfeld, P., 332
Bernick, S., 413-425
Berry, L. J., 266-274
Bertalanffy, F. D., 58, 62, 109, 116, 119
Bessman, S. P., 377, 380
Best, C. H., 424
Better, N., 131
Bierman, E. L., 398, 403, 412
Biggs, M. W., 421, 425
Bilbey, D. L. J., 61, 62, 96, 196, 219, 222, 232, 239
Billiau, A., 402
Billiteri, A., 411
Biozzi, G., 5, 6, 16, 17, 25,

Biozzi (continuation)
33, 59, 62, 72, 96, 97, 106, 132, 195, 197, 198, 202, 277, 283, 284, 291, 292, 301, 313, 402, 404, 411, 424, 425, 502
Bishop, J., 39
Black-Schaffer, B., 300, 311-313
Blattberg, B., 293-299
Blaustein, A., 255
Blickens, D. A., 57, 402, 432
Bliznakov, E. G., 243-255, 265
Bloch, E. H., 33
Bloom, B., 425
Bluhm, G. B., 357-368, 501
Bly, C. G., 56
Boivan, A., 277, 283
Bolis, L., 197-202
Bollman, J. L., 402
Bond, V. P., 380
Bonnin, 161, 162
Bonventre, P. F., 52, 57, 300, 311-313
Borecky, L., 332
Borek, F., 433, 441
Borgstrom, B., 399, 401, 403
Borekley, B. J., 332
Borman, A., 238, 241
Borzelleca, J. F., 264
Boyd, G. A., 411, 412
Boyden, S., 147, 149, 162, 164, 174, 452, 467, 471
Boyer, F., 275-284
Boyse, E. A., 84
Bradley, G. P., 411
Bradley, S. E., 411
Bragdon, J. H. 398, 401, 418, 424
Brandes, D., 106
Brandt, P. W., 96, 97
Braude, A. I., 378, 380
Brauer, R. W. 413, 424
Braun, W., 274, 284
Bray, G. A., 4, 17
Brennan, M. J., 380
Bricauk, H., 468-483
Brieger, H., 109, 117-119
Bright, R., 441
Brill, R. M., 367
Briscoe, J. C., 115, 119
Brodie, B. B., 241
Brot, N., 403
Broustet, P., 468-483
Brown, B. A., 97
Brucer, M., 411
Bubenik, J., 254
Bucher, T., 56
Buckler, F., 332
Bullough, W. S., 233, 241
Bunch, G. A., 131, 132
Bunim, J. J., 241
Buras, N. S., 161, 162
Burns, W. A., 146
Burnstein, M., 443, 445, 450
Burstone, M. S., 106, 131, 145
Burwell, R. G., 131
Bush, I. E., 236-238, 241
Butler, J., 433-441
Butler, W. T., 354
Byers, S., 384, 402, 411, 421, 425, 432, 443, 450, 487

Cain, J. C., 402
Cammarano, P., 344
Campbell, P. A., 343
Cannon, P. R., 344
Cantrell, K., 332
Capocaccia, M., 220
Cappell, D. F., 58, 62
Cappelli, G., 411
Cardinale, M., 300-314
Carleton, H. M., 115, 119
Carozza, F. A., Jr., 291
Carpenter, P. L., 164, 173
Carr, I., 98-107
Carswell, E. A., 84
Casarett, L. J., 108-120, 163-174
Casarett, M. G., 108-120
Casley-Smith, J. R., 220
Castle, W. B., 161, 162
Castro-Murillo, E., 367
Chaikovv, I. L., 403, 421, 425
Chaikoff, I. L., 53, 57
Chambers, J. E., 45
Chandler, A. B., 484, 487, 490
Chaparas, S. D., 255
Charles, L. M., 196, 222, 239
Charlier, H., 283
Chase, H. B., 196
Chase, R. E., 17, 274
Chase, W. E., 344
Cheatham, R. M., 131
Chedid, L., 56, 275-284
Chernew, I., 378, 380
Chessick, R. D., 131
Chevremont, M., 132
Christakis, G. J., 412
Citi, S., 411
Clarke, D. A., 84, 196
Clarke, E., 402
Clitherow, J. W., 132
Cochran, K. W., 331
Cochrane, C. G., 432
Cohen, L. A., 424
Cohen, M., 34-45
Cohn, Z. A., 56, 106, 133, 144-146, 164, 173, 186, 187
Coll, 201
Collins, R. D., 274
Colwell, L. S., 274
Conconi, F., 491
Constanides, P., 441
Cook, G. M. W., 172, 174
Coons, A. H., 57, 354
Cooper, C. W., 33
Cooper, G. N., 49, 56, 106, 107, 188, 195, 254, 264
Cordingley, J. L., 58-62, 196, 222, 239
Cornelius, C. E., 57
Cottrell, T. S., 96
Courtice, F. C., 399, 403
Coutinho, C. B., 264
Cowdry, E. V., 45
Cox, R. A., 331
Coyle, J. F., 412
Crabbe, J., 232, 240
Crawford, T., 484, 487
Cremer, N., 271, 291
Cress, D. C., 492-502
Crockett, R., 468-483
Cronheim, G., 432
Crooke, J. C., 131
Crosthwaite, J. L., 174
Crowley, J. H., 380
Cruchard, A., 354
Cruickshank, A. H., 378, 380
Cuendet, A., 17, 97
Culbertson, Y. T., 411
Cumming, R. H., 161, 162
Curry, J. J., 411

Cutbush, M., 161, 162
Cutting, W., 331
Czuppon, A., 441

Dagley, S., 355
D'Agostini, N., 131
Daido, S., 119
Dallocchio, M., 468-483
Dalton, A. J., 45, 116, 120
Daniel, T., 354
Dannenberg, A. M., Jr., 106, 133, 145
Dauben, G. W., 425
David, H., 484, 487
Davidson, E., 254
Davis, B. J., 131
Davis, E. V., 213
Davis, K. J., 232, 240
Day, A. J., 107, 132, 412
DeBoer, C. J., 332
DeDuve, C., 106, 198, 199, 202
Degna, A. T., 219
Dekruif, P. H., 292
Delaloye, B., 411
DeNicola, P., 491
Desaulles, P., 223, 239
DeSomer, P., 402
DiCarlo, F. J., 56, 188, 190, 196, 264, 265
Diegenbach, P. C., 131
DiGaddo, M., 235, 241
DiLuzio, N. R., 16, 17, 33, 53, 54, 57, 106, 107, 202, 264, 382-403, 409, 412, 413, 424, 432, 441
Divertie, M. B., 119
Dixon, K. C., 412
Dixon, M., 131
Doaust, R., 384, 401
Dobson, E. L., 14, 15, 17, 24, 63-73, 97, 287, 288, 292, 402, 411, 413, 424
Dodd, M. C., 30, 33, 97
Dole, V. P., 383, 401
Donn, A., 97
Dorfman, R. F., 131
Dougherty, T. F., 56, 265, 397, 403
Downie, H. G., 490
Dreyer, W., 344
Druce, C. G., 196
Dubin, D. T., 355
Dubnick, B., 56, 265
Duff, G. L., 424
Duguid, J. B., 490
Dumont, L., 131

Eastham, J. R., 425
Ebert, R. H., 232, 233, 240, 241
Edgren, B., 53, 57, 399, 403
Eilert, M. L., 424
Einheber, A., 146
Elberg, S. S., 284
Elkert, A. T., 355
Elko, E. E., 402
Ellerker, A. R., 131
Elliott, A. Y., 328, 331
Ellison, R. R., 412
Elsbach, P., 96, 132
Emmel, V. M., 45
Ende, E., 18-24
Enders, J. F., 286, 292
English, R., 255
Eppstein, S. H., 241
Epstein, B., 117, 119
Epstein, M. H., 106
Erlanger, B. F., 433, 441
Etinger-Tulcyznika, R., 164, 173
Evans, D. G., 203-213
Evans, G. L., 255
Evrard, E., 402
Exum, E. D., 355

Falb, R. D., 33
Falkner, R., 411
Fariss, B., 145, 213
Farkas, K., 441
Farnham, A. E., 145, 213
Farrar, W. E., 265
Fauvert, R., 411
Fawcett, D. W., 96, 106, 403
Fedorko, M. E., 106, 146, 187
Feigelson, M., 274
Feigelson, P., 274
Felts, J. M., 400, 403
Feltz, G. T., 331
Fenn, W. O., 16, 164, 172, 174, 292, 411
Ferin, J., 117, 120
Feuerstein, J., 56
Fidge, N. H., 107, 132
Field, J. B., 378, 381
Fields, J., 331
Filkins, J. P., 17, 51, 56, 265, 274
Fillios, L. C., 418, 424
Finch, S. C., 369, 378, 380
Fine, J., 131, 264
Finland, M., 291, 292
Finnegan, C., 196
Finney, C. R., 17, 63-73, 97, 402, 411
Fish, P. A., 383, 401
Fisher, M., 120
Fishman, M., 342, 380
Fitch, F. W., 343
Flemens, R., 33
Flora, R. W., 274
Florey, H. W., 233, 241, 487
Folkes, J. P., 57
Foltyn, O., 331
Forman, W. B., 501, 502
Foster, D. O., 274
Fox, A. E., 251, 255
Flemming, C., 195, 196
Flemming, K. B. P., 188-196
Frank, E. D., 131
Frankel, H. H., 424, 425
Fratta, M., 235, 241
Fred, R. K., 1-17, 57
Fredrickson, D. S., 399, 401, 403
Freed, F. C., 233, 235, 240
Freedman, H. H., 264, 274, 284, 291
Freeman, J. A., 146, 213
Freeman, M. T., 354
Freeman, S., 385, 402
French, J. E., 57, 396, 398, 399, 401, 403, 412, 484, 485, 487
Freund, J., 109, 118
Fried, J., 238, 241
Frieman, M., 397, 402, 411, 421, 425, 431, 432, 443, 450, 487
Friedman, R. M., 332
Froesch, E. R., 242
Fruitstone, M., 329, 332
Fugmann, R. A., 255
Fuhrman, G. F., 174
Fujita, T., 432
Fukuda, T., 265
Fukui, G. M., 300-314
Furst, A., 331

Furusawa, E., 331

Gabrielli, E. R., 16, 20, 24, 55-57, 378, 380
Gage, S. H., 383, 401
Gaines, S., 254
Gale, E. F., 57
Gallo, G., 501,
Gandji, F. A., 468-483
Ganong, W. F., 242
Garvin, J. E., 173, 174
Gasso, G., 411
Gatter, R. A., 367
George, E. P., 401
George, S. O., 411
Gerebtzoff, M. A., 131
Gergely, J., 441, 450
Germuth, F. G., 432, 467
Gero, S., 441
Gerok. W., 56
Gershfeld, N. L., 97
Geyer, B. P., 402
Gibb, F. R., 120
Gibbs, J. A., 17
Gillespie, R. E., 196
Gilman, P. A., 24
Glasstone, S., 172, 174
Glende, E. A., Jr., 274
Glenn, E. M., 233, 241
Glover, F. L., 213
Glusenkamp, G., 33
Glynn, M. F., 484, 487
Goevel, W. F., 332
Gofman, J. W., 431
Goldfien, A., 238, 242
Goldstein, M. N., 81
Golfien, A., 401
Gonzalez-Ojeda, D., 145
Good, R. A., 96, 274, 291, 369, 380
Goodman, D. S., 384, 397, 401
Goodman, H. M., 344
Gordis, E., 403
Gordon, A. S., 274
Gordon, E. S., 235, 241
Gordon, G. B., 164, 173
Gordon, J., 164, 173, 443, 450
Gordon, R. S., 398, 401
Gorin, M. H., 33
Gorrer, P. A., 84
Goth, A., 232, 240
Gottlieb, A. A., 340, 341, 344
Gould-Hurst, P. R. S., 107, 412
Graack, B., 196
Grabar, P., 502
Grampa, G., 214-220
Granzer, E., 172, 174
Gray, W., 344
Green, C., 400, 403
Greengard, O., 274
Greer, S. J., 487
Greisman, S. E., 391
Grindlay, J. H., 402
Grode, G. A., 33
Gross, P. R., 274
Groult, N., 451-467
Guerra, S. L., 241
Guest, M. M., 501
Guimaraes, J. P., 217, 220
Gulick, Z. R., 332
Gulliver, G., 383, 401
Gunderson, C. H., 343

Hackensellner, H. A., 484, 487
Hagerman, D. D., 233, 240
Hahn, P. F., 411
Hall, J. A., 380
Halpern, B. N., 2, 16, 17, 24, 33, 62, 72, 96, 97, 106, 132, 195, 198, 202, 283, 284, 291, 292, 301, 313, 386, 402, 411, 413, 421, 424, 425, 505
Hamburger, H. J., 164, 166, 172, 173
Hamerman, D., 368
Hamlin, J. T., III, 383, 401, 403
Hammerstrom, R. A., 380
Hammond, W. S., 333-344
Hampton, J. C., 96, 220, 403
Hanback, L. D., 264
Hand, R. A., 484, 487, 490
Hanson, R. W., 332
Harman, D., 432
Harper, N. J., 132
Harris, H., 148, 162
Harris, J. G., 16
Hartroft, W. S., 418, 424
Haskins, W. T., 284
Haurowitz, F., 56
Haust, M. D., 490
Havel, R. J., 399, 401
Hawn, C. V., 467
Hayes, F. N., 17
Haynes, L. J., 56, 196, 264, 265
Hayworth, P., 255
Heard, D. H., 33
Heath, F. F., 131
Hechter, O., 97
Heftmann, E., 97
Heilman, D. H., 376, 380
Heise, E. R., 133-146, 212, 213
Heller, J. H., 56, 96, 132, 197, 202, 243-255, 264, 332, 412
Heller, M. S., 254, 264
Helms, J., 46-57
Henon, B. K., 131
Henry, R. L., 502
Heymann, H., 332
Heyssel, R. M., 291
Higgenbotham, R., 56, 328, 331
Higgins, J. A., 400, 403
Hill, B. M., 292
Hilleman, M. R., 109, 118
Hills, J. D., 291
Hillyard, L. A., 57
Hinz, C. F., Jr., 292
Hirsch, E. F., 433, 441
Hirsch, J. D., 17, 72, 97, 402
Hirsch, J. G., 106, 146, 187, 292
Hoenig, E. M., 18-24
Hoffman, A., 354
Hoffman, R. G., 263
Hofman, J. W., 442, 450
Hofstee, B. H. J., 138, 145
Högn, E. O., 235, 241
Hohorst, H. J., 56
Hojman, D., 424
Holladay, D. R., 344
Holland, J. F., 331
Hollander, J. L., 367, 368
Holle, G., 400, 403
Holman, J., 240
Holt, S. J., 131
Holter, H., 96
Hood, L., 344
Hosokawa, K., 355
Houston, B., 106
Houston, J., 402

Howard, J. G., 277, 283
Hueper, W. C., 419, 424
Huffman, S., 424
Hull, R. N., 331
Hummell, J. P., 331

Iglewski, B. H., 333-344
Iio, M., 96
Imai, Y., 396, 403
Ingelfinger, F., 411
Irwin, D., 61, 62
Ishiko, S., 119
Issacs, A., 331
Ivemark, B., 399, 403

Jackson, A. L., 255
Jacoby, D., 264, 274
Jacoby, F., 84
Jaffe, R. H., 46, 56, 384, 401 413, 423
Jakab, L., 441
Jandl, J. H., 17, 161, 162
Janeway, C. A., 467
Janigan, D. T., 34, 45
Janoff, A., 265
Jenkin, C. R., 17, 66, 72, 96, 147, 162, 284, 291, 292
Jesaitis, M. A., 332
Joel, P. B., 233, 240
Johnson, A. G., 254, 285
Johnson, I. S., 254, 331
Johnson, J., 331, 502
Johnson, L., 120
Johnson, P., 33
Johnston, M. E., 411
Jones, A. R., 161, 162
Jones, H. B., 292
Jones, R., 403
Jones, R. J., 424
Jones, R. S., 56
Joossens, J. V., 402
Jordan, G., 411
Jordan, P., 399, 403
Juras, D., 343

Kakano, M., 284
Kaliss, N., 254
Kampschmidt, R. F., 56, 71, 73
Kapral, A., 106
Karnovsky, M. L., 93, 96, 97, 145, 203, 212, 213, 233, 240, 370, 380
Karrer, H. E., 96, 116, 119
Karthigasu, K., 147, 162
Kass, E. H., 250, 255
Katchalsky, A., 173, 174
Katz, M., 292
Kaye, G. I., 97
Keene, W. R., 17, 131
Kelly, L. S., 14, 15, 17, 63-73, 97, 402
Kenney, F. T., 274
Kessel, R. W. I., 197-202
Kibrick, S., 332
Kim, 264, 291
Kimbrough, C., 371, 379
Kinberg, D. V., 96
King, D. W., 164, 173
Kinsley, J. W., 106, 145
Kiser, J., 487
Kitamaru, H., 116, 119
Kitay, J. I., 233, 241
Kivy-Rosenberg, E., 16
Kiyasu, D. Y., 425
Kleinschmidt, W. J., 315, 329, 331, 332
Klimov, A. N., 442-450
Kojima, M., 396, 403
Kniker, W. T., 432
Knisely, M. H., 33
Knox, W. E., 274
Kobayashi, T., 265
Koelle, G. B., 122, 131
Koenig, M. G., 291
Koldovsky, P., 254
Krahl, V. E., 115, 119
Krakoff, I. H., 412
Kreutz, F. H., 56
Kritchesky, D., 412
Kroma, E., 195
Kuhar, S., 331
Kull, F. J., 274
Kunkel, H. G., 412

LaBelle, C. W., 109, 117-119
Lackoviv, V., 332
Ladman, A. J., 402
Lamerton, L. F., 217, 220
Lancaster, M. G., 174
Landaburu, R. H., 502
Landy, M., 132, 251, 254, 255, 284, 292
Langendorff, M., 196
Langer, B., 118
LaPaglia, S., 490
Lardy, H. A., 274
Laufer, A., 109, 116, 118
Laurell, C. B., 401
Lautsch, E. V., 419, 424
Lavelle, J. M., 331
LaVia, M. F., 333-344
Lavis, S., 18-24
Leach, L. J., 109, 119
Leake, E. S., 133-146, 213
Leblond, C. P., 109, 116, 119
Lee, A., 107
Lee, L., 25, 33, 492, 501
Lee, M. O., 264
Lee, S. H. S., 332
Leigh, H. M., 241
Leininger, R. I., 33
LeMinor, L., 292
Lemperle, G., 256-265
Lenegre, J., 451-467
Lentz, P, E., 262, 265
Lester, G., 97
Levine, R., 377, 380
Levy, H., 332
Levy, L., 426-432
Levy, M. N., 293-299
Lieberman, S., 441
Liebhaber, H., 331
Lillie, R. D., 371, 380
Lin, E. C. C., 274
Lindner, E., 233, 240
Lipmann, F., 355
Lipo, J. M., 265
Litchfield, J. T., Jr., 301, 314
Lockwood, W. R., 106
Lohss, F., 450
Lossow, W. J., 403
Loud, A. V., 96
Loutit, 159, 162
Low, F. N., 116, 119
Lovelock, F. E., 32, 33
Lovyagina, T. N., 450
Lubitz, J. M., 265
Lucke, B., 97, 164, 173
Lurie, M. B., 106
Lwoff, A., 283

Mabry, D. S., 97
MacCallum, D. K., 425
Mach, B., 344, 355
Mackaness, G. B., 211, 213
Magerlein, B. J., 241

Malinow, M. R., 418, 424
Mallett, N., 97
Manca, M., 491
Manenti, F., 491
Mann, F. C., 397, 403
Mann, G. V., 424
Marcus, S., 56
Margaretten, W., 96, 220
Markowitz, C., 397, 403
Marples, E. A., 131
Marro, F., 201, 202
Martin, D. S., 255
Mason, H. S., 237, 241
Mast, C., 331
Mauping, B., 490
Maurer, P. H., 287, 292
Mayes, P. A., 400, 403
McCandless, E. L., 412
McCarty, D. J., Jr., 367, 368
McCluskey, R. T., 96, 492, 501
McCollester, D. L., 403
McCutcheon, M., 97, 148, 162, 164, 173
McCutcheon, S. A., 501
McDonald, L., 490
McFarland, W., 376, 380
McKenna, J. M., 274
McKhan, C. F., 377, 380
McLimans, W. F., 213
McMillan, G. C., 424
McNeill, H. W., 255
Meade, R. C., 3, 17
Mehrishi, J. N., 171, 172, 174
Meier, R., 223, 239
Meister, P. D., 241
Melly, M. A., 291
Mene, G., 33
Merigan, T. C., 329, 332
Meritt, B. C., 240
Mesrobeanu, L., 283
Metzger, G. V., 108-120, 163-174
Meyer, E. J., 24
Michael, G., 264
Michael, J. G., 254, 284
Michaels, B., 332
Mickelsen, O., 418, 424
Migita, T., 408, 411
Mignard, V. A., 413-425
Milholland, R. J., 274
Miller, C. P., 196
Miller, E., 45
Miller, L. L., 47, 56
Miller, W. L., 233, 241
Milley, P. S., 109, 111, 116-118
Mills, D., 403, 412
Milner, K. C., 284
Milofsky, E., 145, 213
Milojevic, S., 233
Mitchard, M., 132
Mitchell, J., 354, 355
Mitzkat, H. J., 56
Mizuno, N., 57
Mlodozeniec, P., 56
Mow, H., 107
Moe, R. E., 131
Mollenhauer, H. H., 45
Mollison, P. L., 161, 162
Monaghan, E. A., 381
Monkhouse, F. C., 33
Monto, R. A., 381
Moore, R. D., 24, 109, 113, 116, 118, 345-356
Moore, S., 4, 17
More, R. H., 490
Morita, T., 175-187
Morre, D. J., 45
Morris, A., 57
Morris, B., 53, 57, 396, 398, 399, 401, 403, 412
Morrow, P. E., 108, 109, 118, 120
Morse, W. I., 242
Mott, P. D., 432
Mounter, L. D., 131
Mouton, D., 96, 106, 132, 195, 283, 291, 292, 411, 502
Movat, H. Z., 484, 487, 490
Moyer, L. S., 33
Mudd, S., 97, 164, 173
Muehbarcher, C., 331
Muench, H., 301, 314
Mumaw, V., 24, 354
Munck, A., 97
Murillo, G. J., 56
Murphy, E., 331, 488, 490
Murphy, J. B., 254
Murray, H. C., 241
Murray, I. M., 66, 72, 96, 285-292
Murray, R. G., 385, 402
Mustard, J. F., 484, 487, 488, 490
Mutungi, N. J., 56
Myers, P., 33
Myrvik, Q. N., 133, 138, 143, 145, 146, 203-213

Nabors, C. J., 56, 265
Nachmansohn, D., 131
Nagaishi, C., 116, 119
Nagler, A. L., 96
Nahamias, A. J., 330, 332
Naito, C., 401
Nakano, M., 274
Nava, C., 491
Nelson, E. L., 161, 162
Nelson, R. A., 292
Nestel, P. J., 398, 403
Nettesheim, P., 175-187
Neufield, F., 164, 173
Neumayr, A., 411
Neuschloss, S. M., 445, 450
Neveu, T., 384, 402, 425
Nicol, T., 56, 58-62, 96, 191, 192, 196, 214, 219, 221-242
Niewiarowski, S., 490
Nisselbaum, J. S., 332
Nitti, F., 283
Noble, E. P., 381
Nolan, J. P., 369, 378, 380
Nomura, M., 355
Noonan, S. M., 369-381
Nordlie, R. C., 274
Normann, S. J., 16, 33, 56, 66, 71-73, 96, 290-292
Northup, P. V., 333-344
Nossal, G. J., 343
Novellie, G. D., 344
Novy, F. G., 291
Noyes, P., 196
Numano, F., 432
Nungester, W. J., 173
Nussenzweig, V., 495, 502

Ochoa, S., 355
O'Gorman, P., 84
Ohorodnik, J. M., 501
Ohringer, L., 431, 432
Okada, M. Y., 119, 265
O'Keefe, L. M., 490
Okishio, T., 450
Old, L. J., 84, 196

Olivecrona, T., 383, 389, 397, 399, 401, 403
Olson, R. E., 384, 401
Ono, K., 403
Oren, R., 133, 145, 203, 213
Ornstein, L., 131
Osawa, S., 57
Osler, A. G., 288, 292
Otaka, E., 57
Ott, F., 450
Ouchi, E., 203, 213
Ovary, Z., 292
Oxman, E., 52, 57
Ozere, R. L., 332

Pagano, J. S., 331
Page, A. R., 369, 380
Paigen, K., 355
Plade, G. E., 96, 134, 213, 356
Palmer, A. C., 131
Palmer, D. L., 292
Panagistis, N., 56
Pappas, G. D., 96, 97
Parant, F., 275-284
Parant, M., 56, 275-284
Pardee, A. B., 355
Parker, H. G., 6, 17, 63, 65, 66, 72, 73
Parks, B. H., 284
Parks, H. F., 96
Paranetto, F., 146
Pasero, G., 491
Pasternak, V. Z., 254, 264
Paterson, J. C. S., 161, 162
Patek, P. R., 413-425
Pautrizel, R., 468-483
Pavillard, E. R. J., 133, 145
Payne, F. E., 331
Payne, T. P. B., 378, 380
Paz, R. A., 233, 241
Pearse, A. G. E., 106, 131
Pease, D. C. 367
Pekin, T. J., Jr., 367
Pellegrino, A., 424
Pequignot, G., 411
Perillie, P. E., 369, 378, 380
Perkins, E. H., 175-187
Peterman, M. L., 356
Peterson, D. H., 237, 241
Peterson, R. E., 237, 241
Pethica, B. A., 174
Petracek, F. J., 432
Petrova-Maslakova, L. G., 442-450
Petti, G., 197-202
Pfuderer, P., 342, 344
Phillips, G. E., 56, 196, 265
Pickering, G., 431
Pillemer, L., 292
Pirani, C. L., 233, 240
Polley, H. F., 237, 238, 241
Poole, J. C. F., 484-487
Poplawski, A., 490
Porterfield, J. S., 33
Powell, H. M., 331
P'Pool, D., 402, 412
Prestidge, L. S., 355
Probst, G. W., 331
Pyzikiewicz, T., 56, 380

Quantock, D. C., 221-242
Quastel, J. H., 202
Quick, A. J., 27, 33
Quintana, C., 368

Rachlin, W., 131
Rake, G. W., 213
Ramo, S., 411
Randall, H. G., 292
Ransom, J. P., 254, 264, 265
Rawson, A. J., 367
Razaka, G., 468-483
Reade, P. C., 220
Rebuck, J. W., 369-381
Reed, L. J., 301, 314
Regelson, W., 315-332
Reichard, S. M., 274
Reinders, W., 292
Reineke, L. M., 241
Reinhardt, W. O., 425
Reiser, R., 399, 403
Renais, J., 451-467
Rendi, R., 355
Renold, E. A., 242
Reynolds, E. S., 45
Rhodes, J. M., 344
Ribi, E., 284
Rich, A., 342, 344
Riddle, J. M., 357-368, 378, 379, 381, 501, 502
Ridout, J. H., 424
Rigdon, R. H., 274
Riggi, S. J., 17, 56, 264, 382-403, 412, 441
Rittenberg, M. S., 264
Robert, C., 56
Roberts, A. R., 56
Roberts, J. C., 431
Roberts, S., 233, 235, 240, 241
Robinson, H. J., 232, 240
Rocha e Silva, M., 232, 240
Rodionova, L. P., 442-450
Rogers, D. E., 291
Rogister, G., 131
Rohlich, P., 403
Rosen, F., 274
Rosenman, R. H., 411, 425, 431
Rosenthal, S. R., 264
Ross, I. S., 117, 119
Ross, O. A., 292
Rossatti, B., 131
Rostgaard, J., 107
Rottem, Z., 331
Rouiller, C., 24, 56
Rowley, D., 17, 66, 72, 96, 164, 173, 284, 291, 343
Rowsell, H. C., 490
Rubens-Duval, A., 234, 241
Rubin, 56
Rudbach, J. A., 284
Rudloff, D., 332
Ruggs, J. C., 109, 118
Ruhenstroth-Bauer, G., 174
Ruol, A., 411
Rupp, J. C., 354
Rutenberg, A. M., 131
Rutenberg, S., 131, 264
Ruzsa, P., 403

Saba, T. M., 16, 33
Sabatini, D. D., 45
Saito, K., 145, 213, 263, 265
Sacquet, E., 283
Salky, N. K., 402, 403, 412
Samaille, J., 450
Sampaio, M. M., 116, 119
Sanders, E., 402
Sanderson, R. P., 255
Saphir, O., 431, 432
Sbarra, A. J., 96, 203, 212, 213, 233, 240
Scebat, L., 451-467, 468, 471, 475

Scharff, M. D., 344
Schayer, R. W., 232, 240
Schepers, G. W. H., 109, 118
Schilling, F. J., 412
Schimassek, H., 46-57
Schimke, R. T., 274
Schlagel, C. A., 233, 241
Schlossman, S., 17
Schmid, W., 57
Schmidt, F. C., 96
Schneebeli, G., 56
Schoenberg, M. D., 20, 24, 57, 109, 113, 116, 118, 345-356
Schotz, D. L., 118
Schotz, M. C., 45
Schrantz, F. S., 274
Schrodt, A. G., 17
Schroeder, M. A., 424
Schueler, F. W., 235, 236, 241
Schueler, W., 223, 239
Schumaker, V. N., 96
Schwartz, 161, 162
Schwartz, B. S., 255
Schwarz, R. S., 344
Schweet, R., 57, 355
Scott, R. F., 403
Scow, R. O., 398, 403
Seaman, G. V. F., 33, 174
Seamans, P. A., 380
Sebestyen, M. M., 16, 17, 402
Seegers, W. H., 501, 502
Seligman, M., 502
Sellers, E. A., 424
Selvaraj, R. J., 213
Selye, H., 266, 274
Serio, M., 411
Severini, A., 219
Sewell, W. T., 115, 119
Shapiro, B., 397, 399, 400, 403
Shear, M. J., 132
Sheldon, W. H., 378, 381
Shepherd, P. A., 403
Sheppard, C. W., 411
Shihama, A. I., 57
Shilo, M., 314
Shimamoto, T., 419, 432
Shipkey, F. H., 45
Shohl, J., 378, 381
Shore, M. L., 1-17, 57, 412
Shorter, R. G., 116, 119
Shrago, E., 274
Sigel, M., 332
Silver, M. J., 490
Silver, N. J., 196, 265
Silverberg, A., 24
Simmonds, W. J., 403
Simon, K. A., 402
Singer, J. M., 18-24
Singhal, R. L., 274
Sinitzina, T. A., 442-450
Siperstein, M. D., 425
Skarnes, R. C., 283, 284
Smiley, R. L., 232, 240
Smith, C. E., 131
Smith, E. E., 131
Smith, J. J., 17, 25, 33, 51, 56, 265, 274
Smith, M. A., 274
Smith, M. R., 232, 240
Smith, W. W., 196
Smuckler, E., 146
Smythe, D. J., 274
Snell, F. M., 16, 24, 55, 57, 232, 239
Snell, J. F., 96
Snell, R. S., 96
Snyder, I. S., 266-274
Solmssen, U. V., 235, 241
Solomon, E., 408, 411
Sorem, G., 251, 255
Sorrels, M. F., 403
Spackman, D. H., 4, 17
Spector, W. G., 233, 234, 241
Spicer, 329
Spiro, D., 96, 220
Sprague, G., 196
Spurlock, B. O., 146, 213
Srivastava, S. K., 274
Staple, E., 412
Stare, F. J., 402, 424
Stavitsky, A. B., 354
Steiglitz, R. A., 17
Stein, W. H., 4, 17
Stein, Y., 397, 399, 400, 403
Steiner, J. W., 109, 118
Stekiel, W. J., 265
Stembridge, V. T., 402
Stepto, R. C., 233, 240
Stevens, G. D., 332
Steinhorner, R., 412
St. George, S., 131, 402, 432
Stiffel, C., 16, 72, 96, 97, 106, 132, 195, 283, 284,
Stiffel (Continuation) 291, 292, 402, 404, 411, 424, 425, 502
Stinebring, W., 274, 332
Stirland, R. M., 501
Stjernholm, R. L., 381
Storey, E., 234, 241
Strander, H., 332
Straumfjord, J., Jr., 331
Strauss, B., 292
Strauss, R., 431
Strong, I., 299
Stryzak, D., 431
Stuart, A. E., 49, 56, 57, 96, 106, 132, 147-162, 188, 195, 254, 264
Sultzer, B. M., 264
Surgeneor, D. M., 33, 97
Suter, E., 263, 265
Sutherland, A. J., 402, 412
Sutherland, K., 233, 240
Sutliff, W. D., 291, 292
Sutton, J. S., 81, 84, 106
Svehag, S. E., 354
Sweeney, E. W., 274
Sykes, J., 355
Szego, C. M., 233, 235, 240, 241
Szekely, J., 441

Takay, M., 57
Takemoto, K. K., 329, 331
Tal, C., 118
Talal, N., 355
Taliaferro, W. H., 344
Talmage, D. W., 344
Taplin, G. V., 196
Tawde, S., 344
Telander, R., 487
Telischi, M., 432
Tennyson, V. M., 97
Terres, G., 255
Tessmer, C. F., 274
Texon, M., 431
Thannhauser, S. J., 402
Thompson, F. C., 164, 173
Thomas, L., 96, 97, 196, 232, 240, 264, 265, 274, 291
Thomas, W. A., 403
Thorbecke, G. J., 264
Thorn, G. W., 242
Thorpe, B. D., 56

Titus, J. L., 119
Todd, F. W., 292
Toman, R., 441
Tompkins, E. H., 412
Toro, I., 403
Torri, A., 491
Trapani, R. J., 132
Trefouel, T., 283
Tria, E., 197, 201, 202
Trounce, J. R., 131
Trump, B., 146
Truding, N., 401
Tsorch, Y., 18-24
Tuccio, L. S., 254, 265
Tullis, J. L., 33, 97
Tunis, M., 331, 332
Turner, F. J., 255

Uhr, J. W., 343, 344
Ullmann, E. G., 275
Upton, A. C., 402
Urbonkova, G., 120

Vaheri, A., 330, 331
Vaheri, D., 331
Vallebona, A., 220
Van Den Bosch, J., 402
Vanderhoff, J. W., 24
Van Oss, C. J., 24
Van Rood, J. J., 343
Vassalli, P., 335, 344, 355, 501
Vatter, A. E., 45, 333-344
Vaughan, R. B., 147, 162
Vazques, D., 355
Vernon-Roberts, B., 56, 196, 219, 221-242
Vester, J. W., 383, 401
Vetter, H., 411
Villee, C. A., 233, 240
Villiaumey, J., 235, 241
Virag, S., 441
Vlckova, A., 120
Von Ehrenstein, G., 344
Waddell, W. R., 385, 402
Wagner, H. N., 96, 408, 411
Wahlquist, M. L., 107, 412
Walburg, A. E., Jr., 175-187
Walcher, D. N., 331
Wallace, J. M., 97
Wallach, D. F., 96
Walter, P. C., 106, 145
Waranvdekar, V. S., 132
Ward, H. K., 286, 292
Ward, I. R., 56
Ware, A. G., 501
Ware, C. C., 196
Warner, G. F., 411
Warner, J. R., 344
Warner, L., 33
Watson, D., 264, 274, 291
Watson, J. D., 355
Watson, M. L., 56
Watson, W. L., 367
Watts, H. F., 431
Webb, E. C., 131
Weber, G., 274, 408, 412
Wedgwood, R. J., 292
Weidanz, W. P., 292
Weinhouse, S., 433, 441
Weintraub, A., 241
Weisberger, A. S., 345-356
Weiser, W. J., 484, 487
Weiss, L., 81, 84, 106
Weissman, G., 97, 232, 240, 264, 265
Werthessen, N. T., 487
West, D., 106
Wheelock, E. E., 317, 331
Whereat, A. F., 412
Whitby, J. L., 254, 284
White, A. E., 355
Whitehouse, F. W., 369-381
Whitehouse, M. W., 412
Wiener, E., 133, 144, 145
Wiener, J., 85-97, 220
Wilcoxon, F., 301, 314
Wild, D. G., 355
Wilens, S. L., 430, 432
Wiley, G. G., 284
Wilkins, D. J., 24, 25-33, 164, 166, 173, 174, 254
Wilkinson, G. K., 107, 412
Williams, M. A., 98-107
Williams, M. C., 403
Williams, T., 131
Willmar, E. N., 97
Wilson, A. T., 284
Wilson, I. B., 131
Winebright, J., 343
Wissler, R. W., 343, 344, 418, 424
Withers, R. F. J., 131
Wiznitzer, T., 131
Wlodawer, P., 401
Wolf, W., 484, 487
Wolfe, S., 354, 355
Wolff, S. M., 432
Wood, W. B., 232, 240, 274
Woods, M. W., 254
Woodside, 116, 120
Wooles, W. R., 57, 106, 264, 402
Wright, C. S., 30, 33, 97
Wright, H. F., 254
Wulff, H. R., 381
Wyngaarden, J. B., 241

Youngner, J., 274, 332

Zambemard, J., 45
Zampi, G., 408
Zierler, K. L., 377, 381
Ziliotto, D., 411
Zilversmit, D. B., 53, 57, 411, 412
Zinsser, H., 287, 292
Zucker-Franklin, D., 367
Zvaifler, N. J., 367
Zweifach, B. W., 96, 196, 265, 274

GPSR Compliance
The European Union's (EU) General Product Safety Regulation (GPSR) is a set of rules that requires consumer products to be safe and our obligations to ensure this.

If you have any concerns about our products, you can contact us on

ProductSafety@springernature.com

In case Publisher is established outside the EU, the EU authorized representative is:

Springer Nature Customer Service Center GmbH
Europaplatz 3
69115 Heidelberg, Germany

www.ingramcontent.com/pod-product-compliance
Ingram Content Group UK Ltd.
Pitfield, Milton Keynes, MK11 3LW, UK
UKHW051325070726
13610UKWH00014B/89

* 9 7 8 1 4 6 8 4 7 7 9 7 9 *